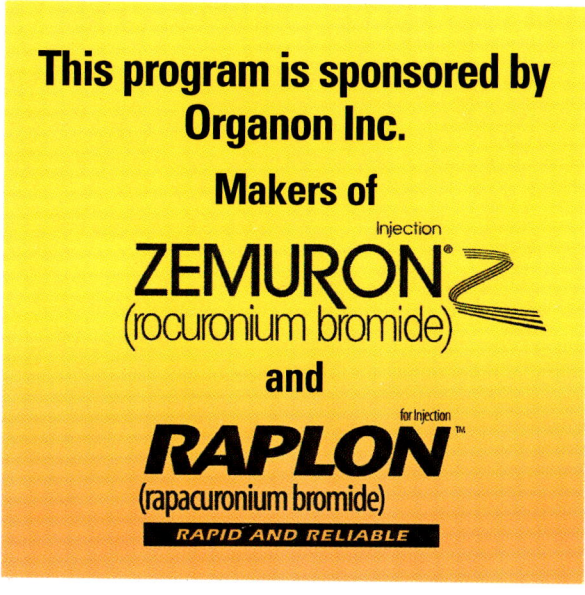

CLINICAL PEDIATRIC ANESTHESIA

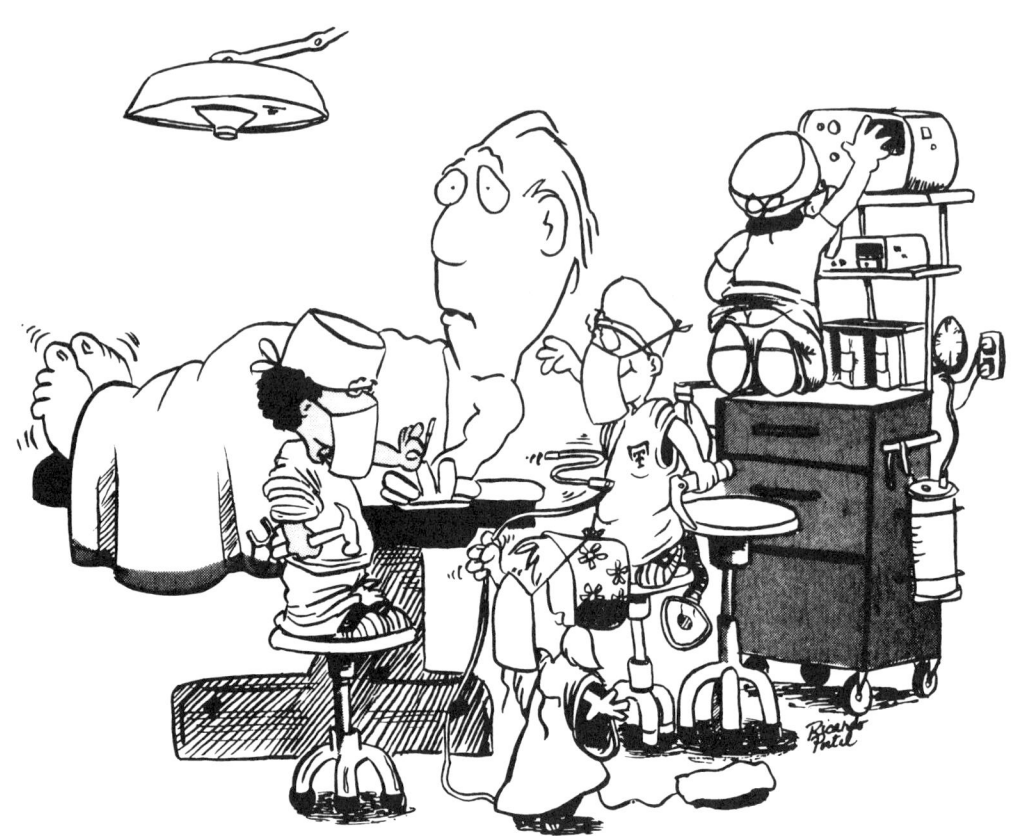

CLINICAL PEDIATRIC ANESTHESIA

Edited by

J. Michael Badgwell, M.D.
*Professor of Anesthesiology and Pediatrics
Chairman, Department of Anesthesiology
University of Nevada School of Medicine
Las Vegas, Nevada*

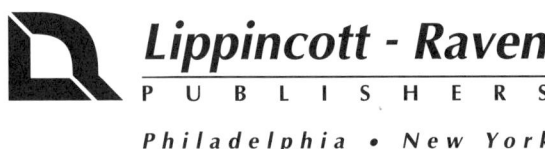

Lippincott - Raven
PUBLISHERS
Philadelphia • New York

Acquisitions Editor: R. Craig Percy
Developmental Editor: Ellen DiFrancesco
Manufacturing Manager: Dennis Teston
Production Manager: Jodi Borgenicht
Production Editor: Christina Zingone
Cover Designer: Patricia Gast
Indexer: Elizabeth Babcock-Atkinson
Compositor: Lippincott–Raven Electronic Production
Printer: Maple Press

© 1997 by Lippincott–Raven Publishers. All rights reserved. This book is protected by copyright. No part of it may be reproduced, stored in a retrieval system, or transmitted, in any form or by any means—electronic, mechanical, photocopy, recording, or otherwise—without the prior written consent of the publisher, except for brief quotations embodied in critical articles and reviews. For information write **Lippincott–Raven Publishers, 227 East Washington Square, Philadelphia, PA 19106-3780.**

Materials appearing in this book prepared by individuals as part of their official duties as U.S. Government employees are not covered by the above-mentioned copyright.

Printed in the United States of America

9 8 7 6 5 4 3 2 1

Library of Congress Cataloging-in-Publication Data

Clinical pediatric anethesia/edited by J. Michael Badgwell.
    p.   cm.
  Includes bibliographical references and index.
  ISBN 0-397-51476-X
  1. Pediatric anesthesia.   I. Badgwell, J. Michael
  [DNLM: 1. Anesthesia—in infancy & childhood.   WO 440 C6415 1997]
RD139.C554   1997
617.9′6798—dc21
DNLM/DLC
For Library of Congress

Care has been taken to confirm the accuracy of the information presented and to describe generally accepted practices. However, the authors, editor, and publisher are not responsible for errors or omissions or for any consequences from application of the information in this book and make no warranty, express or implied, with respect to the contents of the publication.

The authors, editor, and publisher have exerted every effort to ensure that drug selection and dosage set forth in this text are in accordance with current recommendations and practice at the time of publication. However, in view of ongoing research, changes in government regulations, and the constant flow of information relating to drug therapy and drug reactions, the reader is urged to check the package insert for each drug for any change in indications and dosage and for added warnings and precautions. This is particularly important when the recommended agent is a new or infrequently employed drug.

Some drugs and medical devices presented in this publication have Food and Drug Administration (FDA) clearance for limited use in restricted research settings. It is the responsibility of the health care provider to ascertain the FDA status of each drug or device planned for use in their clinical practice.

To Lynn, Ashley, and Christy

"How the mother is to be pitied
Who hath handsome daughters!"
—John Gay

Contents

Contributing Authors ix
Preface xi
Acknowledgments xiv

1. Preoperative Evaluation 1
   Lynda J. Means

2. Induction of Anesthesia 15
   J. Michael Badgwell

3. Peripheral and Central Vascular Access and Invasive Monitoring 49
   J. Michael Badgwell, Robert S. Holzman, and William S. Schechter

4. Tracheal Tube and Laryngeal Mask Placement in Routine and Difficult Airways 77
   J. Michael Badgwell

5. Delivery and Monitoring of Alveolar Ventilation 113
   J. Michael Badgwell

6. General Anesthesia Maintenance, Emergence, and Tracheal Extubation 145
   Ira S. Landsman, Peter J. Davis, and J. Michael Badgwell

7. Anesthesia for the Neonate 163
   Steven C. Hall

8. Anesthesia for the Ex-Premature and Ex-Extracorporeal Membrane Oxygenated Infant 195
   Frederic A. Berry and J. Michael Badgwell

9. Perioperative Fluid Management 213
   Eugene B. Freid and J. Michael Badgwell

10. Perioperative Pain Management 227
    J. Michael Badgwell, Joseph P. Cravero, Brenda C. McClain, Linda Jo Rice, and Melissa M. McLeod

11. Anesthesia for Procedures in and around the Airway 267
    Lynne Ferrari

12. Anesthesia for Infants and Children With Congenital Heart Disease 295
    J. Michael Badgwell and Louis W. Elkins

13. Pediatric Neuroanesthesia: Beyond the Theory 339
    Bruno Bissonnette

14. Common and Uncommon Coexisting Diseases That Complicate
Pediatric Anesthesia 381
Ann G. Bailey and J. Michael Badgwell

15. Management of the Child with Major Trauma 413
Aleksandra J. Mazurek and J. Michael Badgwell

16. Sedation, Analgesia, and Anesthesia for Painful or Frightening Procedures
Outside the Operating Room 435
Lawrence Roy

17. Postanesthesia Care Issues 461
Robert D. Valley

Parting Shot 477
J. Michael Badgwell

Subject Index 479

Contributing Authors

J. Michael Badgwell, M.D.
Professor of Anesthesiology and Pediatrics
Chairman, Department of Anesthesiology
University of Nevada School of Medicine
2040 West Charleston Boulevard, Suite 601
Las Vegas, Nevada 89102

Ann G. Bailey, M.D.
Associate Professor of Anesthesiology and
  Pediatrics
Department of Anesthesiology
University of North Carolina School of Medicine
CB# 7010, 223 Burnett-Womack Building
Chapel Hill, North Carolina 27599-7010

Frederic A. Berry, M.D.
Professor of Anesthesiology and Pediatrics
Department of Anesthesia
University of Virginia Health Sciences Center
Children's Medical Center
P.O. Box 10010
Charlottesville, Virginia 22906-0010

Bruno Bissonnette, M.D., F.R.C.P.C.
Professor of Anesthesia
University of Toronto Faculty of Medicine
1 King's College Circle
Toronto, Ontario, Canada M5S 1A8
Director, Division of Neurosurgical Anesthesia
Department of Anesthesia
The Hospital for Sick Children
555 University Avenue
Toronto, Ontario, Canada, M5G 1X8

Joseph P. Cravero, M.D.
Assistant Professor
Department of Anesthesia and Pediatrics
Dartmouth Hitchcock Medical Center
One Medical Center Drive
Lebanon, New Hampshire 03756

Peter J. Davis, M.D.
Professor of Anesthesiology and Pediatrics
Department of Anesthesiology and Critical Care
  Medicine
University of Pittsburgh School of Medicine
Children's Hospital of Pittsburgh
3705 Fifth Avenue
Pittsburgh, Pennsylvania 15213-2583

Louis W. Elkins, M.D.
Cardiovascular Surgeon
Arkansas Cardiovascular Surgery Associates
9601 Lile Drive, Suite 200
Little Rock, Arkansas 72205

Lynne Ferrari, M.D.
Medical Director, Preoperative Services
Associate in Anesthesia
Children's Hospital
300 Longwood Avenue
Boston, Massachusetts 02115
Assistant Professor of Anesthesia
Harvard Medical School
25 Shattuck Street
Boston, Massachusetts 02115

Eugene B. Freid, M.D.
Associate Professor of Anesthesiology and
  Pediatrics
Department of Anesthesiology
University of North Carolina School of Medicine
CB 7010, 223 Burnett-Womack Building
Chapel Hill, North Carolina 27599-7010

Steven C. Hall, M.D., F.A.A.P.
Arthur C. King Professor of Pediatric
  Anesthesiology
Professor of Anesthesiology
Northwestern University Medical School
303 East Chicago Avenue
Chicago, Illinois 60611-3008
Anesthesiologist-in-Chief
Children's Memorial Hospital
2300 Children's Plaza
Chicago, Illinois 60614

Robert S. Holzman, M.D.
Associate Professor of Anesthesia
Harvard Medical School
25 Shattuck Street
Boston, Massachusetts 02115
Senior Associate in Anesthesia
Children's Hospital
300 Longwood Avenue
Boston, Massachusetts 02115

Ira S. Landsman, M.D.
Assistant Professor of Anesthesiology and Pediatrics
Department of Anesthesiology and Critical Care
   Medicine
University of Pittsburgh School of Medicine
Children's Hospital of Pittsburgh
3705 Fifth Avenue
Pittsburgh, Pennsylvania 15213-2583

Aleksandra J. Mazurek, M.D.
Assistant Professor
Department of Anesthesia, #19
Northwestern University Medical School
303 East Chicago Avenue
Chicago, Illinois 60611-3008
Children's Memorial Hospital
2300 Children's Plaza
Chicago, Illinois 60614

Brenda C. McClain, M.D., D.A.B.P.M.
Assistant Professor
Department of Anesthesiology and Pediatrics
Vanderbilt University Medical Center
T-0118 Medical Center North
Nashville, Tennessee 37232

Melissa M. McLeod, M.D.
Assistant Professor
Department of Anesthesiology
Eastern Virginia Medical School
Children's Hospital of the King's Daughters
601 Chldren's Lane
Norfolk, Virginia 23507

Lynda J. Means, M.D.
Associate Professor of Anesthesia and Surgery
Department of Anesthesia
Indiana University School of Medicine
1120 South Drive
Indianapolis, Indiana 46202-5114
Riley Hospital for Children
702 Barnhill Drive
Indianapolis, Indiana 46202-5200

Linda Jo Rice, M.D.
Professor of Clinical Anesthesia
University of South Florida
12901 Bruce B. Downs Boulevard
Tampa, Florida 33612-4799
Director of Pain Management
All Children's Hospital
565 21st Avenue, North East
St. Petersburg, Florida 33704

Lawrence Roy, B.S.L., M.D., F.R.C.P.C.
Associate Professor
Department of Anesthesia
University of Toronto
   Faculty of Medicine
1 King's College Circle
Toronto, Ontario, Canada M5S 1A8
Senior Anesthetist
Department of Anesthesia
Hospital for Sick Children
555 University Avenue, Suite 2211
Toronto, Ontario, Canada, M5G 1X8

William S. Schechter, M.D.
Assistant Professor of Anesthesiology
   and Pediatrics
Columbia University
College of Physicians and Surgeons
622 West 168th Street
New York, New York 10032

Robert D. Valley, M.D.
Associate Professor of Anesthesiology
   and Pediatrics
Department of Anesthesiology
University of North Carolina
   School of Medicine
CB#7010, 223 Burnett-Womack Building
Chapel Hill, North Carolina 27599-7010

Preface

"I love being a writer. What I can't stand is the paperwork."
—Peter DeVries

Egad! Not another anesthesia textbook! Enough is enough already! "Why another?" you may rightly ask. However, if we trace the origin of the present work, you may view our efforts more charitably. When the publisher came to us in October of 1994 asking us if we needed another textbook on pediatric anesthesia, we irreverently mentioned that perhaps we could write a book called *Pediatric Anesthesia for the Uninterested*, fashioned after that critically unacclaimed and rather ignoble book called *Anesthesia for the Uninterested*, written by John D. Tolmie and Alexander A. Birch and published in 1986 by Aspen Press. The aforementioned publisher left us alone, and we thought we were successful in our discouragement. Two months later, to our surprise and vexation, we received a call saying, "Yes, we would like to publish *Pediatric Anesthesia for the Uninterested*." "Wow!" we said. We paused. We scratched our collective head. Perhaps, with a little more sophistication and a little more maturity and with all the best pediatric anesthesiologists as authors, an informal but highly informative book might be just what we downtrodden anesthesiologists need. Therefore, we embarked on the effort. It became our goal to produce something refreshing and new. We wanted to take the tired old truths of pediatric anesthesia and make them jet with new life. If the information presented arouses the occasional smile, all the better.

"If you are just capable of being miserable and making other people miserable, you're not a great actor [or writer]. If you can make them laugh, too, that's another matter."
—Robertson Davies

For whom is this book written? We hope that this book finds its way into many different hands. For instance, we hope that the book proves useful to those in training and to those "fully trained," to the general anesthesiologist, who only occasionally is required to do pediatric anesthesia, and to bonafide pediatric experts. We have designed the book to provide an opportunity for readers to rub elbows, in an informal manner, with our esteemed clinician-authors. We've designed the book's format to allow the experts to show how they really do it. We want to expose our expert's practice—practices known to be built on science, tempered by years of experience. We hope that the book becomes useful for a wide variety of clinicians — from those in training to those who consider themselves fully trained. It is our fondest desire that the book serve as an accurate guide for all who practice pediatric anesthesia. We have made every attempt to make it beneficial for anyone who provides anesthetic care to infants and children.

"Inherently each of us has the substance within to achieve whatever our goals and dreams define. What is missing from each of us is the training, education, knowledge, and insight to utilize what we already have."
—Mark Twain

Except as a guide to a deeper insight into the authors' expertise, this will not be a comprehensive reference book. Please bear in mind as you read, however, that information presented is not static, it only reflects what is currently done in pediatric anesthesia. This information will change in time as future generations of pediatric anesthesiologists pick up the trade.

> "Books...are an elemental model of how culture is perpetuated, the wisdom of the tribe passed on to posterity to be added to, edited, and modified by subsequent generations."
> —Robert Andrews

This book is presented in an informal writing style and will not, however, underestimate you as a reader (or as a clinician). Therefore, although we'll be informal in our approach to the material, we will not "dumb it down". Nevertheless, we are sure you'd like things cleared up as much as possible. We feel that we can clear things up more quickly with an informal approach.

> "My aim is to put down on paper what I see and what I feel is the best and simplest way."
> —Ernest Hemingway

On your behalf, we have asked the contributing authors to reveal a deeper insight than normally would be expected in contributing to a textbook of this nature. To accomplish this lofty goal, we've asked them to loosen up and have fun in presenting their information. We've asked them to tell us what they actually do. There are several things *to look for* in this book: look for it to be very clinical and "how-to-do-it" (without sacrificing the science, of course). We have attempted to boil down science and practice to their clinical essence.

> "One of the most important things about writing is to boil it down and not bore the hell out of everybody."
> —Robertson Davies

As you may have noticed, there are many quotable quotes in this book. We have taken undue effort to place them only where they seem appropriate. Although we don't want to distract you from the learning process, we have assumed (right or wrong) a responsibility to entertain as well as inform you. As a result, quotes should fit the text. There are many pictures, illustrations, and even cartoons.

There are several things *not to look for* in this book: Don't look for tedious explanations or theoretical ways to do things. Don't look for deep reference lists. On the other hand, you'll be glad to read you needn't look for blather regarding a comprehensive analysis of each and every controversy. We have not neglected to include, however, several flies in the facial ointment of pediatric anesthesia convention. In addition, please don't look for absolute consistency in writing style from chapter to chapter. We had fully intended to smooth out the wet concrete of each chapter into one smooth sidewalk, but we ran out of time. There is, however, consistency of content with few redundancies and contradictions from chapter to chapter. For example, a chapter on equipment submitted by Bob Holzman and William Schechter contained a virtual encyclopedia of information on the subject but had to be dissected and added in bits to selected chapters rather than risk presenting the same material twice.

The book is arranged under chapters that reflect the gamut of pediatric anesthesia experience. Topics in this book have been chosen because they matter. Chapters are written by people who matter. Although this is current stuff, authors address cutting-edge issues as important now as they were for Ayre's and Jackson-Rees. We presume the chosen authors collectively constitute the shapers of our modern pediatric anesthesia landscape. We further presume they can get their points across concisely. In fact, if contributors weren't laconic, we scissored.

> "Life is too short for a long story."
> —Lady Mary Wortley Montagu

An informal format has allowed us to venture far beyond the confines of the conventional anesthesia textbook, bringing to light insights from those authors whom we may have only presumed to know. In the welter of unfiltered information unleashed by documented experience and research, it is easy to lose sight of how authentic anesthesiologists can fertilize our thoughts not with a lot of manure, but rather with bold descriptions of how they actually practice.

In summary, we would like you to have fun reading this book. This book is for your enjoyment, as well as for your education.

> "People do not get 'heavy' with wisdom. They get light. The wiser you become, the lighter you become. This is an unsolicited testimonial for lightheartedness...I suggest you pay attention."
>
> —Tom Robbins

We realize that criticism of scholarly writing is usually more favorable if that writing is highly formal. There seems to be a great belief among critics that there is something very fine about being miserable and something rather second-rate about being happy. In writing this book, we learned what good writers have known: serious writing is relatively easy; it is difficult to be successfully light-hearted on the written page. Nevertheless, we made the effort. We wanted the book to reflect the enjoyment we derive from what we do.

> "It's hard enough to write a good drama, it's much harder to write a good comedy, and it's hardest of all to write a drama with comedy, which is what life is."
>
> —Jack Lemmon

Furthermore, we presume that lying in wait out there is a small but loyal opposition consisting of the uniformed, the uninterested, and the scornful. To the Loyal Opposition, let us plead forgiveness by saying that we've made an all-out effort for this book to be highly informative, but we're also hoping that you find this book to be, well, fun. We hope the information presented will stand out from the existing landscape, compel a second or third look, and, in the long run, lie deep in the reader's memory to be drawn upon when the need arises.

> "These words dropped into my childish mind as if you should accidentally drop a ring into a deep well. I did not think of them much at the time, but there came a day in my life when the ring was fished up out of the well, good as new."
>
> —Harriet Beecher Stowe

It is our fondest desire that, after reading this book the information contained will be your own, will become part of you, and will help you to practice safe and enjoyable pediatric anesthesia.

> "All good books are alike in that they are truer than if they had really happened, and after you are finished reading one, you will feel that all that happened to you and afterwards it all belongs to you..."
>
> —Ernest Hemingway

J. MICHAEL BADGWELL, M.D.

Acknowledgments

The editor and authors acknowledge the dedicated people who made this book possible. First, we must recognize our teachers. Of course, there were the attendings and faculty that taught us through the years, but in the case of this book, our most recent and most valuable teachers have been our patients and our anesthesiology residents. Yes, indeed, their search to rise above ignorance served as a gristmill that ground us in to what we are today. Hopefully, the results of their questions (i.e., our answers) have made it to the pages of this book.

A few others deserve special praise and recognition. First, and certainly foremost, we must single out Sandra Castro, Dr. Badgwell's administrative assistant who, in the strictest sense of the word, "wrote" the book. Believe us, without Sandra the book would never have been. Sandra typed, word processed, organized, collected, called, and on and on. But, more importantly, Sandra is brilliant and intuitive. Therefore, if you find parts of this book to be brilliant, more than likely it is a reflection of Sandra's contribution.

Also deserving of our gratitude and acknowledgment are Gabor Racz, M.D., and Randy Hickle, M.D. Gabor, as Chairman of the Department of Anesthesiology at Texas Tech University Health Sciences Center, made certain Dr. Badgwell had the time and resources to finish the project. Randy, through his patronage and funding, assured that time was made available for Dr. Badgwell to put the book together.

We, of course, congratulate Ricardo Postel, the illustrator, for delivering exactly the cartoon figures we requested. All it took for Ric was the mention of a concept and the figure materialized. The more serious illustrations were drawn by the intrepid and unflappable Meadow Green. Each of our illustrators undertook their efforts as a labor of love, and it shows.

Steven Hall, M.D., Chief of Anesthesia at the Chicago Children's Hospital, deserves a very special mention. Steve has been a constant source of encouragement and inspiration for the Editor and has spent many hours poring over these pages in critical analysis. Although his efforts were truly deserving of Co-Editor status, Steve eschewed that title but fulfilled the role nevertheless.

Finally, no set of acknowledgments would be complete without thanking our cast of editors from Lippincott–Raven, led by Craig Percy, the Executive Editor. Craig has been at our side from the beginning, facilitating each and every move. Ellen DiFrancesco, our Developmental Editor; Andrea Williams, Mr. Percy's Administrative Assistant; and Christina Zingone, the Production Editor deserve our praise, recognition, and commendation. A very special thank you goes to Christina who spent many extra hours poring over the final product to make sure it would be as close to perfect as possible.

In conclusion, we give credit to mentors who've steadfastly guided us. Although we can't list them all, we would like to single out one for special recognition and gratitude: Robert E. Creighton, M.D., of the Hospital for Sick Children in Toronto. It was this magnificent iconoclast who has taught many to think for themselves. With apologies to Bob for falling short of his standards for self-thinking, we present this book as a representation of our progress so far.

CLINICAL PEDIATRIC ANESTHESIA

1
Preoperative Evaluation

Lynda J. Means

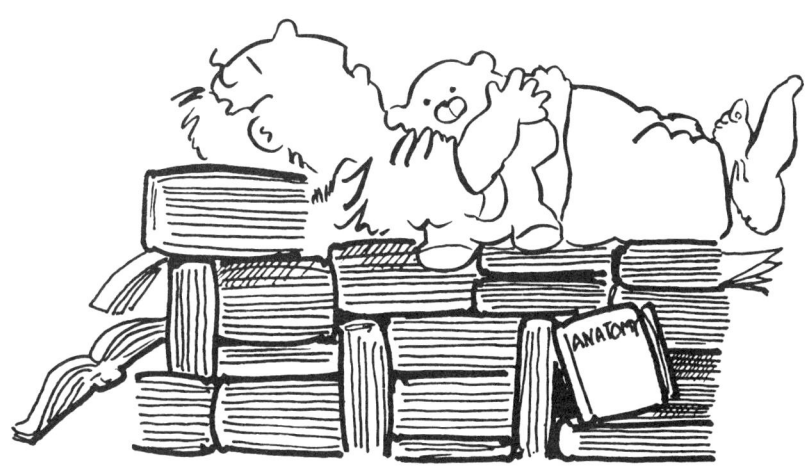

"When action grows unprofitable, gather information; when information grows unprofitable, sleep."
—Ursula K. Le Guin

Pediatric anesthesia, whether outpatient or inpatient, is a continuum of clinical care. This continuum begins with the preoperative evaluation and continues through considerations of the fasting interval, premedication, induction of anesthesia, maintenance of anesthesia, emergence from anesthesia, postoperative analgesia, and care of the child in the postanesthesia care unit or intensive care unit. Information gathered during the preoperative evaluation influences decisions made during the remainder of anesthesia care.

This chapter emphasizes the components of a careful and thorough preoperative evaluation for children scheduled for operative procedures or for sedation outside the operating room.

MEETING THE FAMILY AND PUTTING THEM AT EASE

Psychological Preparation of the Child and Family

The anesthetic preoperative evaluation not only includes the acquisition of medical information and assessment of the child's physiologic status, but also offers a brief opportunity to help alleviate the child's and the family's anxieties about impending anesthesia and surgery.

Much has been written about postoperative behavioral disturbances in children, although there are few prospective, blinded, controlled studies with large numbers of patients that have examined behavioral outcomes and preoperative interventions. There is consensus that children between the ages of 1 and 3 years, who have been previously hospitalized

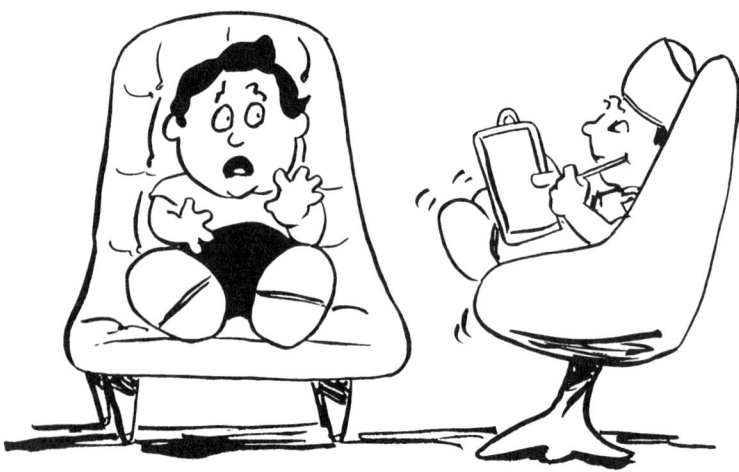

and who have had stormy anesthetic inductions, are at risk for developing postoperative behavior disturbances (1). Unfortunately, there is no consensus as to which preoperative interventions will guarantee the avoidance of such behaviors. The benefit and liability of parental presence at the time of induction or preoperative medication in reducing behavioral changes are hotly debated. However, the anxiolytic effect of the anesthesiologist's preoperative interview is well documented (2).

A skillfully conducted interview, which gathers medical and psychosocial information, conveys concern and respect, and affords an opportunity to ask questions, may significantly reduce preoperative anxiety even if conducted immediately before anesthesia (3). The anesthesiologist should be cognitive of the age and intellectual development of children and pose questions and responses to the child accordingly. Phrases such as "put to sleep," which may revive unpleasant memories of Fido's last visit to the veterinarian, should be avoided. The interview should preferably be conducted with the anesthesiologist sitting or kneeling, since this conveys time devoted to the family in an unhurried fashion and brings one down to the level of the child in an unintimidating fashion.

Many hospitals have developed "child-friendly" environments as part of the preoperative program with coloring books, tours, videos, child life experts, and play therapy. Allowing children to take a favorite toy, blanket, or other "lovie" into the operating rooms also serves to comfort the child.

ELICITING IMPORTANT INFORMATION

Medical History and Review of Organ Systems

"We have not all had the good fortune to be ladies. We have not all been gentlemen, or poets, or statesmen; but when the toast works down to the babies, we stand on common ground."

—Mark Twain

Many children presenting for minor or routine surgical procedures are in good health and pose no special problems from confounding medical conditions. However, at times healthy children present for surgery as the result of illness (e.g., appendicitis) or with a concurrent illness (e.g,, upper respiratory infection), which necessitates a detailed history of onset, duration, symptoms, and degree of incapacitation to assess physiologic compromise. Children with complex medical conditions who present for seemingly minor surgical procedures such as otoplasty can pose a challenge for even the most experienced anesthesiologist. The anesthesiologist evaluating a

TABLE 1. *Potential medical problems associated with admission to neonatal intensive care unit*

Medical or surgical condition	Secondary condition	Anesthetic implications
Anemia	Decreased oxygen carrying capacity	Postoperative apnea, especially in the neonate with a hematocrit <30%
Diaphragmatic hernia	Persistent pulmonary hypertension of the newborn; hypoplastic lungs; congenital heart disease; small abdominal cavity	Pulmonary hypertension; impaired pulmonary and respiratory function; limit ventilation pressures to avoid pneumothorax; surgical repair may occur in neonatal intensive care unit while patient receiving extracorporeal membrane oxygenation
Esophageal atresia	Tracheoesophageal fistula (see below)	Esophageal dysmobility
Myelodysplasia	Hydrocephalus; urogenital disease	Extreme heat and evaporative losses if large lesion; positioning difficult; latex allergy with repeat exposures to latex products
Necrotizing entercolitis	Short gut syndrome	Fluid, electrolyte imbalance; large third-space fluid shifts; heat and evaporative losses great
Omphalocele and gastroschisis	Other congenital defects, especially midline defects in patients with omphalocele, notably cardiac; small abdominal cavity	Fluid, electrolyte imbalance; respiratory compromise with closure of defect secondary to tight abdominal closure or may require "silo" for closure; major heat loss
Prematurity	Pulmonary insufficiency; patient ductus arteriosus and congestive heart failure; intraventricular hemorrhage; inguinal hernia; retinopathy of prematurity	Pulmonary compromise; at risk for oxygen toxicity; heat and evaporative losses great; meticulous fluid management; postoperative apnea
Tracheoesophageal fistula	50% have associated congenital defects, primarily cardiac and musculoskeletal	Pulmonary soiling; tracheomalacia; possible ventilation compromise if gas diverted from lungs through fistula

child must not only elicit important facts that reflect the degree of current hemodynamic, respiratory, renal, or intravascular volume status, but also inquire about factors that are unique to the pediatric patient and play an important role in the perioperative period.

Significant past medical history in many patients begins in the perinatal period. A history of admission to a neonatal intensive care unit suggests potential problems that may continue far beyond the perinatal period (Table 1). Of special concern is the potential development of postoperative apnea in former preterm infants **(see Chapter 8)**. Coté and associates (4) examined data from eight prospective studies that investigated the incidence of apnea after inguinal herniorrhaphy in former preterm infants. The authors determined that (a) apnea was strongly and inversely related to both gestation age and postconceptional age; (b) an associated risk factor was continuing apnea at home; (c) small-for-gestation-age infants seemed to be somewhat protected from apnea; and (d) anemia was a significant risk factor. No consistent policy regarding the postoperative disposition of these patients could be determined. Therefore, each physician and institution must evaluate each patient on an individual basis.

Medications and Allergies

Parents and children should be queried as to current and previously ingested medications because these can have a profound impact on the conduct of anesthesia (Table 2). Patient compliance should be investigated.

4 CHAPTER 1: PREOPERATIVE EVALUATION

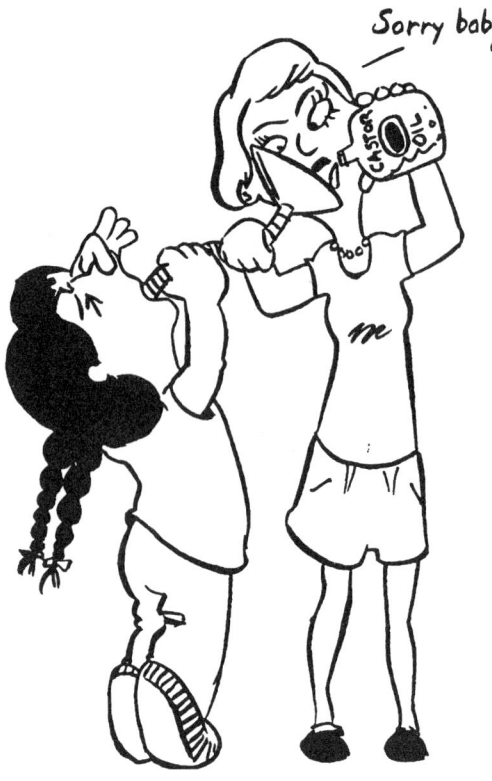

Often parents become more honest in this area if the physician expresses understanding that it is very difficult to always get children to take medication.

It is important to ask about allergies that the child may have not only to drugs, but also to other substances such as soy products, eggs, or rubber products. There have been numerous case reports of anaphylaxis to rubber or latex during anesthesia (5). At-risk populations include children with myelodysplasia and those with congenital urologic abnormalities. These patients should be carefully screened for sensitivities to common rubber-containing products (e.g., balloons, rubber gloves, or rubber toys), and every attempt should be made to avoid exposure while the child is in the hospital.

Previous Experience with Anesthesia

"Every time history repeats itself the price goes up."
—Anonymous

If the child had a previous experience with anesthesia, it is important to carefully inquire whether there were any complications or unpleasant encounters. Did the child experience separation anxiety, nausea or vomiting, or inadequate analgesia? Was there a prolonged emergence or postextubation croup? Was the perioperative experience as pleasant for the family as could be expected? If not, what were the apparent or perceived reasons for an unpleasant experience? An open discussion of events can offer explanations and assurances that the anesthesiologist will attempt to do everything possible to make this operative experience a more pleasant one. It can also help

TABLE 2. *Medications affecting anesthetic management*

Medication	Anesthetic implications
Anticonvulsants	Drug-induced enzyme induction or liver dysfunction; may be hepatotoxic and cause blood dyscrasia; increases nondepolarizing muscle relaxant requirements
Aminophylline	Severe dysrhythmias may occur when used with halothane.
Aspirin	Platelet dysfunction
Chemotherapeutic agents	Immunosuppression
Busulfan (Myleran)	Pulmonary toxicity; decreased plasma cholinesterase levels
Carmustine (BCNU)	Pulmonary toxicity
Cyclophosphamide (Cytoxan)	Decreased plasma cholinesterase levels; alveolitis with low continuous dose
6-Mercaptopurine (6-MP)	Cholestatic jaundice
Doxorubicin (Adriamycin) and daunorubicin (Daunomycin)	Cardiotoxicity: ECG changes; congestive heart failure secondary to diffuse cardiomyopathy at doses > 550 mg/m^2
Bleomycin (Blenoxane)	Pulmonary fibrosis
Vincristine (Oncovin)	Neuropathies
Nonsteroidal anti-inflammatory drugs	Platelet dysfunction

the anesthesiologist to attempt to avoid previous unpleasant experiences, such as removing an anxious and screaming preschool-aged child from parents without first considering a preoperative medication. The use of oral midazolam (0.5 mg/kg, given 20 minutes before separation from parents) allows most children to be relaxed and to separate smoothly from parents (6,7). Parents should be warned that their child may become clumsy or a bit ataxic and should be protected from potential falls or other traumas after the administration of a preoperative medication.

Family History

"Happy the people whose annals are vacant."
—Thomas Carlyle

The clinician should seek information regarding anesthetic-related complications, such as prolonged weakness or paralysis after an anesthetic (cholinesterase deficiency) or malignant hyperthermia. The general population may not be familiar with the phrase "malignant hyperthermia," but may respond affirmatively if asked whether a relative experienced a rapid temperature elevation, became rigid, or had an unanticipated admission to the intensive care unit after anesthesia. If the family history suggests cholinesterase deficiency, the neuromuscular blocking drugs metabolized by cholinesterase, succinylcholine and mivacurium, can be avoided.

CHILD AND PARENTAL CONCERNS

Risks of Anesthesia

"To fear the worst oft cures the worst."
—William Shakespeare

Perhaps the most crucial part of the preoperative evaluation is that which allows the parents time to ask questions. One of the most common concerns expressed by parents is that they have heard "the anesthetic is the most dangerous part of the operation." To reassure parents, one can mention the use of highly technologic monitors and explain that, as the anesthesiologist, your presence is continuous to ensure the safety of the child.

When explaining risks of anesthesia to parents, avoid quoting figures from pre-pulse oximetry morbidity and mortality studies evaluating children (the only ones available). These figures do not represent the real risks for children today or for the particular child and are unnecessarily frightening to families. Analysis of combined adult and pediatric data from the American Society of Anesthesiologists Closed Claims Project clearly shows a decrease in respiratory system damaging events (e.g., inadequate ventilation or oxygenation, difficult tracheal intubation, and esophageal intubation), brain damage, and death when claims from 1975 to 1978 were compared with those submitted after 1990 ($P \leq .01$) (8). These trends coincide with the ASA Standards for Basic Anesthetic Monitoring, which includes pulse oximetry (as of January 1, 1990) and capnography (as of January 1, 1991). To put this in perspective for the parents, one can mention that their child's risk of suffering injury in an automobile accident while riding to the hospital is greater than the risk of the child suffering injury during anesthesia.[a] Whatever "risk figure" you use, be certain to explain to the parents that every precaution will be taken to ensure a safe and uneventful anesthetic for their child.

Finally, in a recent *New York Times* article, the author suggested that "given two equally competent physicians, pick the one with a smile and optimistic disposition" (9).

SYSTEM EVALUATION

Airway Evaluation

The history should include questions regarding respiratory effort, snoring, stridor,

---

[a] Ed. Note (JMB): "I once heard the grandfather of pediatric anesthesia, Robert M. Smith, say before a large group that he told parents there was less than a one-in-a-million chance something might go wrong with the child during anesthesia. Needless, to say, I've used this 'statistic' frequently. If it's good enough for Bob Smith's patients, it's good enough for mine."

quality of speech, and cough. Loud snoring, sleep disturbance, mouth breathing, and nasal stuffiness are suggestive of significant tonsillar or adenoid hypertrophy. Such children may pose a challenge during inhalation induction owing to partial airway obstruction. The child with a history of a "barky" or seal-like cough during episodes of respiratory tract infections may be more prone to postextubation croup. Many children with craniofacial syndromes not only present with airway abnormalities that pose a challenge to intubation (Fig. 1), but also have other organ system abnormalities (Table 3). Thorough examination and assessment of the airway can often predict a difficult intubation and allow time for careful preparation. Although useful in predicting the difficult intubation in adult patients, it is uncertain whether the Mallampati airway classification is applicable in children (10). Physical examination of the airway should include the following:

- Identification of obvious anatomic malformations
- Evaluation of mandibular shape and evidence of previous reconstruction
- Assessment of ability to open mouth, subluxate mandible, and extend neck
- Observation of relative size of tongue to oral cavity and for presence of high-arched and narrow palate
- Estimation of hyoid-mandible distance
- Evaluation of child's voice

An example of the usefulness of voice evaluation would be in finding laryngeal papillomas in a child with progression from normal voice characteristics to hoarseness to aphonia to respiratory distress.

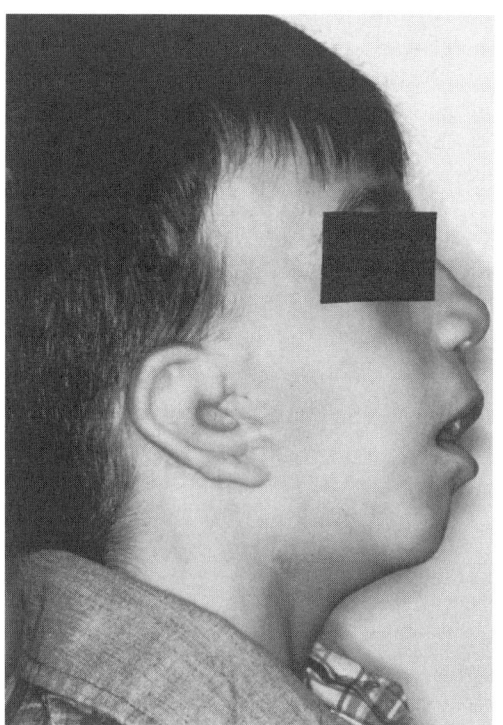 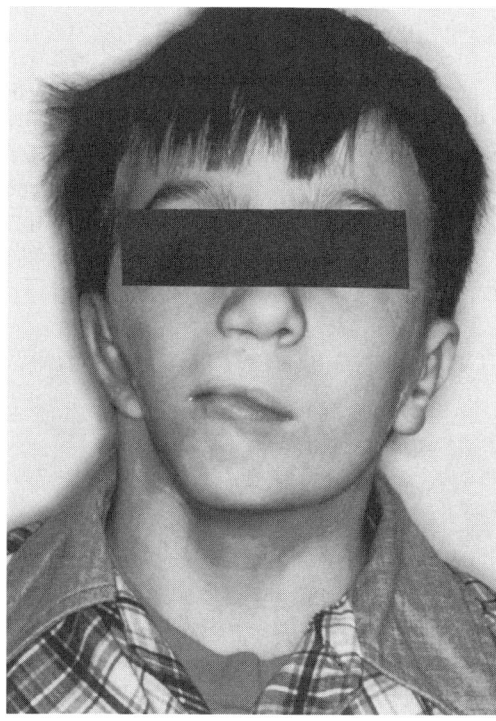

FIG. 1. (A) A 7-year-old child is scheduled for otoplasty as an outpatient. **(B)** Physical examination reveals that access to the airway may be difficult owing to mandibular hypoplasia and deformity.

TABLE 3. *Craniofacial deformities and associated conditions*

Name	Craniofacial deformities	Associated conditions	Anesthetic implications
Apert's syndrome	Craniosynostosis, especially coronal suture; hypoplastic midface	Polysyndactyly, especially second, third, and fourth fingers; may be mentally compromised	Difficult intravenous access
Crouzon's disease	Craniosynostosis, hypoplastic maxilla, hypertelorism, exophthalmos	Conductive hearing loss; may be mentally compromised	May be obligate mouth breather secondary to upper airway obstruction
Goldenhar's syndrome	Unilateral mandibular hypoplasia, cleft palate, micrognathia	Vertebral anomalies	May be difficult intubation
Hemifacial microsomia	Unilateral ear anomalies, unilateral hypoplasia of the mandibular condyle and ramus		May be difficult intubation
Moebius sequence	Micrognathia and limited mandibular movement (sixth and seventh cranial nerve palsy)	May have more extensive cranial nerve involvement with ptosis and limited tongue movement	Difficult intubation
Pfeiffer's syndrome	Brachycephaly; hypoplastic maxilla	Broad thumbs and great toes; syndactyly; may be mentally compromised	
Pierre Robin anomalad	Mandibular hypoplasia, micrognathia, glossoptosis, cleft palate	Otherwise normal	Difficult intubation initially as infant, but patients exhibit mandibular "catch-up" growth as toddlers
Treacher Collins syndrome	Mandibular hypoplasia, hypoplastic zygomatic arches, malformation of external ear	Hearing compromise	Difficult intubation; may occasionally require tracheostomy for respiratory

Cardiovascular Evaluation

The child who presents for anesthesia and surgery with a previously undiagnosed cardiac murmur poses a diagnostic challenge. If the history reveals obvious or suspected information that supports the diagnosis of cardiovascular abnormality (e.g., family history of congenital heart disease, failure to thrive, limited exercise tolerance, frequent respiratory problems) and if the situation permits, cardiac consultation should be obtained. Equally problematic is evaluation of a murmur that may be "innocent" or physiologic (11). Innocent murmurs are heard in up to 50% of normal pediatric patients at some point during childhood. The cause of these murmurs is usually turbulent blood flow through any of the great vessels. Features that commonly differentiate innocent from pathologic murmurs are listed in Table 4. If there is uncertainty regarding the significance of a murmur and if time allows, a consultation with a cardiologist is desirable. For patients with congenital heart disease, prophylaxis against subacute bacterial endocarditis is necessary. Guidelines from the American Heart Association are outlined in Tables 5 and 6 (12).[b]

TABLE 4. *General criteria that distinguish innocent from pathologic cardiac murmurs*

Innocent murmurs	Pathologic murmurs
Occur early in systole	Occur late in systole
Short in duration	Pansystolic
Low intensity	Very loud
Short in duration	Continuous
Crescendo-decrescendo	All diastolic
Poorly transmitted	

---

[b]Ed. Note (JMB): This information is also presented in **Chapter 12** in an expanded form. We feel the information is important enough to be presented twice.

TABLE 5. Endocarditis prophylaxis

I. Standard regimen for dental/oral/upper respiratory tract procedures in patients at risk (including those with prosthetic heart valves and other high-risk patients)
   Amoxicillin 50 mg/kg (max. 3 g) orally 1 h before procedure, then 25 mg/kg (max. 1.5 g) 6 h after initial dose
   For amoxicillin-/penicillin-allergic patients:
   Erythromycin ethylsuccinate 20 mg/kg (max. 1 g) orally before and 10 mg/kg (max. 0.5 g) orally 6 h after procedure
   OR
   Clindamycin 10 mg/kg (max. 300 mg) orally 1 h before procedure and 5 mg/kg (max. 150 mg) 6 h after initial dose
II. Alternate prophylactic regimens for dental/oral/upper respiratory tract procedures in patients at risk
   For patients unable to take oral medications:
   Ampicillin 50 mg/kg IV or IM (max. 2 g) 30 min before procedure, then ampicillin 25 mg/kg IV or IM or amoxicillin 25 mg/kg orally 6 h after initial dose
   For ampicillin-/amoxicillin-/penicillin–allergic patients unable to take oral medications:
   Clindamycin 10 mg/kg (max. 300 mg) IV 30 min before procedure and 5 mg/kg (max. 150 mg) IV (or orally) 6 h after initial dose
III. Regimen for genitourinary (GU)/gastrointestinal (GI) procedure patients or patients considered to be at high risk who are not candidates for the standard regimen for dental/oral/upper respiratory tract procedures
   Ampicillin 50 mg/kg (max. 2 g) IV (or IM) plus gentamicin 2 mg/kg (max. 80 mg) IV (or IM) 30 min before procedure, followed by amoxicillin 25 mg/kg (max. 1.5 g) orally 6 h after the initial dose. Alternately, the parenteral regimen may be repeated 8 h after the initial dose.
   For amoxicillin-/ampicillin-/penicillin–allergic patients:
   Vancomycin 20 mg/kg (max. 1 g) IV administered over 1 h, starting 1 h before procedure; no repeat dose necessary for dental/oral/upper respiratory tract procedures; may be repeated once 8 h after initial dose for GU/GI procedures
IV. Alternate oral regimen for low-risk patients undergoing GU/GI procedures
   Amoxicillin 50 mg/kg (max. 3 g) orally 1 h before procedure, then 25 mg/kg (max. 1.5 g) 6 h after procedure

IM, intramuscular; IV, intravenous.
In patients with compromised renal function, it may be necessary to modify or omit the second dose of gentamicin or vancomycin.
Adapted from Dajani et al, ref. 12, with permission.

TABLE 6. When is endocarditis prophylaxis not recommended?

Cardiac conditions	Dental or surgical conditions
Isolated secundum atrial septal defect (ASD)	Endotracheal intubation
Ventricular septal defect, secundum ASD, and patent ductus arteriosus 6 months after repair and without residua	Dental procedures that do not result in bleeding
Mitral valve prolapse with normal valvular structure and without regurgitation	Intraoral injection of local anesthetics except intraligamentary injections
Innocent or physiologic murmurs	Cardiac catheterization
Previous Kawasaki syndrome without valvular dysfunction	Endoscopy with or without gastrointestinal biopsy
Previous rheumatic fever without valvular dysfunction	Bronchoscopy with a flexible bronchoscope, with or without bronchoscopy
Cardiac pacemakers and defibrillators	Tympanostomy tube insertion

Adapted from Dajani et al, ref. 12, with permission.

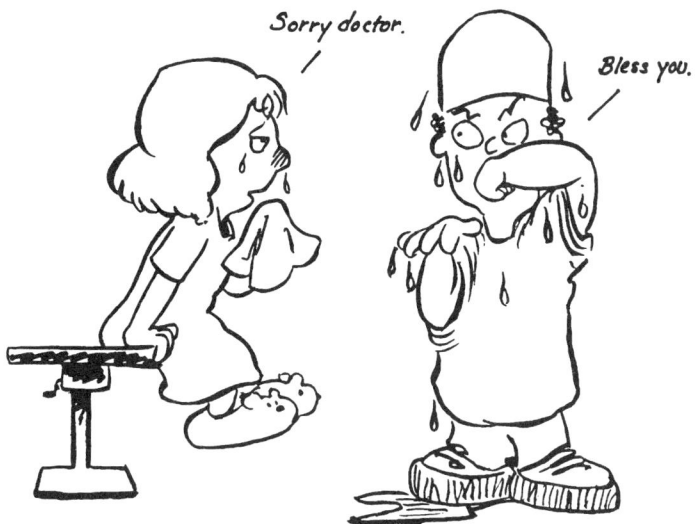

The Child with a Runny Nose

"We are so fond of one another because our ailments are the same."
—Jonathan Swift

The child with a runny nose and possible upper respiratory infection (URI) can present a clinical dilemma regarding whether to postpone the operative procedure. There is no one way to resolve this dilemma.[c]

In fact, there is a wide range of opinions and approaches to this clinical problem (13,14). Tait and Knight (15) have reported that when comparing children with and without viral URI symptoms undergoing myringotomy and tympanostomy, there was no increased morbidity in children with URI symptoms. On the other hand, other authors have pointed out that the potential complications facing a child with a URI are not trivial. Children with respiratory infections have heightened sensitivity of their airways, as well as increased secretions, both of which may lead to laryngospasm, bronchospasm, coughing, and breath-holding, which may ultimately lead to hypoxia (16–20). Furthermore, children with respiratory infections have decreased mucocillary flow and are at risk for atelectasis (21).

Generally speaking, the child with a runny nose who has a core temperature of < 38°C, no cough, no other signs or symptoms of acute illness (e.g., normal appetite and activity) and whose rhinorrhea is "this way all of the time" has a noninfectious runny nose and is unlikely to develop complications. On the other hand, the child with a fever of > 38°C or who has a cough or other systemic signs or symptoms of illness or whose nasal discharge is purulent may have an infectious URI.

"We are such docile creatures normally that it takes a virus to jolt us out of life's routine."
—E.B. White

When considering whether or not to proceed, the anesthesiologist, with the child's surgeon, must weigh the risk-to-benefit ratio of proceeding with a surgical procedure in a child who is not in optimal health. It is obvious that emergency surgery must proceed. However, in an otherwise healthy child who is in the recovery phase of an acute viral illness and whose symptoms are not worsening, proceeding with anesthesia and surgery is reasonable. The child who presents with fever, worsening cough, or history of general

---

[c]Ed. Note (JMB): This book presents more than one way to manage this dilemma. Turn to **Chapter 14** for Ann Bailey's guidelines for management of the child with a URI.

malaise, and is scheduled for an elective procedure should be rescheduled (based on return to normal lung function) in 4 to 6 weeks. There is consensus, however, that for a period of time in the perioperative period, the child with a URI may have lower than normal saturation and that time to desaturation may be less (22). Therefore, in all phases of anesthesia care, monitoring with pulse oximetry is needed, and supplementary oxygen is likely to be required.

PERTINENT LABORATORY EVALUATION

In recent years, the value of screening tests in otherwise healthy surgical patients has been questioned (23). Preoperative laboratory tests are now most often used for specific diagnostic purposes or to establish important baseline values (e.g., hemoglobin [Hb] level determination in anticipation of major blood loss). Although there are no uniform guidelines for the use of preoperative laboratory tests, the following discussion of specific tests addresses the most commonly asked questions.

Hemoglobin Concentration

It is unlikely that mild anemia will have any discernible impact on the course of anesthesia or will dictate a change in perioperative management in an otherwise healthy child (24,25). Anemia has been reported in up to 2% of pediatric surgical patients (26). Most commonly, these have been reported as mild anemias (Hb level ≥9.5 g/dl), which can be detected only with blood testing. Thus, routine Hb screening is unnecessary for otherwise healthy children (27,28). A preoperative Hb determination should be carried out when significant anemia (<9 g/dl) is very likely (e.g., in infants <1 year, former preterm infants, and patients with chronic illness) or to establish a baseline in anticipation of significant surgical blood loss (29). Anemia (hematocrit <30%) is a significant risk factor for postoperative apnea in former preterm infants, and it has been suggested that elective surgery be delayed until the infant's hematocrit is >30% (30).

In patients with sickle cell disease (SCD; including sickle cell anemia, sickle Hb C disease, and the sickle thalassemias), the optimal level of sickle Hb to avoid perioperative complications is unknown. In a retrospective study of pediatric patients, Griffin and Buchanan (31) concluded that preoperative transfusions might be avoided in children with SCD who undergo most minor elective surgical procedures. Patients undergoing thoracotomy, laparotomy, or tonsillectomy and adenoidectomy are at risk of developing postoperative complications and would benefit from an evaluation for preoperative transfusion. Recent results from two large multicenter studies have led to new recommendations for the perioperative transfusion management of such patients. The Preoperative Transfusion in Sickle Cell Disease Study Group investigated the outcomes of patients randomly assigned to either an aggressive or a conservative transfusion regimen (32). The current preoperative transfusion method of choice in elective surgery is a conservative transfusion practice designed to raise the Hb to 10 g/dl without regard for the resultant Hb S level (32). This is in contrast to a former more aggressive transfusion regimen intended to decrease the Hb S level to < 30%.

The Cooperative Study of Sickle Cell Disease Group (33) has found that surgical procedures can be performed more safely in patients with SCD than previously reported (34). For minor procedures (e.g., inguinal hernia repair and myringotomy), many patients did not receive transfusions and complication rates were low. Overall, morbidity was 0.3%. Complications were found to be more common after regional anesthesia, but researchers attributed this to the higher rates of complications in SCD patients undergoing obstetric procedures and not necessarily to the technique (primarily epidural analgesia or anesthesia). They state that "the role of transfusion in the perioperative period remains to be defined, but data do suggest that not all patients undergoing surgery should routinely receive blood transfusions" (34). Because the preoperative transfusion practice remains controversial, perioperative evaluation and management of patients with SCD must be done in conjunction with the patient's hematologist and surgeon to optimize outcome. Risk status, Hb phenotype, surgical procedure, and past medical history with emphasis on pulmonary complications and past hospitalizations should be thoroughly assessed and considered when planning transfusion and anesthetic management. Past history of pulmonary problems, older age, and a greater number of previous hospitalizations are more common in patients who subsequently develop acute chest syndrome or painful crisis in the postoperative period.

Pregnancy Testing

"Our bodies are shaped to bear children and our lives are a working out of the process of creation."
—Phyllis McGinley

Adolescents may not disclose their pregnancy for a variety of reasons, such as fear, distrust, ignorance, or denial. Concern exists regarding the adverse effects that anesthesia, surgery, or radiographic exposure may have on the fetus. Azzam and associates reported their findings from a 2-year period of mandatory pregnancy testing in postmenarchal surgical adolescents at a children's hospital (35). Of 412 patients age 10.5 to 20 years, none younger than age 15 years had a positive urine pregnancy test. Five of the young women ≥15 years had a positive test (2.4%). As a result, two of the surgeries were postponed, one was conducted under local anesthesia without sedation, one patient's condition was medically managed, and in one patient the operation was performed without nitrous oxide under general anesthesia.

The authors conclude from the resulting data and from consultation with a corporate law firm that "a policy of mandatory pregnancy testing in pediatric patients ≥15 years is advisable. Specific written consent is not necessary, but proper notification processes must be established." An accompanying editorial questioned these conclusions based on the concept of patient autonomy (self-directing freedom), the concept of distributive justice (limited resources should be managed in a fashion that most benefits society), and knowledge that there is no increased incidence of congenital anomalies associated with a single exposure to modern inhaled anesthetics (36).

Evidence supports increased fetal demise with first-trimester exposure to general anesthetics and pelvic surgical procedures (37,38). Whether pregnancy screening of all females of childbearing age prior to surgical procedures is routine or selective is a matter of policy of the individual facility. As a minimum, however, patients must be informed of the purpose and implications of results obtained from the urine specimen.

Urinalysis, Chest Radiographic Examination, and Serum Electrolytes

Routine preoperative urinalysis, chest radiographs, and serum electrolytes are not necessary as part of the preoperative evaluation. These tests should be obtained only when there is historical or physical evidence to warrant such.

Coagulation Screening

Although previously undiagnosed coagulopathy could lead to serious perioperative morbidity (39,40), screening tests have weak predictive value for the risk of surgical bleeding in patients who have no history of abnormal bleeding (41–43). A history in either the patient or family is useful in selecting patients for further diagnostic testing. A history of excessive bruising is often reported, is frequently a matter of parental perception, and is reported in patients with and without bleeding disorders, particularly in children with light

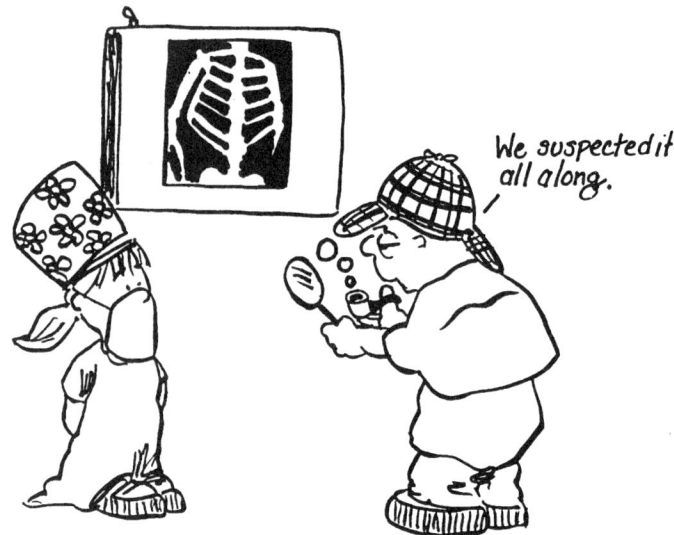

complexions (44). A history of large bruises, hematoma, or simultaneous bruising on several parts of the body is more suggestive of pathology. Unusual forms of bleeding such as hematochezia, frequent and prolonged epistaxis, or unusual bleeding after minor trauma (e.g., dental extraction) are also suggestive of a clotting disorder.

In patients in whom a hemostatic defect is suspected by history, the diagnostic yield of tests is greater than when they are used for screening an asymptomatic population (45). Therefore, testing should be considered in patients in whom either history or medical conditions suggest a possible hemostatic defect (45). In patients undergoing surgery in whom the procedure itself could cause hemostatic perturbations (e.g., cardiopulmonary bypass), when the coagulation system is particularly needed for adequate hemostasis (e.g. tonsillectomy), and in patients for whom even minimal postoperative bleeding could be critical (e.g., during neurosurgery), laboratory evaluation of the coagulation system should be obtained.

REFERENCES

1. McGraw T: Preparing children for the operating room: psychological issues. Can J Anaesth 1994;41:1094–1103.
2. Egbert LD, Battit GE, Turndorf N, Beecher HK: The value of the preoperative visit by the anesthetist. JAMA 1963;185:553–555.
3. Arellano R, Cruise C, Chung F: Timing of the anesthetist's preoperative outpatient interview. Anesth Analg 1989;68:645–648.
4. Coté CJ, Zaslavsky A, Downes JJ, et al: Postoperative apnea in former preterm infants after inguinal herniorrhaphy. Anesthesiology 1995;82:809–822.
5. Means LJ, Rescorla FJ: Latex anaphylaxis: report of occurrence in two pediatric surgical patients and review of the literature. J Pediatr Surg 1995;30:748–751.
6. McMillan CO, Spahr-Schopfer IA, Sikich N, et al: Premedication of children with oral midazolam. Can J Anaesth 1992;39:545–550.
7. Levine MF, Spahr-Schopfer IA, Hartley E, et al: Oral midazolam premedication in children: the minimum time interval for separation from parents. Can J Anaesth 1993;40:726–729.
8. Cheny FW: The ASA closed claims project: lessons learned. In: 1995 Annual Refresher Course Lectures. American Society of Anesthesiologists, 422.
9. Wade N: The spin doctors. New York Times Magazine. January 7, 1996.
10. Kopp VJ, Bailey A, Valley RD: Utility of the Mallampati classification for predicting difficult intubation in pediatric patients. Anesthesiology 1995;83:A1147.
11. Rosenthal A: How to distinguish between innocent and pathologic murmurs in childhood. Pediatr Clin North Am 1984;31:1229–1240.
12. Dajani AS, Bisno AL, Chung KJ, et al: Prevention of bacterial endocarditis: recommendations by the American Heart Association. JAMA 1990;264:2919–2922.
13. Betts EK, Schreiner MS, Cameron C: Should children with upper respiratory tract infections receive general anesthesia for elective surgical procedures? Anesthesiol Rev 1994;21:139.
14. Tait AR, Reynolds PI, Gutstein HB: Factors that influence the anesthesiologist's decision to cancel elective surgery for the child with an upper respiratory tract infection. J Clin Anesthesiol 1995;7:491–499.

15. Tait AR, Knight PR: The effects of general anesthesia on upper respiratory tract infections in children. *Anesthesiology* 1987;67:930–935.
16. Empey DW, Laitinen LA, Jacobs L, et al: Mechanisms of bronchial hyperreactivity in normal subjects after upper respiratory tract infections. *Am Rev Respir Dis* 1976;113:131–139.
17. Olsson GL, Hallen B: Laryngospasm during anaesthesia: A computer-aided incidence study in 136,929 patients. *Acta Anaesthesiol* Scand 1984;28:567–575.
18. Olsson GL: Bronchospasm during anaesthesia: a computer-aided incidence study of 136,929 patients. *Acta Anaesthesiol* Scand 1987;31:244–252.
19. Rolf N, Cote CJ: Frequency and severity of desaturation events during general anesthesia in children with and without upper respiratory infections. *J Clin Anesthesiol* 1992;4:200–203.
20. DeSoto H, Patel RI, Soliman IE, Hannallah RS: Changes in oxygen saturation following general anesthesia in children with upper respiratory infection signs and symptoms undergoing otolaryngological procedures. Anesthesiology 1988;68:276–279.
21. Carson JL, Collier AM, Hu SS: Acquired ciliary defects in nasal epithelium of children with acute viral upper respiratory infections. *N Engl J Med* 1985;312:463–468.
22. Kinouchi K, Tanigami H, Tashiro C, et al: Duration of apnea in anesthetized infants and children required for desaturation of hemoglobin to 95%: the influence of upper respiratory infections. *Anesthesiology* 1992;77:1105–1107.
23. Macpherson DS: Preoperative laboratory testing: should any tests be "routine" before surgery? *Med Clin North Am* 1993;77:289–308.
24. National Institutes of Health. Consensus conference: perioperative red blood cell transfusion. *JAMA* 1988;260:2700–2703.
25. Roy WL, Lerman J, McIntyre BG: Is preoperative haemoglobin testing justified in children undergoing minor elective surgery? *Can J Anaesthesiol* 1991;38:700–703.
26. O'Conner ME, Drasner K: Preoperative laboratory testing of children undergoing elective surgery. *Anesth Analg* 1990;70:176–180.
27. Baron MJ, Gunter J, White P: Is the pediatric preoperative hematocrit determination necessary? *South Med J* 1992;85:1187–1189.
28. Berry FA: Preoperative assessment and general management of outpatients. *Int Anesthesiol Clin* 1982;20:3–15.
29. Steward DJ: Screening tests before surgery in children. *Can J Anaesthesiol* 1991;38:693–695.
30. Welborn LG, Hannallah RS, Luban NL, et al: Anemia and postoperative apnea in former preterm infants. *Anesthesiology* 1991;74:1003–1006.
31. Griffin TC, Buchanan GR: Elective surgery in children with sickle cell disease without preoperative blood transfusion. *J Pediatr Surg* 1993;28:681–685.
32. Vichinsky EP, Haberkern CM, Neumayr L, et al: A comparison of conservative and aggressive transfusion regimens in the perioperative management of sickle cell disease. *N Engl J Med* 1995;333:206–213.
33. Koshy M, Weiner SJ, Miller ST, et al: Surgery and anesthesia in sickle cell disease. *Blood* 1995;86:3676–3684.
34. Platt OS, Brambilla DJ, Rosse WF, et al: Mortality in sickle cell disease: life expectancy and risk factors for early death. *N Engl J Med* 1994;330:1639–1644.
35. Azzam FJ, Padda GS, DeBoard JW, Krock JL, Kolterman SM: Preoperative pregnancy testing in adolescents. *Anesth Analg* 1996;82:4.
36. Duncan PG, Pope WD: Medical ethics and legal standards. *Anesth Analg* 1996;82:1–3, 1996.
37. Duncan PG, Pope WD, Cohen MM, Greer N: Fetal risk of anesthesia and surgery during pregnancy. *Anesthesiology* 1986;64:790–794.
38. Brodsky JB, Cohen EN, Brown BW Jr, et al: Surgery during pregnancy and fetal outcome. *Am J Obstet Gynecol* 1980;138:1165–1167.
39. Janvier G, Winnock S, Freyburger G: Value of the activated partial thromboplastin time for preoperative detection of coagulation disorders not revealed by a specific questionnaire. [Letter]. *Anesthesiology* 1991;75:920–921.
40. Bolger WE, Parsons DS, Potempa L: Preoperative hemostatic assessment of the adenotonsillectomy patient. *Otolaryngol Head Neck Surg* 1990;103:396–405.
41. Burk CD, Miller L, Handler SD, Cohen AR: Preoperative history and coagulation screening in children undergoing tonsillectomy. *Pediatrics* 1992;89:691–695.
42. Suchman AL, Mushlin AI: How well does the activated partial thromboplastin time predict postoperative hemorrhage? *JAMA* 1986;256:750–753.
43. Rodgers RP, Levin J: A critical reappraisal of the bleeding time. *Semin Thromb Hemost* 1990;16:1–20.
44. Nosek-Cenkowska B, Cheang MS, Pizzi NJ, et al: Bleeding/bruising symptomatology in children with and without bleeding disorders. *Thromb Haemost* 1991;65:237–241.
45. Rapaport SI: Preoperative hemostatic evaluation: which tests, if any? *Blood* 1983;61:229–231.

2

Induction of Anesthesia

J. Michael Badgwell

The induction of anesthesia in infants and children can be rewarding and even pleasant. This chapter provides information to help make induction a pleasant experience.

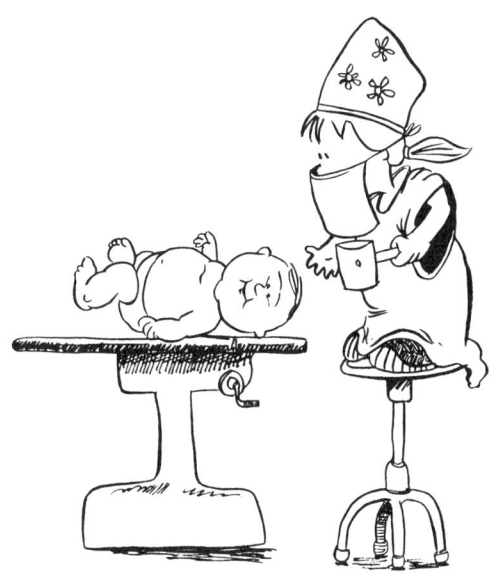

PREPARING THE ROOM

The use of a simple mnemonic, "I AM The MD," reminds one of the things that need to be arranged before the induction of anesthesia. These letters stand for *I*ntravenous, *A*irway, *M*achines, *T*emperature, *M*onitors, and *D*rugs. Preparation of equipment for intravenous access is discussed in **Chapter 3**, for airways in **Chapter 4**, and for anesthesia machines, breathing circuits, ventilators, and respiratory monitors in **Chapter 5**.

It is important that equipment be set up in the exact order indicated by the mnemonic. For instance, intravenous (IV) equipment is set up first, followed by airway equipment, and then machines, monitors, and drugs. Then, if an emergency situation suddenly erupts (e.g., a severely traumatized child), the most essential items are available first.

NONINVASIVE MONITORING IN THE PEDIATRIC PATIENT

"There are worse occupations in this world than feeling a [child's] pulse."
—Laurence Sterne

Precordial Stethoscope

Modern technology has provided us with a wealth of monitoring devices sufficient to inundate the pediatric surgical patient. However, the time-honored precordial stethoscope is the simplest tool available for continuous monitoring in pediatric anesthesia practice. The precordial stethoscope was made popular by Dr. Robert Smith during his years of practice at the Children's Hospital in Boston and is now considered a standard of care in pediatric anesthesia textbooks (1,2).

Placed over the left sternal border at the second or third intercostal space, the precordial stethoscope is used to evaluate heart rate and heart tones and to detect the presence of heart murmurs and air emboli. The clinician should be able to assess qualitative changes in heart tones, from "crisp" at the start of induction to "muffled" as the child's depth of

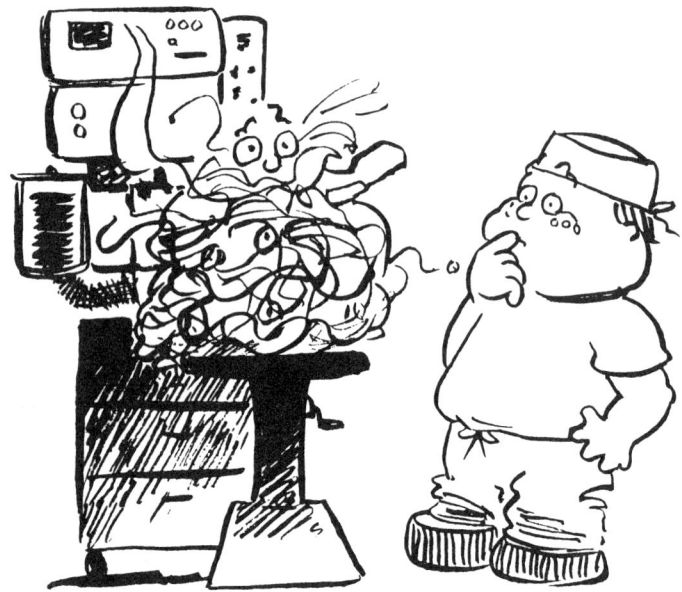

anesthesia increases and cardiac output falls.[a]

Although ventilation may be assessed with the precordial stethoscope, it does not adequately distinguish between esophageal and endotracheal intubation nor can it accurately detect endobronchial intubation. For these reasons, a binaural stethoscope and auscultation over the lung fields and stomach is always used to confirm precordial stethoscope information. In the final analysis, the precordial stethoscope's greatest value may be that it requires and maintains contact between patient and anesthesiologist.

Despite its many limitations, the precordial stethoscope is useful in a variety of circumstances. It is simple and unobtrusive to apply during inhalation induction of anesthesia in children. For example, a precordial stethoscope may be placed early in the induction (before other monitors), avoiding the placement of electrocardiogram (ECG) electrodes and other monitors that often disturb anxious children. In addition, the precordial stethoscope is useful during the transportation of children from induction rooms to the operating theater or from the theater to the recovery room, when other portable monitors are impractical or unavailable. Used during emergence from anesthesia, the precordial stethoscope may help in the detection of laryngospasm, upper airway obstruction, or croup.

Esophageal Stethoscope

The esophageal stethoscope may be used after the child's trachea is intubated. This device consists of a soft catheter with distal perforations covered with a cuff. The esophageal stethoscope may not be as helpful as a left-placed precordial stethoscope in differentiating endobronchial intubation. Nevertheless, an esophageal stethoscope may be used when a precordial stethoscope is impractical because of the site of surgery or for the purpose of facilitating temperature monitoring when a thermistor has been incorporated into the probe.

Electrocardiogram

Continuous ECG monitoring provides valuable information regarding heart rate and

---

[a]Ed. Note (JMB): Caution is advised, however, as these so-called muffled heart tones are subtle and may not be detectable until over a 50% reduction in cardiac output has occurred (3).

rhythm and should be used in pediatric surgical patients whenever possible. Although there are distinct differences between infant and adult ECGs, the most significant difference is that due to right axis shift in the infant; that is, the R wave is most pronounced in lead III in the infant in contrast to lead II in the adult. ECG may be used effectively to determine both rhythm disturbances and heart rate. Normal limits of heart rate for children vary by age (Table 1).

ECG allows the clinician to diagnose dysrhythmias such as heart block, supraventricular tachycardias, and premature atrial and ventricular contractions. The latter dysrhythmias are usually benign in children, resulting from the interaction of either endogenous or exogenous epinephrine and the halogenated anesthetics. Dysrhythmias should not be dismissed, however, even when blood pressure (BP) is stable, but should heighten an index of suspicion for the existence of other problems, such as inadequate oxygenation or ventilation or early malignant hyperthermia.

ECG may also be used to detect electrolyte abnormalities in children. Infants and children requiring massive transfusion of blood products are prone to increases in serum potassium (from old banked blood) and decreases in serum calcium concentrations (occurring as a result of the high citrate content of blood products). These problems are frequently seen in children undergoing liver transplantation, craniofacial reconstruction, and removal of large vascular tumors. Hyperkalemia produces a characteristic peaked T wave, whereas hypocalcemia produces a prolonged QT interval.

TABLE 1. *The relationship of age to heart rate*

Age	Mean heart rate (beats /min)
0–24 hours	120
1–7 days	135
8–30 days	160
3–12 months	140
1–3 years	125
3–5 years	100
8–12 years	80
2–16 years	75

Although rare in the pediatric population, ischemic changes can occur in normal children as well as in children with congenital heart disease (3). Therefore, the ST segment should be observed in pediatric surgical patients whenever possible.

As in adults, an adequate heart rate does not always imply adequate tissue perfusion. Used by itself, the ECG will not detect significant reductions in cardiac output (4). In children, loss of sinus rhythm is a late finding in cardiac depression, particularly when it is due to an overdose of a halogenated anesthetic. Therefore, ECG should always be used in conjunction with other monitors that detect changes in perfusion and BP. When doing a regional anesthetic technique, lead II is optimal for detection of local anesthetic toxicity (T-wave elevation) (5).

Neuromuscular Blockade Monitoring

A twitch monitor is applied to pediatric patients who receive muscle relaxants. Pediatric electrodes are placed along the ulnar nerve at the wrist (Fig. 1) or one of the nerves in the leg (Fig. 2). Extremity placement is preferable to placement on the face near the eye, since monitoring the twitch around the orbicularis oris muscles may underestimate muscle relaxation and overestimate the reversal of muscle relaxant.

Blood Pressure Monitoring

As with cardiac rate, BP in infants and children is age-dependent (Table 2). Because of its ease of operation and accuracy, automated oscillometry (e.g., Dinamap, Critikon, Tampa, FL) has virtually taken over as the primary BP monitor. A misconception is that a certain portion of the cuff must be placed directly over an artery for accurate measurement. Because the cuff acts as a signal sensor of pressure oscillations under the entire cuff, placement of the cuff directly over an artery is unnecessary.

The automated cuff is deflated in increments and compares two cardiac cycles at each deflation. If noise levels are high (from

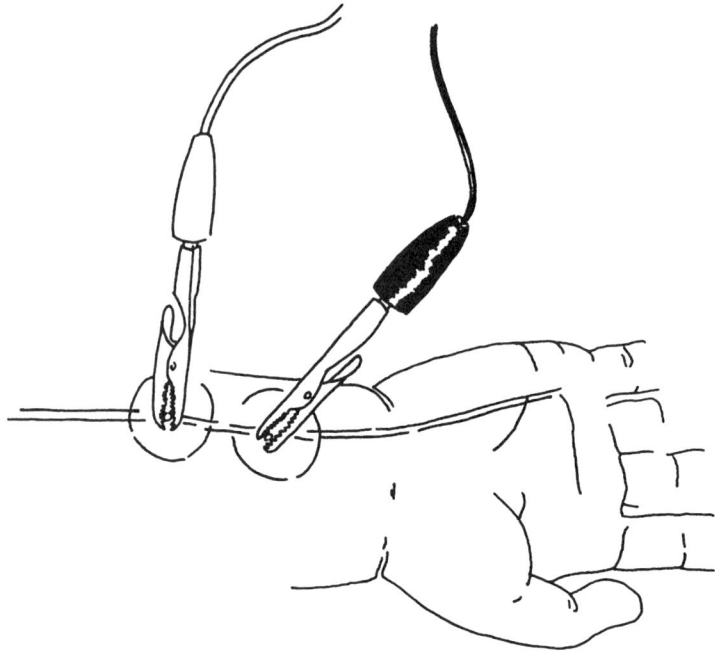

FIG. 1. Electrode placement for neuromuscular stimulation at the wrist.

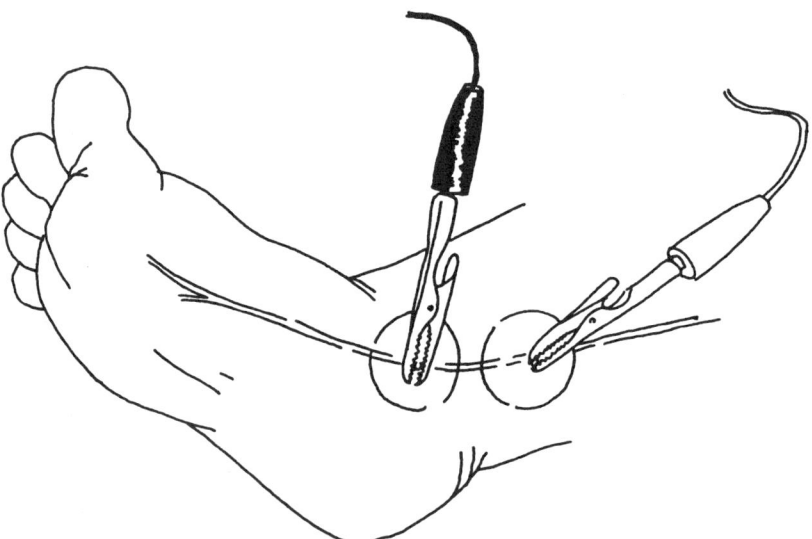

FIG. 2. Electrode placement for neuromuscular stimulation at the ankle.

TABLE 2. *The relationship of age to blood pressure*

Age	Normal blood pressure (mm Hg)	
	Mean systolic	Mean diastolic
0–12 hours (preterm)	50	35
0–12 hours (full-term)	65	45
4 days	75	50
6 weeks	95	55
1 year	95	60
2 years	100	65
9 years	105	70
12 years	115	75

child's movement during measurement), successive cardiac cycles are compared until two comparable cycles are recorded at a given inflation pressure. If noise levels are low (from lack of cuff movement during measurement), then deflation of the cuff proceeds more rapidly. This explains the differences in time it may take to measure a BP in struggling compared with nonstruggling children during the course of an anesthetic induction.

Accuracy of automated BP devices depends on several factors. Foremost is the use of an appropriately sized cuff. The cuff width should be 50% of the circumference or 120% of the diameter of the limb (6,7). A cuff that is too narrow may produce larger errors (overestimated BP) than one that is too wide (underestimated BP). We recommend using a cuff that is at least two thirds the distance between the child's axilla and antecubital fossa. In infants and children, normal BP varies with age.

Automated Blood Pressure Measurement in the Neonate

BP measured by automated oscillometry is accurate in very-low-birth-weight infants if the mean arterial pressure is above 40 mm Hg (8, 9). For mean arterial pressures under 40 mm Hg, automated monitors may give readings above those determined by the intra-arterial method. Therefore, a low reading (<40 mm Hg) in a neonate may critically underestimate the degree of hypotension that is actually present. Awareness of this fact is helpful to guide therapy in neonates who may develop cardiac depression during induction **(see Increasing the Inspired Concentrations of Halothane and Sevoflurane)**.

TEMPERATURE MONITORING AND MAINTENANCE

Core body temperature is continuously measured using either a rectal, nasopharyngeal, esophageal, bladder, or axillary probe. Skin temperature (e.g., measured using a "stick-on" patch) is not usually an accurate reflection of core body temperature and may give information leading to misguided management of body temperature.

Intraoperative hypothermia is deleterious for a host of reasons, most notably because hypothermia causes the following:

- Release of catabolic stress hormones
- Impaired cardiopulmonary resuscitation if the child develops cardiac arrest
- Impaired platelet function
- Poor behavior in the postanesthesia care unit

Infants and children have a relatively large surface area-to-weight ratio and become hypothermic more quickly than adults after the induction of anesthesia, especially if preventive measures are not taken. Children, like adults, undergo 90% of their heat loss through the skin (10). This fact presents a compelling argument for using one of the newer forced-air warming devices. These warming devices are made ready in advance. Then, when the child comes into the room, the blanket is placed on top and around the child (Bair Hugger, Augustine Medical; Pediatric Quilt, Baxter) or under the child (Warm Touch, Mallinckrodt Medical; Fig. 3). With each of these blankets, warm air is forced over the child's skin, providing a positive heat flux that warms the child's skin and maintains core temperature (11). A recent observation was that when forced-air warm-

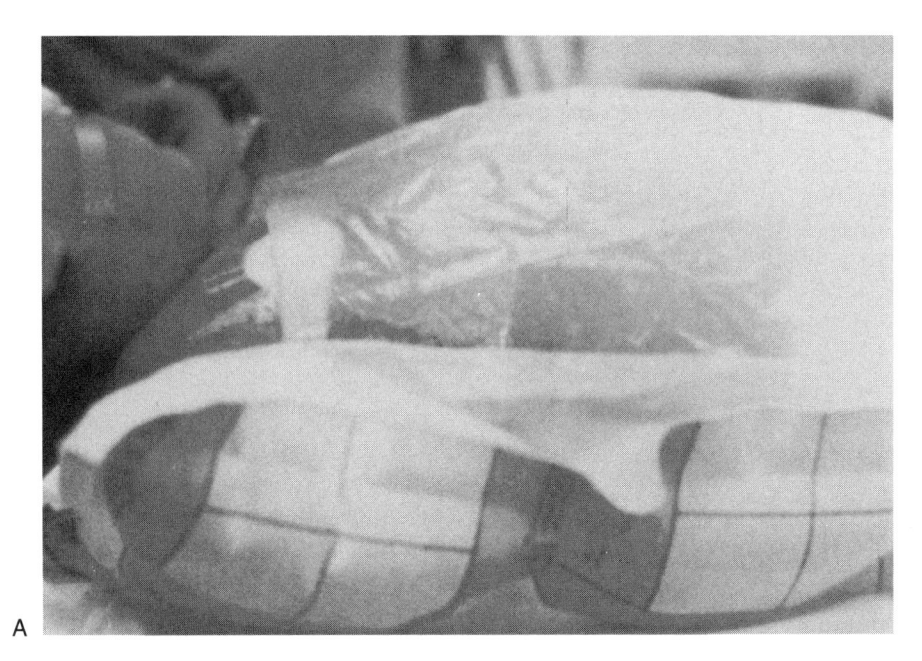

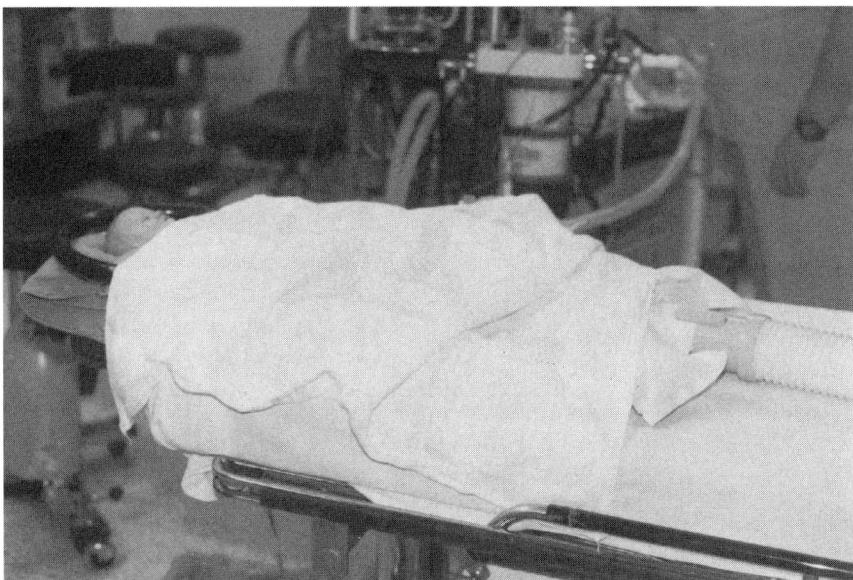

FIG. 3. (A) During a waiting period before the surgical procedure begins, an infant is lying on a forced-air warming blanket covered with a clear plastic sheet. **(B)** In another child on a forced-air blanket, note the placement of the air entry nozzle into the end of the blanket. Burns have been reported when this air entry nozzle is used to blow air under the blanket without using the manufactured warming blanket.

ers are used, infants and children may stay warm in an often-cool operating room (12).[b]

Drugs

There are only three or four drugs (in addition to emergency resuscitation drugs) that I actually draw up before the induction of anesthesia: sodium thiopental, atropine, succinylcholine, and, if I plan to use it, a single nondepolarizing muscle relaxant. If atropine is to be given, a mixture of 4 ml of thiopental with 1 ml of atropine (0.4 mg/ml) yields 20 mg/ml for thiopental and 0.08 mg/ml atropine. Then, if 5 mg/kg thiopental is given, 0.02 mg/kg atropine follows along. Atropine is administered if succinylcholine is administered as part of the induction sequence. Furthermore, succinylcholine should always be made available in case the child develops laryngospasm. Whereas the routine use of atropine is a point of minor controversy in pediatric anesthesia, it is not controversial to have a syringe containing atropine available for emergencies when anesthetizing all children. Bradycardia is always a possibility.[c]

Muscle Relaxants

Succinylcholine

The routine use of succinylcholine in children and adolescents was recently labelled as contraindicated by the Food and Drug Administration (FDA) (package insert for succinylcholine, Burroughs Wellcome, November 1992) and then later changed to a box warning (package insert for succinylcholine; Burroughs Wellcome, November 1994). These measures came about as the result of reported cases of hyperkalemic cardiac arrest in male children with undiagnosed Duchenne's muscular dystrophy. Succinylcholine is still the drug of choice for use in the child who develops laryngospasm or for use in a rapid sequence induction (e.g., for use in patients with full stomach). I draw up undiluted succinylcholine, 20 mg/kg, in a 3-ml or 5-ml syringe for children, and I have ready a 10 mg/ml solution of succinylcholine in a 3-ml syringe for infants. Sudden cardiac arrest after succinylcholine is, until proved otherwise, due to increased potassium in a patient with undiagnosed myopathy treatable by $CaCl_2$ (10 mg/kg). If succinylcholine triggers malignant hypothermia syndrome, the signs and symptoms can develop quickly, but the presenting signs are rigidity, tachycardia, dysrhythmias, and hypercapnia, not sudden cardiac arrest.

Nondepolarizing Muscle Relaxants

In pediatric anesthesia, it was once (and may still be in some places) fairly common practice to do an inhalation induction of children followed by an IV catheter insertion and then succinylcholine administration and endotracheal intubation. To avoid the complications and controversy of succinylcholine, many pediatric anesthesiologists have replaced succinylcholine with a nondepolarizing muscle relaxant (Table 3).

The choice of a nondepolarizing muscle relaxant depends on the following:

- Desired rapidity of onset
- Estimated duration of action
- Side effects one wishes to avoid
- Side effects one wishes to achieve

For example, if spontaneous ventilation in a patient is planned, the trachea may be intubated with mivacurium, an agent with short duration of action. By contrast, if fentanyl, which causes bradycardia, is used, pancuronium, which causes tachycardia, would be the desired neuromuscular blocking agent. To avoid histamine release, vecuronium or rocuronium would be chosen in a volume-depleted child. A child in shock should not receive one of the histamine releasers mivac-

---

[b]Ed. Note (JMB): This environmental management strategy allows both optimal patient care and a pleasant workspace for medical personnel.

[c]Ed. Note (JMB): Bradycardia is usually the result of a treatable cause (e.g., hypoxemia). Likewise, premature ventricular contractions (PVCs) that occur frequently during induction are usually the result of hypercarbia, light anesthesia, and catecholamines and are easily treatable by corrective measures (e.g., hyperventilation or deeping anesthesia).

TABLE 3. Available nondepolarizing muscle relaxants

	Rocuronium bromide	Vecuronium bromide	Atracurium besylate	Mivacurium chloride	Pancuronium bromide
Onset	Rapid	Intermediate (decreased age ~ faster onset) (14)	Intermediate	Intermediate	Intermediate
Duration	Intermediate	Intermediate	Intermediate	Short	Long
Dose for intubation (mg/kg)	0.6	0.1–0.4	0.3–0.4 (1 mo–2 yrs under halothane) 0.5 (>2 yrs)	0.2–0.6 (administer over 5–15 sec [over 60 sec in histamine-sensitive patients])	0.06–0.1
Intubation time[a]	30–60 sec (13)	Dose (mg/kg) Time (min) 0.1 ~1.5 (15) 0.25 1.0–1.5 0.4 0.5–1.0 (16)	1.5–2.5 min (17,18)	1.5–2.0 min	2–3 min

[a]Times to good or excellent intubating conditions.

urium or atracurium. Following are a few words and tips about the various agents.

Atracurium. Atracurium may be prepared in a 1 mg/ml dilution (convenient for use in most infants and children). Atracurium may become relatively inactive after a long shelf-life at room temperature. Therefore, it is usually best to obtain fresh atracurium from the refrigerator before each use.

Vecuronium. Vecuronium requires reconstitution and is drawn up ahead of time and diluted appropriately. Decreasing age is associated with a fast onset of action of vecuronium (14). A faster onset is also associated with larger doses, but a larger dose will cause longer duration of action.

Rocuronium. Rocuronium is gaining increasing popularity as a relatively fast-acting neuromuscular muscle relaxant. Although it is not as fast as succinylcholine, it does offer faster onset than the other neuromuscular relaxants (13). Good-to-excellent intubating conditions after rocuronium 0.6 mg/kg can be obtained within 30 to 60 seconds in young children. If necessary, intramuscular (IM) rocuronium may be administered to permit tracheal intubation in infants and children (e.g., when one wishes to avoid succinylcholine in an infant or child with laryngospasm when a suitable vein is inaccessible). Deltoid (but not quadriceps) injection of 1.0 mg/kg rocuronium IM permits tracheal intubation in lightly anesthetized infants at 2.5 minutes and children (1.8 mg/kg) at 3 minutes (19). These doses result in paralysis exceeding 1 hour and may possibly limit usefulness of IM rocuronium for brief procedures.

BEFORE INDUCTION BEGINS

Fasting

There is no increased risk of gastric content aspiration in children who are allowed to ingest unlimited amounts of clear liquids (apple juice, water, clear gelatin, sugar water) up to 2 hours before anesthetic induction (20–24) (**see Chapter 9**). A regimen that provides fluids 2 hours before surgery will help to keep the child relatively well hydrated and help to prevent hypotension during induction.

Premedication

Midazolam

Pharmacologic advances have provided the practitioner with a variety of medications to be used for preoperative sedation/analgesia in children. Midazolam, however, has become the most commonly used pharmacologic agent for preoperative medication in these patients.[d] Midazolam has been instilled,

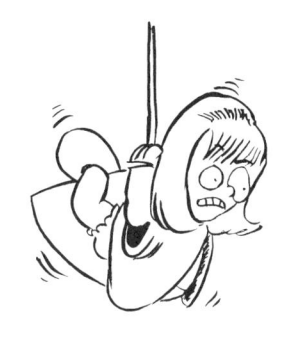

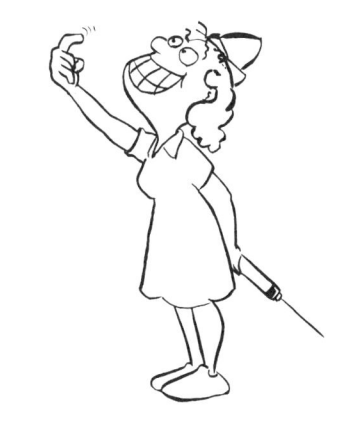

---

[d]Ed. Note (JMB): In the *Physician's Desk Reference,* one finds that most medications (including midazolam orally) are not "approved" for pediatric application! This usually indicates that the appropriate double-blind randomized study required for labeling by the FDA was never carried out. This does not, however, prohibit the practitioner from using the medication provided that the practitioner is familiar with the drug or has acquired training in its use (25).

inserted, or injected (IV and IM) into almost every conceivable orifice (26–32). It is my preference, however, to administer this drug orally (0.5 mg/kg). Larger doses (0.75 mg/kg) fail to provide superior sedation and may prolong the postoperative sedation period. Midazolam has a very bad aftertaste. To mask this bad taste, just about everything has been used as a vehicle for administration. I use simple grape elixir from the pharmacy or mix it with pediatric acetaminophen or ibuprofen elixir. The latter drug is appropriate if administration of a nonsteroidal anti-inflammatory agent (NSAID) is warranted and is not contraindicated (e.g., NSAIDs are contraindicated before tonsillectomy because they may impair coagulation).

Oral Transmucosal Fentanyl Citrate

Although oral transmucosal fentanyl citrate (OTFC; Fentanyl Oralet) is most helpful as an analgesic medication for children without IVs who are undergoing painful procedures (e.g., burn dressing changes), this formulation has found limited usefulness as a premedication before surgical procedures in children. Nevertheless, it can be used. For example, if a child (>3 years) has significant pain preoperatively or if significant pain is expected postoperatively (especially if the child's trachea will remain intubated), then OTFC may be indicated to provide preoperative sedation and analgesia. Because respiratory depression may occur both pre- and postoperatively after the use of this formulation, the child should be monitored with pulse oximetry after the drug's administration. In addition, nausea and vomiting may also occur pre- or postoperatively after administration of OTFC. For these reasons, oral midazolam is more often a better surgical premedication than OTFC.

In summary, if the child is to remain intubated, or is expected to have significant pain postoperatively, especially if regional analgesia or intraoperative opioids are avoided, it is appropriate to administer OTFC preoperatively (15 µg/kg).

Considerations by Age

Children can be subdivided into four groups according to their generally expected behavior during the induction period. From 0 to 6 months of age, children are in the "golden age of blissful ignorance." At this age, they separate easily from parents and usually lie calmly on the table or in a nurse's arms awaiting their graceful induction of anesthesia.

However, when children reach a certain age (usually about 9 months), they become very much their parents' children, and separation anxiety is a primary fear during their hospitalization. When children reach the age of about 4 to 6 years (up until about age 12), they enter into the "age of reason." At this age, children may choose their induction method—either IV or inhalation anesthesia. Adolescent children become "supermen" and "superwomen" on the outside, but underneath may be very frightened and, above all, very modest.

THE INDUCTION PROCEDURE

The Induction Room (Where Parents Can Be Present)

At some institutions (e.g., the author's), a special room is frequently used in which parents may be present during the induction of anesthesia. Parents can be present during inhalation induction until the child first loses consciousness (Fig. 4). The parents are accompanied back to the waiting room, while IV cannulation, intubation, and the rest of the induction are completed.

Parent selection and education of parents are very important in this process (33). Unduly anxious parents are usually not good candidates to be present during induction. Parents should be told or shown precisely what to expect during the induction sequence so that they are not frightened by such things as partial airway obstruction. Infants less than 1 year of age are rarely suitable candidates for parental presence at induction.

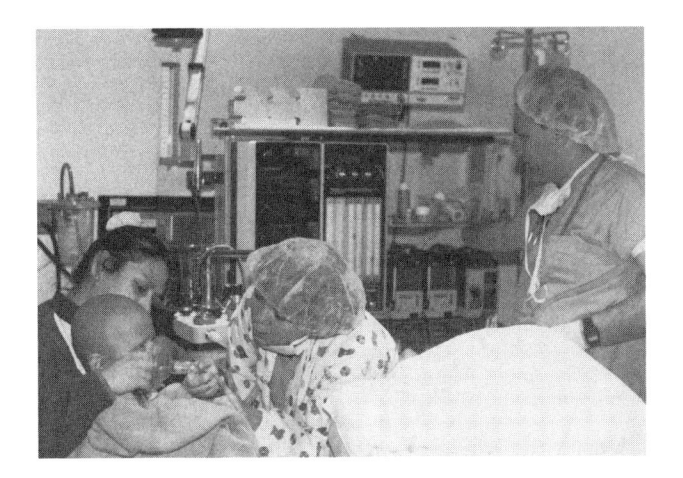

FIG. 4. Parents are often allowed into the operating room or a special "induction" room during the child's induction of anesthesia. Note that the child is on the parent's lap, and one clinician is adjusting the inspired concentration of anesthetic gases while the other is helping the mother to apply the mask. As the child goes off to sleep, one clinician will assume control of the patient and moves the child over to the bed, paying particular attention to preserving patency of the child's airway.

The Operating Room

Before induction, the room and all its equipment are prepared with the child's comfort in mind. For instance, the face mask can be made more enticing by swabbing the inside of the mask with flavoring. Almost every artificial flavor, including piña colada for more sophisticated children, is available at the grocery store. Before the patient is brought in, the room is warmed. The room that is uncomfortably warm for an adult is more than likely just right for the infant or child. Later, after application of a forced-air warmer **(see Temperature Monitoring and Maintenance)** and surgical draping, the room may be cooled (12). Persons in the room should be instructed that mask induction of anesthesia is about to begin so that they may discontinue any chatter or banging of equipment.

Bringing the Patient to the Operating Room

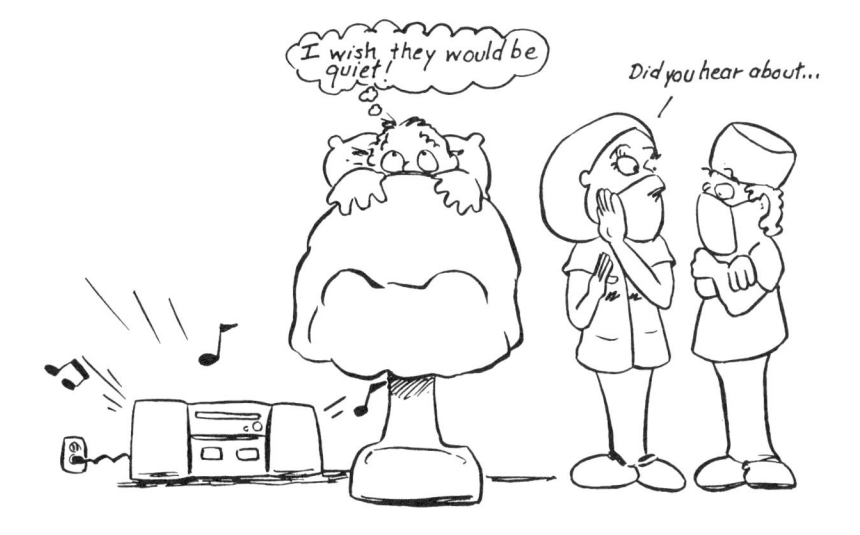

Patients may be brought to the operating room on a gurney, or they may be carried in by a nurse, physician, or parent. In some institutions, the patients actually walk or ride in a wagon to the operating room. Patients can be told that they are being brought into a spaceship or being taken for a ride at their favorite amusement park. This "ride" can be continued on the electric adjustable bed where the patient can be tilted and moved up and down. A ploy I have used is to tell the children that there are puppy dogs loose in the room and we are going to go look for them. For reasons yet unknown, this trick usually seems to work.

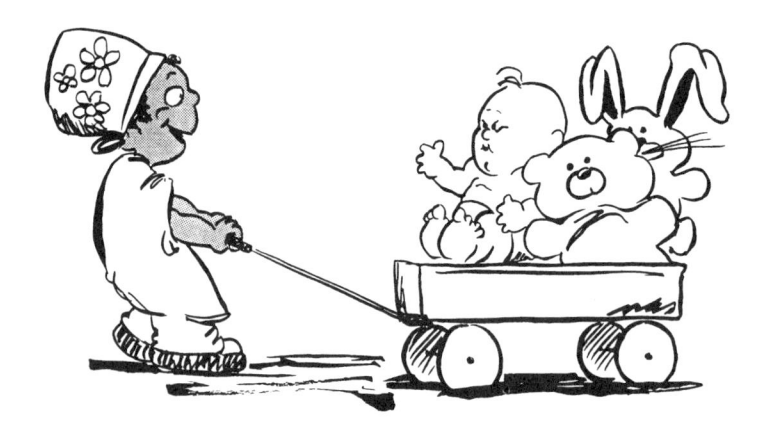

Placing the Child on the Surgical Bed

Usually, children are better off with a mask induction if they are allowed to sit on the surgical bed rather than being forced to lie down on it. The patient is placed on the table in a position with the back against the physician's abdomen (Fig. 5). In this way, children are not slammed flat on the surgical bed, but are allowed to preserve a small vestige of dignity and self-control. Monitors can be applied if the child is agreeable, but often only a pulse oximeter is "allowed." In the sedated child, however, it is usually a very simple matter to apply the required monitors. One can speak of applying "muscle testers" (BP cuffs), ECG "lie detectors" ("better watch what you say"), and "ET band-aids" (pulse oximeters) (Fig. 6).

Mask Application

There are various ways to get the child to accept the face mask. Children can be told that they are jet pilots about to use a special jet pilot mask. They can be told that they will be blowing up a balloon. They can play the Cap-

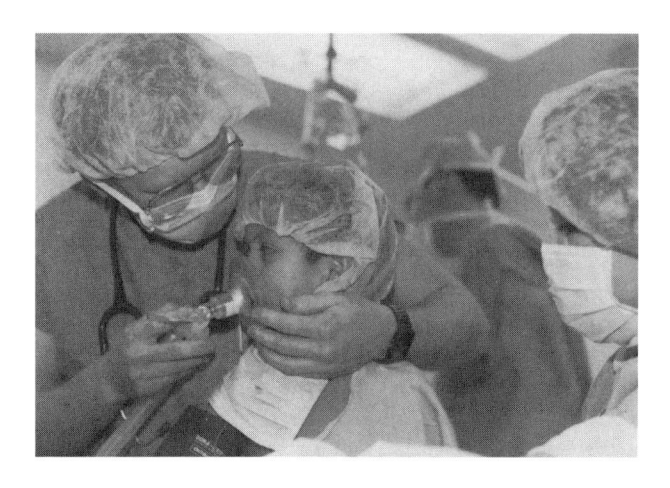

FIG. 5. The child is allowed to sit for the induction of his anesthetic. The child's back is up against the clinician's abdomen, allowing the child to feel less restrained than if slammed down on the table. As the child goes off to sleep, he is gently lowered to the table.

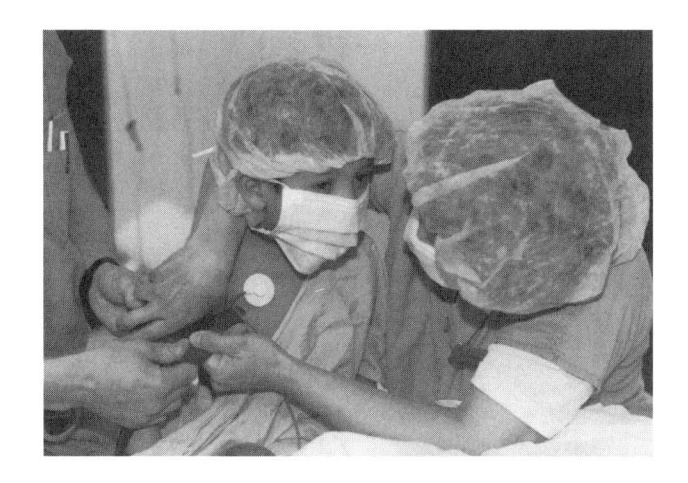

FIG. 6. Monitors are usually applied before the induction of anesthesia.

tain Capno video game, where they breathe through the face mask and make a squiggly line (their capnographic trace) on the video screen. Children can even be shown cartoons (played on standard operating room video equipment) as they drift off to sleep (Fig. 7).

One can also use reverse psychology. You can say, "Gee, I'm going to breathe this very special space gas, but you can't have any right now." After a few breaths, you say, "Gee, you know I really wish you could breathe some of this, but we don't know whether you can have any or not." Finally, "Well, okay, you can have some of this nice-smelling gas." This tactic may backfire, especially if you actually sniff the gas. The oc-

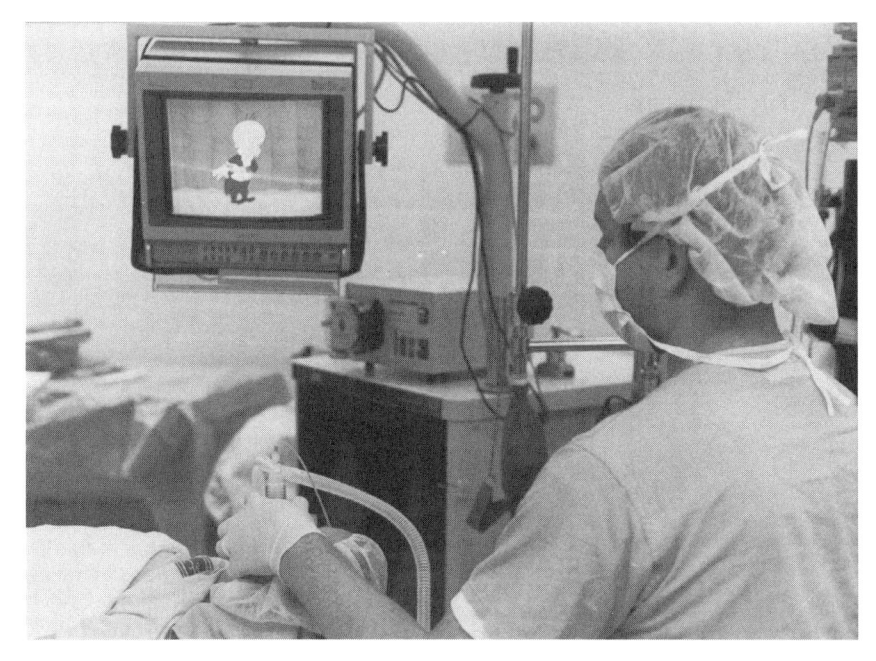

FIG. 7. As a distraction during the induction of anesthesia, the child is positioned so that a cartoon may be viewed.

casional child may say, "Okay, I can't have any. Good, I don't want any...." You'll just have to accept the occasional failure of reverse psychology, eat your words, and go on to something else.

Frequently, the patient will more calmly respond to an authority figure other than an imposing anesthesiologist. At my institution, often one or more of the nursing personnel or anesthesia technicians helps with mask in-

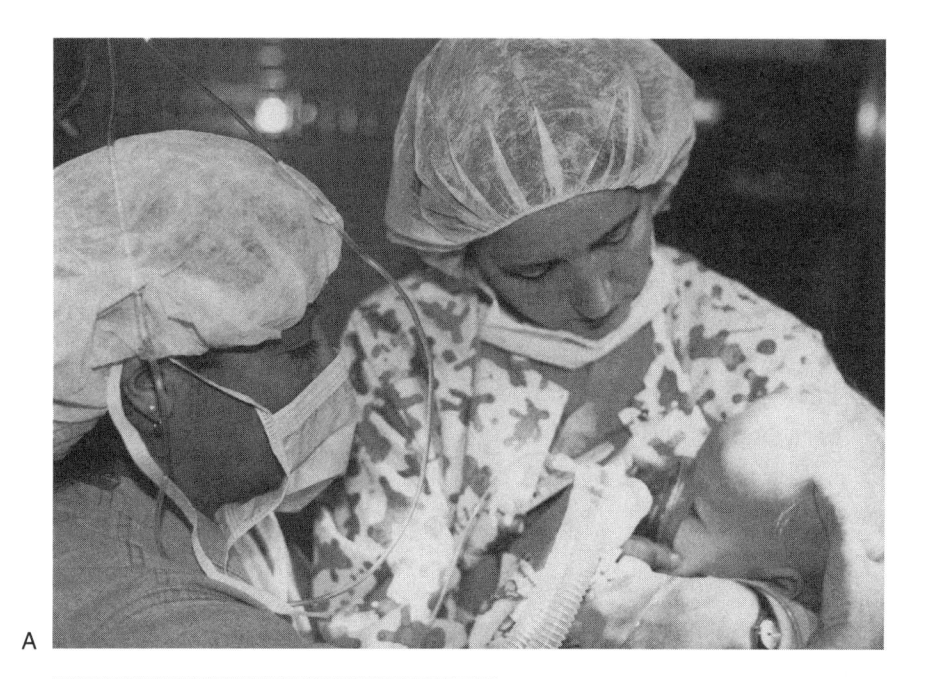

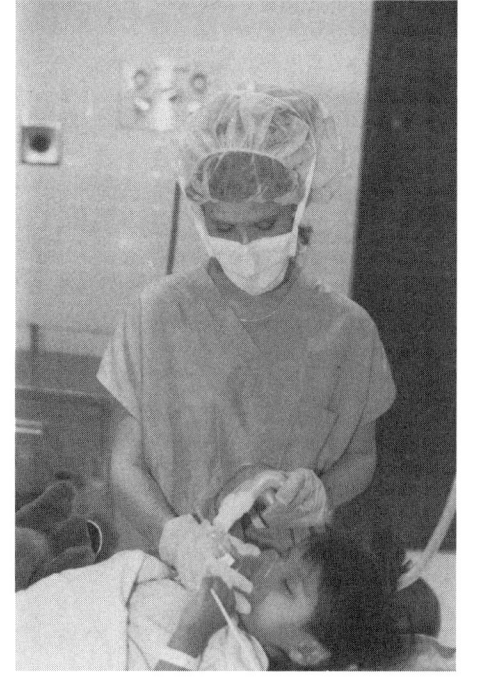

FIG. 8. (A) To initiate the induction of anesthesia in a frightened infant or child, nursing personnel may act as an extension of the supervising clinician by cradling the infant or child and holding the mask gently to the child's face. As soon as the child is "stunned," the clinician accepts the patient and continues the induction. This transfer takes place well before the patient may develop the inevitable airway obstruction (see text). **(B)** An older child accepts a face mask from a friendly "surrogate mommy figure" during the induction of anesthesia. As in **A**, the clinician takes over when the child first "drifts off."

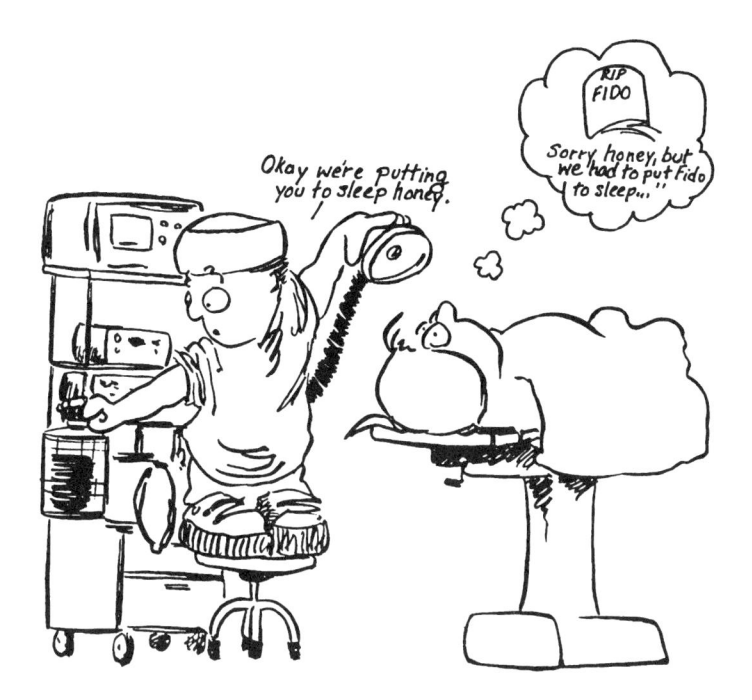

duction by speaking reassuringly while gently cradling the child and holding the mask on the child's face (Fig. 8). This friendly person has helped us to induce anesthesia smoothly and in a caring fashion. It should be noted that the anesthesiologist is still in control of the induction of anesthesia and supervises any personnel helping with the induction. It usually does not take long for the child to become "out of it" enough to be unaware that the clinician has taken over.

The *Art* of the Inhalation Induction

Always *sit* for the induction of anesthesia in children.[e] After the child accepts the face mask, you can say that he or she will begin breathing some "funny-smelling gas" or gas that "smells like mommy's perfume" (Fig. 9). Be careful not to use the words "put to sleep," because these words may have a negative connotation. A rambling banter can begin now, which, if done properly, will border on embarrassment for the anesthesiologist (the clinician's ego is set aside for the time being). It doesn't matter what is said in the spiel, but that it is said in a smooth non-threatening tone to provide reassurance and comfort.

What follows is an example of this rambling, but meaningful and effective, banter. It is meant to show how a typical mask induction might go.

"Okay, Johnny, now that you're a jet pilot and you have a face mask, you're going to be breathing some funny-smelling gas. You want to breath it in and out. Take some very deep breaths and blow up this balloon...the funny one over there. You can blow that up, and if it starts smelling too funny you can just blow the gas away. Take a deep breath and blow the gas away. That's it, take some nice deep breaths and what you'll notice is that as you breathe this very special gas you'll be getting very, very sleepy. It's going to make you feel like you're getting very, very drowsy. Your eyelids are getting very heavy and you're going to feel funny but that's how you should feel. That's a very normal feeling and you're doing just fine. You may feel as if you're

---

[e]Ed. Note (JMB): The First Law of Conservation of Energy (modified from Peter Byles) is: Never run when you can jog, never jog when you can walk, never walk when you can stand, never stand when you can sit, never sit when you can lie, and never lie awake when you can lie asleep.

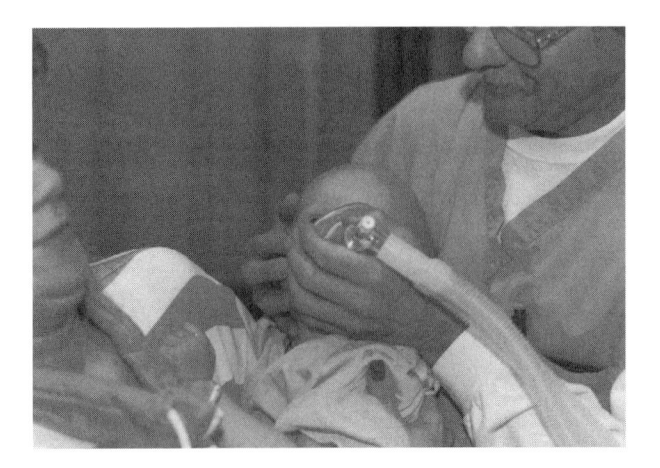

FIG. 9. As the child accepts the face mask and drifts off to sleep, an anesthetic monologue is begun with the child by telling the child that he will be breathing funny-smelling gas or gas that smells like Mommy's perfume. As can be seen from this picture, Mommy gives us the distinct impression that her perfume has never smelled this bad.

floating or drifting high above the clouds. You see pink puffy clouds and purple smoke. Your body is going to get very light; you're going to be drifting, drifting, and you're getting very sleepy. Now you may be feeling funny and that's how you should feel because this special air makes you feel very funny. You're doing just fine. You're getting very sleepy as you breathe more and more. Take some deep breaths, the sandman is going to come and drop some sand in your eyes and you're going to get very sleepy. You're going to notice that you're feeling funny but that's how you should feel. Just close your eyes and go along with the feeling, and close your eyes and imagine that you're in a place that you like very much. You're very comfortable and warm and everything is fine."

"Now the gas is going to change smells a little bit. It's going to start smelling like mommy's perfume or maybe it's going to start smelling like mutant ninja toe-jam or maybe it's going to start smelling like tennis shoes that have been in the back of your closet for a long time. You know how bad those smell, so it's going to start smelling kind of funny. If you don't like it, just blow it away because it's making you very sleepy. This is very good air. It's a very special air that we have just for you that we pipe in from Ozona, Texas. It's so nice. It's just like grandma used to bake. It's making you very sleepy. You are now going into a very deep sleep and nothing can hurt you. You'll feel no pain and no ouchies when you're in this very deep sleep."

Note that nothing said is too silly. A gentle tone of voice and continuous monotone are all that is important. Also, don't ask questions. Children can't breathe deeply and speak at the same time. By contrast, the clinician should maintain constant verbal (and tactile) contact with the patient. Most important, the statements "...you're doing okay..." and "...that's the way you should feel..." are frequently repeated. Children need to be told that this strangely foreign feeling is actually a normal feeling for them at the time. Otherwise, they may perceive this as something very frightening. They might even think they are dying. I have found that this easy-going banter allows most children to get through the hyperexcitable period (stage 2) and, in most cases, creates a very smooth induction of anesthesia.

As the anesthetic induction begins, the clinician dials in a mixture of 70% N_2O/30% O_2 and begins the gradual induction of anesthesia. While the child drifts off to sleep, the concentration of halothane or sevoflurane is gradually increased **(see Increasing the Inspired Concentrations of Halothane and Sevoflurane)**.

Face Mask Application

Proper face mask application is very important to maintain airway patency during the induction of anesthesia in infants and children (Figs. 10 and 11). An inflatable pillow-type face mask is placed gently on the child's face, and the anesthesiologist's mid-

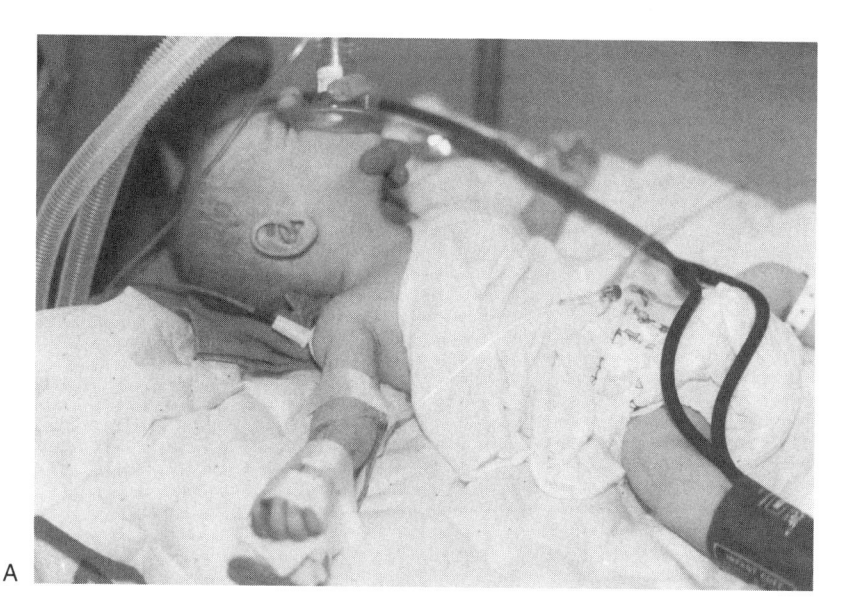

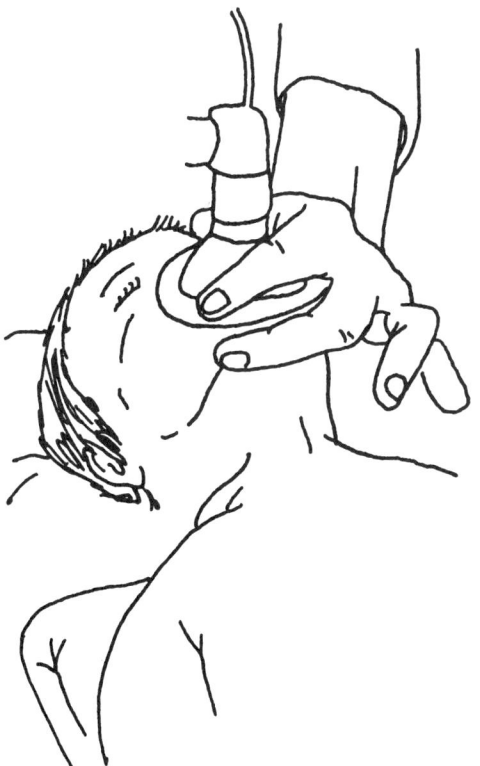

FIG. 10. (A) Proper face mask application is important to maintain airway patency during the induction of anesthesia in infants. **(B)** It is very important to place the middle or ring finger along the ramus of the mandible and to keep the other fingers off the soft airway structures overlying the larynx and glottic opening.

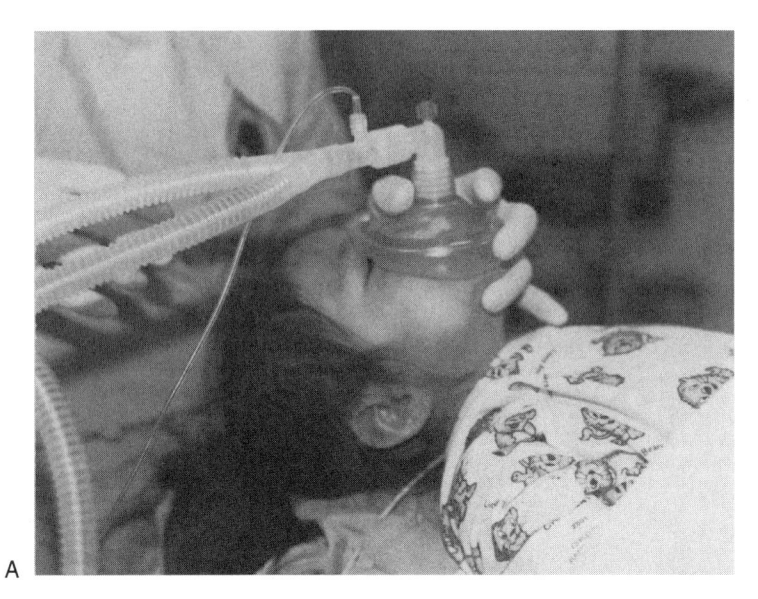

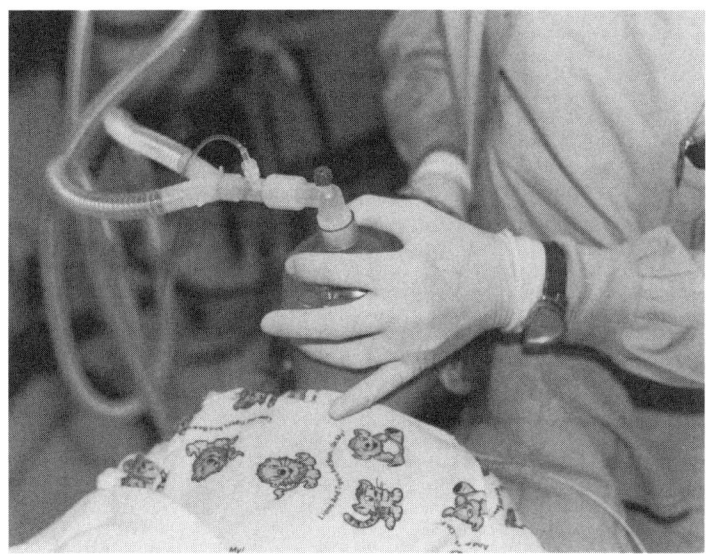

FIG. 11. (A) Appropriate mask application is shown, with the clinician's ring finger along the ramus of the mandible and the little finger well off the supraglottic structures. (B) Another view of proper mask application. Jaw thrust is achieved by the clinician pulling backward with the weight of his body and large muscles of the shoulder. This maneuver allows the clinician to use a grip that is relaxing for the fine muscles of the hand and forearm. This relaxed hand grip is relatively stress-free and allows mask application for long periods of time without undue fatigue.

dle or ring finger is placed along the chin and anterior ramus of the child's mandible (Fig. 12). The palm of the hand is then placed gently against the child's cheek, and chin-lift/anterior jaw thrust is accomplished by applying upper and backward traction on the chin/jaw. This technique involves pulling with the weight of the body and large muscles of the shoulder, thereby preventing muscular fatigue of small, fine muscles of the hand and forearm. One should take care to avoid digital pressure in the region of the submental triangle, which could push the child's tongue up to the roof of the mouth and cause the airway to obstruct. If positive-pressure ventilation (PPV) is needed, a small leak at the mask-cheek interface is allowed (actually, desirable) to prevent excessive gas from entering the stomach (Fig. 13). Eventually, as the child gets sleepier, variable degrees of airway obstruction will develop despite expert mask application. When airway obstruction occurs, a different mask application, the "survival position," is applied **(see Anatomic Airway Obstruction)**.

The *Science* of the Inhalation Induction

Choice of Agents

Halothane is relatively nonirritating to airways and provides smooth induction characteristics compared with isoflurane and desflurane. Halothane has been the most commonly used agent for induction of anesthesia in children for nearly four decades. Disadvantages of halothane include its high solubility in blood and tissues (leading to slow wash-out) and cardiac toxicity (leading to dysrhythmias and bradycardias, as well as cardiorespiratory depression).

Sevoflurane, a newer agent with fewer side effects has successfully challenged halothane's dominant role in pediatric anesthesia (34). It is unique among the ether series of inhalation anesthetics in that it does not trigger airway reflex responses during inhalation induction in infants and children. This attribute together with its low blood and tissue solubilities and cardiorespiratory stability make sevoflurane a suitable alternative for halothane. Because sevoflurane does not trigger airway reflex responses, it may allow more rapid increases in inspired concentrations during induction of anesthesia and therefore may allow more rapid anesthetic induction than does halothane. A side-by-side analysis of induction, recovery, and safety characteristics of halothane and sevoflurane is provided in the following text.

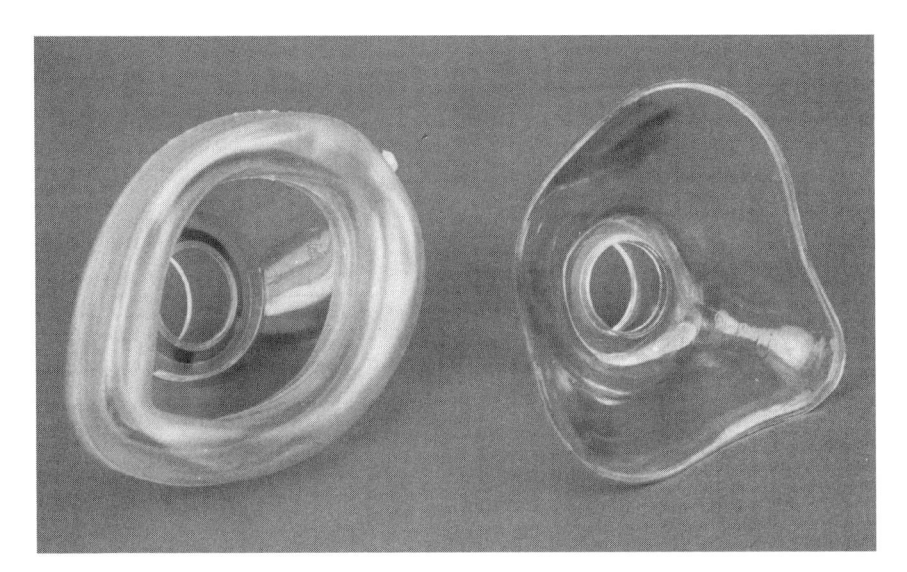

FIG. 12. A "pillow" face mask *(left)* and a Rendell-Baker-Soucek mask *(right)* compared. The lower dead space of the Rendell-Baker-Soucek mask is an advantage for small infants and children who are breathing spontaneously, while a tight mask seal is more easily obtained with the cushioned mask. During the inhalation induction of anesthesia, better fit has a higher priority than the rather insignificant dead-space issue. Therefore, pillow masks are most often used for the induction of anesthesia in infants and children. (Reprinted with permission from M. Sosis, M.D., Ph.D. ed., *Anesthesia Equipment Manual*, Lippincott–Raven Publishers, in press.)

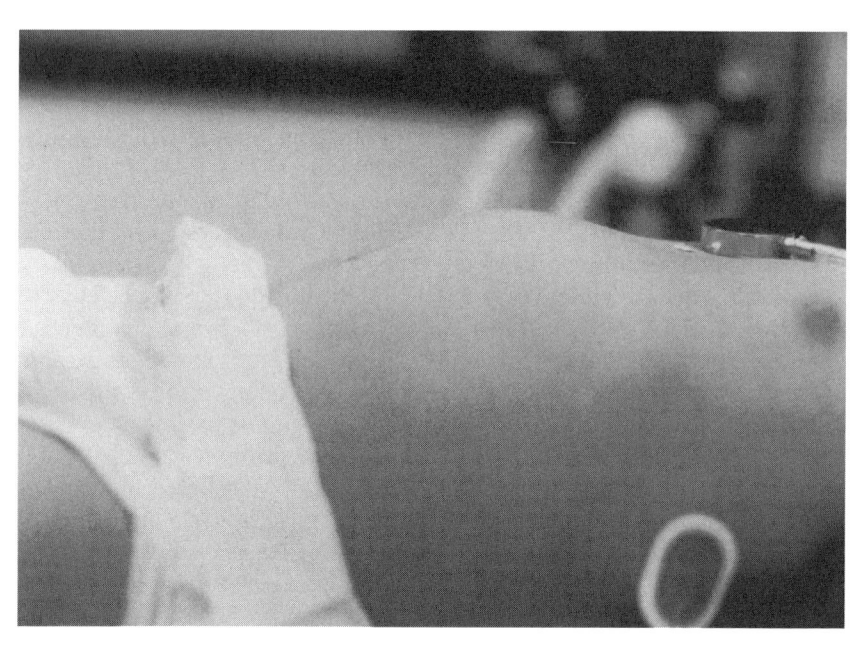

FIG. 13. A child with a belly full of gas after a routine mask induction. Gastric distention may be reduced by avoiding positive-pressure ventilation (PPV) during the induction of anesthesia. If PPV is needed, a small leak at the mask cuff/cheek interface may be allowed, provided the child is adequately ventilated. This small leak allows gas to escape to the room rather than fill the child's stomach.

Increasing the Inspired Concentrations of Halothane and Sevoflurane

To begin induction of anesthesia with either gas, it is helpful to dial in high fresh gas flows (fresh gas flow, 7 to 10 L/min). High fresh gas flows facilitate rapid changes in inspired concentrations and allow for a more rapid induction of anesthesia. With either agent, the inspired concentration is increased in stepwise increments every three to four breaths. With halothane, the increments are 0.5% to 1.0%, and for sevoflurane these increments are 1.5% to 2.0%.[f]

Based on relative minimum alveolar concentration (MAC) values of these agents, 4% halothane is equivalent to approximately 8% sevoflurane. Knowing this 4:8 relationship is helpful when determining maximum inspired concentrations of these agents (~3% to 4% in children spontaneously breathing halothane and ~7% to 8% in those spontaneously breathing sevoflurane). Remember that MAC is only a relative concept (35). Volatile anesthetic agents are titrated in a dose-response curve aimed not only at inducing anesthesia, but, more importantly, at preventing cardiovascular depression (see **Avoiding Overdose of Volatile Anesthetic Agents**).

Induction Characteristics of Halothane versus Sevoflurane

The time from application of the face mask until the loss of eyelash reflex is not clinically faster for sevoflurane (1.3 minutes) than for halothane (~1.6 minutes) (34).

---

[f]Ed. Note (JMB): As I gain more experience with sevoflurane, I find myself increasing the inspired concentration much more rapidly during inhalation induction. In fact, a typical sevoflurane technique is to allow the child to breathe 70% N$_2$O/30% O$_2$ for a minute or so and then introduce sevoflurane at 8% inspired concentration—almost like a single breath technique.

Side effects of the volatile anesthetic agents include the following:

- Coughing
- Breath-holding
- Laryngospasm
- Bronchospasm
- Secretions
- Excitement
- Vomiting

The latter side effects are similar during induction with both halothane and sevoflurane (34). By contrast, cardiovascular events, including bradycardia, can be expected to occur less frequently with sevoflurane than with halothane. The cardiovascular depressant effects and ECG disturbances (PVCs, nodal rhythm, premature atrial contractions, bradycardia, and decreased cardiac output) that occur with halothane are well known. Sevoflurane is not, however, totally lacking in cardiovascular effects, and minor ECG disturbances may occur with the use of this agent (34).

Nevertheless, there is a trade-off for the lower incidence of cardiovascular events with sevoflurane. Agitation and excitement may occur more frequently during induction of sevoflurane than during halothane induction. However, this observation is based on data from unpremedicated patients. It is possible that agitation and excitement can be attenuated during sevoflurane induction by premedication of children with sedative agents (e.g., midazolam).

In summation, as observed in ambulatory surgery patients, the induction, recovery, and safety characteristics of sevoflurane in children are comparable to those of halothane (34).

> "Sevoflurane is a suitable alternative to halothane for use in children undergoing minor ambulatory surgery."
> —Lerman et al (34)[g]

---

[g]Ed. Note (JMB): Stated another way: Halothane is a suitable alternative to sevoflurane for use in children undergoing minor ambulatory surgery.

Avoiding Overdose of Volatile Anesthetic Agents

A major cause of morbidity and mortality is anesthetic overdose during an otherwise straightforward inhalational anesthetic administered to a healthy infant or child. In this patient, a confluence of factors contribute to the relative ease by which anesthetic overdose is achieved. Most important, the uptake of inhalation anesthetics and associated loss of consciousness are more rapid in infants and small children than in adults owing to major differences between adults and infants in alveolar ventilation, body composition, and distribution of cardiac output. For example:

- Infants breathe faster, have higher alveolar ventilation, and have smaller functional residual capacity to minute ventilation ratios than do adults, leading to faster wash-in and wash-out of inhalation anesthetic.
- Infants have less muscle mass and fat with proportionally more blood flow to vessel-rich organs such as the heart, brain, and liver.
- Infant organs (including brain and heart) have shorter time constants.

As a result of the latter factors, alveolar pressures of volatile agent increase more rapidly in pediatric patients than in adults for the same induction time (36). Therefore, the neonate's brain and heart become saturated with inhalation agent faster than the adult's brain and heart.

In addition, cardiovascular depression may occur in infants who receive PPV with a relatively high concentration of volatile agent (37,38). The cardiovascular depressant effect of controlled ventilation on the rate of wash-in of volatile agent must not be underestimated (39). Spontaneous ventilation is an effective negative feedback mechanism to autoregulate the depth of anesthesia during an inhalational anesthetic. Volatile anesthetic agents in spontaneously breathing infants will depress the respiratory control center (causing uptake to cease) well before they will depress cardiac tissue. By contrast, controlled ventilation allows volatile agents to bypass the negative feedback effect of spontaneous ventilation, leading to a downward spiral of cardiac depression. Depressed cardiac output decreases the uptake of anesthetic from the alveolus and further increases the alveolar anesthetic partial pressure. Increases in the alveolar anesthetic partial pressure further depress cardiac output, and so on. If untreated, this downward spiral will continue until circulation collapses.

To provide conditions for tracheal intubation, the clinician must be prepared with a plan using either deep anesthesia or light anesthesia and a muscle relaxant. To accomplish laryngoscopy and intubation in infants and children using deep anesthesia, about 1.2% end-tidal halothane (or 1.3 MAC) is required (40). We should be concerned, however, that "breathing the patient down" with an inhalation agent to sufficient levels to allow intubation puts the infant or child at risk for cardiac depression and hypotension. To prevent this from happening, a rational approach might be the early use of muscle relaxants (Fig. 14). To do this, an IV cannula is inserted as soon as possible during inhalation induction. After the IV cannula is inserted, a nondepolarizing muscle relaxant is given to provide conditions for tracheal intubation. For the reasons already discussed, it may be considered prudent to avoid succinylcholine as the choice for muscle relaxant to prevent potential complications (e.g., masseter spasm, hyperkalemic cardiac arrest, and malignant hyperthermia).

If IV access is delayed, the clinician has the choice of tracheal intubation under deep volatile anesthesia or to inject IM succinylcholine or IM rocuronium. If the child's airway is patent and the child has stable hemodynamics and continues to breathe spontaneously, it may be appropriate to deepen the anesthetic, give IM atropine, and then intubate the trachea. If the child has partial or complete airway obstruction, is not breathing spontaneously, or has unstable hemodynamics (e.g., bradycardia, hypotension), it is more appropriate to give an IM muscle relaxant and IM atropine, turn off the volatile agent manually, ventilate with 100% O_2, and intubate the trachea when conditions permit.

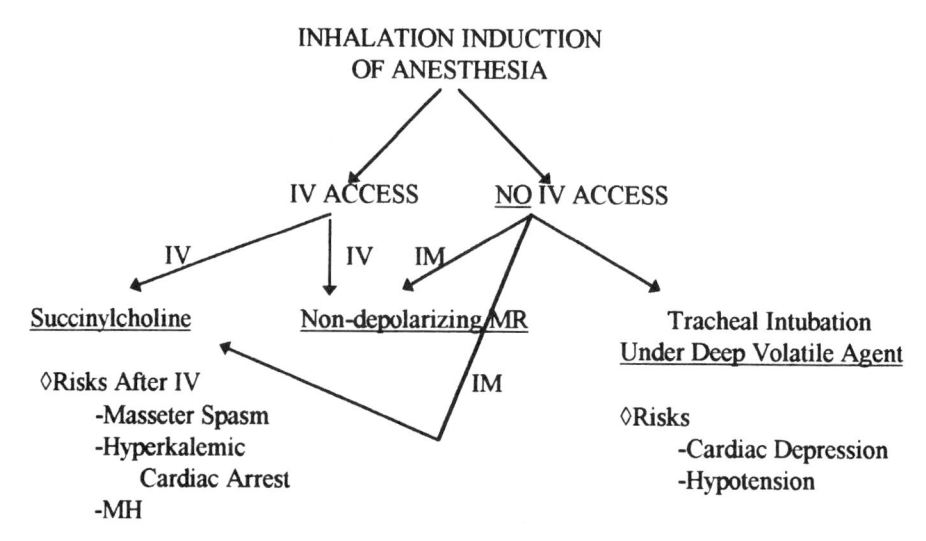

FIG. 14. An algorithm for the rational use of muscle relaxants during inhalation induction of anesthesia (see text).

The following tips are provided to help prevent overdose of volatile anesthetic agents in infants and children:

- Allow spontaneous ventilation at high inspired concentrations of volatile agent. (It is all relative, but generally speaking ≥2.0% MAC inspired agent is considered high.)

- Avoid controlled ventilation and high inspired concentrations of volatile agent.

- Avoid prolonged preoperative fasting intervals to prevent the child from becoming dehydrated and subsequently hypotensive.

- Establish IV access early in the induction sequence.

- If there is a problem starting an IV:
  - Allow spontaneous ventilation of minimally effective inspired concentrations of volatile agent until a vein is cannulated.
  - Consider IM injection of muscle relaxant.

Upper Airway Obstruction during Induction

Anatomic Airway Obstruction

As a result of relaxation of airway muscles involved in regulating upper airway caliber, *all children's airways obstruct during inhalational induction of anesthesia.* Upper airway inspiratory muscles in children are very sensitive to the depressant effect of volatile agents. For example, the genioglossus muscle (which normally increases the caliber of the pharynx by displacing the tongue anteriorly during inspiration) and other pharyngeal and laryngeal abductor muscles are easily depressed by relatively light levels of anesthesia, resulting in loss of airway patency (41,42). To make matters worse, inspiratory activity of the genioglossus muscle is more sensitive to halothane at a given concentration than is the diaphragm (43). This differential sensitivity leads to an increase in thoracoabdominal incoordination and labored breathing ("paradoxical respiration") (44).

Although usually obvious, upper airway obstruction that occurs in infants and young children is not always apparent clinically. Children often play "possum" (i.e., hold their breath and pretend to be asleep). Application of the "survival position" (see following text) and the insertion of a plastic oral airway **(see Chapter 4)** usually promote spontaneous ventilation and relieve the partial upper airway obstruction.

The survival position is a modification of the traditional jaw-thrust/chin-lift maneuver (Fig. 15).

The Survival Position

- Fingers remain on the bony prominences of the face.

- Using the tips of the index and ring fingers, jaw thrust is applied bilaterally to the ascending ramus of the mandible immediately behind the pinna of the ear (at the most cephalad level, abutting the mastoid process, not to the angle of the jaw).

- Using the thumbs, downward pressure is applied to the face mask creating tight seal.

- The jaw and chin are rotated downward, further enhancing patency of the airway by opening the mouth.

When done properly, the latter maneuver actually dislocates the ascending ramus anteriorly while rotating the temporomandibular joint counterclockwise and forcing the chin downward and the mouth open (Fig. 16). There are other benefits to this maneuver. For example. soft tissue is lifted off the hypopharynx and back wall of the pharynx, further improving patency of the supraglottic airway. In addition, the survival position provides a mild nociceptive stimulus that may stimulate spontaneous ventilation and a more rapid induction of anesthesia, particularly in the child who is playing "possum".

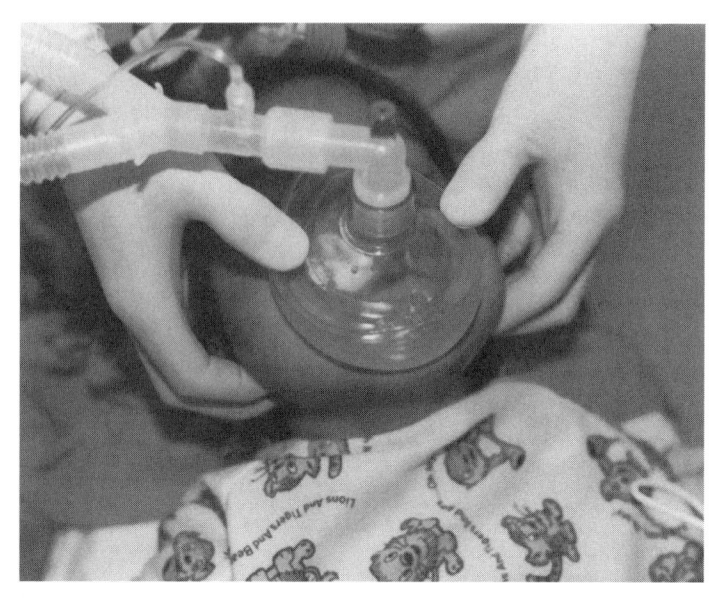

FIG. 15. The survival position is a modification of the traditional jaw-thrust/chin-lift maneuver. Note that the tips of the index and ring fingers are applied to the ascending ramus of the mandible behind the pinnae of the ear, applying jaw thrust bilaterally. The thumbs apply downward pressure to the facemask creating a tight seal. The jaw and chin are rotated downward, further enhancing patency of the airway by opening the mouth.

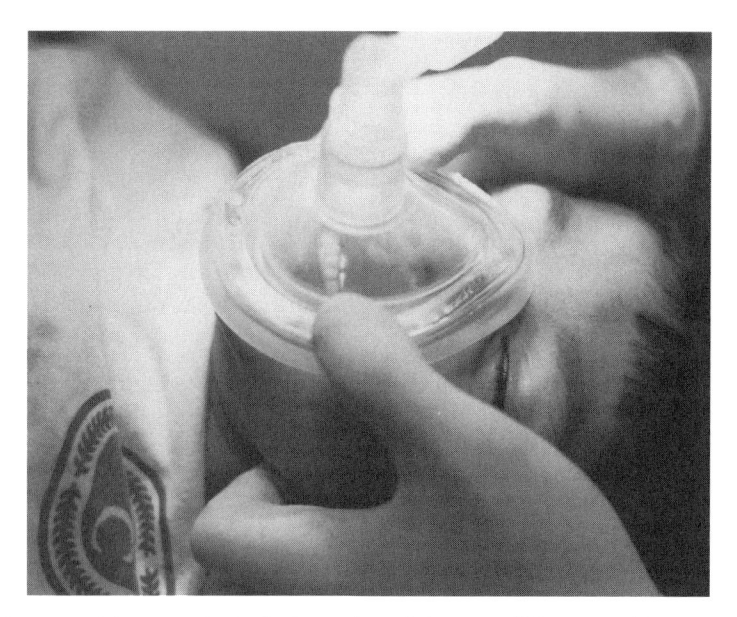

FIG. 16. The downward (counterclockwise) rotation of the mandible around the temporomandibular joint achieving improved airway patency when using the survival position.

Laryngospasm

When anatomic airway obstruction can be ruled out and the child still has airway obstruction, it is likely that laryngospasm has developed. The incidence of laryngospasm is 8.7 of 1000 patients in the total population and 17.4 of 1000 in patients age 0 to 9 years (45). Patients 1 to 3 months old have three times the incidence of laryngospasm compared with that of any other age group. Although most instances of laryngospasm resolve without serious complications, about 5 of 1000 patients who experience laryngospasm may have cardiac arrest (46).

Pathophysiology

Laryngospasm involves apposition of structures at three levels: the supraglottic folds, the false vocal cords, and the true vocal cords. A dual mechanism closes the larynx during laryngospasm: a shutter effect involving the vocal cords and a ball-valve effect involving the false cords and redundant supraglottic tissues, owing to shortening of the thyrohyoid muscle (45).

As the translaryngeal pressure gradient increases during inspiration, soft tissues of the supraglottic region are drawn into the laryngeal inlet. After laryngospasm develops, it can become a prolonged process because of a continuous contraction of abdominal muscles, expiratory effort, and continuing closure of the larynx. In a sense, laryngospasm may be considered as an extreme form of cough (47). *No matter what we call it, laryngospasm may be sustained and may become progressively worse as supraglottic tissues fold over the vocal cords during forceful inspiratory efforts.*

Etiology

Laryngospasm occurs as a response to stimulation of visceral nerve endings in the pelvis, abdomen, thorax, or larynx. The following are risk factors for laryngospasm:

- Age (see earlier in text)
- Extubation of the trachea
- Presence of a nasogastric tube or oral airway
- Endoscopy or esophagoscopy
- Upper respiratory infections
- Light anesthesia

Whereas light levels of any volatile anesthetic agent can predispose toward laryngospasm during the induction of anesthesia, isoflurane and desflurane are associated with the highest risk. For this reason, halothane and sevoflurane are used as induction agents in children. Any airway manipulation (e.g., laryngoscopy, suction, intubation) should commence only when the child is either wide awake or deeply anesthetized.

Management

The treatment of laryngospasm depends on whether airway obstruction is complete or incomplete (Fig. 17). The single diagnostic feature that distinguishes complete from incomplete airway obstruction is very simply the absence or presence of sound. If there are inspiratory or expiratory squeaks, sounds, grunts, or whistles, then chances are that the child has incomplete airway obstruction. Airway obstruction of either type requires initial treatment with a patency preserving maneuver such as the survival position or a modified jaw-thrust/chin-lift maneuver.

> "In skating over thin ice, our safety is in our speed."
> —Ralph Waldo Emerson

Because incomplete airway obstruction may rapidly become complete, signs and symptoms of obstruction (e.g., tracheal tug, paradoxical respiration) should be treated aggressively. The first maneuver is to apply gentle positive pressure with 100% O_2 by face mask. An effective technique to deliver gentle positive pressure is to "flutter the bag."[h] In this technique, the reservoir bag is very rapidly squeezed and released in a staccato rhythm

---

[h]Ed. Note (JMB): Credit for development of this technique must go to Dr. John Ryan, one of the giants in pediatric anesthesia. Undoubtedly, countless babies' lives have been saved using this bag flutter technique.

```
                    ┌─────────────────────┐
                    │ INCOMPLETE AIRWAY   │
                    │    OBSTRUCTION      │
                    └──────────┬──────────┘
                               │
                               ▼
              ┌──────────────────────────────┐
              │  APPLY GENTLE POSITIVE       │
              │  PRESSURE WITH 100% OXYGEN   │
              │  SURVIVAL POSITION           │
              │  ("FLUTTER THE BAG")         │
              └──────────────────────────────┘
                   │            │
           IMPROVED│            │NO IMPROVEMENT    ┌──────────────────────────┐
                   │            └─────────────────▶│ DEEPEN ANESTHESIA WITH   │
                   ▼                               │ INTRAVENOUS THIOPENTAL   │
        ┌──────────────────────────────┐           │ STABILIZE THE AIRWAY AND │
        │ ELIMINATE NOXIOUS STIMULUS   │           │ RESUME ANAESTHETIC       │
        │ INCREASE OR DECREASE CONC.   │           └──────────────────────────┘
        │ OF VOLATILE AGENT            │
        └──────────────────────────────┘
                   │            │
           IMPROVED│            │NO IMPROVEMENT    ┌──────────────────────────┐
                   │            └─────────────────▶│ IV SUCCINYLCHOLINE +     │
                   ▼                               │ ATROPINE VENTILATE WITH  │
        ┌──────────────────────────────┐           │ 100% OXYGEN AND INTUBATE │
        │ STABILIZE PATIENT AND        │           │ WITH E.T. TUBE           │
        │ RESUME ANAESTHETIC           │           └──────────────────────────┘
        └──────────────────────────────┘
```

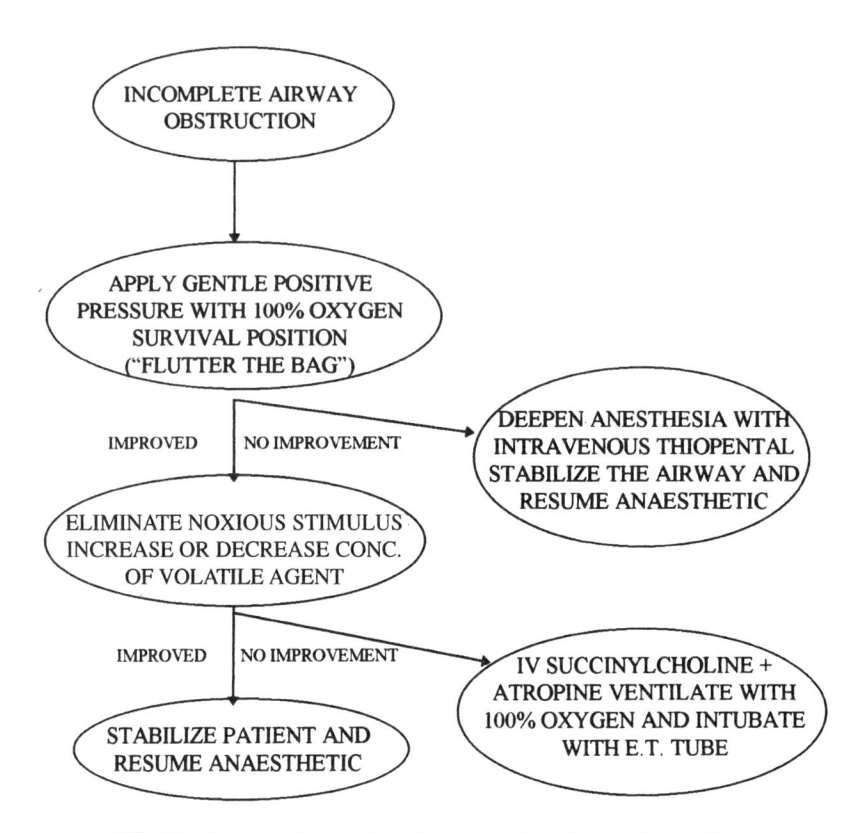

FIG. 17. An algorithm to treat incomplete airway obstruction. (Reprinted with permission, from ref. 47.)

very similar to what one would see with atrial flutter of the heart. In essence, one performs a manual high frequency oscillatory ventilation with this technique. If airway obstruction improves using the flutter technique, the concentration of volatile agents may be increased or decreased as necessary and flutter ventilation continued or normal manual ventilation resumed. If the patient further improves, anesthesia and normal ventilation may be resumed.

If there is no improvement after PPV, one may deepen the anesthetic (e.g., IV thiopental), remove the noxious stimulus, and further stabilize the airway. If there is no improvement after deepening anesthesia or eliminating the noxious stimulus, then IV succinylcholine plus atropine may be indicated.

Complete airway obstruction shares many of the clinical signs with incomplete obstruction—tracheal tug, indrawing of the chest wall, and marked abdominal respiration. The absence of respiratory sounds, however, is the hallmark of complete laryngospasm. Positive pressure cannot "break" laryngospasm in the presence of complete airway obstruction and may in fact worsen laryngospasm by forcing supraglottic tissues downward to occlude the glottic opening. "Overuse" of the high-pressure flush valve to fill the breathing circuit and anesthetic bag may dilute anesthetic gases and lead to a lighter plane of anesthesia in the child. In addition, high pressure applied to the airway may force gas down the esophagus and into the stomach, reducing ventilation even more.

The treatment of complete airway obstruction is intended to lengthen the thyrohyoid muscle and unfold the soft supraglottic tissue (Fig. 18). In the survival position a (two-person technique), one person holds the mask tightly to the face and stretches the jaw (and larynx)

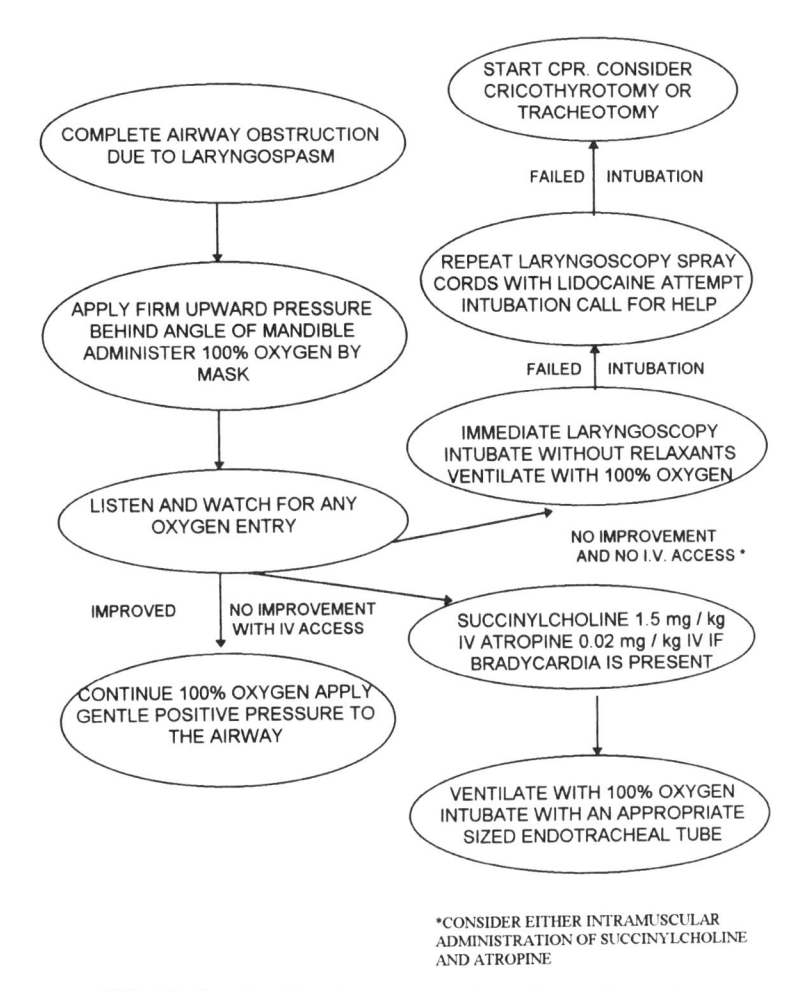

```
                    START CPR. CONSIDER
                    CRICOTHYROTOMY OR
                       TRACHEOTOMY

                        FAILED │ INTUBATION

                    REPEAT LARYNGOSCOPY SPRAY
COMPLETE AIRWAY OBSTRUCTION    CORDS WITH LIDOCAINE ATTEMPT
   DUE TO LARYNGOSPASM          INTUBATION CALL FOR HELP

                        FAILED │ INTUBATION

APPLY FIRM UPWARD PRESSURE     IMMEDIATE LARYNGOSCOPY
 BEHIND ANGLE OF MANDIBLE      INTUBATE WITHOUT RELAXANTS
 ADMINISTER 100% OXYGEN BY     VENTILATE WITH 100% OXYGEN
          MASK
                                  NO IMPROVEMENT
                                  AND NO I.V. ACCESS *
  LISTEN AND WATCH FOR ANY
       OXYGEN ENTRY
                               SUCCINYLCHOLINE 1.5 mg / kg
    IMPROVED  NO IMPROVEMENT   IV ATROPINE 0.02 mg / kg IV IF
              WITH IV ACCESS    BRADYCARDIA IS PRESENT

CONTINUE 100% OXYGEN APPLY
GENTLE POSITIVE PRESSURE TO
       THE AIRWAY              VENTILATE WITH 100% OXYGEN
                               INTUBATE WITH AN APPROPRIATE
                                 SIZED ENDOTRACHEAL TUBE
```

*CONSIDER EITHER INTRAMUSCULAR
ADMINISTRATION OF SUCCINYLCHOLINE
AND ATROPINE

FIG. 18. An algorithm to treat complete airway obstruction. (Reprinted with permission, from ref. 47.)

while the other person applies gentle PPV. If the "mask-holding" person hears or feels the movement of air past vocal cords, airway obstruction (at least for the time being) is relieved. If no air can be "squeaked in," further maneuvers are necessary. If the child has IV access, then IV succinylcholine, 1.5 mg/kg, may be given along with atropine, 0.02 mg/kg. If laryngospasm occurs without IV access, IM succinylcholine, 4 mg/kg, is recommended (48). If succinylcholine is contraindicated (e.g., in a child with Duchenne's muscular dystrophy), rocuronium may be given to facilitate ventilation and intubation (19). Intralingual atropine and succinylcholine are not rec-

ommended in children anesthetized with halothane, nitrous oxide/oxygen because ventricular dysrhythmias may occur (49). If laryngospasm is sustained and a child becomes extremely hypoxic, it may be necessary to intubate without muscle relaxation. This may be preferable to waiting for the effects of succinylcholine in a child who has laryngospasm and who is bradycardic. Under these extreme conditions, the vocal folds may be sprayed directly with lidocaine to relax the larynx and facilitate intubation (46). If, after all these measures the airway has not been secured, then cricothyrotomy or emergency tracheostomy may be required.

INTRAVENOUS INDUCTION OF ANESTHESIA

Routine

Certainly, using an IV induction of anesthesia is a fairly sure way to avoid both the cardiac depressant effect of the volatile agents and airway complications associated with inhalation induction (**see earlier in text**). In children younger than 1 year of age, it is the author's preference to induce anesthesia intravenously whenever possible. Although anesthesia can be induced in small infants using an inhalational technique, the potential for airway complications is magnified in these patients.

The technique for IV induction is simple, fast, and relatively painless (especially if EMLA cream has been used). Either a 25-gauge butterfly needle with extension tubing or a 22-gauge or a 24-gauge IV catheter is inserted into a vein and the clinician injects bolus doses of the IV induction agents (e.g., thiopental [5 mg/kg], atropine [0.02 mg/kg], and succinylcholine [2 mg/kg]). If IV cannulation is unsuccessful after two attempts, it may be more humane to postpone the IV and do an inhalation induction, accepting the increased potential for complications and dealing with them if they occur. Unfortunately, there are some cases in which a catheter must be inserted and an IV induction of anesthesia initiated. Furthermore, there are some instances in which an IV catheter is strongly recommended during an inhalation induction (e.g., a freely running IV is reassuring during an inhalation induction in a child with a "difficult" airway).

Rapid-Sequence Intravenous Induction

Full-Stomach, No "Open-Eye" Considerations

To prevent pulmonary aspiration of gastric contents in a child with a full stomach, a rapid-sequence IV induction with cricoid pressure is recommended. The editors are aware of a growing trend among some pediatric anesthesiologists not to use cricoid pressure during the sequence of rapid induction. Airway distortion leading to difficult or failed intubation is only one of the reasons offered as justification to "skip" cricoid pressure during rapid sequence induction in infants and children. I believe, however, that cricoid pressure is an important element of the rapid sequence induction and should be applied.[i] In summation, I feel the rapid sequence should include the following:

- Preoxygenation with 100% O_2 by face mask
- IV administration of the following:
  - Thiopental (5 mg/kg)
  - Atropine (0.02 mg/kg), if succinylcholine used
  - Rapidly acting muscle relaxant
    - Succinylcholine (2 mg/kg) or
    - Rocuronium (0.6 mg/kg)
- Cricoid pressure

In some circumstances, it may be appropriate to induce anesthesia via face mask in a child with a full stomach (**see Difficult Airway and Open-Eye, Full Stomach Considerations**). In general, this is a judgment call and depends on the experience of the clinician. If mask induction is performed in a child with a full stomach, cricoid pressure is applied throughout the induction and the child is allowed to breathe spontaneously (Fig. 19). In addition, these children are "induced" in the head-down lateral position, if possible.

Full-Stomach, Open-Eye Considerations

In the child who has suffered a penetrating eye injury and has a full stomach (Fig. 20), our goals during induction are the following:

- To protect the child's airway
- To prevent acid aspiration

---

[i] Ed. Note (JMB): As is the case for difficult airways, perhaps our training should include performing cricoid pressure on routine cases so that we can perform it well in the full-stomach situation.

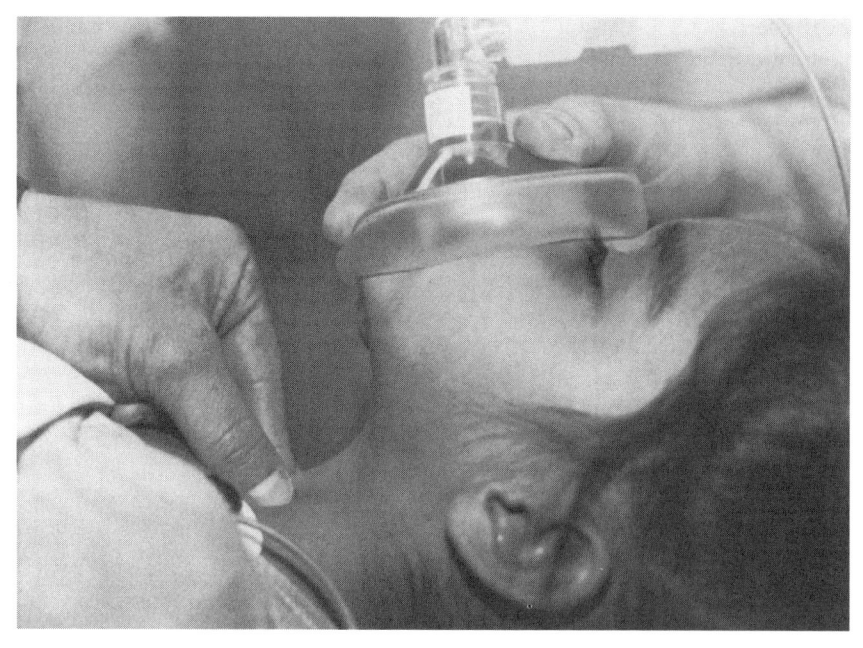

FIG. 19. Application of cricoid pressure in a child during the induction of anesthesia. If applied with the appropriate downward pressure, patency of the airway is maintained and simultaneously the lungs are protected from the aspiration of gastric contents.

- To maintain normal intraocular pressure during induction to prevent extrusion of ocular contents

Because these goals are somewhat mutually exclusive, they create one of the most debated challenges in anesthesia practice. To help resolve this challenge, these questions are asked of the surgeon.

- Is the stomach really full?

- Is the eye truly open?
- How big is the laceration?
- Can the eye be saved?

Then, decisions become easier. For example, if the eye cannot be saved, intraocular pressure increase may no longer be an issue. Furthermore, the risk of extrusion of ocular contents depends on the magnitude of the increase in intraocular pressure and the size of the laceration

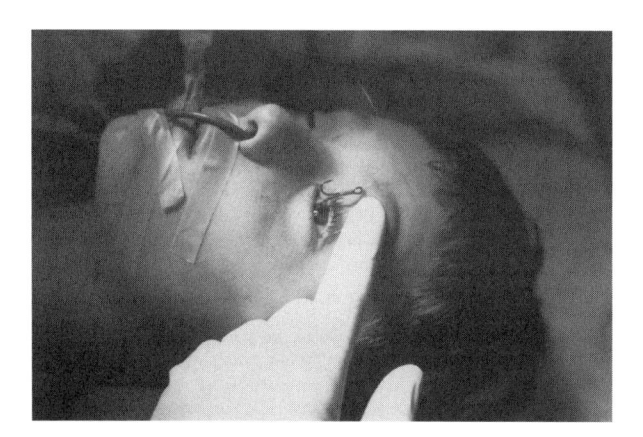

FIG. 20. A 6-year-old child with a treble fish hook lodged in the eye.

in the globe. The risk for extrusion varies directly with the fourth power of the radius of the corneal tear for a given intraocular pressure. Therefore, extrusion is much less likely in a child with a needle puncture compared with a full-length corneal laceration.

In the child with an open-eye injury and full stomach, I recommend a rapid-sequence IV induction except in circumstances in which a difficult airway is anticipated. In the latter case, an inhalational induction may be required **(see Difficult Airway and Open-Eye, Full-Stomach Considerations)**. A rapid sequence induction should begin with application of the appropriate monitors, preoxygenation[j] for 3 minutes, administration of drugs, application of cricoid pressure after loss of the eyelash reflex, and tracheal intubation within 1 minute of administration of the induction agent (50). A drug sequence (51) proven to avoid significant increase in intraocular pressure consists of the following:

- Lidocaine, 1.5 mg/kg
- Pancuronium, 0.15 mg/kg, or rocuronium, 0.6 mg/kg
- IV solution flush, 3 to 5 ml
- Thiopental, 5 to 7 mg/kg
- Atropine, 0.02 mg/kg

IV lidocaine is administered over a 20- to 30-second period and at least 90 seconds before muscle relaxant. Pancuronium, 0.15 mg/kg, will depress the twitch response 95% within 90 seconds, will provide good to excellent intubating conditions in 60 seconds, and will not increase intraocular pressure in children (51). High-dose atracurium has not found favor because of the risk of histamine release and the ensuing systemic hypotension. High-dose vecuronium (0.4 mg/kg) has a very rapid onset of action (39 ± 11 seconds); however, as with pancuronium, the duration of action is long (75 ± 10 minutes) (52). Rocuronium (0.6 mg/kg) may be a suitable alternative to pancuronium when a shorter duration of action is desired (60 ± 15 minutes). After muscle relaxant administration, the child is asked to hold up an arm. When the earliest sign of weakness appears (e.g., child's arm drops) or when a maximum time of 20 seconds has elapsed, thiopental and atropine are administered.

The choice of a nondepolarizing muscle relaxant rather than succinylcholine is related to the size of the laceration. Succinylcholine is suitable if the child has a small laceration of the eye (<4 mm in length). In this case, the induction drug sequence may be modified to include succinylcholine. If, on the other hand, the injury is a larger laceration (>4 mm in length), a nondepolarizing relaxant such as pancuronium (0.15 mg/kg), vecuronium (0.4 mg/kg), or rocuronium (0.6 µg/kg) is used.[k]

Difficult Airway and Open-Eye, Full-Stomach Considerations

If a child with an open-eye injury is complicated because of being a difficult intubation, then priority should be directed away from the eyeball and toward maintenance of the airway during induction. Anesthesia should be induced by an inhalational induction with the patient in the decubitus position. Cricoid pressure should be applied after loss of consciousness. Anesthesia may be maintained by one of several techniques depending on the anesthesiologist and the estimated duration of surgery. Nitrous oxide, oxygen, and halothane constitute

---

[j]Ed. Note (JMB): A traumatic preoxygenation in a struggling child may do more harm than good in the child with an open eye injury. Therefore, preoxygenation may need to be modified or even avoided in this circumstance.

"There is a point where methods devour themselves."
—Frantz Fanon

[k]Ed. Note (JMB): Despite the well-known effect of succinylcholine on intraocular pressure, it continues to be used with little apparent risk by some anesthesiologists in patients with penetrating eye injuries that are >4 mm in length (53). How can we explain the safe use of succinylcholine in these circumstances? The increase in intraocular pressure after succinylcholine is similar to that measured after tracheal intubation and is markedly less than the increase associated with crying, coughing, and straining (54). In other words, most kids will have already put themselves through an eyeball content stress test. The pressure increase induced by succinylcholine pales in comparison.

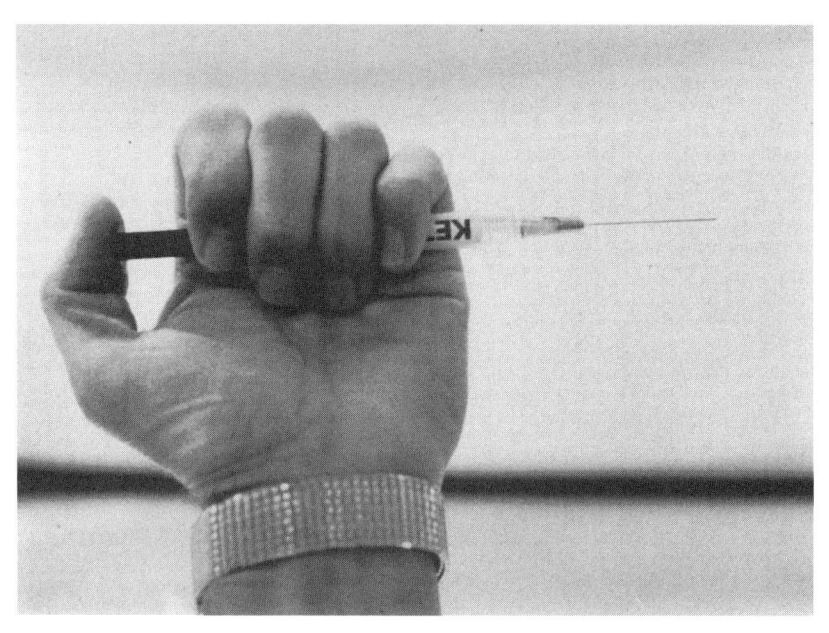

FIG. 21. The Fritz Berry ("top-gun") grip on the ketamine syringe ready for intramuscular injection through the patient's gown into the deltoid muscle.

the most commonly used anesthetic techniques in children, although IV anesthesia (propofol or midazolam combined with fentanyl) supplemented by nitrous oxide in oxygen may be preferred to minimize the duration of neuromuscular blockade. At the completion of anesthesia, the neuromuscular blockade should be reversed (when at least two twitches of the train of four are present). The child may be extubated when the gag reflex has returned and spontaneous respiration has resumed. All children should be extubated in the lateral decubitus position. Since these children still have full stomachs at the completion of surgery, we do not believe there is sufficient indication to extubate them during a deep level of anesthesia.

INTRAMUSCULAR INDUCTION OF ANESTHESIA

The IM induction is hardly ever used any more, but there are two circumstances in which it is still useful: (a) in the child with congenital heart disease before line placement and (b) in the hysterical child without an IV who won't hold still for a mask induction.

About the only drug used in the situation is ketamine. Ketamine preserves cardiac contractility and BP (at least in normovolemic patients), and after IM injection it provides a motionless child within 1 minute or so. IM dosage varies from a stunning dose of 3 mg/kg to a full anesthetic dose of 8 mg/kg. Ketamine may be given through the child's gown sleeve into the deltoid muscle via the Fritz Berry technique (Fig. 21).

"A child is a temporarily disabled and stunted version of a larger person, whom you will someday know. Your job is to help them overcome the disabilities associated with their size and inexperience so that they get on with being that larger person."

—Barbara Ehrenreich

REFERENCES

1. Smith RM: *Anesthesia for infants and children.* St. Louis: Mosby, 1959:92.
2. Gregory GA: *Pediatric anesthesia,* 2nd ed. New York: Churchill Livingstone, 1989:478.
3. Bell C, Rimar S, Barash P: Intraoperative ST segment changes consistent with myocardial ischemia in the neonate: a report of three cases. *Anesthesiology* 1989;71: 601–604.

4. Cartabuke RS, Davidson PJ, Warner LO: Is premedication with oral glycopyrrolate as effective as oral atropine in attenuating cardiovascular depression in infants receiving halothane for induction of anesthesia? *Anesth Analg* 1991;73:271–274.
5. Freid EB, Bailey AG, Valley RD: Electrocardiographic and hemodynamic changes associated with unintentional intravascular injection of bupivacaine with epinephrine in infants. *Anesthesiology* 1993;79:394–398.
6. Kimble KJ, Darnall RA Jr, Yelderman M: An automated oscillometric technique for estimating mean arterial pressure in critically ill newborns. *Anesthesiology* 1981;54:423–425.
7. Park MK, Kawabori I: Need for an improved standard for blood pressure cuff size. The size should be related to the diameter of the arm. *Clin Pediatr* 1976;15:784.
8. Diprose GK, Evens DH, Archer LN: Dinamap fails to detect hypotension in very low birthweight infants. *Arch Dis Child* 1984;138:775–778.
9. Wareham JA, Haugh LD, Yeager SB, Horbar JD: Prediction of arterial blood pressure in the premature neonate using the oscillometric method. *Am J Dis Child* 1987;141:1108–1110.
10. Miller G, Badgwell JM, Heinrich R, Curry B: Cutaneous heat loss exceeds respiratory heat loss in anesthetized children. *Anesthesiology* 1993;79:A1170.
11. Kurz A, Kurz M, Poeschl G, et al: Forced-air warming maintains intraoperative normothermia better than circulating-water mattresses. *Anesth Analg* 1993;77:89–95.
12. Badgwell JM, Durham NL, Lacey S, McLeod M: Forced air warming blankets maintain normothermia in infants during anesthesia. *Anesthesiology* 1995;83:A1175.
13. Scheiber G, Ribeiro FC, Marichal A, et al: Intubating conditions and onset of action after rocuronium, vecuronium, and atracurium in young children. *Anesth Analg* 1996;83:320–324.
14. Koscielniak-Nielsen ZJ, Bevan JC, Popovic V, et al: Onset of maximum neuromuscular block following succinylcholine or vecuronium in four age groups. *Anesthesiology* 1993;79:229–234.
15. Ferres CJ, Crean PM, Mirakhur RK: An evaluation of ONC 45 (vecuronium) in paediatric anaesthesia. *Anaesthesia* 1983;38:943–947.
16. Sloan MH, Lerman J, Bissonnette B: Pharmacodynamics of high-dose vecuronium in children during balanced anesthesia. *Anesthesiology* 1991;74:656–659.
17. Lavery GG, Mirakhur RK: Atracurium besylate in paediatric anaesthesia. *Anaesthesia* 1984;39:1243–1246.
18. Goudsouzian N, Liu LM, Gionfriddo M, Rudd GD: Neuromuscular effects of atracurium in infants and children. *Anesthesiology* 1985;62:75–79.
19. Reynolds LM, Lau M, Brown R, et al: Intramuscular rocuronium in infants and children: dose-ranging and tracheal intubating conditions. *Anesthesiology* 1996;85:231–239.
20. Coté CJ: NPO after midnight for children: a reappraisal. *Anesthesiology* 1990;72:589–592.
21. Sandhar BK, Goresky GV, Maltby JR, Shaffer EA: Effect of oral liquids and ranitidine on gastric fluid volume and pH in children undergoing outpatient surgery. *Anesthesiology* 1989;71:327–330.
22. Schreiner MS, Triebwasser A, Keon TP: Ingestion of liquids compared with preoperative fasting in pediatric outpatients. *Anesthesiology* 1990;72:593–597.
23. Splinter WM, Stewart JA, Muir JG: The effect of preoperative apple juice on gastric contents, thirst and hunger in children. *Can J Anaesth* 1989;36:55–58.
24. O Hare B, Lerman J, Endo J, Cutz E: Acute lung injury after instillation of human breast milk or infant formula into rabbits lungs. *Anesthesiology* 1996;84:1386–1391.
25. American Academy of Pediatrics Committee on Drugs Policy Statement: Unapproved uses of approved drugs: the physician, the package insert, and the Food and Drug Administration: subject review. *Pediatrics* 1996;98:143–145.
26. Salonen M, Kanto J, Iisalo E, Himberg JJ: Midazolam as an induction agent in children: a pharmacokinetic and clinical study. *Anesth Analg* 1987;66:625–628.
27. Saarnivaara L, Lindgren L, Klemola UM: Comparison of chloral hydrate and midazolam by mouth as premedicants in children undergoing otolaryngological surgery. *Br J Anaesth* 1988;61:390–396.
28. Karl HW, Rosenberger JL, Larach MG, Ruffle JM: Transmucosal administration of midazolam for premedication of pediatric patients: comparison of the nasal and sublingual routes. *Anesthesiology* 1993;78:885–891.
29. Karl HW, Keifer AT, Rosenberger JL, et al: Comparison of the safety and efficacy of intranasal midazolam or sufentanil for preinduction of anesthesia in pediatric patients. *Anesthesiology* 1992;76:209–215.
30. De Jong PC, Verburg MP: Comparison of rectal to intramuscular administration of midazolam and atropine for premedication of children. *Acta Anaesthesiol Scand* 1988;32:485–489.
31. Rita L, Seleny FL, Mazurek A, Rabins SY: Intramuscular midazolam for pediatric preanesthetic sedation: a double-blind controlled study with morphine. *Anesthesiology* 1985;63:528–531.
32. Spear RM, Yaster M, Berkowitz ID, et al: Preinduction of anesthesia in children with rectally administered midazolam. *Anesthesiology* 1991;74:670–674.
33. Kain ZN, Mayes LC, Caramico LA, et al: Parental presence during induction of anesthesia: a randomized controlled trial. *Anesthesiology* 1996;84:1060–1067.
34. Lerman J, Davis PJ, Welborn LG, et al: Induction, recovery, and safety characteristics of sevoflurane in children undergoing ambulatory surgery. A comparison with halothane. *Anesthesiology* 1996;84:1332–1340.
35. Lerman J, Robinson S, Willis MM, Gregory GA: Anesthetic requirements for halothane in young children 0–1 month and 1–6 months of age. *Anesthesiology* 1983;59:421–424.
36. Salanitre E, Rackow H: The pulmonary exchange of nitrous oxide and halothane in infants and children. *Anesthesiology* 1969;30:388–394.
37. Salem MR, Bennett EJ, Schweiss JF, et al: Cardiac arrest related to anesthesia: contributing factors in infants and children. *JAMA* 1975;233:238–241.
38. Diaz JH, Lockhart CH: Is halothane really safe in infancy? *Anesthesiology* 1979;51:A313.
39. Gibbons RT, Steffey EP, Eger EI II: The effect of spontaneous versus controlled ventilation on the rate of rise of alveolar halothane concentration in dogs. *Anesth Analg* 1977;56:32–34.
40. Yakaitis RW, Blitt CD, Angiulo JP: End-tidal halothane concentration for endotracheal intubation. *Anesthesiology* 1977;47:386–388.
41. Remmers JE, deGroot WJ, Sauerland EK, Anch AM: Pathogenesis of upper airway occlusion during sleep. *J Appl Physiol* 1978;44:931–938.

42. Brouillette RT, Thach BT: A neuromuscular mechanism maintaining extrathoracic airway patency. *J Appl Physiol* 1979;46:772–779.
43. Ochiai R, Guthrie RD, Motoyama EK: Effects of varying concentrations of halothane on the activity of the genioglossus, intercostals, and diaphragm in cats: an electromyographic study. *Anesthesiology* 1989;70:812–816.
44. Motoyama E, Maekawa N, Kamikawa K: Inspiratory muscle incoordination and upper airway obstruction in children during inhalation anesthesia. *Anesthesiology* 1995;83:A1187.
45. Olsson GL, Hallen B: Laryngospasm during anaesthesia. A computer-aided incidence study in 136,929 patients. *Acta Anaesthesiol Scand* 1984;28:567–575.
46. Fink BR: The etiology and treatment of laryngeal spasm. *Anesthesiology* 1956;17:567–575.
47. Roy WL, Lerman J: Laryngospasm in paediatric anaesthesia. *Can J Anaesth* 1988;35:93–98.
48. Liu LM, DeCook TH, Goudsouzian NG, et al: Dose response to intramuscular succinylcholine in children. *Anesthesiology* 1981;55:599–602.
49. Mazze RI, Dunbar RW: Intralingual succinylcholine administration in children: an alternative to intravenous and intramuscular routes? *Anesth Analg* 1968;47:605–615.
50. Lerman J, Kiskis AA: Lidocaine attenuates the intraocular pressure response to rapid intubation in children. *Can Anaesth Soc J* 1985;32:339–345.
51. Cunliffe M, Lerman J, McLeod ME, Burrows FA: Neuromuscular blockade for rapid tracheal intubation in children: comparison of succinylcholine and pancuronium. *Can Anaesth Soc J* 1986;33:760–764.
52. Sloan MH, Lerman J, Bissonnette B: Pharmacodynamics of high dose vecuronium in children during balanced anesthesia. *Anesthesiology* 1991;74:656–659.
53. Libonati MM, Leahy JJ, Ellison N: The use of succinylcholine in open eye surgery. *Anesthesiology* 1985;62:637–640.
54. Drenger B, Pe'er J, BenEzra D, et al: The effect of intravenous lidocaine on the increase in intraocular pressure induced by tracheal intubation. *Anesth Analg* 1985;64:1211–1213.

Clinical Pediatric Anesthesia, edited by
J.M. Badgwell. Lippincott–Raven Publishers,
Philadelphia © 1997.

3
Peripheral and Central Vascular Access and Invasive Monitoring

J. Michael Badgwell, Robert S. Holzman, William S. Schechter

"In art economy is always beauty."
—Henry James

As in art, anesthesia is most beautiful when it is most economical. John Relton, a senior anesthetist at the Hospital for Sick Children in Toronto, teaches young trainees that there are only two requisites for a successful pediatric anesthetic: a first-class intravenous (IV) access and a first-class airway.

Whereas this is the truth in probably 90% of cases or more, there are some cases in which a first-class arterial line or a first-class central venous cannula is needed as well. This chapter provides information to establish life-supporting "lines" in pediatric patients.

PERIPHERAL INTRAVENOUS ACCESS

Peripheral IV access in infants and children can present a challenge. As with any challenge of this nature, the first step is to arrange the necessary equipment beforehand. IV administration sets are prepared and filled before the case begins. Sets for pediatric patients have a graduated drip chamber for quantifying and limiting the amount of fluid delivered.

Intravenous Fluid Filters

Blood

Although adult blood filtering systems are acceptable for pediatric use, the priming volume for these filters is usually excessive in very small infants. Small-volume microaggregate filters have been developed but may lead to significant red cell destruction (1,2). Furthermore, although it is necessary in children (as in adults) to filter (using a 170-µm filter), measure, and warm administered red blood cells, it is not necessary to filter cells with a very small pore filter (e.g., a 20 to 40 µm filter) (3).

Air

IV line air filters are available (Pall Set Saver Extended Life, Pall Biomedical, Inc, Puerto Rico) and should be used. The use of IV air filters is encouraged, since the incidence of small ventricular septal defects or patency of the foramen ovale is not uncommon in the first year of life. These children, and those with repaired or unrepaired congenital heart disease with intracardiac communications, are at risk for paradoxical air embolism (4). For these reasons, meticulous care should be taken to remove air bubbles from IV lines in all pediatric patients, whether or not an air filter is used.

Intravenous Infusion Pumps and Rate Controllers

Pumps designed to provide precise quantities of IV medications and continuous infusion for regional anesthesia are common in the pediatric operating room. Syringe pumps deliver precise volumes of an infusate under pressure from a filled syringe attached to a carrier and clamp, which is driven by a motorized screw (5). These pumps are ideal for pediatric care, especially with the increasing practice of continuous IV anesthesia. Facility with calculations in µg/kg/min for children or conversion tables conveniently available to the anesthetist are urged for practical daily use.

IV Equipment Kidney Basin

For convenience and accessibility, equipment needed for IV placement may be placed in a small kidney basin. Placed in the basin are 22-gauge and 24-gauge catheters, a small tourniquet, alcohol swabs, tape, 4 × 4 gauze pads, and a small arm board (Fig. 1). The apparatus is self-contained and is easily transportable to the IV site.

Are Two Relatively Small IV Catheters Better Than One Large One?

Two separate infusions through small cannulas outperform a single large-bore catheter when high flow from an infusion system is required (6). This may be particularly applicable to pediatric patients with veins so small as to only allow 24-gauge catheters. The size of the cannula is an important consideration in infants and children. Although a 24-gauge cannula is appropriate for many infants, the fascia in some parts of the body (i.e., dorsum of the foot) may cause a flimsy 24-gauge cannula to buckle. Most veins in both infants and children will accept a 22-gauge cannula. In fact, when cannulation is difficult, a slightly larger cannula may be more successful.

PERIPHERAL INTRAVENOUS INSERTION TECHNIQUES

It is surprising that the most difficult IV access is not always in the neonate but more frequently in the infant between 3 and 12 months of age. In the neonate with scant amounts of fat in the subcutaneous skin layer, the skin is somewhat transparent and venous cannulation may be fairly easy. By contrast, in the pudgy 1-year-old infant veins are often not so visible (or even palpable). Nevertheless, to successfully cannulate veins in any pediatric age group, the clinician must keep several rules in mind:

- Know the anatomy of the venous distribution.
- Always begin with the most distal venous site and proceed proximally.
- Never attempt IV access proximal to the site of a preexisting cannula.
- Make conditions optimal.

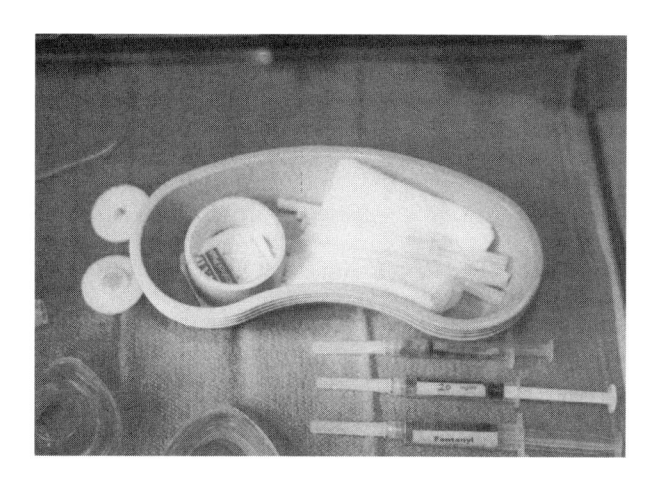

FIG. 1. A kidney basin containing IV catheters, 4 × 4 gauze pads, tape, and alcohol swabs are prepared so that all necessary equipment may be taken to the IV insertion site.

Although these rules may seem obvious, many attempt their first venous cannulation in a proximal vein that appears large, rather than in a smaller distal tributary. The net effect of failing to cannulate the larger proximal trunk is that all the sites including those that are distal are lost because the failed cannulation produces a proximal hematoma. If a larger IV than one already in place is needed, it is best to cannulate another vein to preserve the existing site. Other tips include (a) avoidance of compromising situations such as having to reach across the abdomen for a vein on the opposite extremity and (b) avoidance of direct strong light on the extremity, since indirect light often casts a shadow over the back of the hand. Although EMLA (eutectic mixture of local anesthetics; EMLA, ASTRA) cream may anesthetize the skin (although it doesn't take away the child's fear component), it is a venoconstrictor and will blanch the skin. Therefore, EMLA cream may actually make venous cannulation more difficult.

More Helpful Hints for Successful IV Cannulation

- After application of a tourniquet or a tight grasp on the arm or leg by your assistant, squeeze the hand or foot to force the blood into the veins.

- Use gravity to pool blood in the extremity by positioning the extremity below the level of the heart. Anxiety and cool temperatures facilitate venous constriction. (To reverse these effects, the extremity may be wrapped in a warm wet towel for several minutes to dilate the veins.)

- Use one of several prime sites for venous cannulation:
  - Dorsum of the hand
  - Volar aspect of the wrist
  - Antecubital
  - Saphenous

Dorsum of the Hand

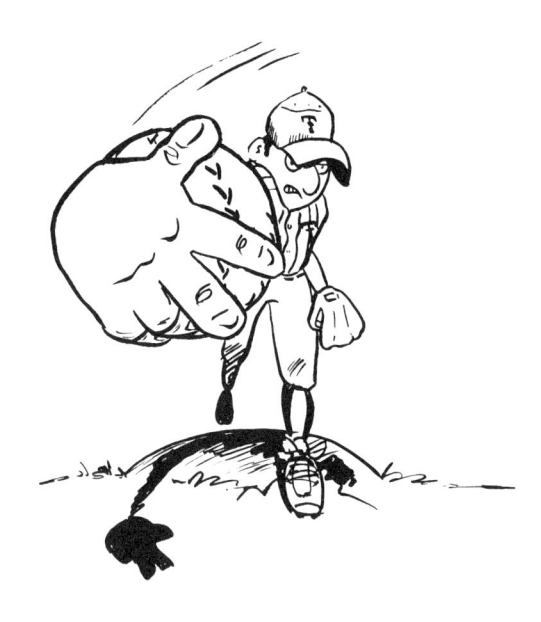

"Whoever wants to know the heart and mind of America had better learn baseball."
—Jacques Barzun

The most common site for venous cannulation in infants and children is the dorsum of the hand. One of the most prominent veins in the hand lies between the fourth and fifth metacarpals, midway along the metacarpal.[a] To successfully cannulate any vein, the skin should be stretched both laterally and longitudinally to prevent the vein from rolling away from the needle. For the dorsal hand veins, this stretching is best accomplished by using the "baseball grip" (Fig. 2) as follows:

- Position your thumb along the child's knuckles.
- Position your fingers across the dorsum of the child's wrist.
- Make sure the child's wrist is flexed to 90 degrees.
- Stretch the child's skin and vein taut.

Direct the bevel upward and puncture the skin directly above the vein (Fig. 3A). It is cru-

---
[a] Ed. Note (JMB): If you don't believe me, take a look at your own hand now.

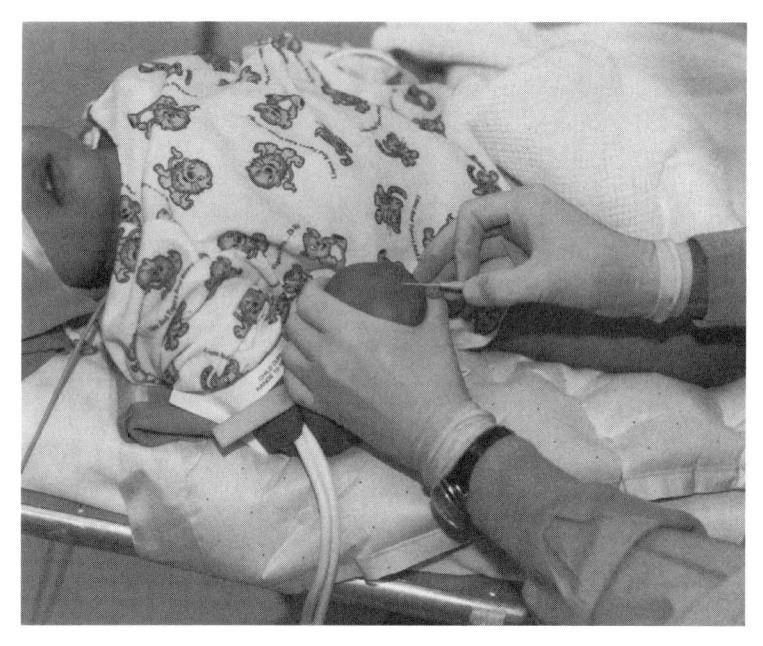

FIG. 2. Using the "baseball grip," IV cannulation is made easily. The skin overlying the dorsum of the child's hand is stretched taut by the clinician's thumb and fingers. The clinician's right middle finger is resting on the child's hand to provide a stable "tripod" effect.

cial that the back wall of the vein is not punctured, so that a hematoma does not occlude the lumen of the vein and prevent successful cannulation. As soon as a venous flashback is observed, the needle is advanced only 1 or 2 mm farther. At this point, the needle should not be withdrawn, but rather fixed. The cannula is threaded up the lumen of the vein with one smooth motion (Fig. 3B). To prevent blood spillage, the needle is withdrawn while the clinician's thumb holds the catheter in place.

Two-Person Dorsal Hand Technique

The two-person technique of IV insertion involves the assistance of someone in the operating room to hold and position the patient's hand while the anesthesiologist (who is simultaneously doing the induction of anesthesia) inserts the IV catheter (Fig. 4). It is important that the assistant (who is acting as the human tourniquet) stretch the skin away from the intended IV site so that the vein is transfixed and will not move. This technique allows the anesthesiologist who is working alone to perform IV cannulation without interrupting inhalation anesthesia.

Volar Aspect of the Hand

In small infants, the only vein available may be found on the volar aspect of the wrist at the midline of the crease (Fig. 5). These veins are extremely close to the skin surface and are thin-walled. Here again, stretching of the skin, in both directions, is the key to successful cannulation.

Antecubital Fossa

In children, as in adults, larger veins, basilic and cephalic, may be found in the antecubital fossa. The basilic vein crosses the antecubital fossa medial to the midline of the antecubital crease and the cephalic vein crosses at the lateral edge of the fossa. In pudgy children, these veins may be no more visible or palpable than any other "hidden" vein. Therefore, another vein (saphenous) deserves early attack in pudgy kids.

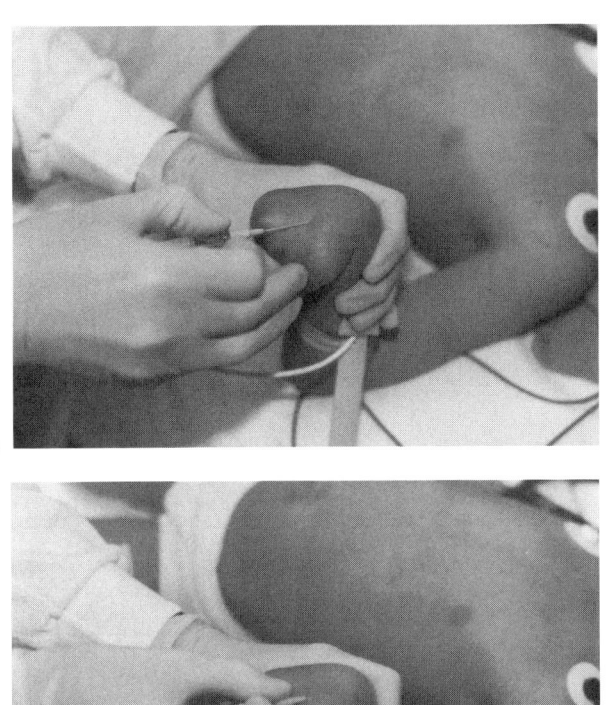

FIG. 3. (A) The needle is advanced until a flash of blood is obtained, and then the needle and catheter are advanced together a few millimeters farther to ensure that the catheter is in the vein. **(B)** With one smooth motion, the needle is retracted and the catheter is advanced over the needle into the vein up to the hub of the catheter. Before the needle is removed from the catheter, the clinician places a thumb over the skin at the tip of the catheter so that no blood will escape. In addition, the tourniquet is removed and the IV tubing is inserted before blood can escape.

Saphenous Veins

Percutaneous. The saphenous vein is the most reliable and constant vein in the human body. This vein crosses the crest of the medial malleolus pointing in the direction of the opposite shoulder (Fig. 6). The key to percutaneous cannulation of the saphenous vein in children is proper hand positioning by the clinician. The fingertip of the index finger is placed on the infant's heel as the thumb pulls the toe downward, stretching the skin and vein over the medial aspect of the ankle (Fig. 7A). This action transfixes the vein and prevents it from rolling. Simply insert the needle through the skin at the base of the malleolus and aim for the child's opposite shoulder. The vein is superficial or deep depending on the child's pudginess factor. The needle is advanced smoothly until a "flashback" is seen (Fig. 7B). The catheter is then passed over the needle and into the vein. If unsuccessful, retract the catheter until a blood return is seen, hook up the IV tubing, and pass the catheter while IV fluids are running (i.e., "float" it in).

Saphenous Vein Cutdown. The saphenous vein may be cannulated under direct vision by

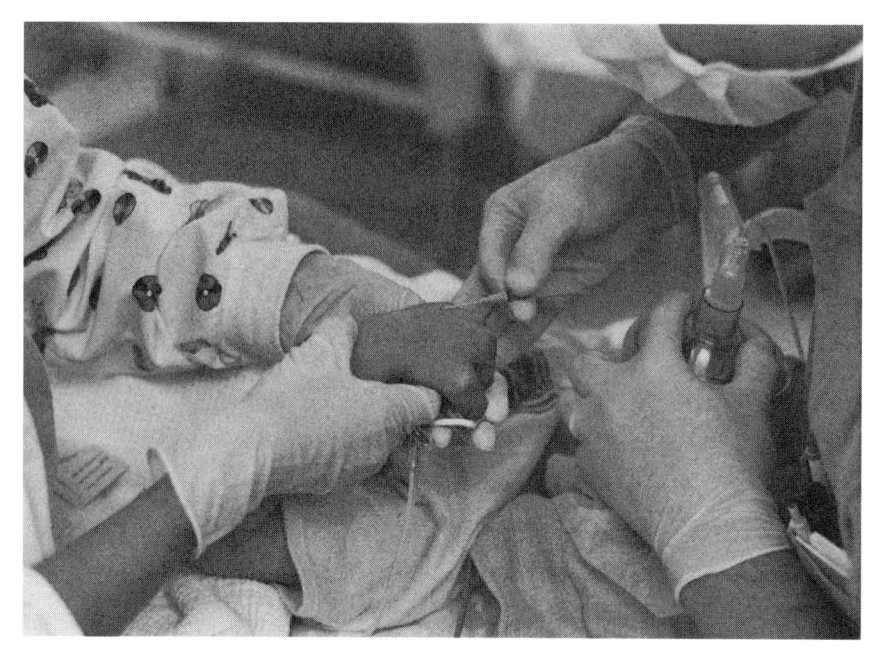

FIG. 4. In the two-person technique of IV insertion, a trained assistant acts as the human tourniquet and stretches the skin taut while presenting the child's extremities to the clinician. Simultaneously, the clinician (with the other hand) is inducing anesthesia by face mask.

surgical cutdown. Simply incise the skin over the vein, retract the vein with a hemostat, and pierce the vein with a catheter/needle (Fig. 6).

Fixation of Peripheral IVs

In many respects, the most critical part of any IV is making sure it stays in place. It is easy to keep an IV secure in a child who is anesthetized and paralyzed. It is not so easy to keep the IV in place when the child is struggling and squirming during emergence. The child may lose his or her IV just when it is needed the most. Adverse events requiring IV access for therapy (e.g., laryngospasm, apnea, aspiration) occur most often during induction and emergence. Therefore, we recommend going overboard when it comes to a secure dressing for the IV (Fig. 8). One of us (JMB) uses several meters of tape and an armboard (or footboard) on every IV. This practice has made him the target of much good-hearted ridicule ("What is that—a short-arm cast?"). Nevertheless, he's never lost an IV in the postanesthesia care unit even in the most vigorous of struggling children, some of whom have needed sedative medication, resuscitative drugs, or succinylcholine for laryngospasm.

WHEN ALL ELSE FAILS

"God Almighty hates a quitter."
—Samuel Fessenden

Femoral Vein Cannulation

If all else fails, venous access may be established by a femoral vein cannulated using the Seldinger technique (Fig. 9)(7). Several different kits are available for femoral vein cannulation, or kits can be assembled from readily available material for use in the Seldinger technique. First, depending on the child's size, either a 20-gauge or a 22-gauge catheter (Deseret Angiocath, Becton-Dickinson Vascular Access, Sandy, UT) is inserted into the vein. In a smaller child, the insertion of a 0.45-mm

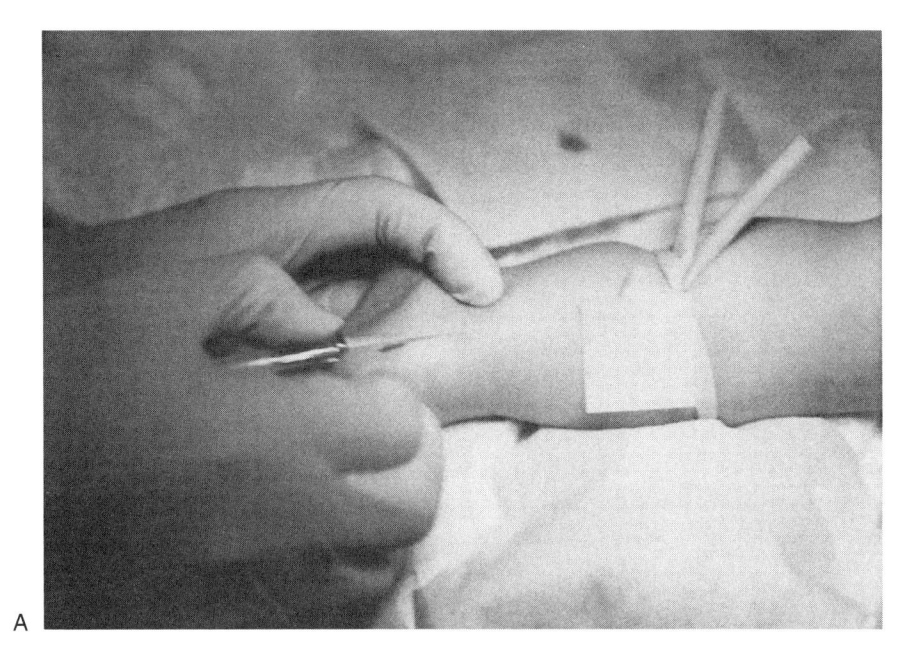

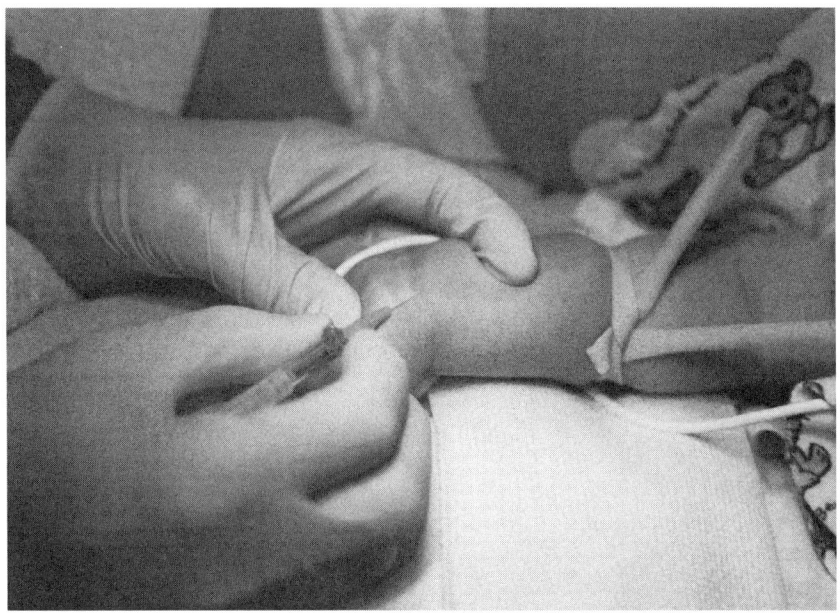

FIG. 5. **(A)** In small infants, the best veins are often found on the volar aspect of the wrist. The principles for successful cannulation are the same as for any venous cannulation. The child's skin is stretched taut by the clinician's thumb and finger, and the catheter advanced until a flashback is seen. **(B)** The needle and catheter are advanced a bit further to ensure catheter placement in the vein. Then, with one motion, the needle is retracted and the catheter advanced.

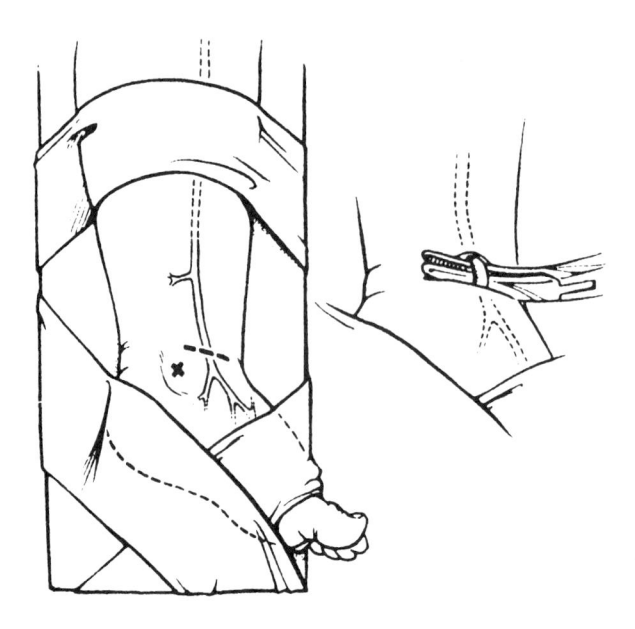

FIG. 6. The saphenous vein is probably the most invariable vein in the human body. It "runs" just in front of the medial malleolus and angles toward the contralateral shoulder. The saphenous vein can be cannulated percutaneously or through a small incision under direct vision. A small curved hemostat is placed under the vein to bring it into proper position for cannulation. (From American Heart Association: *Textbook of Pediatric Advanced Life Support,* Dallas, AHA, 1994, with permission, copyright American Heart Association.)

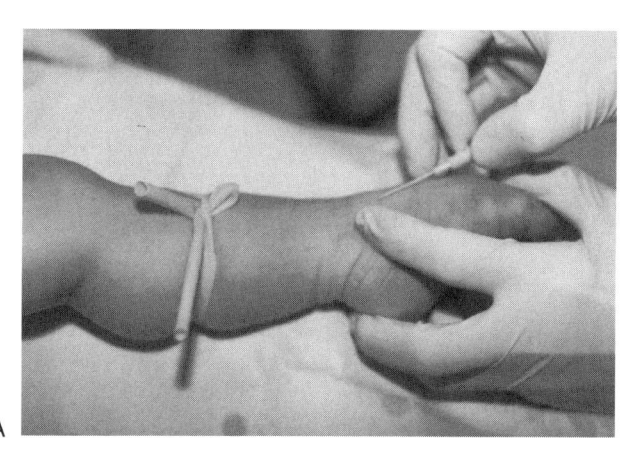

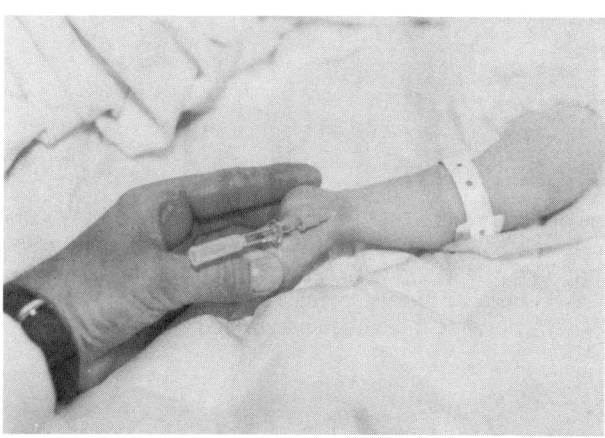

FIG. 7. **(A)** In proper positioning for saphenous vein cannulation, the child's toes are retracted downward with the clinician's thumb while the fingertips stabilize the heel. The needle is inserted at the base of the medial malleolus and advanced toward the contralateral shoulder. **(B)** The proper grip is again shown. Note that the toe is pulled downward and the heel maintained with the clinician's index finger. The catheter is advanced until there is a flashback and then the needle is removed. Often, the saphenous vein cannot be palpated. However, by knowing the exact location of the vein, the procedure can be done "blindly." The key to successful cannulation lies in advancing the cannula a few millimeters more after the flashback is observed. If one goes through and through the vessel, one may back into the vessel, hook up the IV, and then advance the catheter while fluids are infusing ("floating-the-catheter").

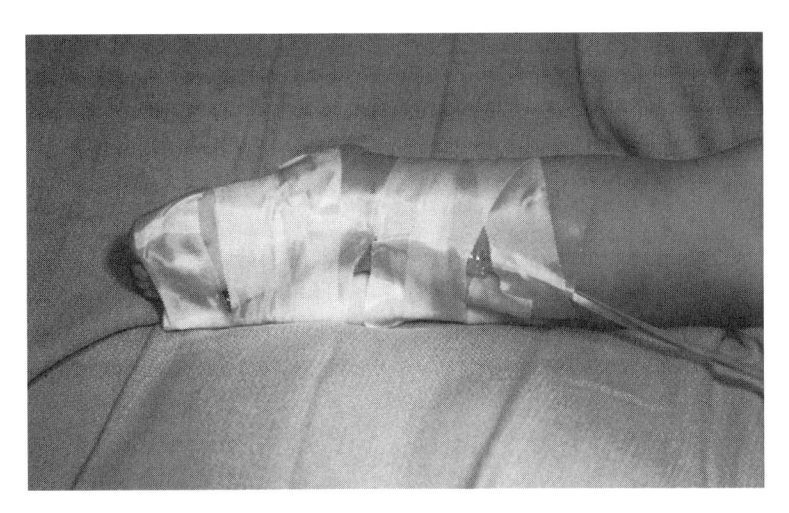

FIG. 8. A well-secured saphenous vein IV in an infant. This infant had an upper respiratory infection and experienced laryngospasm after extubation. Despite the child's thrashing and squirming, the IV stayed in place, allowing injection of IV succinylcholine to treat the laryngospasm.

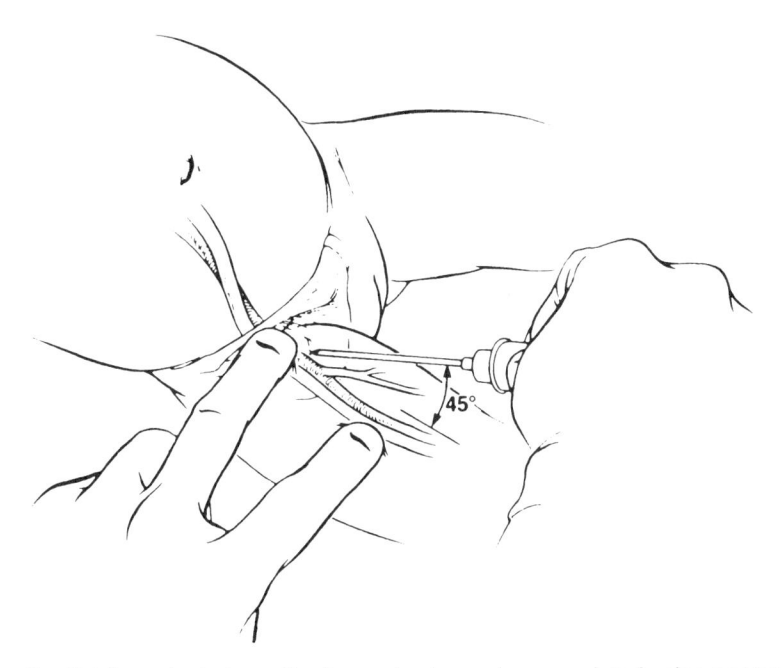

FIG. 9. Using the Seldinger technique, the femoral vein can be cannulated using appropriately sized catheters. These same anatomic landmarks are important in femoral artery cannulation for arterial monitoring. (From American Heart Association: *Textbook of Pediatric Advanced Life Support,* Dallas, AHA, 1994, with permission, copyright American Heart Association.)

spring guidewire (Arrow Duoflex, Reading, PA) then allows insertion of a 20-gauge catheter and will then allow a 0.635-mm spring guidewire and the insertion of almost any sized catheter including a 7F catheter (Rapid Infusion Catheter exchange Set, Arrow Duoflex) for very rapid infusions. One advantage of a femoral vein cannula is that it may be used for central venous monitoring (**see Central Venous Pressure Monitoring**) as well as for fluid administration.

Intraosseous Needle Insertion

As a last resort (usually), vascular access may be achieved through an intraosseous needle (8). This is recommended primarily for children younger than 6 years of age because they still have red bone marrow. The marrow cavity can be accessed regardless of intravascular volume status because the vascular net inside the bone is supported by the bone structure and does not collapse with volume depletion. In this technique, a bone marrow needle (No. 15 Jamshidi, Baxter Healthcare Corporation, Valencia, CA) or a No. 14 through 18 Cook intraosseous infusion needle (Cook Critical Care, Bloomington, IN) (Fig. 10A) is percutaneously inserted into the flat portion of the proximal tibia (Fig. 10B). Entry is made in the tibial plateau 1½ cm below the knee joint and 2 cm medial to the tibial tuberosity. The special bone marrow–stiletted needle is inserted with a rotary motion into the bone until the cavity is reached. The depth of the needle insertion should be planned before placement. If it is advanced too far, the needle will penetrate the posterior cortex and will not allow infusion. The needle should be firmly set in the bone. Often, bone marrow may be aspirated to confirm the placement. A syringe or IV line can be attached, and if it runs easily, placement is confirmed. Slight extravasation around the placement site should not prevent use of the needle. The catheter can serve as a conduit for all IV fluids and drugs.

Crystalloids, blood products, and drugs may be given. Fluids may be infused by intraosseous route at rates up to 40 mL/min (using 300 mm Hg pressure). Contraindications to intraosseous insertion are a broken bone or a previous unsuccessful attempt at insertion (9). The most common complications of intraosseous infusion are osteomyelitis, bone fractures, and compartment syndrome (10). Although the intraosseous technique is a major innovation in resuscitation of the pediatric patient, it is only a temporary measure until intravascular volume is replenished and permanent access to the circulation is gained. Because it may be lifesaving, an intraosseous needle is recommended for every crash cart and is a part of the necessary equipment in every operating room.

CENTRAL VEIN CANNULATION

The following are the most common *indications* for the insertion of a central venous cannula:

- Monitoring central venous pressure
- Venous access during major surgery with massive fluid shifts or blood loss
- Cardiac surgery
- Procedures that carry a high risk of venous air embolism
- When inotropic drugs may be necessary

There are no absolute *contraindications* to central venous cannulation. However, relative contraindications exist when there is sepsis, infection, or broken skin at the site of insertion, or an additional risk of pneumothorax (e.g., in status asthmaticus).

Insertion Methods

As in adults, insertion sites include the internal jugular (high, low, or posterior approach), external jugular, subclavian (infraclavicular or supraclavicular approach), femoral, basilic, and axillary. The most common method used for successful placement of the central venous line is the Seldinger technique (7), which can be used for inser-

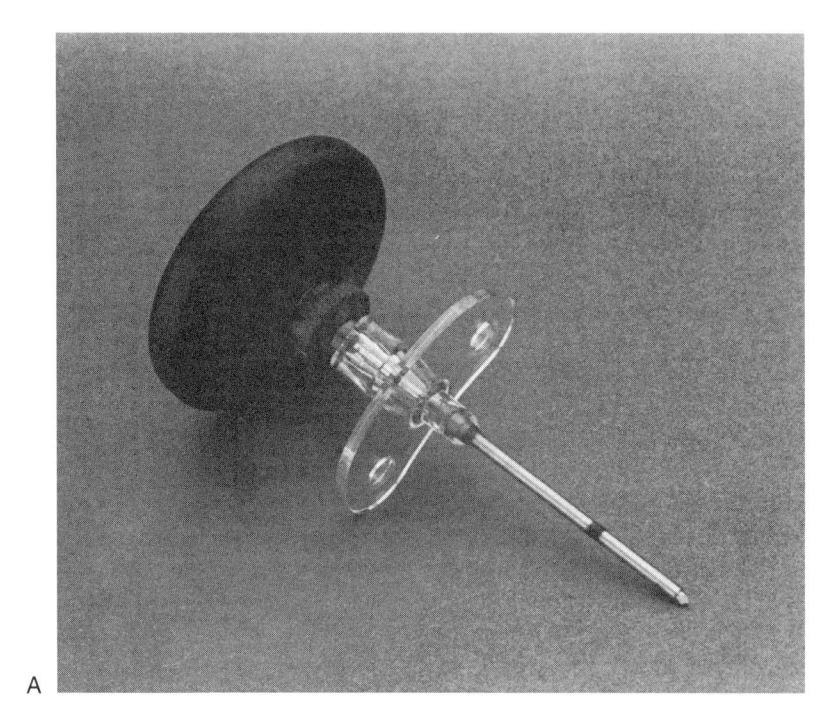

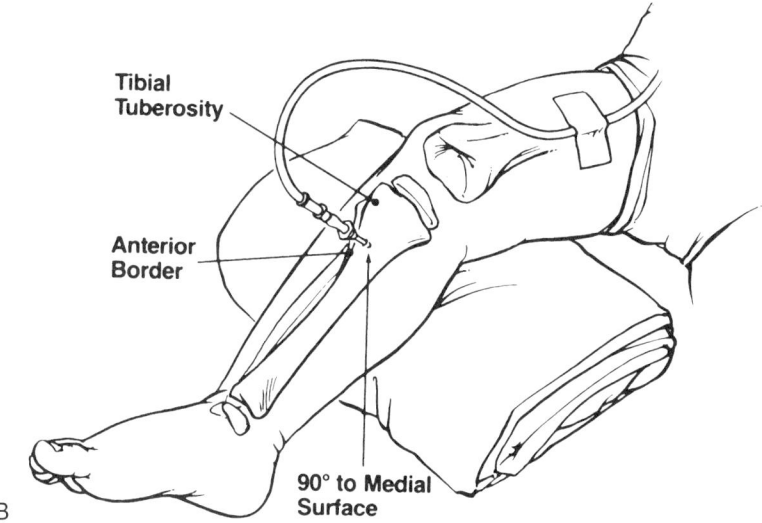

FIG. 10. **(A)** A Cook intraosseous infusion needle (see text for details) (Courtesy Cook Catheter Company). **(B)** For intraosseous infusions, a bone marrow needle or specially made intraosseous needle is inserted into the tibial plateau (just medial and down from tibial the tuberosity). The catheter is then secured and IV solutions and medications may be administered. (From American Heart Association: *Textbook of Pediatric Advanced Life Support,* Dallas, AHA, 1994; with permission, copyright American Heart Association.)

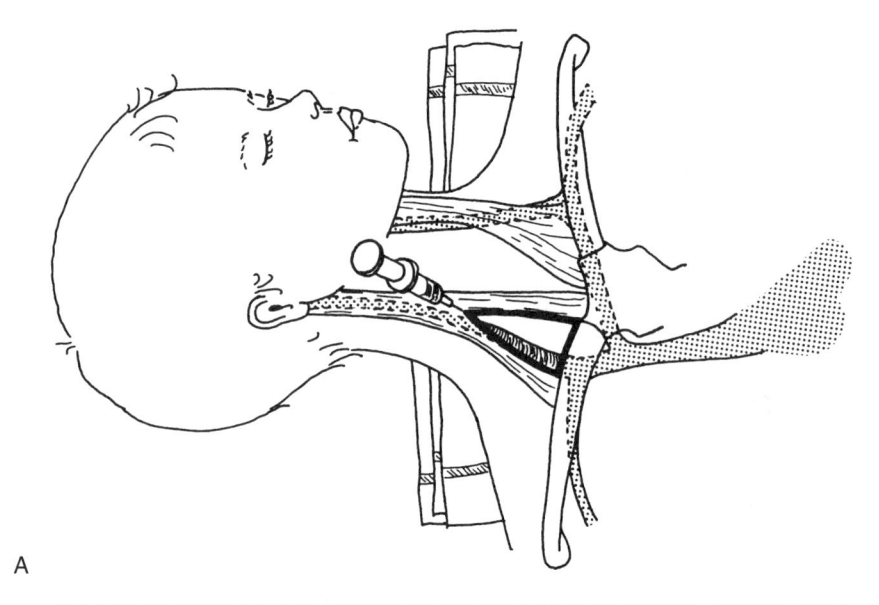

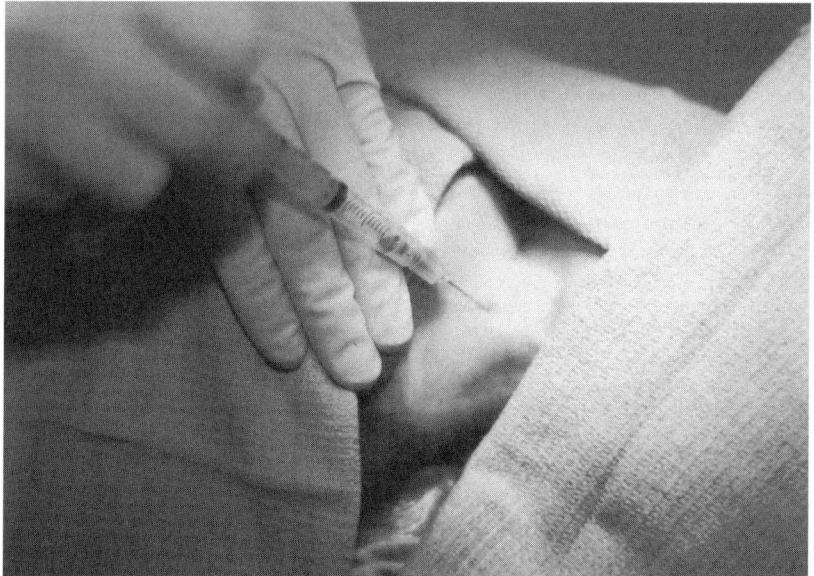

FIG. 11. **(A)** The internal jugular vein courses just to the medial aspect of the clavicular head of the sternocleidomastoid muscle. The high approach for internal jugular cannulation involves inserting a needle at the apex of a triangle formed by the two heads of the sternocleidomastoid muscle. **(B)** One of the keys for successful cannulation of the internal jugular vein involves retraction of the skin cephalad. The needle is inserted at the apex of the triangle described above (**A**). Gradual aspiration is applied until blood flashback is observed. Cannulation of the internal jugular is often best accomplished by backing into the vessel. The needle and catheter seem to "rebound" into the vein that had been compressed by the initial forward puncture.

tion of single-, double-, and triple-lumen catheters.

Internal Jugular Vein Cannulation (High Approach)

The child is positioned on a table in Trendelenburg's position with towels placed under the shoulders. This positioning is very important because it allows more direct access to anatomic landmarks (Fig. 11A). Skin overlying the jugular vein is retracted cephalad by the clinician's fingers, and the needle is inserted at a 45-degree angle through the skin at a point overlying the upper apex of a triangle formed by the two heads of the sternocleidomastoid muscle and the clavicle (Fig. 11B). Vessel location may be identified using an ultrasound vascular access guidance device (Site Rite II, Dymax Corporation, Pittsburgh, PA). With or without ultrasound guidance, the needle is directed toward the ipsilateral nipple with gentle aspiration of a syringe until a slight "give" is felt and blood flashes back into the syringe as the jugular vein is entered. Often at this point, aspiration of blood is not successful (even though a flashback was initially seen). What may have happened is a "through-and-through" puncture of both venous walls.

"Salvage" may be accomplished by "backing into" the vein and aspirating again. After successful aspiration of blood, the syringe is removed and a guidewire is passed. The goal of catheter insertion is to place the tip at the junction of the vena cava and the right atrium. To achieve this goal, a catheter of appropriate length is chosen (Table 1) and depth of insertion estimated by holding the catheter above the child to assess where the tip will terminate. It is important not to cut the catheter to length with scissors because the resultant sharp tip may perforate the atrium or vena cava.

Subclavian Vein Cannulation

Subclavian vein cannulation involves passage of a catheter inserted at a 30-degree angle though the skin inferior to the clavicle at a point where it bows at about one half to two thirds of its length from the sternoclavicular junction (Fig. 12). The needle is aimed at the sternal notch and advanced while "hugging" the clavicle and continuously aspirating. When the needle enters the subclavian vein, blood is aspirated, the syringe disconnected, and a guidewire inserted. A catheter is then inserted using the Seldinger technique.

Complications of Central Venous Insertion

"I see mysteries and complications wherever I look, and I have never met a steadily logical person."
—Martha Gellhorn

Complications may be related to placement of the central venous cannula in general (e.g., inadvertent arterial puncture with subsequent hematoma), or, more specifically, complications may be related to the catheter tip (e.g., perforation of the heart or a vessel wall) (Fig. 13). A catheter tip resting against the heart or a great vessel may in time cause it to erode and perforate. Perforation of the heart or great vessel within the mediastinum may lead to

TABLE 1. *Standard catheter length available for pediatric use[a]*

French size	Length	Venous access size	Recommended patient weight (kg)
4.0 / 5.0[b]	5 cm (2 in)[b]	IJ, EJ	<10
4.0/5.0[c]	8 cm (3 ft/8 in)[c]	IJ, EJ	10–40
4.0 / 5.0	12 cm (~ 5 in)	Right subclavian	10–40
4.0/5.0	15 cm (~6 in)	Left subclavian	10–40

[a]Cook Central Venous Catheter Sets, Cook, Inc, Bloomington, IN 47402.
[b]Double Lumen Central Venous Catheter Tray Reorder C-UPLMY-S01-PED
[c]Double Lumen Central Venous Catheter Tray Reorder C-UPLM-401J

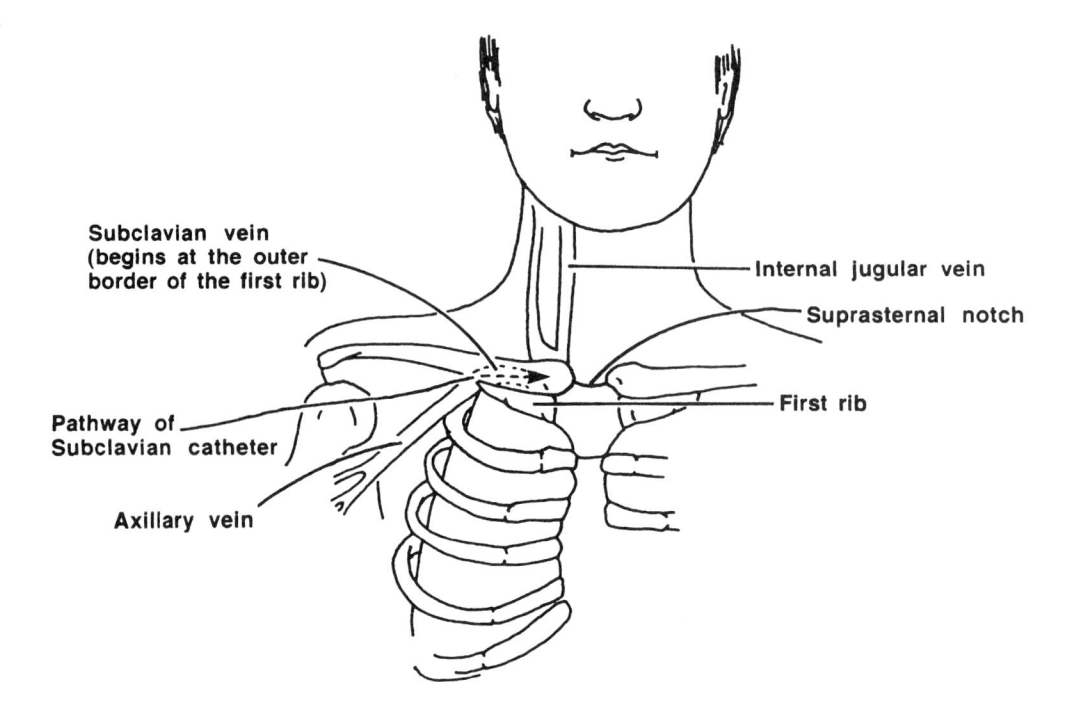

FIG. 12. Important anatomic landmarks for successful cannulation of the subclavian vein. A catheter is inserted through the skin inferior to the clavicle at a point where it bows at about one half to two thirds of its length from the sternoclavicular junction (e.g., a bit more lateral than shown in this figure).

hemothorax or cardiac tamponade. It is therefore important to eliminate factors that may predispose to perforation. Tips of currently available catheters are made of soft pliable material designed to avoid perforation. Therefore, these catheters should not be "cut to fit," since this will create a sharp cutting edge. Rather, a catheter of appropriate length should be prepared initially.

The location and angle of the catheter tip to the vessel wall should be carefully checked radiographically. An incident angle of the catheter tip to the vessel wall of > 40 degrees is more likely to cause perforation (11). Another critical factor that can predispose to perforation is the choice of puncture site. The left subclavian and left jugular veins should be avoided when practical. In adults, 80% of perforations due to erosions occur when these vessels are used (12).

Central Venous Pressure Monitoring

Central venous pressure (CVP) is measured at the junction of the vena cava and the right atrium. As in adults, measurements are used to assess the status of circulatory blood volume and the function of the right ventricle. The value of CVP is usually measured as a mean at the end of respiration. The normal values for CVP vary with age; however, a range of 3 to 12 cm H_2O is accepted for most healthy infants and young children. However, a trend in measurements is often more useful in the therapeutic management of children than an absolute value. In addition, the measurement of CVP may be influenced by spontaneous or controlled ventilation, crying, or position of the patient. As in adults, the CVP is "zeroed" with the transducer or at the level of the atria.

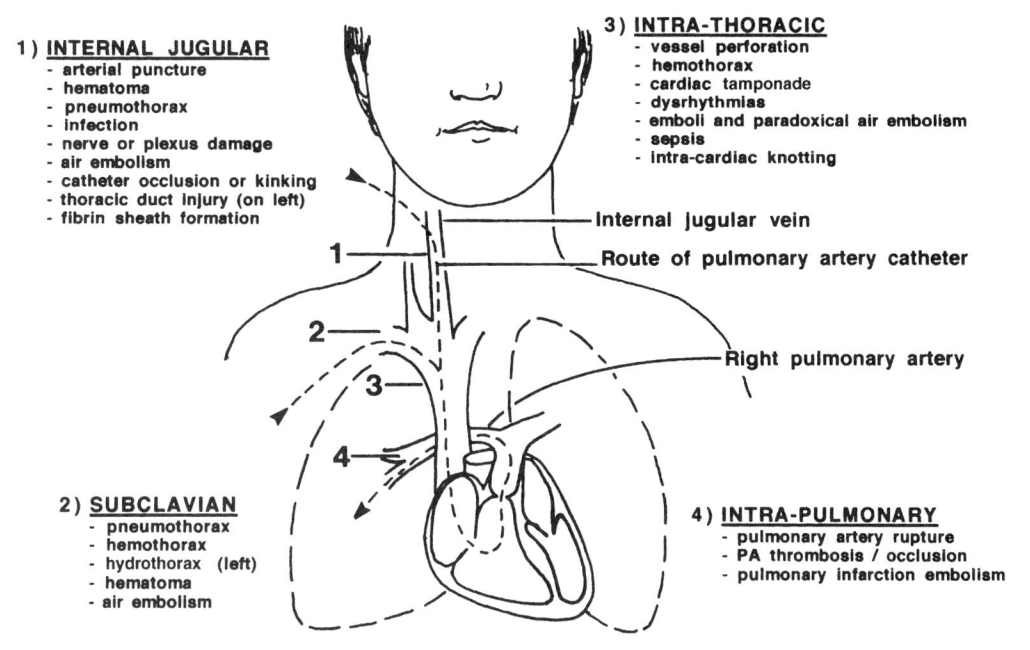

FIG. 13. Potential complications of central vascular cannulation. (Modified and redrawn with permission, Millar CL, Burrows FA: Invasive Monitoring in the Pediatric Patient. In *International Anesthesiology Clinics: Anesthesia Equipment for Infants and Children*. Ed.: Pullerits J and Holzman RS. Summer 1992/Vol. 30, p. 99.)

PULMONARY ARTERIAL FLOTATION CATHETERS

Because of advances in technology that allow the addition of thermistors, oximeters, and pacing ports to its tip, the flow-directed pulmonary catheter is now used in many different clinical situations in children. The use of pulmonary arterial flotation catheters has provided an opportunity to quantify, monitor, and modify the hemodynamic status of the patient during a variety of therapeutic maneuvers.

Indications

Pulmonary artery flotation catheters may be indicated in a many clinical circumstances. This type of catheter may be particularly helpful in the pediatric cardiac patient, especially in the presence or anticipation of left ventricular dysfunction **(see Chapter 12)**. Pulmonary artery flotation catheters are used to guide management in the manipulation of preload and afterload with fluids or pharmacologic agents and for the assessment of cardiac output when global cardiac function is known to be impaired. They may also be helpful in the management of children with cardiogenic and septic shock and when maintenance of normal systemic vascular resistance and cardiac performance may influence outcome (Table 2).

Finally, pulmonary artery flotation catheters may be used to monitor oxygen carrying capacity in an attempt to optimize the supply and delivery of oxygen to tissues and to measure mixed venous oxygen saturation (SvO_2). SvO_2 can be measured by withdrawing a blood sample through the pulmonary artery flotation catheter or by fiberoptic oximetry. The normal SvO_2 is 75% (Fig. 14) and a decrease of 5% to 10% is considered significant. Low arterial oxygen saturation (SaO_2), low cardiac output, low hemoglobin concentration, or elevated oxygen consumption will result in a decline in SvO_2.

TABLE 2. *Pulmonary artery catheterization data*

Procedure	Normal value
Measured data	
Pulmonary artery pressure (PAP)	15–30/4–12 mm Hg
Pulmonary capillary wedge pressure (PCWP)	5–12 mm Hg
Cardiac output (CO)	Varies with patient size
Central venous pressure (CVP)	3–12 mm Hg
Mixed venous oxygen tension (MVO$_2$)	35–45 mm Hg
Calculated data	
Cardiac index (CI) = $\dfrac{CO}{BSA}$	3.0–1.0 L/min/m^2
Systemic vascular resistance index = $\dfrac{(\overline{SAP} - CVP) \times 80}{CI}$	800–1200 dynes/sec/cm^{-5}
Pulmonary vascular resistance index = $\dfrac{(\overline{PAP} - PCWP) \times 80}{CI}$	50–200 dynes/sec/cm^{-5}
Oxygen consumption = CO(AVO$_{2\text{content difference}}$)	110–150 ml/min/m^2

AV, arteriovenous; BSA, body surface area; $\overline{SAP}$, mean systemic arterial pressure; $\overline{PAP}$, mean pulmonary artery pressure.

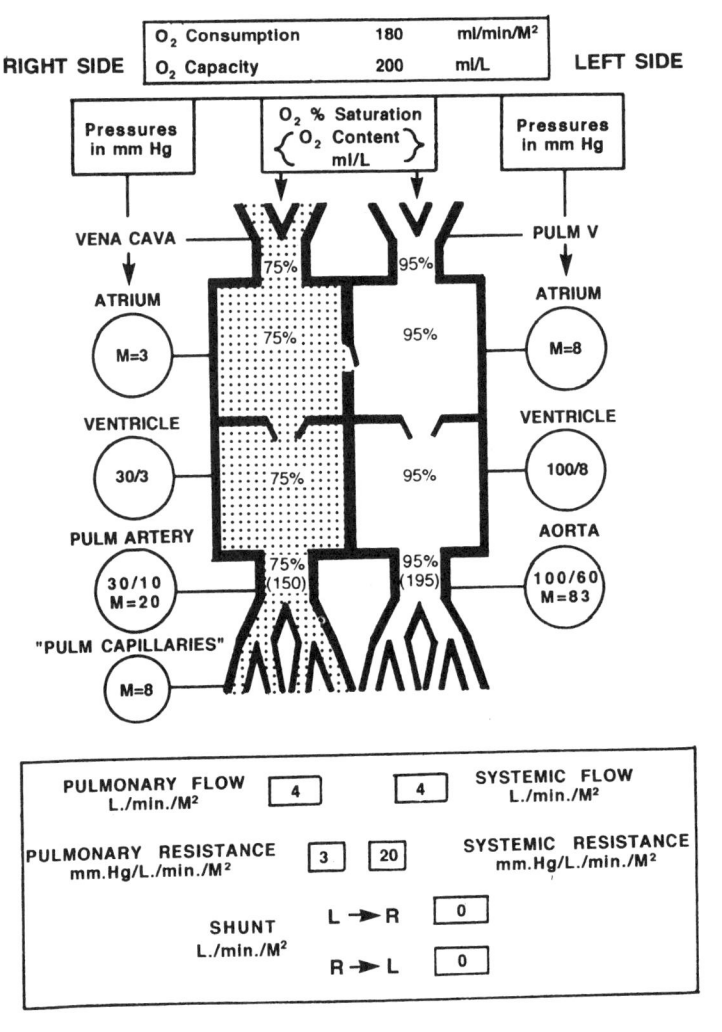

FIG. 14. Normal variables important in the interpretation of pulmonary artery catheter data. (Reprinted with permission, from Nadas AD, Fyler D: *Pediatric Cardiology*. 3rd Ed., 1972, p. 459.)

Contraindications

Insertion of a pulmonary artery catheter is associated with a relatively high risk for complications. Therefore, benefits must be weighed against the risks of insertion. Contraindications may be absolute or relative and are interpreted with the clinical situation:

- An intra- or extracardiac defect may result in an aberrant catheter course, incorrect interpretation of the data, or an increased risk of systemic emboli.
- The presence of a coagulopathy or severe thrombocytopenia is only a relative contraindication; in these situations, the use of a peripheral insertion site may be possible.
- Sepsis or broken skin at the site of insertion is a more serious contraindication.
- Dysrhythmias caused by the passage of the catheter through the heart may compromise the patient's condition.
- Children with preexisting conduction defects (e.g., left bundle-branch block) may develop complete heart block.

Sites of Insertion

Sites for insertion of the pulmonary artery catheter are those used for central venous access: internal jugular vein, subclavian vein, femoral or basilic. In the child weighing less than 15 kg, insertion into the femoral vein may be easier technically. Catheter sizes and length are age related (Table 3):

TABLE 3. *Guidelines for correct pulmonary artery catheter size in pediatric patients*

Age of patient (y)	Catheter size (Fr)	Catheter length in cm (right atrium port to tip)
Newborn–3 y	5	10
3–8	5	15
8–14	7	20
>14	7	30

Insertion Methods

Insertion of a pulmonary artery flotation catheter is similar to that of a standard central venous catheter. There are two methods of establishing correct placement of the catheter in the pulmonary vascular tree: pressure waveforms and fluoroscopy. As in adults, the more common method used is to display pressure waveforms. The distal lumen of the catheter is connected to the pressure-monitoring device that displays the characteristic waveform of the vessels and cardiac chambers through which the catheter tip passes. Alternatively, when the child is small (less than 15 kg) or cardiac output is low, the use of fluoroscopic placement may be preferred. A chest radiograph is performed after every insertion to check the placement of the catheter and to exclude pneumothorax.

Complications

Complications of pulmonary artery monitoring includes the complications associated with internal jugular or subclavian vein catheter insertion as well as the following additional potential complications (Fig. 13):

- Endocarditis
- Valve damage
- Balloon rupture
- Intracardiac tangles and knots
- Inaccurate pressure measurements in presence of congenital heart lesions **(see Chapter 12)**

INSERTION OF ARTERIAL CATHETERS

Percutaneous Placement

Virtually all peripheral arteries have been used for cannulation, the most common being the radial or femoral arteries (13,14). Other arteries amenable to cannulation include the

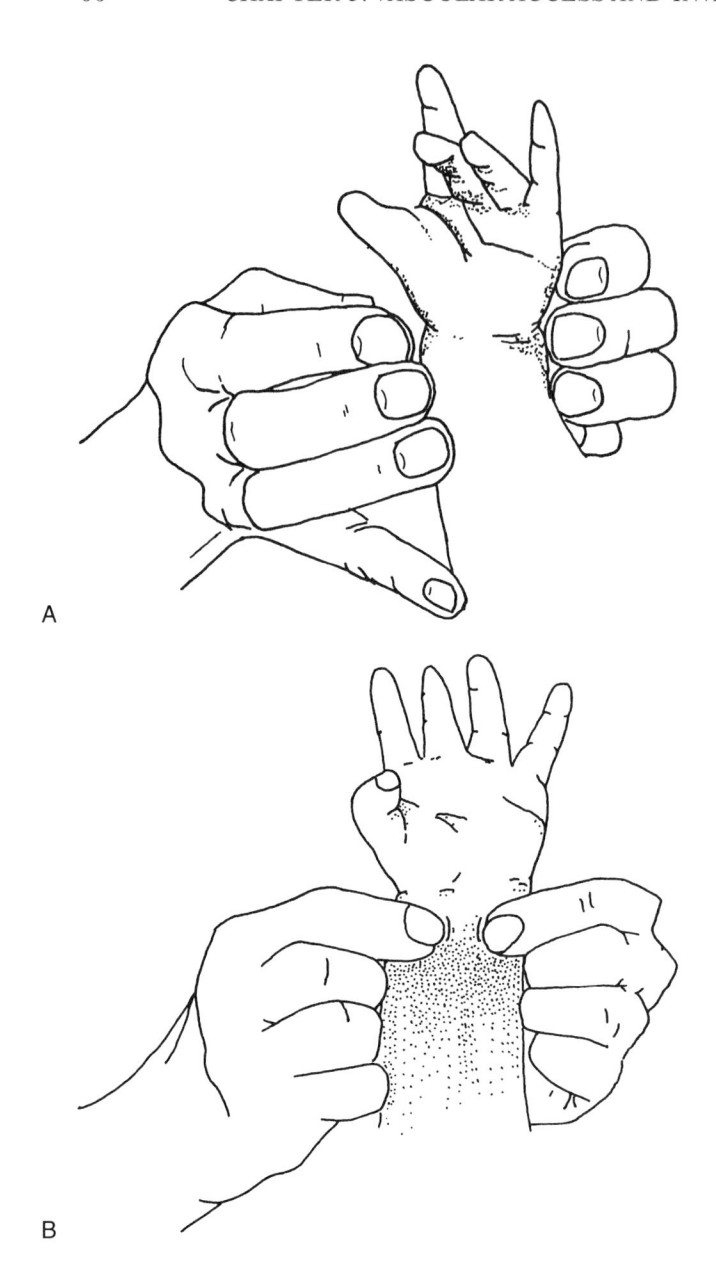

FIG. 15. Allen's test may be performed in children **(A)** by occluding both the radial and ulnar arteries **(B)**

ulnar, brachial, axillary (15), dorsalis pedis, posterior tibial, and superficial temporal (16) vessels, and the umbilical artery in newborns. Before insertion is attempted, an Allen's test for collateral circulation is recommended (Fig. 15)(17). Practically speaking, however, it may be difficult to perform an Allen's test on a very young or uncooperative patient.

Radial Artery

Percutaneous catheter placement in a radial artery can be accomplished using one of several methods. The most common method is direct arterial puncture with the catheter fed over the needle (Fig. 16). In preparation for insertion, the child's extremity is immobilized by taping the extremity securely to a board.

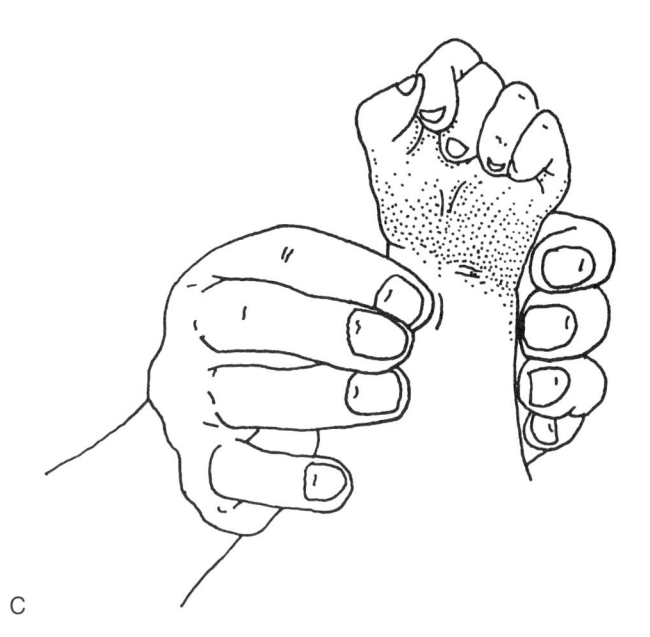

and then observing for reperfusion after the ulnar artery pressure is released **(C)**.

Alternatively, a Seldinger technique modified for small infants uses a 15-cm straight angiographic guidewire 0.4 mm in outer diameter placed through a 22-gauge catheter inserted into the artery by backing into the artery after a through-and-through puncture (Fig. 17). In this technique, the catheter is advanced over the wire and secured.

Fixation. The arterial catheter is connected to a T-connector with a short segment of tubing. With this apparatus, arterial access is available through a rubber port directly on the catheter preventing the need to aspirate large volumes of blood with each sample. Fixation of the cannula can be achieved with tape, sutures, or sterile dressing. Splinting the wrist with a padded board reduces the likelihood that movement of the wrist will interfere with the pressure tracing. Disconnection of the cannula from the connecting tubing could result in a major hemorrhage and exsanguination of the patient. This mishap would be immediately evident as a loss of pressure tracing.

Arterial Locating Techniques. In preterm and newborn infants, the use of a cold (fiberoptic) light source shone through the wrist from below makes it possible to visualize the artery as it pulsates in the wrist (18,19). In difficult cases in older children, a Doppler flow transducer may be useful for localizing a pulsating artery that is hard to palpate.

Femoral Artery

Landmarks for the femoral artery are identified as for the femoral vein (Fig. 18; Fig. 9). Using the Seldinger technique, a needle and then wire are inserted into the femoral artery followed by the insertion of a 22- or 20-gauge catheter.

Surgical Cutdown

A surgical cutdown of the radial artery may be the preferred option in patients in whom percutaneous placement in the radial or femoral artery is likely to be difficult or has failed previously. The incidence of vessel thrombosis, however, is higher with surgical cutdown (20). Several techniques are available for cutdown. One technique involves a longitudinal or transverse incision of the skin over the radial artery and the placement of proximal and distal ties around the artery.

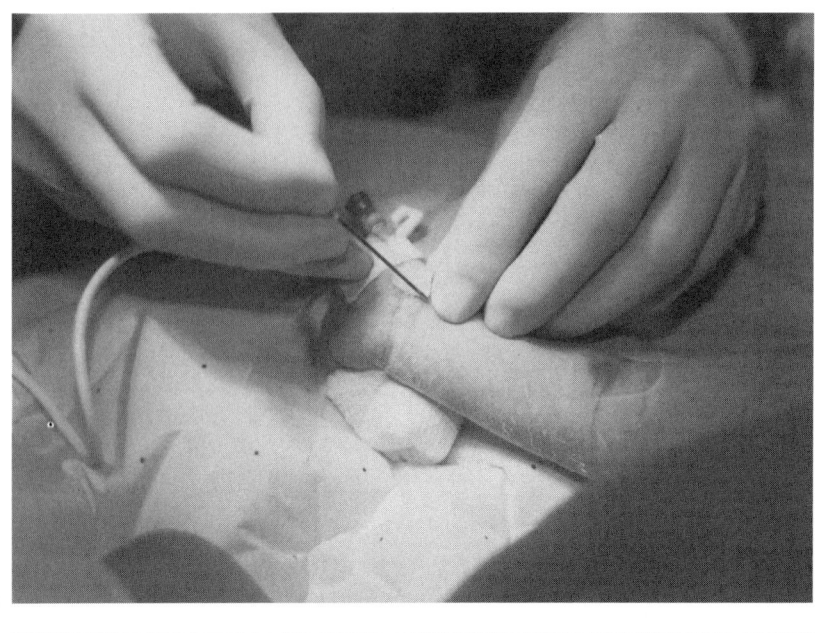

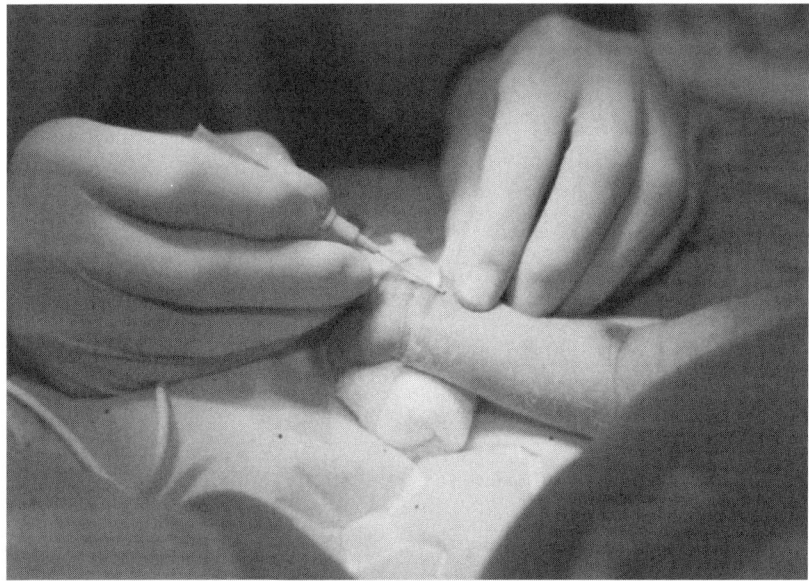

FIG. 16. Percutaneous radial artery catheterization. **(A)** First, the radial artery is identified and the overlying skin is pierced with an 18-gauge needle. **(B)** A catheter/needle is inserted at about a 30-degree angle through the skin incision.

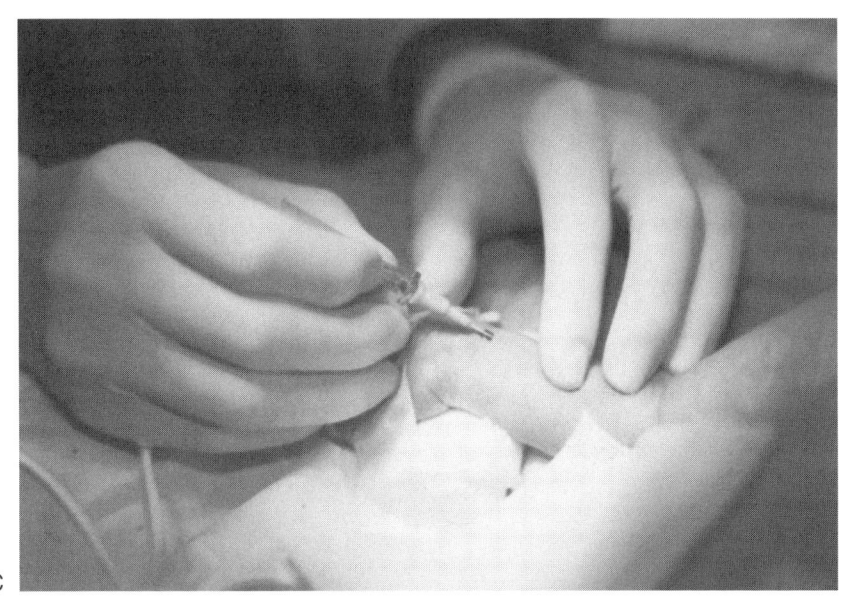

(C) The needle and catheter are advanced until a flashback is observed. After flashback, the needle is advanced approximately 1 mm more with the catheter to ensure that the catheter will be well within the artery. The needle is then slowly withdrawn and the catheter advanced further into the artery.

Under direct vision, the artery is pierced with a needle and catheter and the cather passed over the needle into the artery (Fig. 19A). The distal tie is moved proximally over the catheter and both proximal and distal ties are tied over the catheter proximal to the arterial incision (Fig. 19B). In a second technique, a small curved hemostat is inserted under the exposed artery, and a needle and catheter are inserted into the artery over the hemostat (Fig. 20).

INTRA-ARTERIAL BLOOD PRESSURE MONITORING

Originally, direct monitoring of arterial blood pressure in pediatrics was restricted by the small size of patients' arteries relative to the diameter of the cannula. Today, the availability of high-quality narrow-gauge cannulas ensure that direct intra-arterial monitoring is not only feasible but widely practiced in pediatric anesthesia.

Indications

The indications for use of intra-arterial pressure monitoring are based primarily on hemodynamic and pulmonary considerations, individual patient and surgical factors, and a risk-to-benefit analysis. Arterial blood pressure is a function of blood volume, cardiac output, and peripheral vascular resistance and may be used as an indication of adequate organ perfusion. Normal values for blood pressure in infants and children vary with age **(see Table 2, Chapter 2)**.

Contraindications

Contraindications to the use of intra-arterial pressure monitoring may be absolute, such as skin infection or inadequate collateral flow, or relative, such as the presence of coagulopathy.

Cannula Materials

The size of the cannula is critical in pediatric patients, especially for ease of insertion

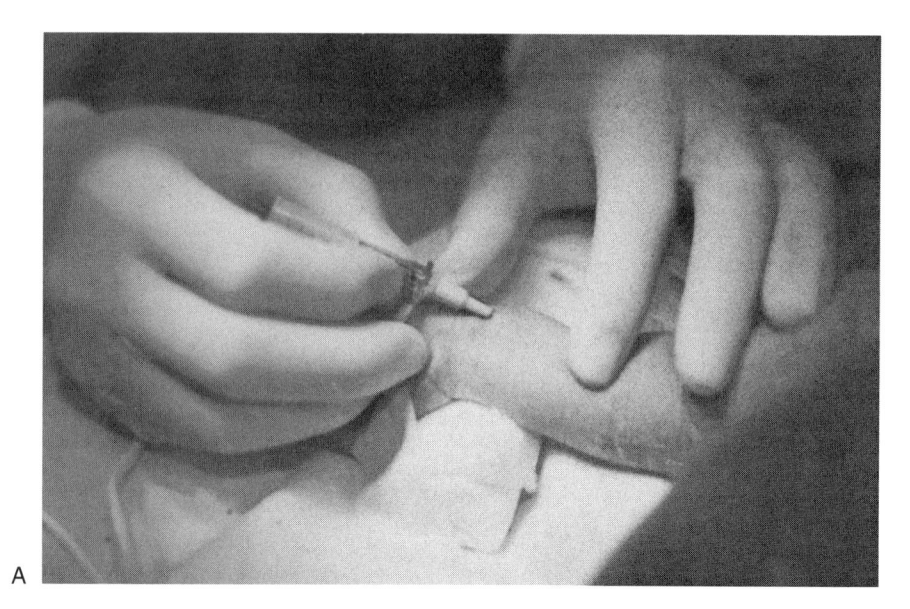

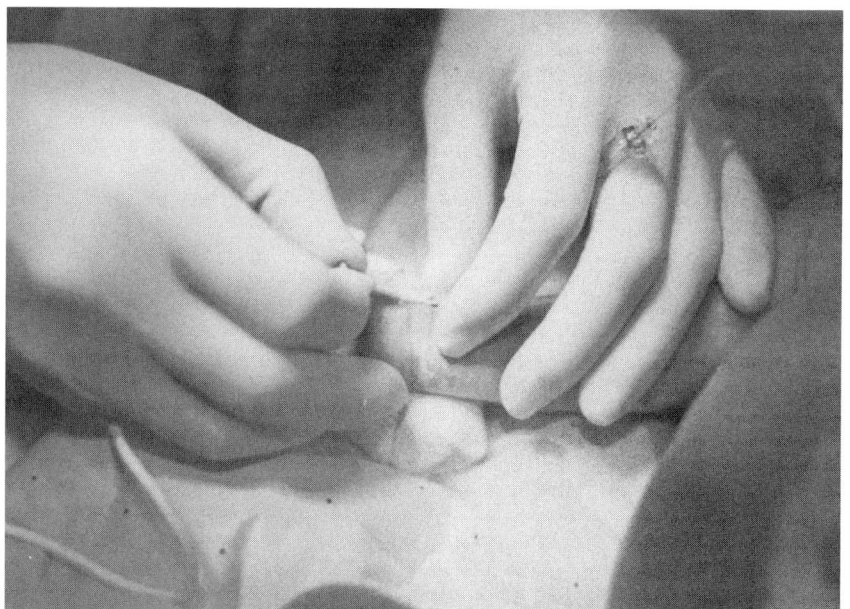

FIG. 17. An alternative technique for radial artery catheterization. **(A)** In this technique, the radial artery is punctured "through and through," using a 22-gauge needle/catheter. **(B)** The needle is removed and the catheter gradually withdrawn until blood flows are through the catheter.

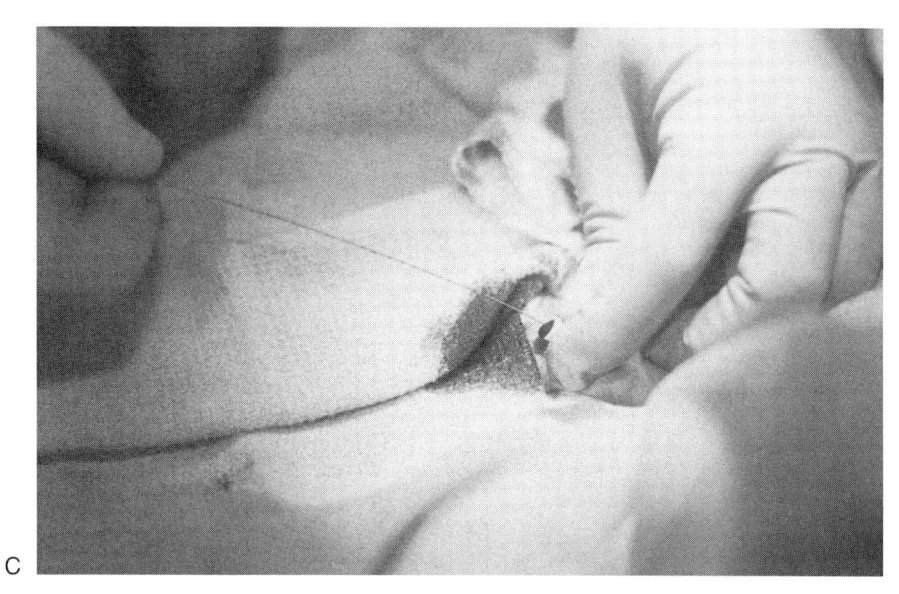

(C) A 0.45-mm diameter spring guidewire (Arrow, No. AW-04018, Reading, PA) is inserted through the catheter and into the artery. The catheter is then slipped over the wire into the artery.

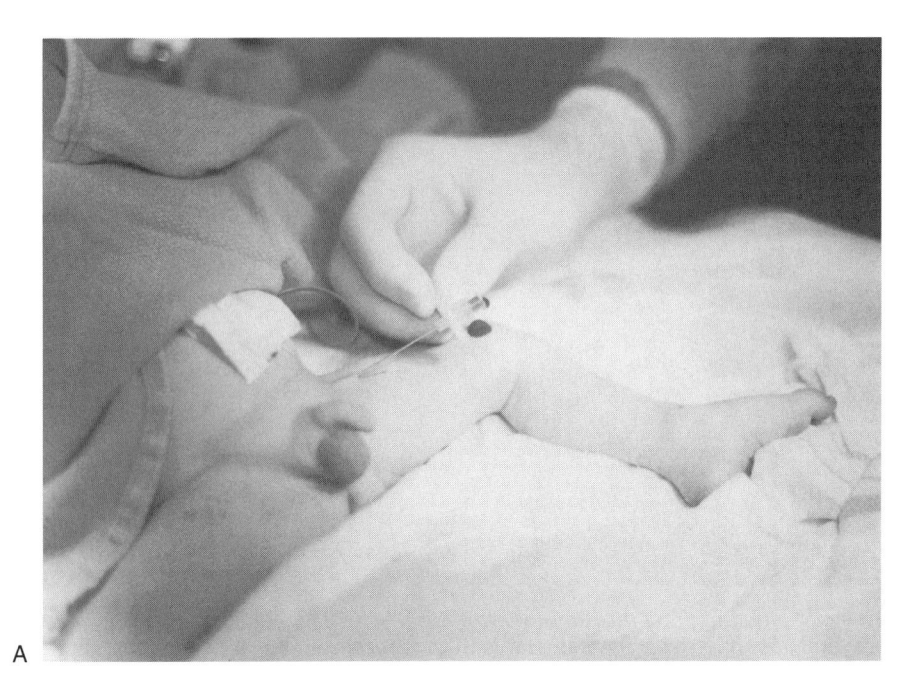

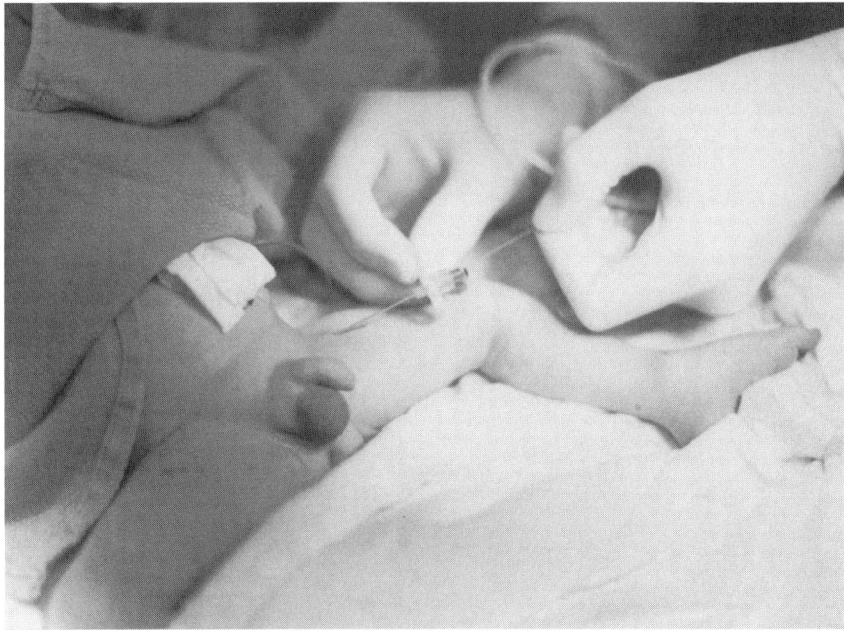

FIG. 18. Femoral artery catheterization. **(A)** A needle is inserted into the femoral artery below the inguinal ligament (to avoid peritoneal perforation). **(B)** When there is a good blood return, a guidewire is inserted through the needle into the vessel, and then an appropriate-sized catheter is placed over the guidewire.

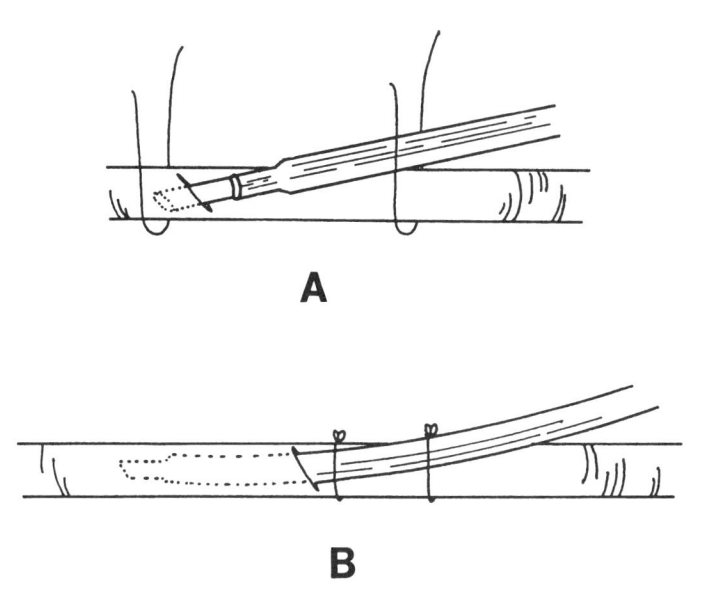

FIG. 19. A technique for surgical cutdown of the radial artery. **(A)** After skin incision and arterial identification, proximal and distal ties are placed around the artery. A needle/catheter is then inserted into the artery under direct vision. **(B)** The needle is withdrawn and the catheter advanced into the artery. The distal tie is then moved to a proximal position to preserve patency of the artery after the catheter is removed.

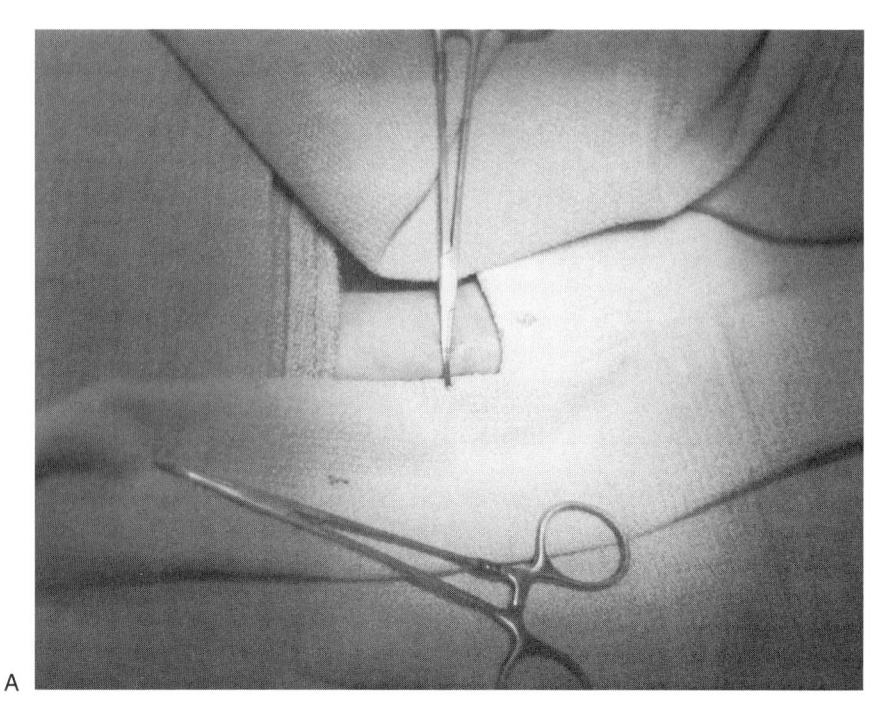

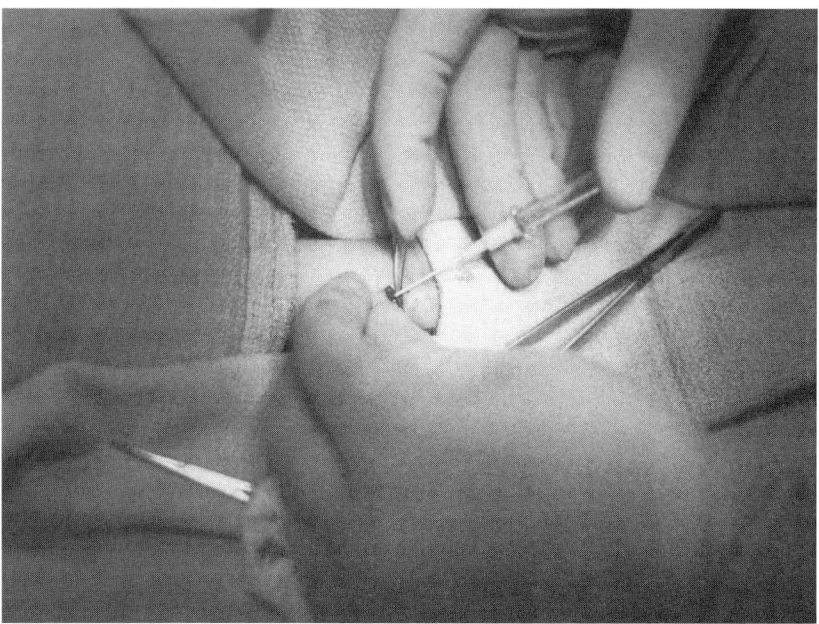

FIG. 20. Another technique of surgical cutdown of the radial artery. **(A)** After incision and localization of the radial artery, a small curved hemostat is placed under the artery. **(B)** A catheter/needle is then inserted under direct vision in the artery. The needle is withdrawn and the catheter advanced. The skin is then sutured and the catheter secured.

and withdrawal of samples. A 24-gauge cannula is recommended for infants weighing less than 3 kg, and 22-gauge catheters are usually appropriate for infants weighing ($\geq$3 kg. Shorter cannulas (3.2 cm) are particularly suitable for younger patients. The small-gauge, nontapered, nonpyrogenic (Teflon) cannulas are less thrombogenic than the polypropylene type (21), whereas those made of polyurethane are less rigid and potentially less traumatic.

REFERENCES

1. Schmidt WF III, Kim HC, Tomassini N, Schwartz, E: RBC destruction caused by a micropore blood filter. *JAMA* 1982;248:1629–1632.
2. Longhurst DM, Gooch WM III, Castillo RA: In vitro evaluation of a pediatric microaggregate blood filter. *Transfusion* 1983;23:170–172.
3. American Society of Anesthesiologists, Committee on Transfusion Medicine: *Question and answers about transfusion practice,* ed. 2 Dallas, American Society of Anesthesiologists Committee on Transfusion, 1992:24.
4. Clayton DG, Evans P, Williams C, Thurlow AC: Paradoxical air embolism during neurosurgery. *Anaesthesiology* 1985;40:981–989.
5. Holzman RS: Intravenous infusion equipment. *Int Anesthesiol Clin* 1992;30:35–50.
6. Goodie DB, Philip JH: An analysis of the effect of venous resistance on the performance of gravity-fed intravenous infusion systems. *J Clin Monit* 1994;10:222–228.
7. Seldinger SI: Catheter replacement of the needle in percutaneous arteriography. *Acta Radiol Diagn* 1953;39:368–376.
8. Fiser DH: Intraosseous infusion. [Review]. *N Engl J Med* 1990;322:1579–1581.
9. Guy J, Haley K, Zuspan SJ: Use of intraosseous infusion in the pediatric trauma patient. *J Pediatr Surg* 1993;28:158–161.
10. Zimmerman JJ, Coyne M, Logsdon M: Implementation of intraosseous infusion technique by aeromedical transport programs. *J Trauma* 1989;29:687–689.
11. Blackshear RH, Gravenstein N: Critical angle of incidence for delayed vessel perforation by central venous catheter: a study of in vivo data. *Ann Emerg Med* 1992;21:242–247.
12. Tocino IM, Watanabe A: Impending catheter perforation of superior vena cava: radiographic recognition. *Am J Roentgenol* 1986;146:487–490.
13. Glenski JA, Beynen FM, Brady J: A prospective evaluation of femoral artery monitoring in pediatric patients. *Anesthesiology* 1987;66:227–229.
14. Graves PW, Davis AL, Maggi JC, Nussbaum E: Femoral artery cannulation for monitoring in critically ill children: prospective study. *Crit Care Med* 1990;18:1363–1366.
15. Lawless S, Orr R: Axillary arterial monitoring of pediatric patients. *Pediatrics* 1989;84:273–275.
16. Prian GW, Wright GB, Rumack CM, O'Meara OP: Apparent cerebral embolization after temporal artery catheterization. *J Pediatr* 1978;93:115–118.
17. Allen EV: Thromboangiitis obliterans: methods of diagnosis of chronic occlusive arterial lesions distal to wrist with illustrative cases. *Am J Med Sci* 1929;178:237–244.
18. Pearse RG: Percutaneous catheterisation of the radial artery in newborn babies using transillumination. *Arch Dis Child* 1978;53:549–554.
19. Cole FS, Todres ID, Shannon DC: Technique for percutaneous cannulation of the radial artery in the newborn infant. *J Pediatr* 1978;92:105–107.
20. Miyasaka K, Edmonds JF, Conn AW: Complications of radial artery lines in the paediatric patient. *Can Anaesth Soc J* 1976;23:9–14.
21. Bedford RF, Major MC: Percutaneous radial-artery cannulation—increased safety using teflon catheters. *Anesthesiology* 1975;42:219–222.

4

Tracheal Tube and Laryngeal Mask Placement in Routine and Difficult Airways

J. Michael Badgwell

MANAGEMENT OF ROUTINE AIRWAYS

Oral Airways

Oral airways of various sizes are made available before the child is anesthetized. An appropriate-sized plastic oral airway is one that, when placed on the side of the child's face, extends from the lips to the ramus of the mandible (Fig. 1). The tip of an oral airway that is too large may (a) push the epiglottis down into the glottic opening, precipitating laryngospasm during light anesthesia, or (b) obstruct the glottic opening altogether (Fig. 2A). The tip of an oral airway that is too small may push the tongue backward and cause further obstruction (Fig. 2B). The correctly sized oral airway maintains space between the tongue and other airway structures (Fig. 3). Insertion of an oral airway is made infinitely easier by using a tongue depressor. Oral airways are not "threaded." Twisting the oral airway into place may cause trauma to soft oral tissues and does not work as well as using a tongue depressor to guide the airway over the tongue (Fig. 4).

Nasopharyngeal Airways

A nasopharyngeal airway is a trumpeted, soft rubber or polyvinyl chloride tube that provides a conduit for gas flow between the tongue and the posterior pharyngeal wall. Responsive patients, such as children awakening from anesthesia with partial airway obstruction, tolerate nasopharyngeal airways better than they tolerate the oral variety. Nasopharyngeal airways are available in sizes 12F to 36F. The 12F nasal airway is the appropriate size for a full-term newborn infant. Before insertion in any infant or child, however, the proper length is estimated by measuring the distance from the tip of the nose to the tragus of the ear (Fig. 5).

The airway is lubricated and inserted through a nostril in a posterior direction perpendicular to the coronal plane and passed gently along the floor of the nasopharynx. The nasal airway may be turned or twisted to follow the pathway of least resistance, but it should never be forced because the airway may damage mucosa or adenoidal tissue, causing epistaxis.

Masks

Plastic, padded, clear masks (e.g., Cushioned Mask, Vital Signs, Totowa, NJ) are preferred because they protect the patient and allow visualization of things going on under the mask such as cyanosis, vomitus, or bleeding. The ideal pediatric mask should fit over the bridge of the nose and the cheeks and chin for an air-tight seal. As a general rule, a mask that is slightly too large is much better than one that is slightly too small. A mask that is too small may actually obstruct the nares and will not allow proper mouth opening when the survival position is applied (see below). Further-

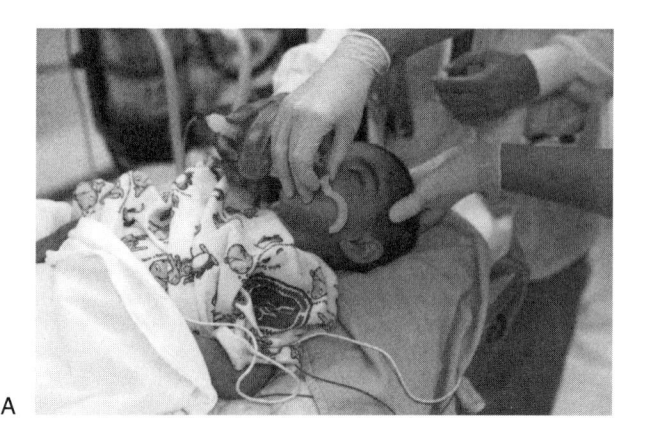

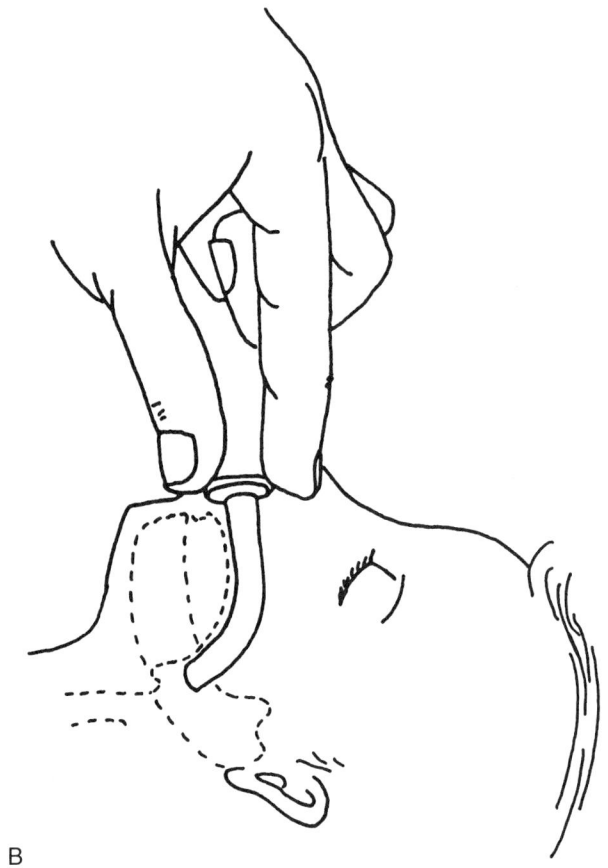

FIG. 1. (A and B) An appropriate-sized plastic oral airway extends from the lips to the ramus of the mandible when placed on the side of the child's face.

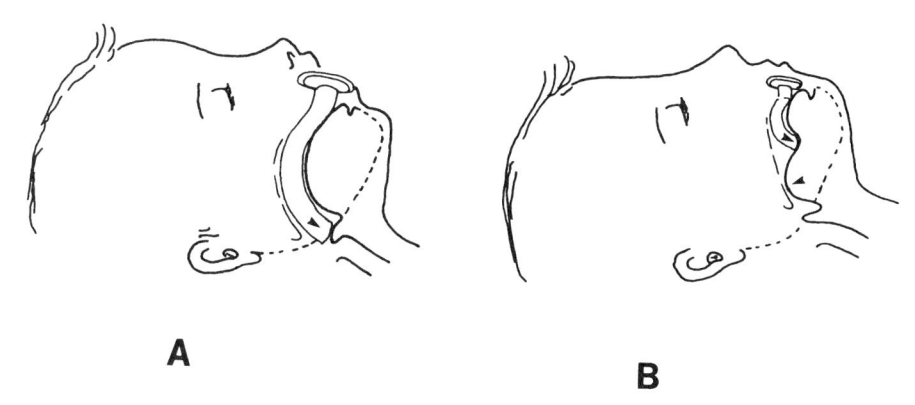

FIG. 2. (A) The tip of an oral airway that is too large may (1) push the epiglottis down into the glottic opening or (2) slide past the epiglottis and obstruct the glottic opening. **(B)** The tip of an oral airway that is too small may push the tongue backward and cause further obstruction.

more, the mask should accommodate an oropharyngeal or nasopharyngeal airway during spontaneous or assisted ventilation. As a practical note, removal of the "spider" (strap holders) present on some masks allows a more comfortable grip on the mask.

Endotracheal Tubes

The appropriately sized endotracheal tube can be chosen using one of the two available formulas:

$$\text{Age} + 4.0/4.0 = \text{ETT size}$$

$$\text{Height (cm)}/20 = \text{ETT size}$$

where ETT is endotracheal tube.

Or, the diameter of the external nares or the distal tip of the child's fifth digit may be used as approximations of the outer diameter of the endotracheal tube. The endotracheal tube that will easily fit through the external nares will fit into the nearest portion of the trachea, the cricoid ring. I recommend that three sizes of endotracheal tubes be made available: (a) the size expected, (b) one size larger, and (c) one size smaller. If oral tracheal intubation is planned, tubes should be cut to the appropriate length (usually at the * on the tube). A rough guide for the approximate depth of endotracheal insertion (e.g., the distance from gingiva to mid-trachea) is to multiply the internal diameter (ID) of the endotracheal tube times three. For example, a 4.0-ID endotracheal tube would be taped to the face with teeth or lips at the 12-cm mark.

Laryngoscope Blades

Several different blades must be ready before the induction of anesthesia in case the initially chosen blade proves to be inadequate. In general, I prefer to initially choose either a Flagg or improved vision (IV) MacIntosh for infants and children (Table 1). The Flagg blade has a wide C-shaped flange (much wider than the Miller) useful in pushing the infant's large tongue out of the way (Fig. 6). The IV MacIntosh blade has a modified curvature on the lateral edges of the blade and allows for an improved vision of the airway structures compared with the older version of the MacIntosh (Fig. 7).

Suction Apparatus

Perhaps the most important equipment to have available are the suction apparatus and suction catheters. It is preferable to have a small pediatric-sized Yankeur suction tip available, as well as a soft suction catheter. Often during the induction of infants and chil-

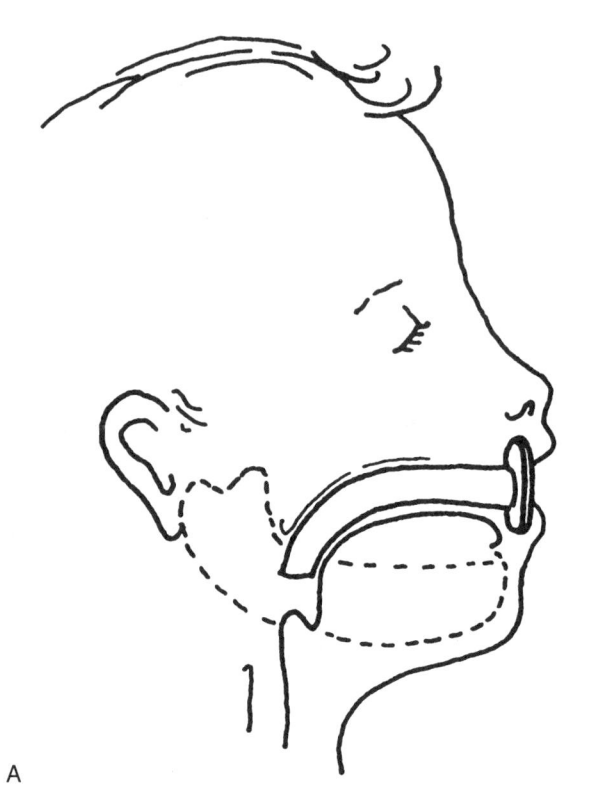

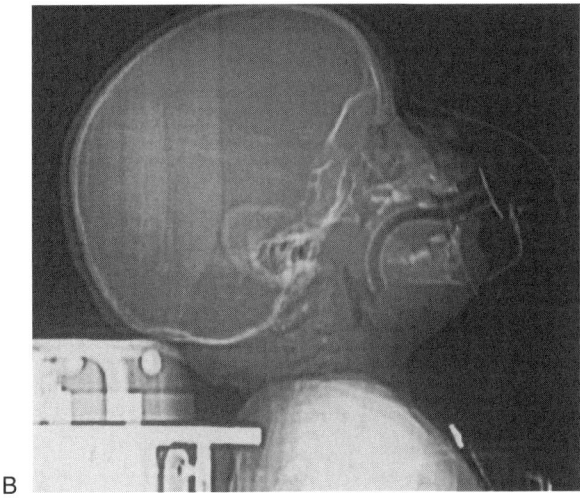

FIG. 3. (A) The appropriate-sized oral airway maintains space between the tongue and other airway structures. **(B)** In this radiograph of a 1-year-old, 10-kg child, the plastic oral airway is shown in position. This oral airway is on the borderline of being too large because it almost touches the epiglottis. Airway patency, however, was maintained throughout a computed tomography scan.

dren, especially during mask induction, an excessive amount of gas is swallowed (or squeezed) into the stomach. To permit adequate ventilation, it may be necessary to aspirate the stomach using the soft suction catheter. If so, it should be done promptly, usually before endotracheal intubation.

Tracheal Tube Placement

"When you see something that is technically sweet, you go ahead and do it and you argue about what to do about it only after you have had your technical success. That is the way it was with the atomic bomb."

—J. Robert Oppenheimer

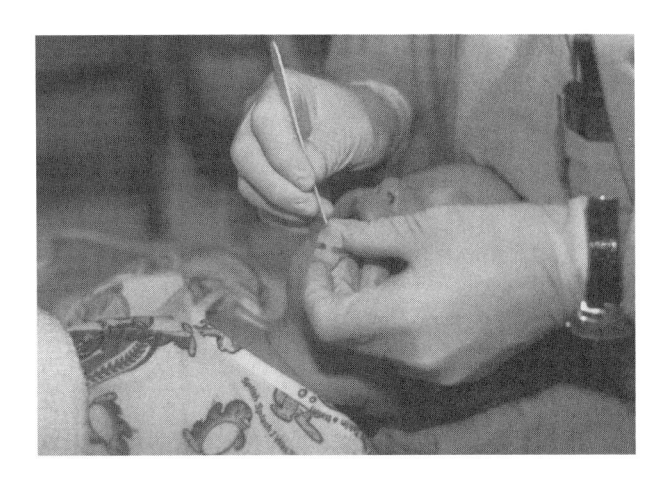

FIG. 4. A tongue depressor is essential in insertion of the plastic oral airway.

Oral Insertion

What follows is an expanded version of the "Creighton technique" for endotracheal intubation of pediatric patients (1). Although useful in all ages of pediatric patients, it is particularly useful in small infants. I have never seen Dr. Creighton fail to intubate even the most difficult of pediatric airways, including small infants with Pierre Robin syndrome, using only a standard laryngoscope and a Flagg 1 blade. If used properly, Dr. Creighton's technique is reliable, repeatable, and almost infallible in both routine and difficult intubations.

> "All presentations, articles, and chapters on the pediatric airway start with a litany of the differences between the infant airway and that of the older child and infants. These include a large head and short neck, the narrow nares, the large tongue, the high glottis, the slanting

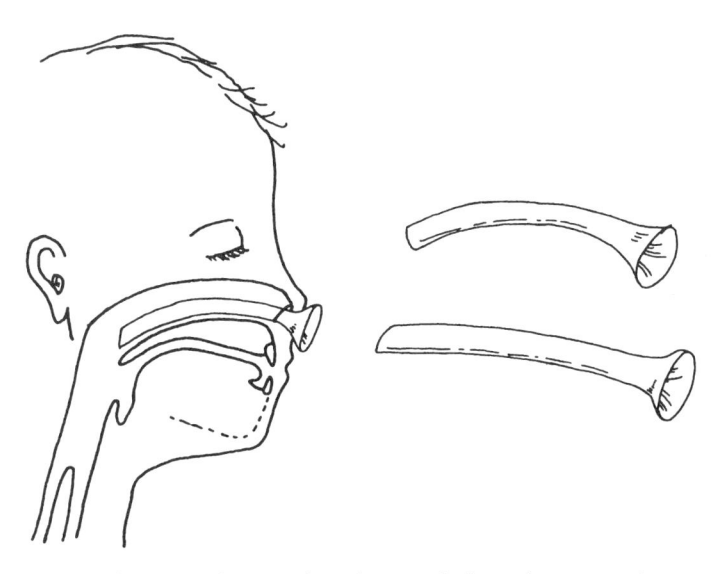

FIG. 5. A nasopharyngeal airway of proper length extends from the external nares to the posterior pharynx without touching the epiglottis or glottic opening.

TABLE 1. Size and type of laryngoscope blades for age

Approximate age (y)	Blade
Premature infants	Miller 0
0 to 2–3	Flagg 1
2–3 to 8	Mac 2
≥8	IV Mac 3

Mac=MacIntosh.

vocal cords, and the narrow epiglottis which is angled away from the axis of the trachea. At first glance, this seems a formidable list of potential difficulties. In practice, there is less than meets the eye in the normal newborn."
—Robert Creighton, MD (1)

Anatomic Airway Differences

The airway of the pediatric patient, particularly the infant, differs anatomically from that of the adult (Fig. 8). One should not get too concerned about the myriad of anatomical airway differences between infants and adults, however; it is really only the large tongue and high-riding epiglottis (it rides high on the tongue) that angles away from the trachea that present clinical considerations.

Equipment

Many intubation problems in pediatric patients arise because clinicians attempt intubation with a curved MacIntosh blade. The truth is that the anatomy of infants requires a straight blade. Therefore, in children less than about 2 to 3 years of age, a Flagg 1 blade, though not widely known, is advantageous over the MacIntosh because the Flagg is straight **(see Laryngoscopic Blades)**. The Flagg blade is advantageous over the straight Miller blade because the wide C-shaped flange of the Flagg blade does a better job of pushing the child's relatively large tongue to the left, holding it there for direct visualization of the glottic opening.

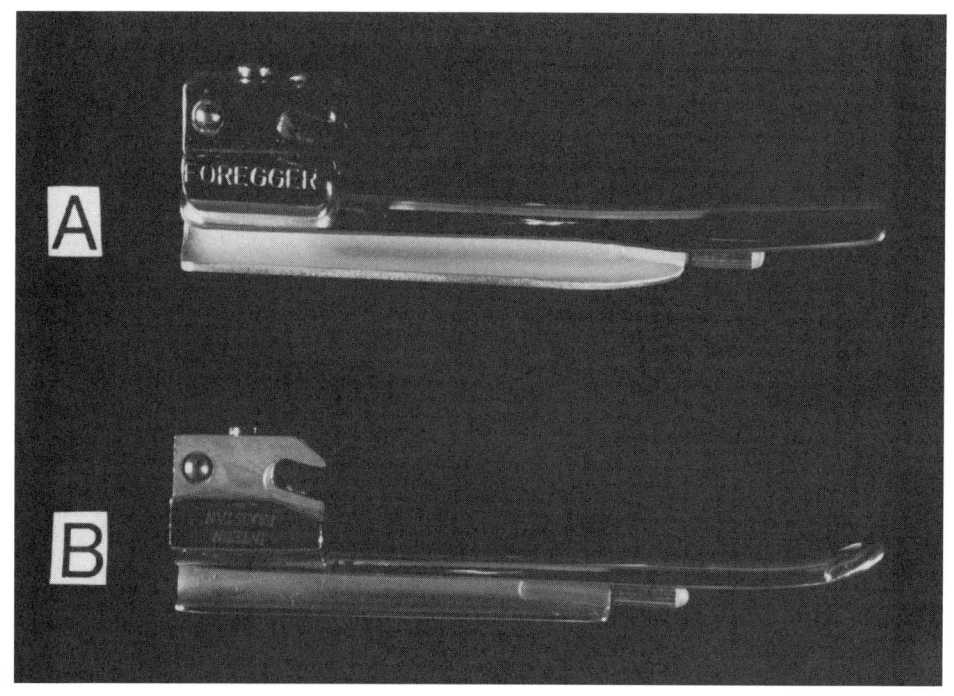

FIG. 6. (Left) A side-by-side comparison of the Flagg **(A)** and Miller **(B)** blades.

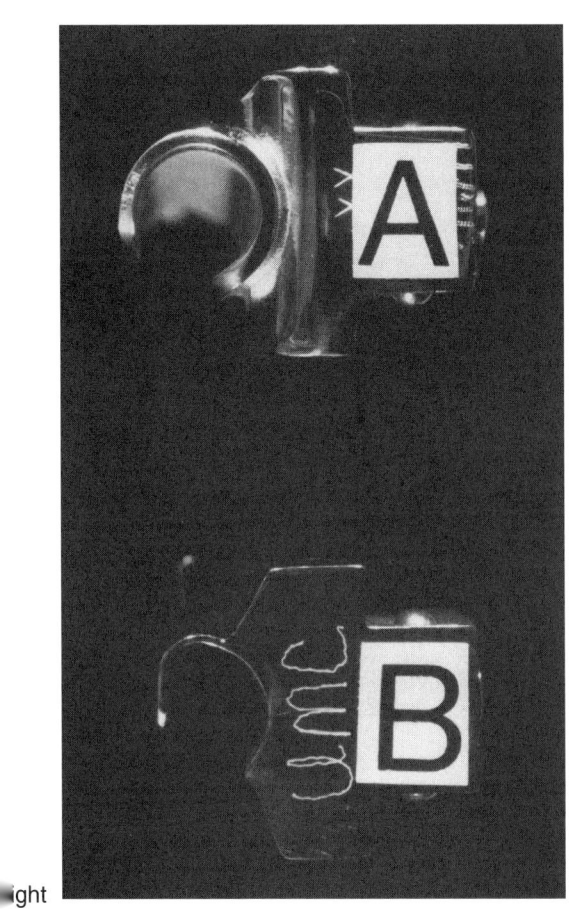

FIG. 6. *Continued.* **(Right)** A wide C-shaped flange of the Flagg blade is advantageous in pediatric anesthesia because the Flagg does a much better job of getting the tongue out of the way than does the Miller blade.

Technique

First, the head is placed in a head ring in the sniff position.[a] If necessary—it is frequently necessary in small infants with big heads—a towel is placed under the shoulders so that the head is in a neutral position, with the neck neither flexed nor extended (Fig. 9). In the next step, the thumb is placed on the child's forehead, the fingertips on the child's occiput, and the child's neck extended (Fig. 10). Neck extension allows the mouth to open, making it accessible for insertion of the laryngoscope blade, and allows the laryngoscope handle room enough to be maneuvered without hitting the chest (Fig. 11). The straight blade of the laryngoscope is placed in the right-hand corner of the mouth lateral to the tongue. The route to the larynx from the base of the tongue forms a much more acute angle in the infant than in the older child and adult and, unless the blade is placed lateral to the tongue, exposure of the glottis will be very difficult.

After placement of the laryngoscope blade into the oral cavity, the head and neck are brought back into neutral position (Fig. 12). *Returning to neutral position is the most important maneuver in the successful intubation of infants.* Intubation is easier in the neutral position because the angle made by the oral and tracheal axes is less acute in the neutral position than if the angle if the child's head is extended (compare the intubational axes in Figs. 9 and 10B). Recall Dr. Creighton's advice that the epiglottis angles away from the axis of the trachea. The epiglottic angle is reduced in the neutral position but angles away more than usual when the head and neck are extended. *Intubation in the neutral position is the major difference in airway management of infants and children versus adults.*

Laryngoscopy in the neutral position requires the laryngoscope blade to be at almost a 90-degree angle to the table top (Fig. 12), not almost parallel with the table top as it would be in an adult. The position of the laryngoscope blade is well to the right of the tongue, pushing the tongue entirely to the left and keeping it out of the way. The tip of the laryngoscope blade then transfixes the tip of the epiglottis, pushing it up against the vallecula, exposing the vocal cords. Using the right hand to push downward on the larynx will bring the cords into view (Fig. 13).[b]

"When one considers the angle between the base of the tongue and the glottic opening, it is obvious that it is much easier to move the glot-

---

[a] Ed. Note (JMB): Dr. Creighton refers to this position as a bird dog on point.

[b] Ed. Note (JMB): It is surprising that the cords usually stay in view after removing downward pressure on the larynx. This occurs for no other reason that I can think of except good clean living.

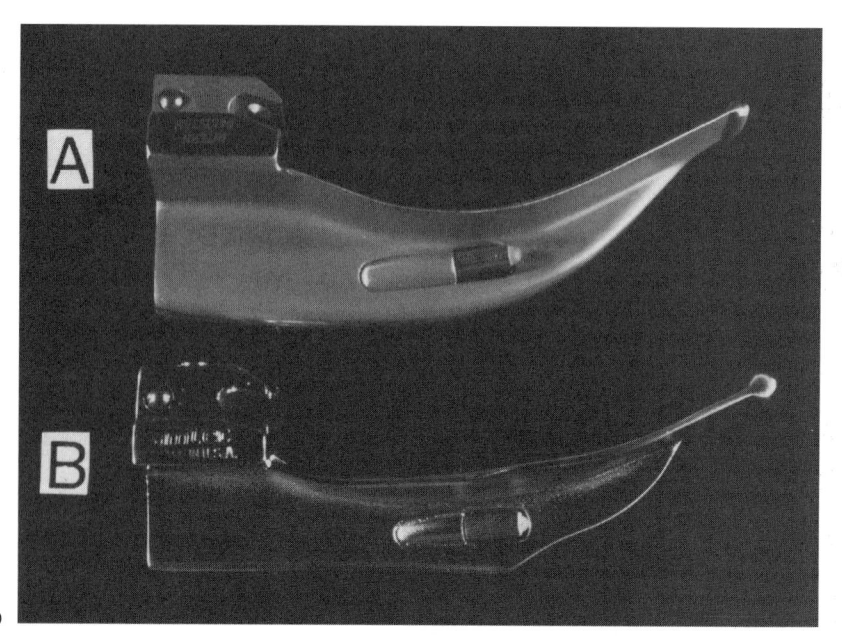

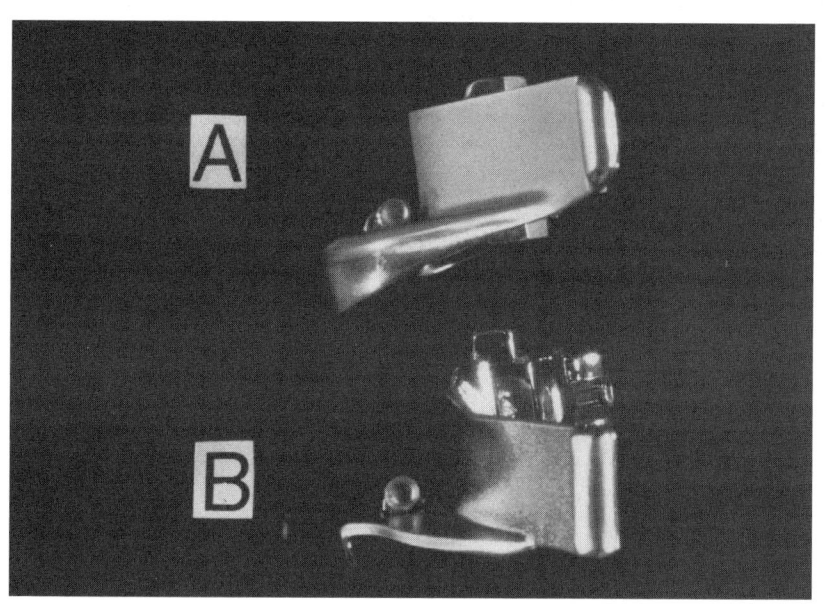

FIG. 7. (Top) A side-by-side comparison of the MacIntosh **(A)** and improved vision (IV) MacIntosh **(B)** blades. **(Bottom)** The modified curvature of the lateral edges of the IV MacIntosh allows for improved vision of the airway structures compared with the flat surface of the older MacIntosh blade.

tic opening posterior and therefore into line with a straight laryngoscope blade than it is to try and iron out the angle between the base of the tongue and the glottic opening by raising the laryngoscope to a position more parallel to the table top."

—Robert Creighton, MD

The endotracheal tube is then inserted into the mouth and passed into the oropharynx with the convexity of the tube on the left side (Fig. 14A). This tube position prevents the hand from blocking vision of airway structures. When the tip of the tube is at the vocal

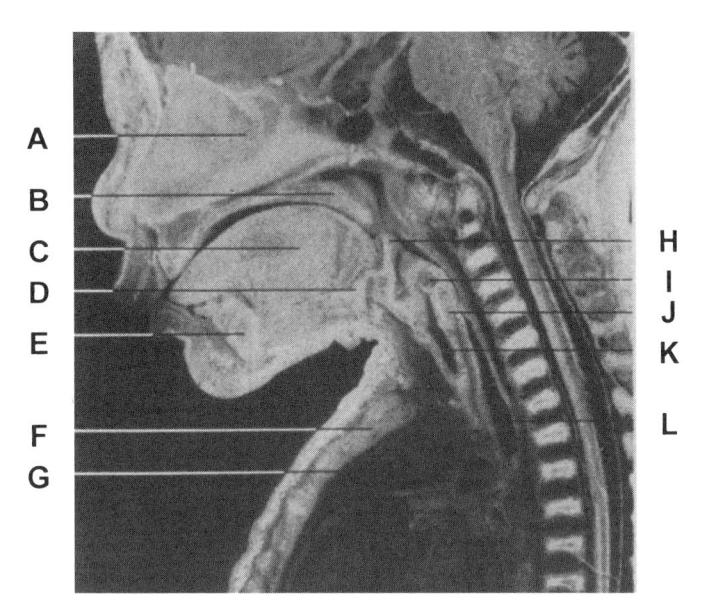

FIG. 8. Sagittal section of the head and neck in an infant cadaver (~10 months of age). *(A)* Ethmoid sinus. *(B)* Soft palate. *(C)* Tongue (the infant tongue is relatively large and completely fills the oral cavity). *(D)* Ascending ramus of mandible. *(E)* Mandible. *(F)* Sternum. *(G)* Thymus gland. *(H)* Epiglottis (high-riding; shown touching the uvula). *(I)* Arytenoid cartilage. *(J)* Cricoid cartilage (narrowest portion of the upper airway. *(K)* Trachea. *(L)* Esophagus. Note that the glottic opening corresponds to C2-C3 (compared with C4-C5 in the adult). The glottis is high in infants (as in dogs) so that the infant can swallow and breathe at the same time (as can dogs). With the development of phonation, the larynx descends and man loses the ability to swallow and breathe simultaneously. With a few exceptions, dogs do not learn to speak, and therefore they maintain this unique ability. (Modified and reprinted with permission, from Rohen JW, Yokochi C: *Color Atlas of Anatomy.* 2nd Ed., 1988, p. 143.

cords, the tube is rotated 90 degrees counterclockwise (so that the convexity is now posterior), then inserted past the vocal cords (see Fig. 14B). After intubation, a soft tampon prepared from 4 × 4 gauze pads may be used to stabilize the endotracheal tube, protect the patient's teeth from the endotracheal tube, and prevent endotracheal tube occlusion from clenched teeth (Fig. 15).

Nasal Insertion

Direct Vision with Child Asleep

Before induction, a suction catheter is placed through a preselected endotracheal tube. In children, the glottic inlet and external nares are approximately equal in diameter. Then, either a mask or intravenous induction may be performed. When adequate anesthesia is achieved, neosynephrine is applied topically to the internal nares to help prevent bleeding. The endotracheal tube is then inserted through the nares and slipped past the nares, tonsils, and adenoid tissue into the posterior pharynx (Fig. 16). The endotracheal tube catheter is suctioned to remove adenoidal or sub-mucosal tissue that may have accumulated during insertion. Alternatively, the suction catheter may be left in the tracheal tube until it is passed through the vocal cords and then suctioned.[c]

From this point on, the technique for laryngoscopy and intubation is essentially the same as for oral intubation. The head is tilted back, the lower lip is swept away with the little finger, and the laryngoscope blade

---

[c]Ed. Note (JMB): Leaving the suction catheter in until after intubation may aid in the insertion of the tracheal tube, minimizing hang-up at the anterior commissure.

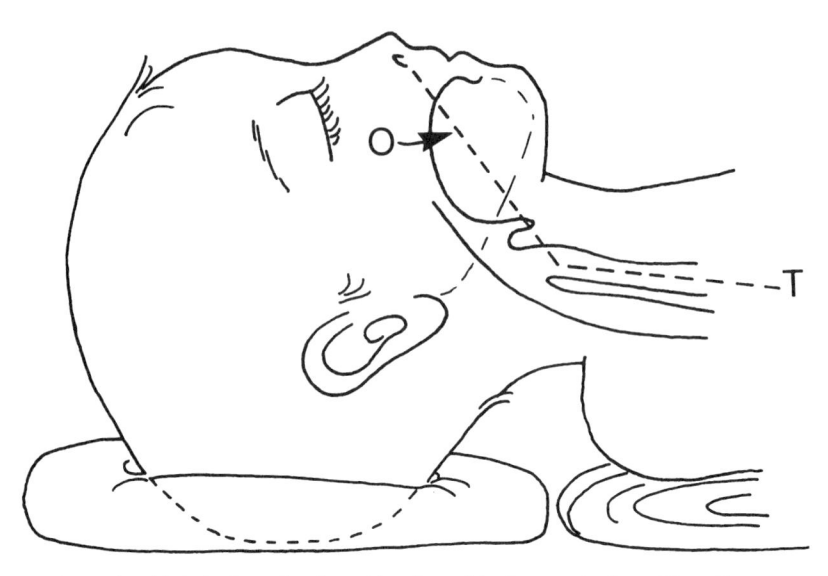

FIG. 9. For endotracheal intubation, the head is placed in the neutral position. Because of the relatively large occiput, a towel is usually required under the shoulders in infants and younger children to achieve proper alignment. In the neutral position, the oropharyngeal and tracheal axes are in the optimal alignment to allow intubation. After extension of the head and neck and insertion of the laryngoscope blade, the head must be brought back into the neutral position to assure successful intubation. T=Tracheal axis, O=Oropharyngeal axis.

is placed in the right side of the mouth and the head is brought back to the neutral position.

The tip of the endotracheal tube is grasped with a Magill's forceps and guided into the glottic opening (Fig. 17). Very frequently, the tip of the endotracheal tube catches or hangs up on the anterior commissure. To treat this, the clinician may do one of three things:

- Tilt the head anteriorly (flexing the neck) to aim the tip of the endotracheal tube into the larynx
- Bend the endotracheal tube tip downward with the Magill's forceps.
- Rotate the endotracheal tube 180 degrees so that the tip points downward.

The tube is taped into place with a small piece of restraining tape, and a turban (created from a blue surgical towel) is applied to the head (Fig. 18). This turban provides a very secure attachment for the endotracheal tube and prevents inadvertent extubation.

Blind Nasal Technique

Blind nasal intubation may be used in children when cervical movement is contraindicated (e.g., the traumatized child with suspected cervical injury). Nevertheless, use of the blind technique in the traumatized child situation may not be the first choice for endotracheal intubation because the tip is more likely to enter the esophagus than the glottis (**see Airway Management in the Traumatized Child with Suspected Cervical Injury**).

Laryngeal Mask Airway

Insertion

The laryngeal mask airway (LMA) is essentially a wide-bore endotracheal tube with an oval, cushioned mask attached at an angle to the tip. The LMA is designed to be positioned blindly so that the masked tip is placed over the epiglottis and larynx to provide a seal around the supraglottic area. It may be suc-

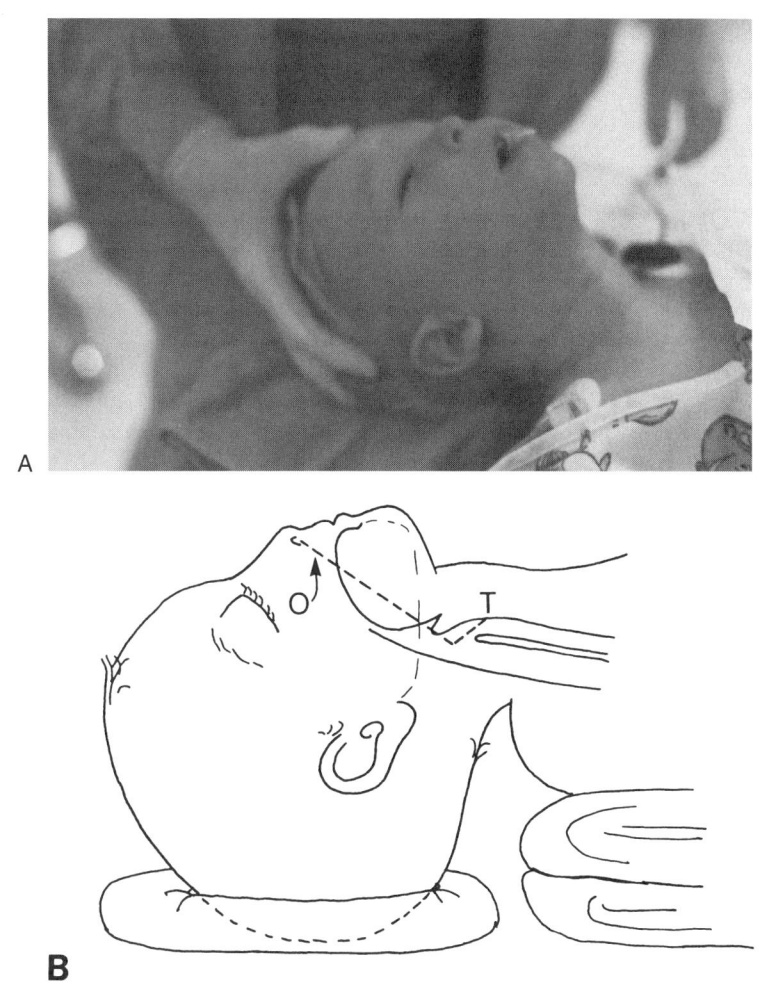

FIG. 10. (A) Before placement of the laryngoscope blade in the child's mouth, the clinician's thumb is placed on the child's forehead, the fingertips are placed on the child's occiput, and the child's neck is extended. Neck extension allows the mouth to open, making it possible for insertion of the laryngoscope blade. **(B)** The extended head and neck position is the least optimal for successful endotracheal intubation in children. In the extended position, the oropharyngeal and tracheal axes form an acute angle that is difficult to intubate. Therefore, before intubation, the child's head and neck must be brought back to the neutral position **(see FIG. 9).**

cessfully used in pediatric patients in whom tracheal intubation is difficult or even impossible (2). Five sizes of LMAs are available in infants and children (Gensia, Inc, San Diego, CA) (Table 2).

The LMA is prepared by aspirating all the air from the mask and lubricating the cuff and tube thoroughly. After the child is anesthetized, the head is extended, the mouth propped open, and the tube passed blindly into the pharynx until resistance is encountered. The LMA is inserted either with a rotational technique (Fig. 19) or with one continuous push with the LMA opening facing anteriorly (Fig. 20). The cuff is inflated and the LMA is observed to ride up slightly. The LMA is then connected to the anesthesia circuit, and several unobstructed breaths confirm proper placement. In many situations, use of the LMA is preferable to holding a face

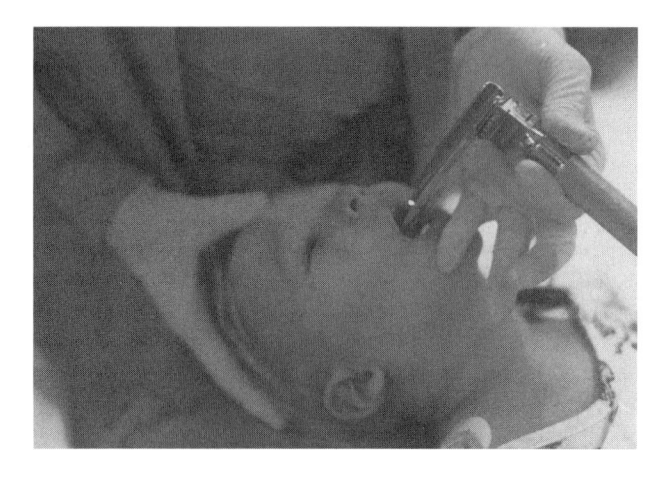

FIG. 11. Neck extension allows the mouth to open and allows space between the child's chest and the laryngoscope handle.

mask on a spontaneously breathing anesthetized patient, especially when the face mask may encroach upon the surgical field. It is also useful in patients who have difficult airways (see following section) when a conventional oral airway fails to provide adequate gas exchange (3).

Pitfalls of LMA Insertion. It should be emphasized that the LMA is only an adjunct to airway management and is not a substitute for tracheal intubation. There are many pitfalls of LMA insertion (Fig. 21). Furthermore, the LMA does not protect the airway from pulmonary aspiration. If a patient were to regurgitate under anesthesia, the bowl of the LMA could prevent escape of regurgitated gastric material and reflect it back into the trachea (4).

MANAGEMENT OF DIFFICULT AIRWAYS

Children are not merely small adults; some are smaller adults than others. Therefore, those with so-called difficult airways are even more problematic than their adult counterparts with airways difficult to intubate. Consequently, not only must airway equipment for the difficult airway be smaller with a wider range of sizes, but a variety of techniques must be available as well. Important advances in the management of the difficult

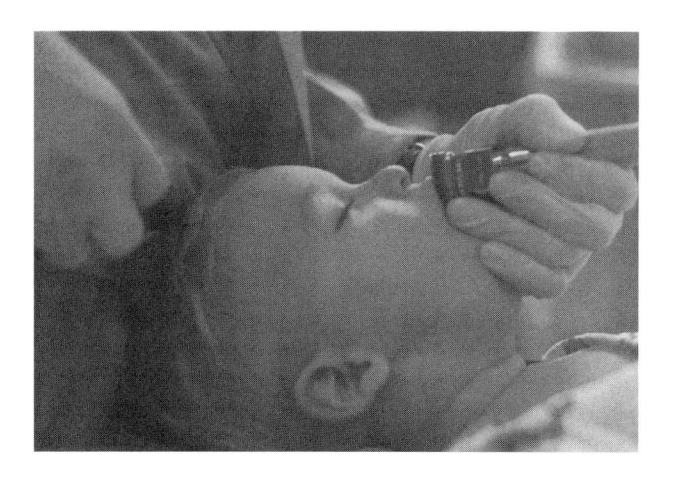

FIG. 12. After placement of laryngoscope blade into the oral cavity, the head and neck are brought back into the neutral position. The clinician's hand, the laryngoscope blade, and the child's chin are now welded together and can be moved together as one unit for optimal visualization of the glottic opening. This one-unit grip also helps to prevent injury to the child owing to a loosely held laryngoscope handle and blade. In infants and children, the laryngoscope blade is almost perpendicular to the table top for optimal visualization of the glottic opening. By contrast, in adults, the blade may be almost parallel with the table top.

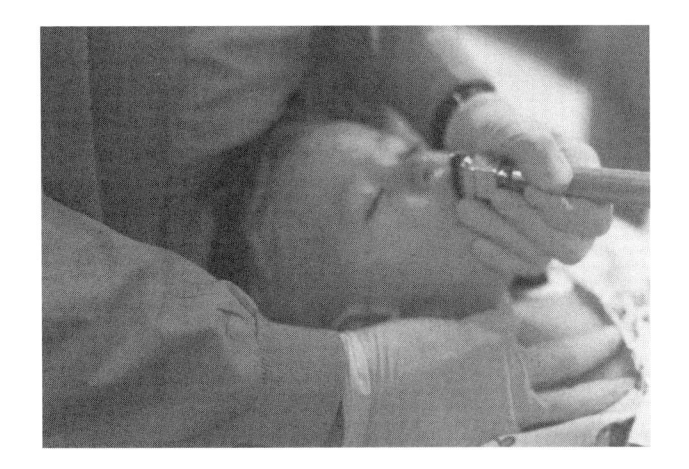

FIG. 13. The laryngoscope blade is inserted well to the right of the tongue, pushing the tongue entirely to the left and keeping it out of the way. The tip of the laryngoscope blade then transfixes the tip of the epiglottis, pushing it up against the vallecula and exposing the vocal cords. The clinician's right hand pushes downward on the larynx to bring the vocal cords into view.

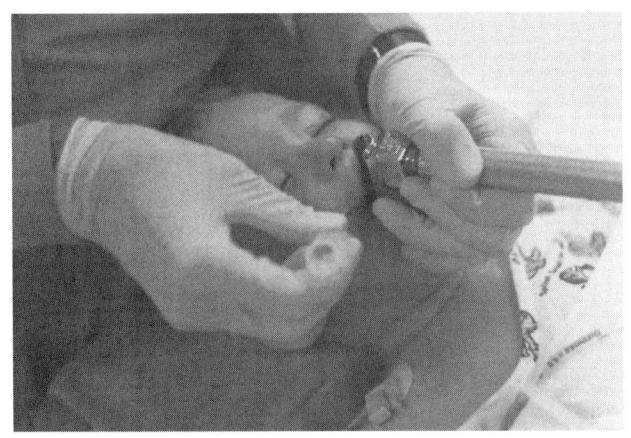

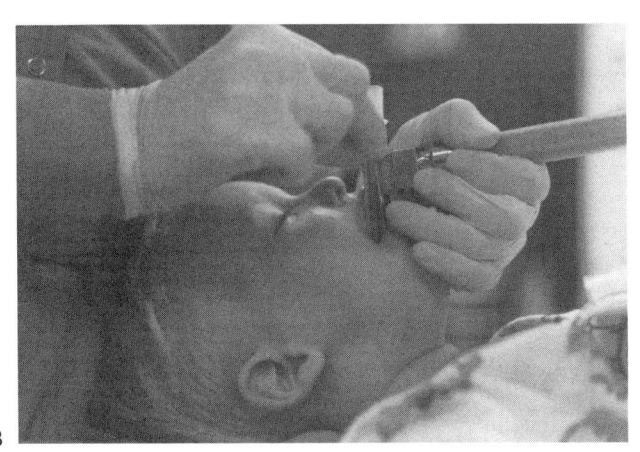

FIG. 14. (A) The endotracheal tube is inserted into the mouth with the convexity of the tube on the left side. **(B)** The endotracheal tube is rotated 90 degrees counterclockwise when the tip approaches the glottic opening. The tube is then inserted through the vocal cords.

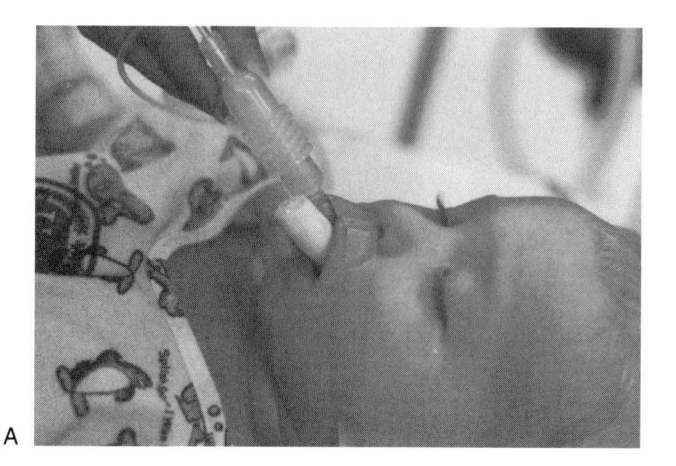

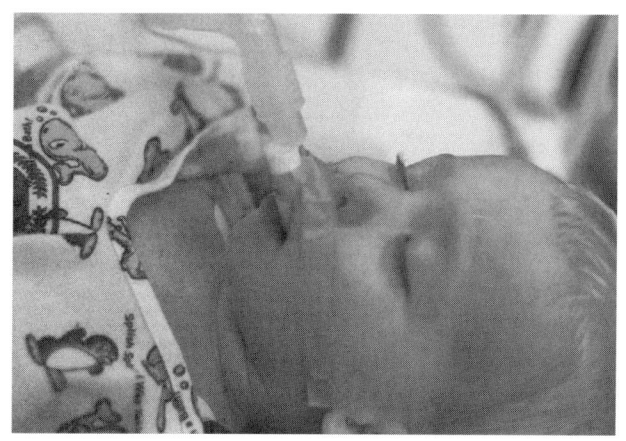

FIG. 15. (A) A soft tampon prepared from 4 × 4 gauze pads is placed in the child's mouth before the tube is finally taped. **(B)** The tampon is used to stabilize the endotracheal tube and protect the patient's teeth. In addition, stimulation of the posterior pharynx (as with a plastic airway) is avoided.

pediatric airway over the past decade include fiberoptic bronchoscopy, the LMA (5), insertion techniques using the LMA (6,7), and the development of smaller lighted stylets (light wands) (8).

Preanesthetic Assessment

"The difficulty in intubation lies entirely with the size of the mandible. If it is smaller than normal, as one finds with Pierre Robin, Treacher Collins and other micrognathic syndromes, intubation may well be difficult, although as the child grows older, intubation problems associated with micrognathia diminish."

—Robert Creighton, MD (1)

In dealing with the pediatric patient with a potentially difficult airway, one must distinguish between (a) the patient who is difficult to manage with a face mask and (b) those in whom tracheal intubation will be difficult. Most children with airway difficulties have a normal laryngeal and tracheal airway, but have a congenital or acquired abnormality affecting *access* to the airway.

The most important anatomic feature of the difficult airway is micrognathia (Fig. 22). Hypoplasia of the jaw decreases the space in which soft tissue can be displaced by the laryngoscope and occurs with congenital disorders such as Pierre Robin, Treacher Collins, and Goldenhar's syndrome (hemifacial microsomia). Macroglossia has the same space-occupying effect as do tumors of the tongue or oropharynx (e.g., cystic hygromas and hemangiomas). The normal measurement of the anterior posterior distance from the inside mentum of the mandible to the hyoid bone is 1½ cm in infants compared with 3 cm in adults. If this distance is less than 1½ cm, a difficult intubation can be predicted. The so-

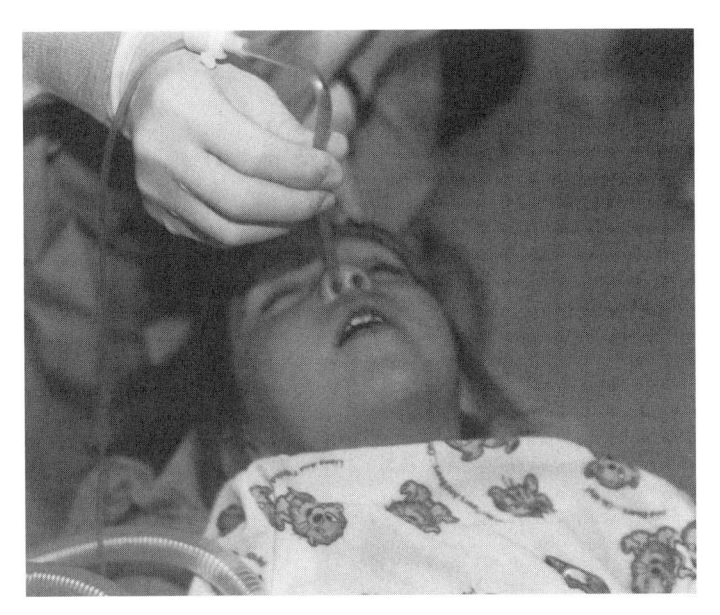

FIG. 16. In nasotracheal intubation of children, the endotracheal tube is inserted through the nares and the head is tilted in the extended position to allow oral laryngoscopy. After the tube is placed through the nares and after insertion of the laryngoscope blade, the head and neck are brought back into the neutral position as in orotracheal intubation.

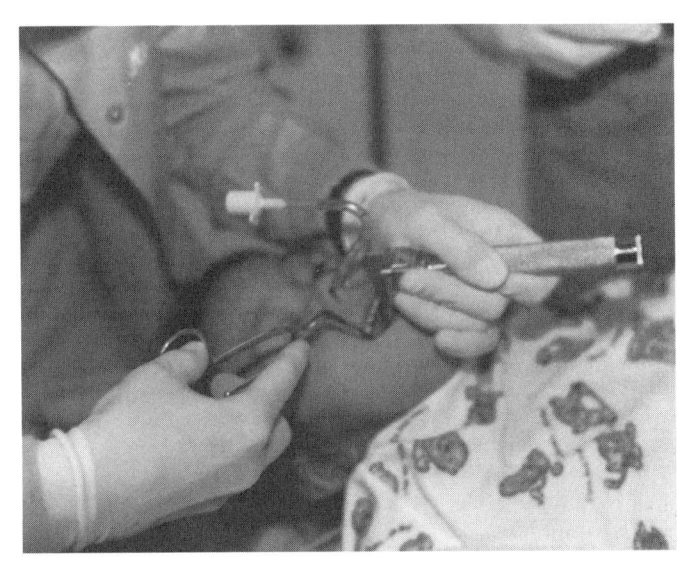

FIG. 17. For nasotracheal intubation, the tip of the endotracheal tube is grasped with Magill's forceps and guided into the glottic opening.

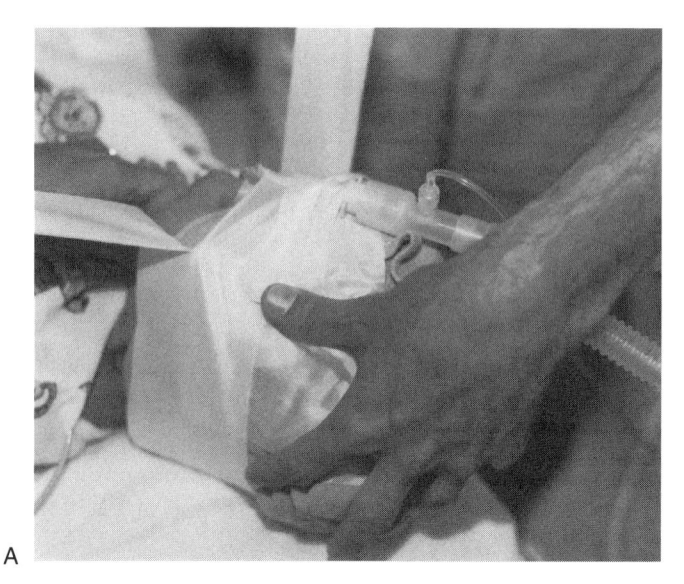

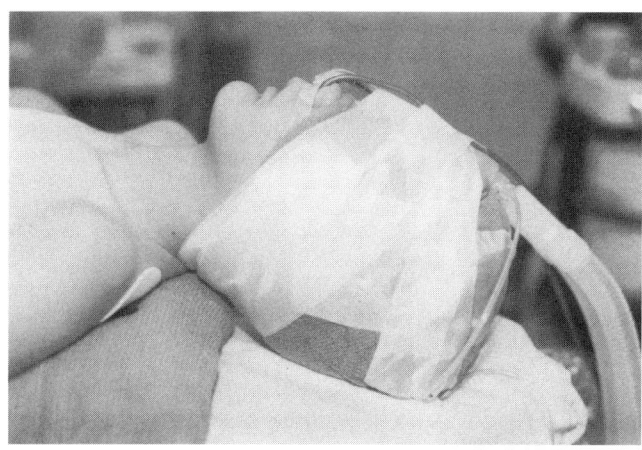

FIG. 18. (A) After nasotracheal intubation, the tube is taped into place around a turban created from a blue surgical towel and then wrapped with broad strips of adhesive tape. **(B)** The final product provides a secure dressing that will protect the patient's face and prevent inadvertent dislodgement of the tube.

called anterior larynx is a misnomer. The larynx is not anatomically anterior. It is merely anterior to the line of vision.

Premedication

Atropine or glycopyrrolate may be beneficial as drying agents, since many patients with difficult airways seem to have excessive secretions that may be compounded if multiple attempts at intubation are needed. Oral or intravenous atropine, 0.02 mg/kg, or glycopyr-

TABLE 2. *The relationship of patient weight to LMA size and cuff inflation*

Mask size	Patient size	Maximum cuff inflation
1	Neonates/infants up to 5 kg	4 ml
1.5	Infants between 5 and 10 kg	7 ml
2	Infants/children up to 20 kg	10 ml
2.5	Children between 20 and 30 kg	14 ml
3	Children and small adults over 30 kg	20 ml

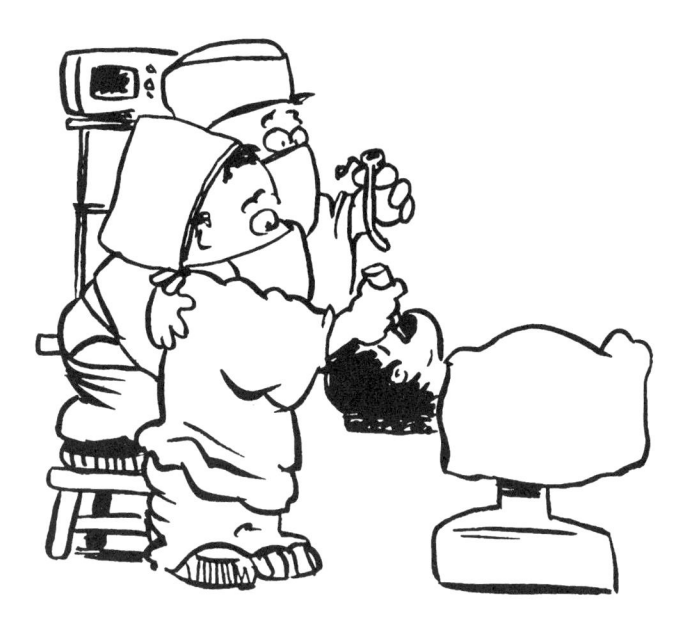

rolate, 0.05 mg/kg, are appropriate dosages. It is probably best to avoid sedatives unless the child can be observed closely.

Induction of Anesthesia

In general, the same principles and precautions for routine induction apply to patients with difficult airways. Airway obstruction and hypoxia can occur with such alarming speed that the surgeon and the emergency airway equipment must be in the operating room before the induction of anesthesia. Only after these personnel and equipment are in the room can induction begin. Inhalational induction with halothane or sevoflurane combined with topical anesthesia is the safest management of the patient with difficult airway. If nitrous oxide is used to speed the induction, it is turned off as soon as possible to ensure the highest possible F_IO_2 to prevent hypoxia if obstruction occurs. Muscle relaxants may be given after it is ensured that the patient is easy to ventilate by face mask.

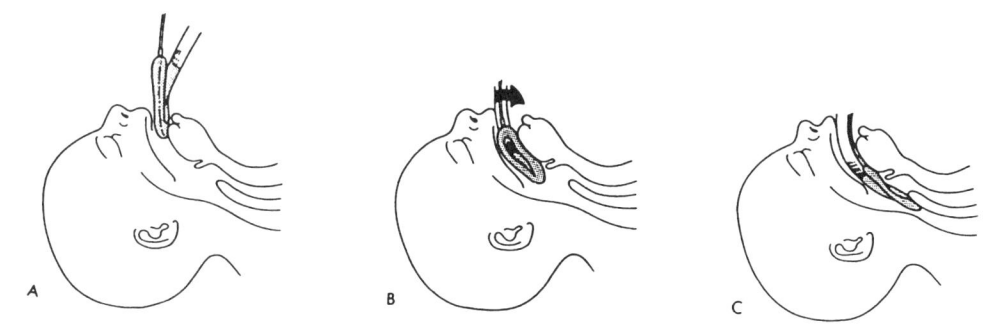

FIG. 19. (A) The laryngeal mask airway (LMA) is inserted with the bevel up into the oropharynx. The LMA is then pushed into the posterior pharynx. **(B)** As the LMA is pushed into the posterior pharynx, it is rotated 90° *(curved arrow)* so that the opening of the LMA apposes the glottic opening. **(C)** The LMA may now be used for spontaneous or controlled ventilation. (Reprinted with permission, from Blackwell Scientific Publishers. Haynes SR, Morton NS: The laryngeal mask airway: a review. *Paediatric Anaesthesia.* 3:65–73, 1993.)

94 CHAPTER 4: TUBE AND MASK PLACEMENT

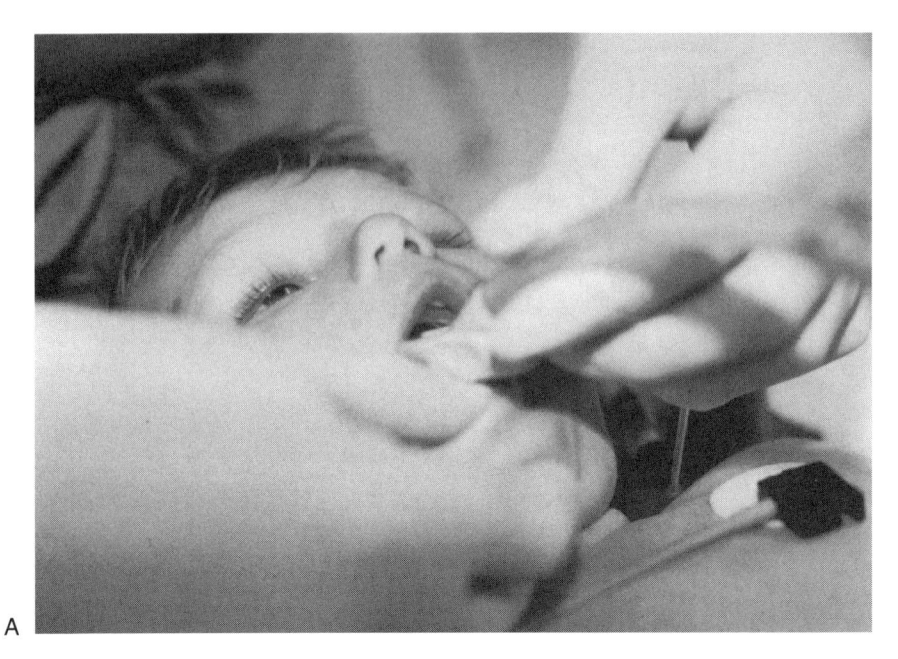

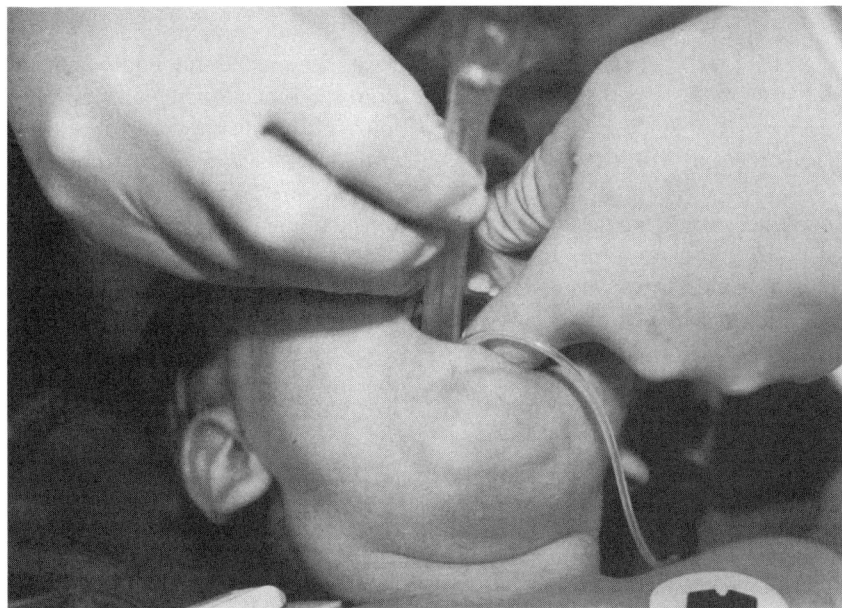

FIG. 20. (A) After testing and deflation of the cuff, the LMA is inserted bevel-down into the mouth of an anesthetized child. **(B)** The laryngeal mask airway (LMA) is pushed with constant pressure into the posterior pharynx and guided with the clinician's finger.

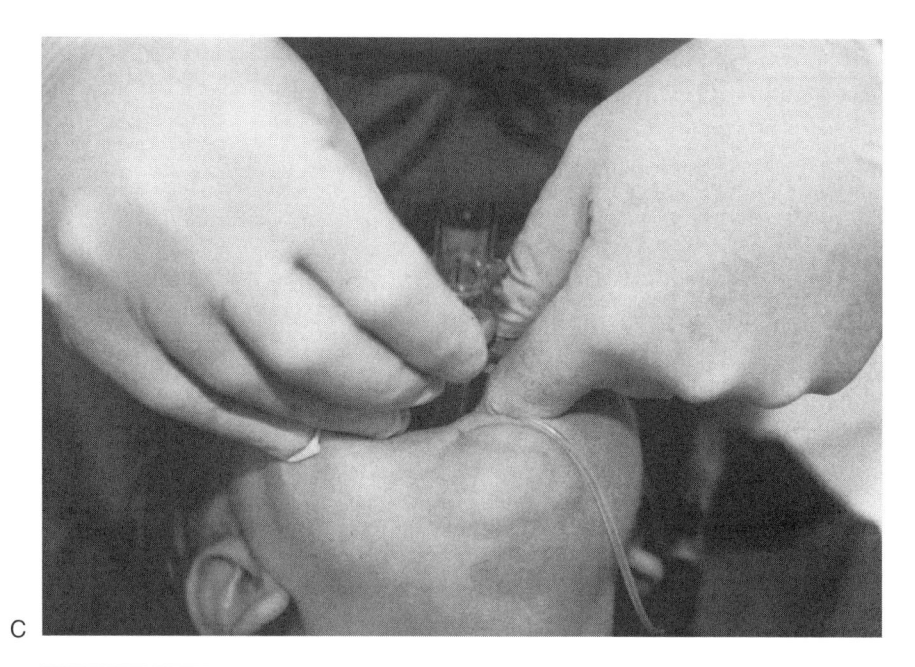

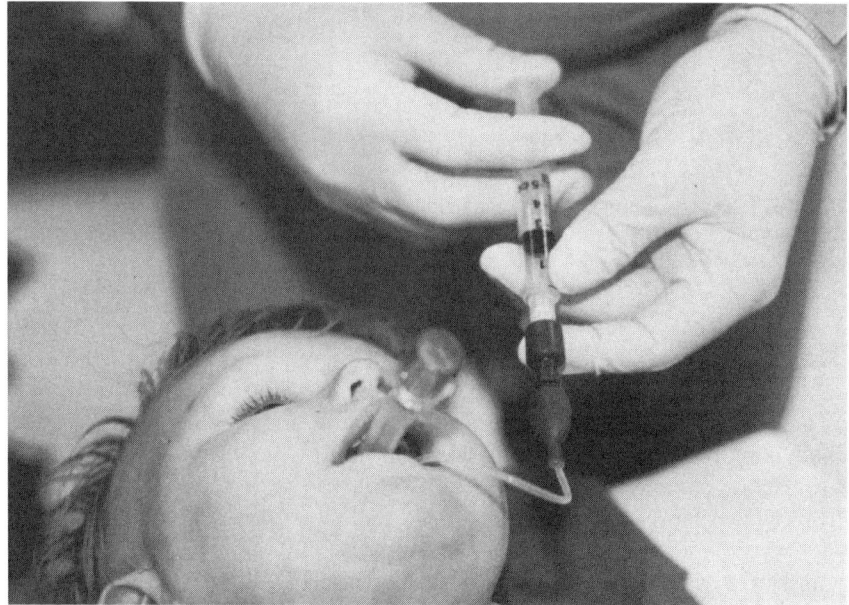

(C) The LMA is further advanced until it covers the glottic opening. **(D)** As it is inflated, the cuff will seat itself over the glottic opening. The LMA will rise slightly as this seating takes place.

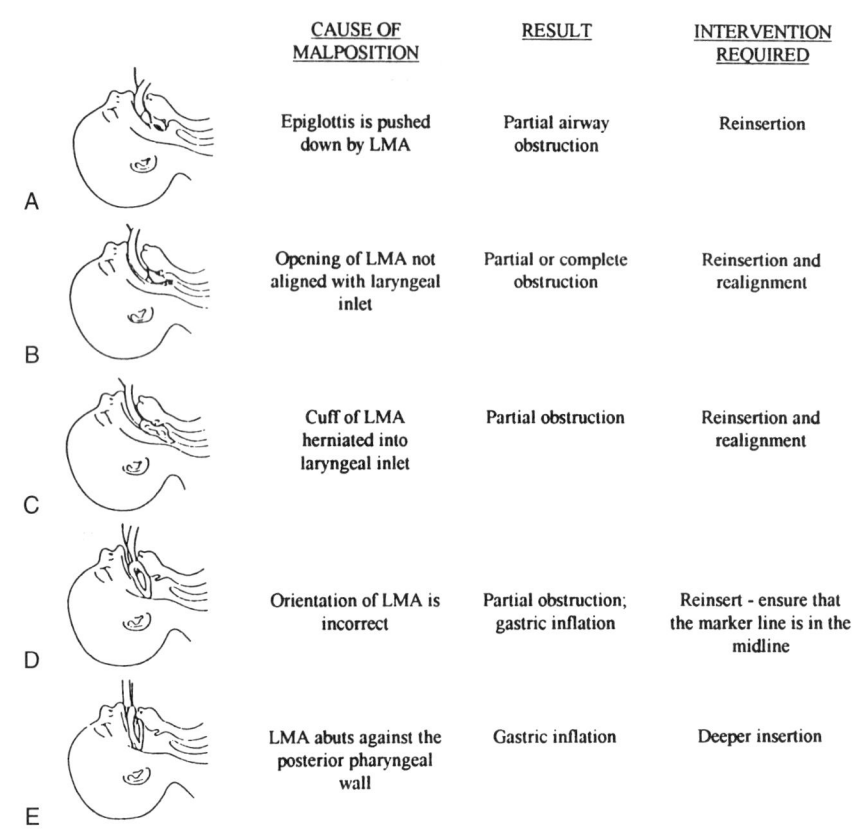

	CAUSE OF MALPOSITION	RESULT	INTERVENTION REQUIRED
A	Epiglottis is pushed down by LMA	Partial airway obstruction	Reinsertion
B	Opening of LMA not aligned with laryngeal inlet	Partial or complete obstruction	Reinsertion and realignment
C	Cuff of LMA herniated into laryngeal inlet	Partial obstruction	Reinsertion and realignment
D	Orientation of LMA is incorrect	Partial obstruction; gastric inflation	Reinsert - ensure that the marker line is in the midline
E	LMA abuts against the posterior pharyngeal wall	Gastric inflation	Deeper insertion

FIG. 21. Pitfalls of laryngeal mask airway insertion. (Reprinted with permission, from Blackwell Scientific Publishers. Haynes SR, Morton NS: The laryngeal mask airway: a review. *Paediatric Anaesthesia* 3:65–73, 1993.)

The Two-Person Technique

Perhaps the simplest and most straightforward method to intubate the difficult pediatric airway is to use a technique referred to variously as two-handed laryngoscopy or simply the "two-person technique" (1). It has proved to be very effective even in the most difficult of intubations. In essence, one person does the laryngoscopy and applies cricoid pressure (hence, two-handed laryngoscopy) while another person inserts the tube (hence, two-person technique).

The patient's head is correctly positioned, and the laryngoscope is placed as previously mentioned for routine laryngoscopy. The laryngoscopist simply applies cricoid pressure and holds it there. In most cases, a portion of the lower laryngeal inlet of the glottis will become visible as the laryngoscopist applies posterior pressure over the larynx with the index and middle fingers (Fig. 23). After a portion of the glottis is exposed, an assistant or nurse can be relied on to pass the endotracheal tube through the vocal cords. Mastering this technique provides the requisite skills to get along without the more complex techniques of intubation (e.g., blind nasal intubation, light wand, retrograde insertion of a wire through the cricoid thyroid membrane) except in rare cases. (Certainly, it will come in handy if a difficult airway needs to be intubated during a power failure.)

It is unwise to become too cavalier, however, with any technique. If an intubation is unexpectedly impossible and the patient may eventually suffer, it is wiser to retire and come back another day.

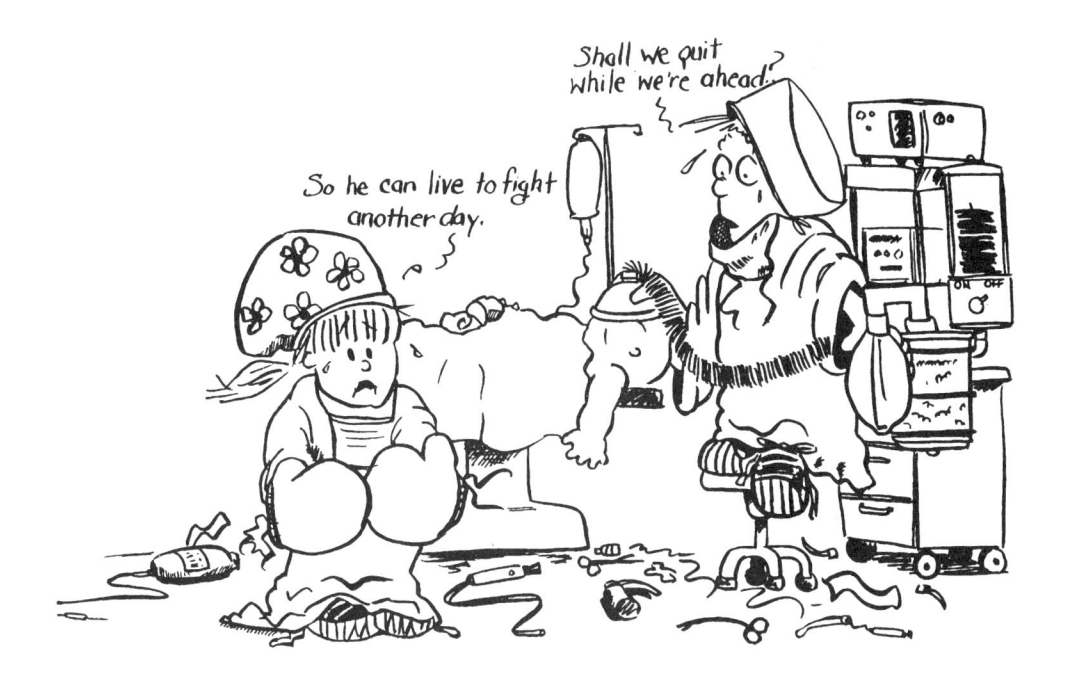

"In the final analysis, if intubation proves difficult and specialized equipment and experienced assistance are not available, it is preferable to discontinue anaesthesia, allow the patient to wake up, and defer surgery until they can be obtained. If they cannot be made available, the patient should be referred to a centre where they are."

—Robert Creighton, MD (1)

Pediatric Light Wands

For many patients with difficult airway access, the light wand (a rigid stylet with a light at the tip) has been a major focus of management (8) (Table 3).

Tracheal intubation with the light wand relies on external visualization of the light in the neck rather than visualization of the larynx or trachea. The tracheas of most patients with limitation of jaw movement or Pierre Robin syndrome and its variants can be intubated using a light wand by means of the oral or the nasal route. A 21-cm reusable fiberoptic light wand (Anesthesia Medical Specialties, Inc, Santa Fe Springs, CA) will accommodate tubes with 3.5 to 4.5 mm ID (Table 4).

With infants, unlike adults, too much light may make it difficult to distinguish between esophageal and tracheal intubation. One manufacturer (Fiberoptic Medical Products, Inc, Allentown, PA) produces a light wand that uses an external light source with a rheostatic control. This approach makes 2.5-mm ID light wands for infants possible and also allows the light output to be optimized for each patient. Many of the commercially available light wands have inadequate rigidity, which prevents the clinician from controlling the direction and movement of the stylet. Rather than preventing airway trauma, an overly flexible stylet is difficult to manipulate and prolongs the time needed to perform an intubation or may make tracheal intubation impossible.

Dr. Mark Shreiner of the Children's Hospital of Philadelphia is the pioneer of light wand intubation. What follows is his impeccable technique for light wand stylet–assisted endotracheal intubation (with permission).

- Lubricate the stylet.
- Cut the tracheal tube, if necessary, so that the lighted stylet remains just inside the tracheal tube. A rubber stopper is useful when using a metal fiberoptic stylet. Removal of the tracheal tube connector is very helpful when using a rigid (metal) lighted stylet.

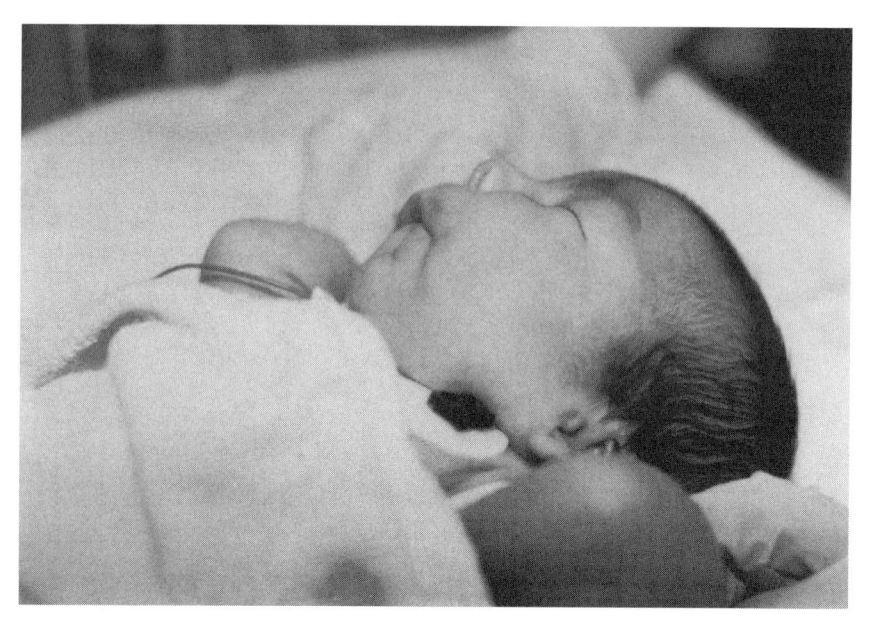

FIG. 22. The clinician's nightmare—an infant with no chin requiring general anesthesia. More than any other condition, micrognathia (as shown here) creates the dreaded difficult airway.

- Shape the stylet-tracheal tube combination into a "hockey stick" configuration. Angles of 90 to 110 degrees appear to work best, but there is a wide range of personal preferences.

- When ready to proceed with tracheal intubation, dim the room lights.

- Introduce the stylet into the oral (or nasal) cavity and seat the stylet under the tongue in the midline with traction elevating the mandible with the left hand. A bright light at the level of the hyoid indicates the stylet is in the vallecula. The light should be just as bright or brighter when placed in the trachea.

- With the light in the midline, advance the stylet, keeping the tip pressing against the anterior aspect of the trachea. The light should remain continuously bright in the midline as it moves caudad. Briefly losing the light and then seeing the bright glow in the midline probably indicates esophageal intubation. This is especially true in infants and small children. The light should remain *continuously* bright.

- If there are problems advancing the stylet, the likely hangup is the epiglottis. Move the stylet back, then down slightly and readvance (visualize in your mind the stylet going under the epiglottis).

- In infants and children, the *feel* of the stylet advancing is just as important as the appearance of the light. A click is often felt when advancing past the epiglottis. Small gentle movements will enable the intubator to locate the stylet in the trachea. Intentionally placing the tube in the esophagus may prove useful as a baseline comparison with the appearance of the light when in the trachea.

- Subglottic narrowing is a cause of failure of the technique. Having a stylet that can accommodate a smaller than predicted tube will prevent failures.

Tips for Light Wand Intubation

- A shoulder roll may help.

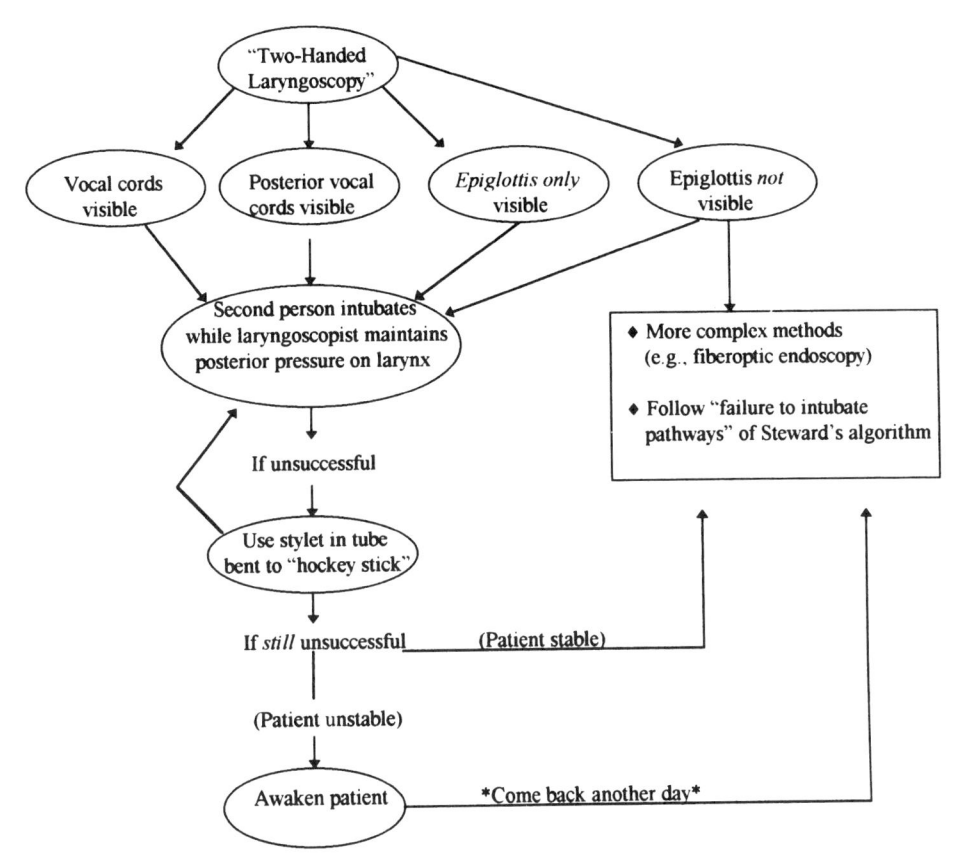

FIG. 23. An algorithm for the proper use of two-handed laryngoscopy in difficult intubations. (Modified and redrawn with permission, Churchill Livingstone, Inc. Berry FA: *Anesthetic Management of Difficult and Routine Pediatric Patients.* 2nd Ed., 1990, p. 187.)

TABLE 3. *Indications and advantages of lighted stylet intubation*

Indications (normal larynx but difficult access to visualize the larynx)	Contraindications
TMJ disease Micrognathia Cervical spine instability Facial trauma	Airway tumor Some airway infectious processes (retropharyngeal abscess)
Advantages	Disadvantages
No need to visualize the larynx Inexpensive Compact Rapid Easily practiced in normal patients Oral or nasal intubation possible Awake or anesthetized patients Unaffected by presence of blood or secretions Easy to clean	Inability to visualize the larynx Room lights dimmed (generally) Most practitioners inexperienced Small size stylets not generally available

Adapted from Cook-Sather SD and Shreiner MS. A simple homemade lighted stylet for neonates and infants: a description and case report of its use in an infant with the Pierre Robin anomalad. *Paediatric Anaesthesia* 1997 (In press).

TABLE 4. Lighted stylets: features, advantages, and disadvantages

Company	Features	Advantages	Disadvantages
Tube-Stat Xomed	Limited reuse, light bulb 25 cm long; cost about $30	Modestly bright, appropriate stiffness	Inadequate length, high failure rate, no infant stylet
Aaron Medical Lighted Intubation Stylet	Limited reuse, light bulb cm long; adult, pediatric, nasal; cost about $30	Bright light; pediatric size (4.0–4.5 mm ID minimum)	Adult stylet inadequate, too stiff and too long, no infant stylet
Fiberoptic Intubation Stilette AMS (Santa Fe Springs, CA)	Reusable, metal jacketed fiber bundle, 33 cm adult, 21 cm pediatric; cost about $75	Light appropriate for children, reusable, thin diameter, adult and pediatric (3.5–4.5 mm ID)	Light inadequate for many adults; light can be too bright for infants; fragile switch (replaceable)
Trachlight Laerdal	Reusable light with limited reuse stylet, retractable stylet; cost $250 + $25/stylet	Best choice for adults or large children, very bright, disposable light sleeve	Expensive; pediatric size(s) still in development
Fiberoptic Medical Products (Allentown, PA)	Variable-size fiber bundles, rheostat-controlled light source (operating room head lamp); cost $90 + disposable sleeve	Brightness adjustable, 2.5 mm ID; adult sizes with appropriate stylets; can augment light output of metal stylets (AMS)	Need for light source, fiberoptic guides tend to be too flexible

ID, internal diameter.
Adapted from Cook-Sather SD and Shreiner MS. A simple homemade lighted stylet for neonates and infants: a description and case report of its use in an infant with the Pierre Robin anomalad. *Paediatric Anaesthesia* 1997 (In press).

- Focus first on getting the stylet down the middle of the tongue, and then focus on the position of the light on the neck.
- In general, do not hold only the handle of the stylet, hold the stylet itself to improve tactile feel.

OTHER EXOTIC BUT USEFUL TECHNIQUES

Fiberoptic Laryngoscopy

Through a Patil-Syracuse Mask

One of the most important keys to fiberoptic laryngoscopy in the pediatric patient is to somehow keep the child asleep and breathing spontaneously while the fiberscope is inserted. This can be accomplished through the use of a specially designed face mask that allows the insertion of the fiberscope through a relatively air-tight port, the Patil-Syracuse mask (Fig. 24). Through this mask, fairly deep anesthesia is maintained in the child, and then the fiberscope is introduced through the port. In addition, positive-pressure ventilation or continuous positive pressure during spontaneous ventilation may be provided. Gentle positive pressure may distend the airways allowing better visualization of the glottic opening.

Through a Laryngeal Mask Airway

Another technique for endotracheal intubation makes use of fiberoptic bronchoscopy through the laryngeal mask airway; a guidewire is then inserted followed by the tracheal tube (6,7) (Fig. 25).

The Bullard Laryngoscope

A technique for the Bullard laryngoscope is described (Fig. 26). First, the selected endotracheal tube is warmed several minutes in heated saline before placing it onto the Bullard laryngoscope. This makes the endotracheal tube more pliable and easier to remove from the stylet. To prevent fogging, one may (a) apply a small amount of defogger to the distal end of

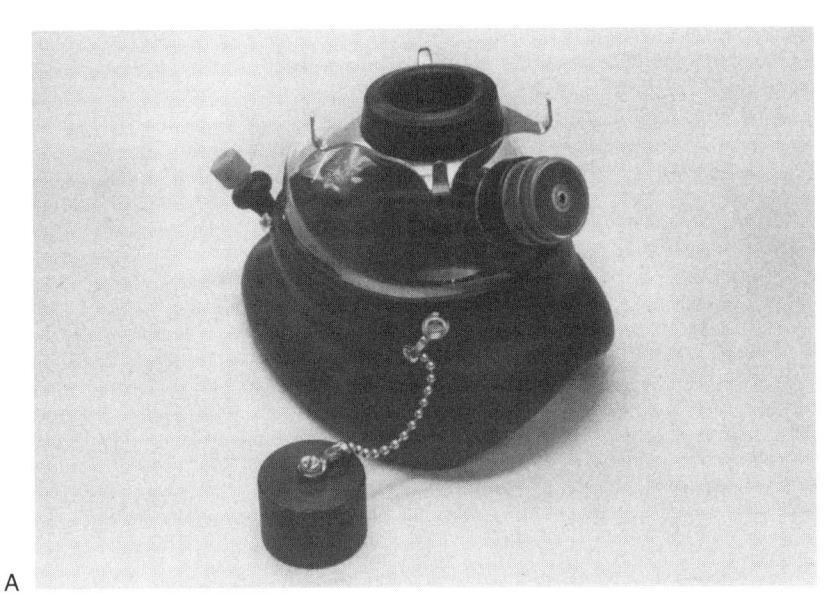

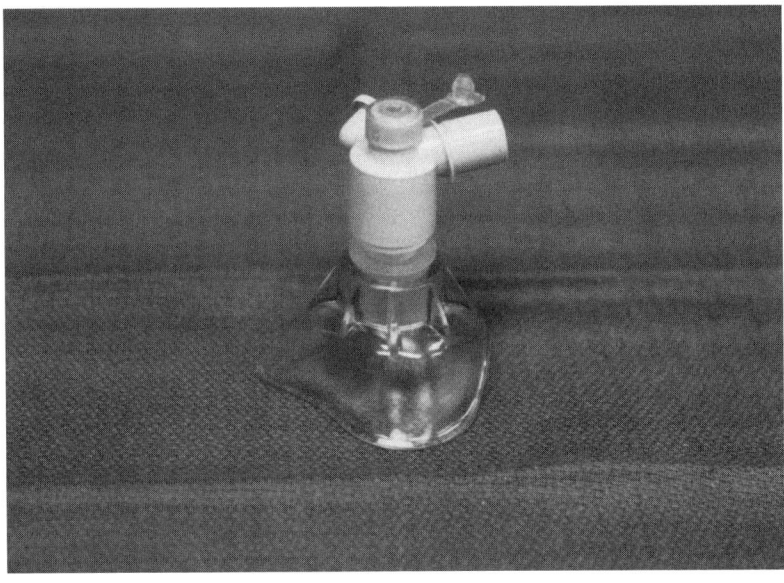

FIG. 24. **(A)** The Patil-Syracuse face mask is available in varying sizes and can be used during spontaneous ventilation while a flexible fiberoptic laryngoscope is inserted through the port. (Reprinted with permission, from Fiberoptic Medical Products, Inc. and Mosby-Year Book, Inc. Patil, Stehling, Zander: *Fiberoptic Endoscopy in Anesthesia*. 1st Ed., 1993, p. 6.) **(B)** A poor-man's Patil-Syracuse may be assembled from readily available parts—a plastic face mask and a bronchoscopic endotracheal tube adaptor.

the laryngoscope or (b) warm the distal end of laryngoscope in warm saline before use. A small amount of lubricant is applied to a gauze pad and spread evenly along the distal portion of the introducing stylet. If the pediatric (long) introducing stylet is to be used, the standard connector must be removed from the pediatric endotracheal tube before it is backloaded over the stylet. Whereas the adult endotracheal tube is positioned such that the distal end of the

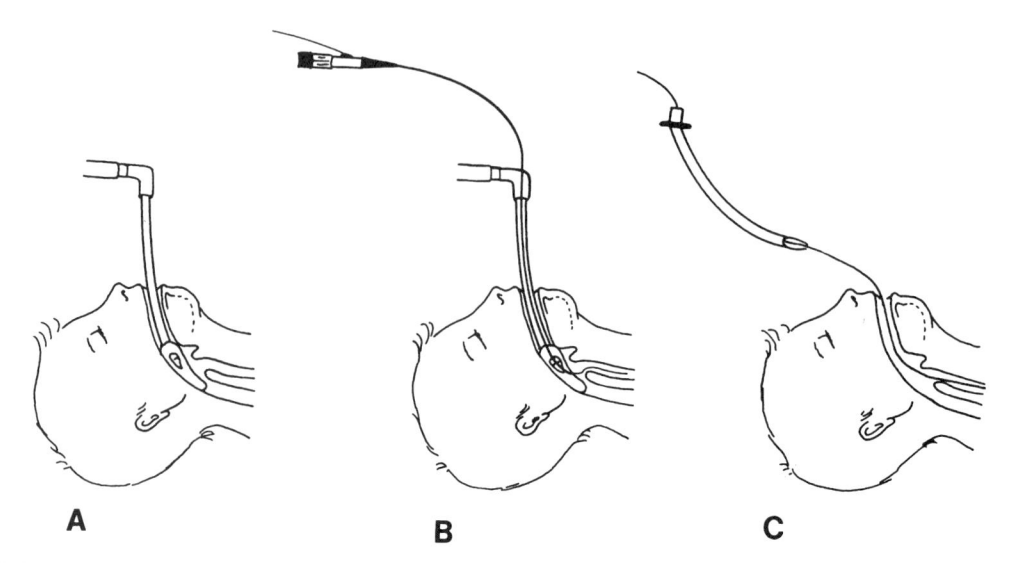

FIG. 25. A useful technique for endotracheal intubation uses the insertion of a laryngeal mask airway (LMA) **(A)**, followed by fiberoptic bronchoscopy through the LMA **(B)**, and then the insertion of a guidewire followed by the tracheal tube **(C)**. (Reprinted with permission, from ref. 6.)

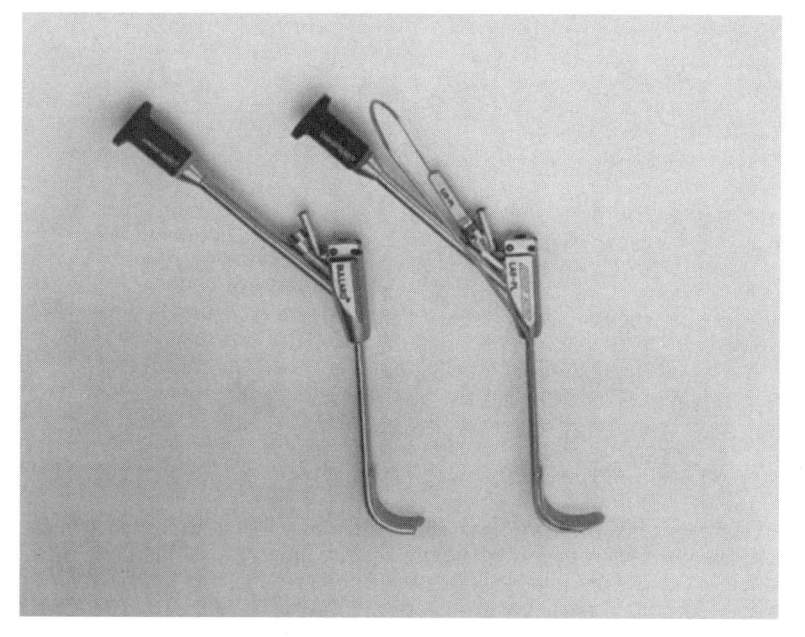

FIG. 26. The Bullard fiberoptic laryngoscope (Circon ACMI, Stamford, CT) is designed as a ladle-shaped rigid blade with a fiberoptic light source and eyepiece. It is available in a pediatric as well as adult size. (Photograph, courtesy of Circon Corporation.)

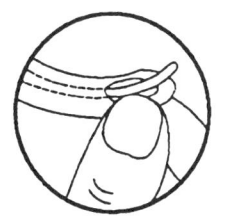

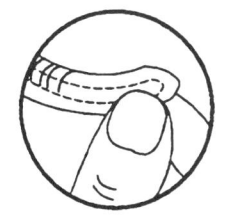

Positioning the LIS-A Adult Stylet Through the ETT

Positioning the LIS-P Pediatric Stylet Through the ETT

FIG. 27. In adult-sized endotracheal tubes, the distal end of the introducing stylet of the Bullard laryngoscope passes through the Murphy eye. By contrast, in pediatric-sized tubes the stylet is positioned near the end, but not protruding through, the tube's central lumen. (Courtesy of Circon Corporation.)

stylet passes through the Murphy eye of the endotracheal tube, the pediatric introducing stylet is positioned such that the stylet is near the end, but *not* protruding through the endotracheal tube's central lumen (Fig. 27).

Proper hand position is important when inserting the Bullard laryngoscope. The thumb of the hand holding the scope should be wrapped around the handle and eyepiece (Fig. 28). The fingertips should rest on the

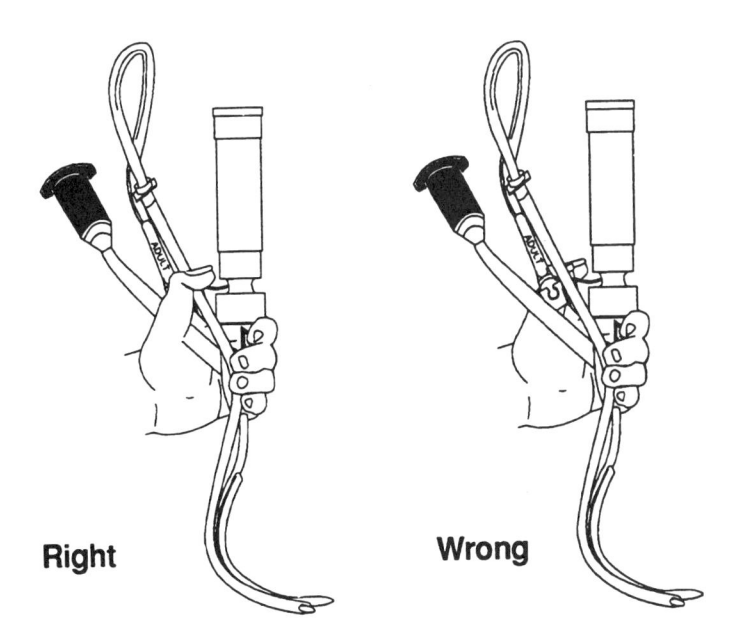

Right   **Wrong**

FIG. 28. The Bullard laryngoscope has been designed for single-handed use with either the left or right hand. Recommended hand position for a proper grip is shown. Proper hand position is most important in using the introducing stylet for intubation. For it to work properly, the thumb of the hand holding the scope should be wrapped around the handle and eyepiece. The fingertips should rest on the stylet/endotracheal tube, holding it against the back of the blade. Orienting the hand such that the fingers are not aiding in the position of the stylet will result in the endotracheal tube being out of position. (Courtesy of Circon Corporation.)

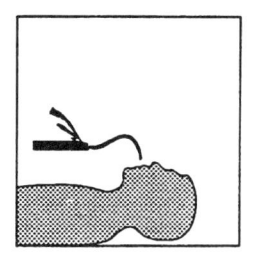

Correct Placement for Introducing the Bullard Laryngoscope

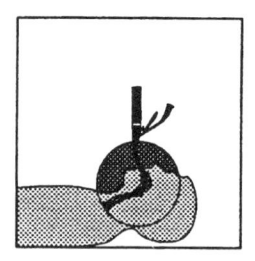

Introducing the Bullard Laryngoscope into the Patient

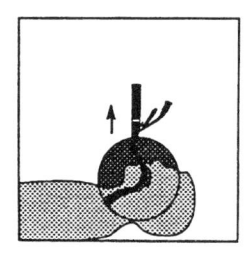

Elevating the Bullard Laryngoscope

FIG. 29. The blade of the Bullard laryngoscope is inserted into the oral cavity, and the laryngoscope is rotated from the horizontal to the vertical position, allowing the anatomically shaped blade to slide around the tongue. Once the laryngoscope is fully vertical, final placement may be facilitated by allowing the blade to drop momentarily to the posterior pharynx. The blade is then elevated against the tongue's dorsal surface. Only minimal upward movement exerted along the axis of the laryngoscope handle is required. This upward movement will result in the blade of the laryngoscope lifting the epiglottis, allowing visualization of the glottic opening. (Courtesy of Circon Corporation.)

stylet/endotracheal tube, holding it against the back of the blade. Orienting the hand such that the fingers are not aiding in the position of the stylet will result in the endotracheal tube being out of position.

The blade of the Bullard laryngoscope is inserted into the oral cavity, and the laryngoscope is rotated from the horizontal to the vertical position, allowing the anatomically shaped blade to slide around the tongue (Fig. 29). After the laryngoscope is fully vertical, final placement may be facilitated by allowing the blade to drop to the posterior pharynx. The blade is then elevated with minimal upward movement while the clinician is looking through the eyepiece. This upward movement results in the blade of the Bullard laryngoscope lifting the epiglottis, allowing visualization of the glottic opening. The endotracheal tube is then slowly advanced toward the glottis while the clinician is viewing through the eyepiece. The endotracheal tube is advanced through the glottis until correctly positioned in the trachea, confirmed visually under endoscopic observation.

After the endotracheal tube is correctly positioned, the Bullard laryngoscope is ready to be removed. The endotracheal tube is stabilized by holding it at its proximal end near the standard connector. While holding the endotracheal tube in place, the laryngoscope blade stylet is removed by slowly rotating the blade out of oropharynx. Final removal of the stylet from the endotracheal tube can be accomplished by lifting the Bullard laryngoscope blade vertically while stabilizing the endotracheal tube. If the pediatric endotracheal tube was used, the standard connector is replaced on it.

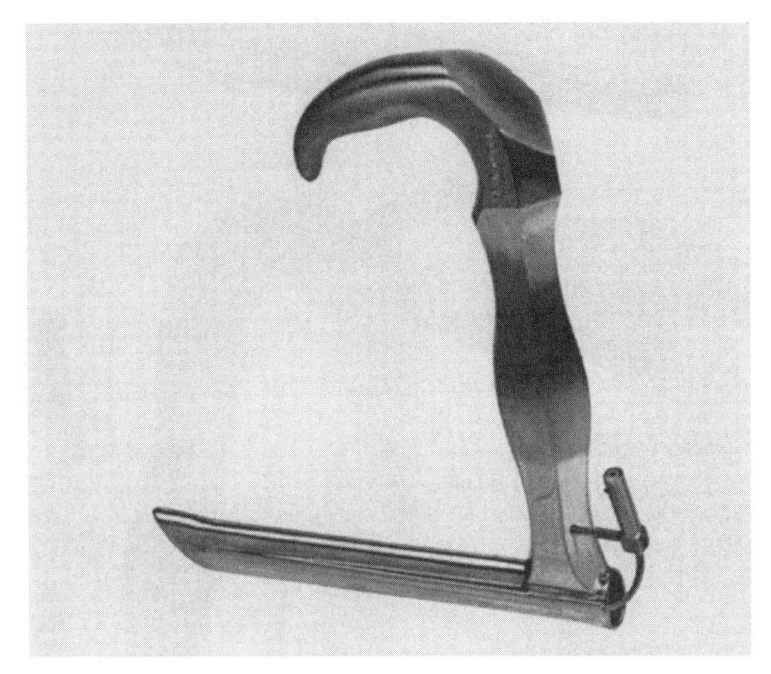

FIG. 30. The anterior commissure laryngoscope.
(Reprinted with permission, from Pilling Weck from the product catalogue.)

The Anterior Commissure Laryngoscope

The anterior commissure laryngoscope technique is borrowed from otolaryngologists, who use the anterior commissure laryngoscope to visualize the cords, trachea, epiglottis, and so on, so that they can do surgery on these structures. If it is good enough for them to operate through, it should be good enough for us to intubate through. The anterior commissure laryngoscope consists of a tubular blade with a fiberoptically illuminated light at the tip (Fig. 30). This blade will displace the tongue and pharyngeal soft tissues and prevent their collapse around the laryngoscope. The tip of the blade is passed directly into the laryngeal inlet. An endotracheal tube (without the adaptor) may then be placed through the tubular blade into the larynx.

WHEN ALL ELSE FAILS

As previously mentioned in a quote from Dr. Creighton, when intubation seems impossible it may be the better part of valor to awake the child so that he or she may live to fight another day. If, however, the child is in dire straits (e.g., is obstructed, cyanotic, and bradycardic) and control of the airway is lost and cannot be reestablished, it may be time for one of the following techniques.

> "In the face of an impossible airway, the anesthesiologist cannot remain frozen performing unsuccessful techniques, but must initiate a different approach."   —Fritz Berry, MD

Rigid Bronchoscopic Intubation With a Hopkins Rod Lens Telescope

The Hopkins rod lens telescope is a rigid metal rod surrounding fiberoptic bundles. An endotracheal tube can be placed over this rod and then inserted into the trachea with direct vision. Most ear, nose, and throat (ENT) specialists are adept at intubating the trachea using this technique. Therefore, one may wish to assemble this equipment (and perhaps an ENT surgeon) before commencing any difficult intubation. If dire circumstances develop, a reliable technique is readily available. The Hopkins rod is found on most, if not all, ENT surgical trays.

Emergency Surgical Airway: Cricothyrotomy

Three approaches to emergency surgical opening of the airway are mentioned in the literature: (a) emergency tracheotomy, (b) emergency cricothyrotomy, and (c) emergency transtracheal ventilation (9). In the experience of most, emergency tracheotomy cannot be performed rapidly enough in dire situations. Likewise, transtracheal jet ventilation is not the answer. Transtracheal jet ventilation is extremely hazardous in children because barotrauma may occur owing to the restricted egress of ventilatory gas (10–13) **(see Chapter 11, Fig. 2)**. Therefore, when endotracheal intubation cannot be accomplished, the most rapid method for oxygenating the patient in an emergency situation (as previously described) is by cricothyrotomy.

Technique

The cricothyroid membrane is identified, and a transverse incision is made down to the cricothyroid membrane (Fig. 31). The cricothyroid membrane is then incised (Fig. 32). A tracheal dilator is inserted to enlarge the opening in the membrane, and a tracheotomy tube or endotracheal tube is inserted. After stabilization of the patient, either a permanent tracheotomy is done and the surgery performed or the cricothyrotomy is used for the operation and immediate postoperative period and then allowed to close. If the patient is not stable, the operation is terminated and performed another day.

Airway Management in the Traumatized Child with Suspected Cervical Injury

Endotracheal intubation in the child after major trauma can be challenging and perplexing. All too often, cervical radiographs are either not available or are never totally "cleared"

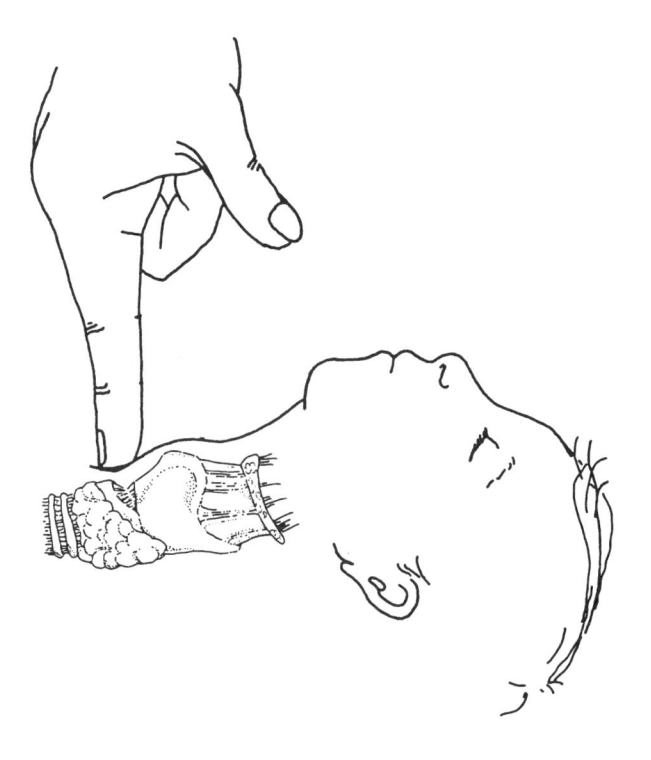

FIG. 31. Before cricothyrotomy, the cricothyroid membrane is identified just below the thyroid cartilage and just above the tracheal rings. (Reprinted with permission from Churchill Livingstone, Inc. Berry FA: *Anesthetic Management of Difficult and Routine Pediatric Patients*. 2nd Ed., 1990, p. 179.)

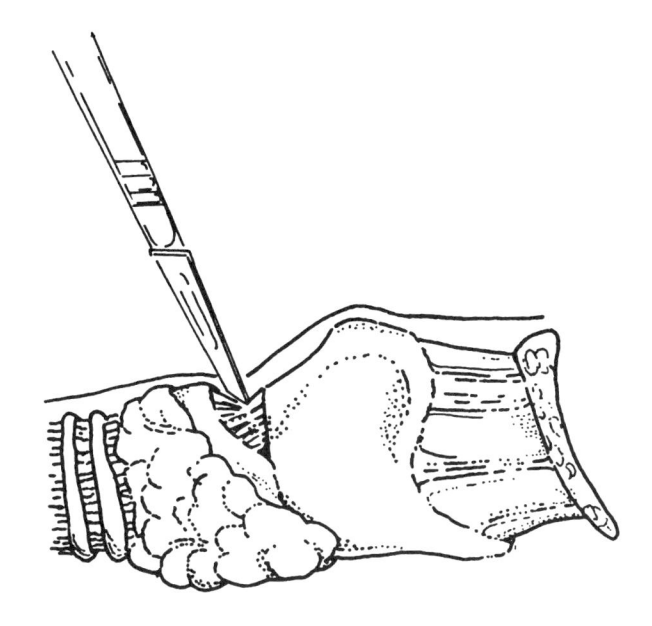

FIG. 32. For cricothyrotomy, the cricothyroid membrane is incised, a tracheal dilator is inserted to enlarge the opening, and a tracheal tube or endotracheal tube is inserted. (Reprinted with permission from Churchill Livingstone, Inc. Berry FA: *Anesthetic Management of Difficult and Routine Pediatric Patients.* 2nd Ed., 1990, p. 179.)

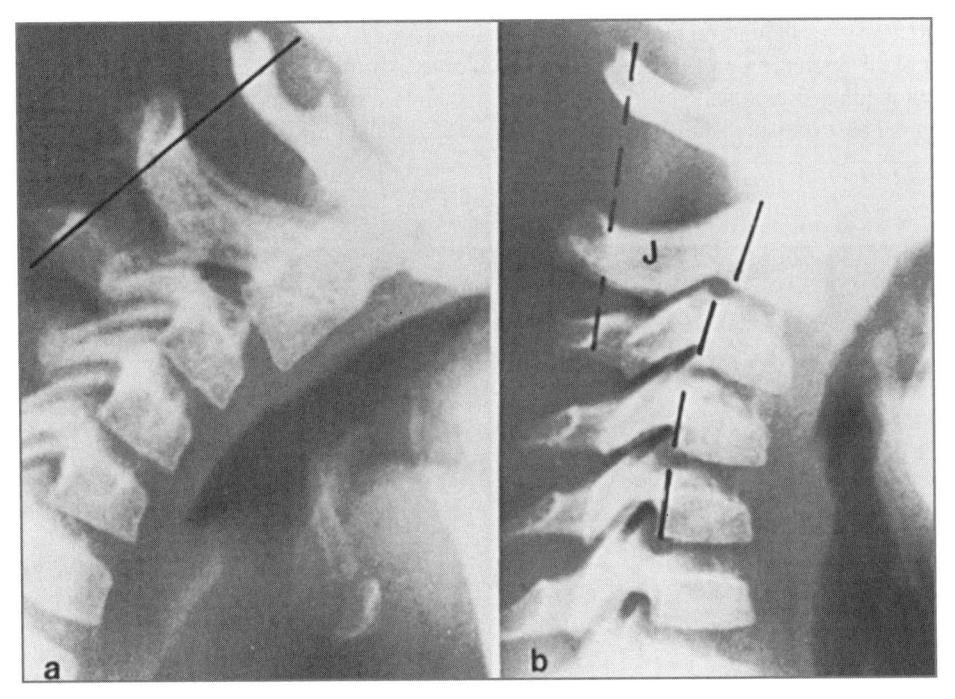

FIG. 33. (a and b) Pseudosubluxation of C2-C3 (apparent, but not real, anterior displacement of C2 on C3) is common in children and, if present, may present a diagnostic dilemma. In this radiograph, pseudosubluxation is present and not true subluxation (as it appears). The body of C2 appears to be anterior to the body of C3 (i.e., the anterior vertebral body line is not intact). However, the dorsal spinous processes and posterior vertebral body line are intact, indicating that true subluxation is not present. (Reprinted with permission, from ref. 14.)

by the radiologist because the radiographs do not include adequate views below C6 or views of the odontoid process (a common site of fracture in children). Furthermore, pseudosubluxation of C2-C3 (anterior displacement of C2 on C3) or C3-C4 is common. If this is present, it could create a diagnostic dilemma (14) (Fig. 33). Furthermore, children can suffer spinal cord injury, yet show no abnormality on the radiograph. Therefore, in most cases, children with closed-head injury are treated as if they have unstable cervical spines.

Unless these children are severely obtunded, intubation without anesthetic agents ("awake intubation") is usually impractical. In addition, laryngoscopy in the awake child is a potent stimulator of intracranial hypertension. Because of the acute nasal-pharyngeal-laryngeal angles in children younger than 8 years old, blind nasotracheal intubation is rarely successful, and it may result in intracranial insertion, if basilar skull fracture is present. Fiberoptic intubation requires prerequisite level of skill and, even in the best of hands and static conditions, it is time-consuming. Therefore, fiberoptic intubation has limited use in acute trauma.

In the anesthetized child whose neck is being held in neutral position by in-line stabilization, oral laryngoscopy under direct vision usually allows successful endotracheal intubation. Use of this technique requires the child's head and neck to be maintained in anatomic alignment with the body by the insertion of the assistant's fingertips under the child's mastoid processes, with gentle stabilization that prevents extension or flexion of the neck (Fig. 34). *During in-line stabilization, no axial traction is applied.* Axial traction may cause further disruption of the cervical spine and should be avoided. The sole purpose of in-line stabilization is to prevent the endoscopist from putting the child's head into flexion or extension. A second assistant should apply cricoid pressure. If the child arrives with a cervical stabilization device in place, it may be carefully removed (while maintaining in-line stabilization) to gain access to the child's larynx. If a younger child's

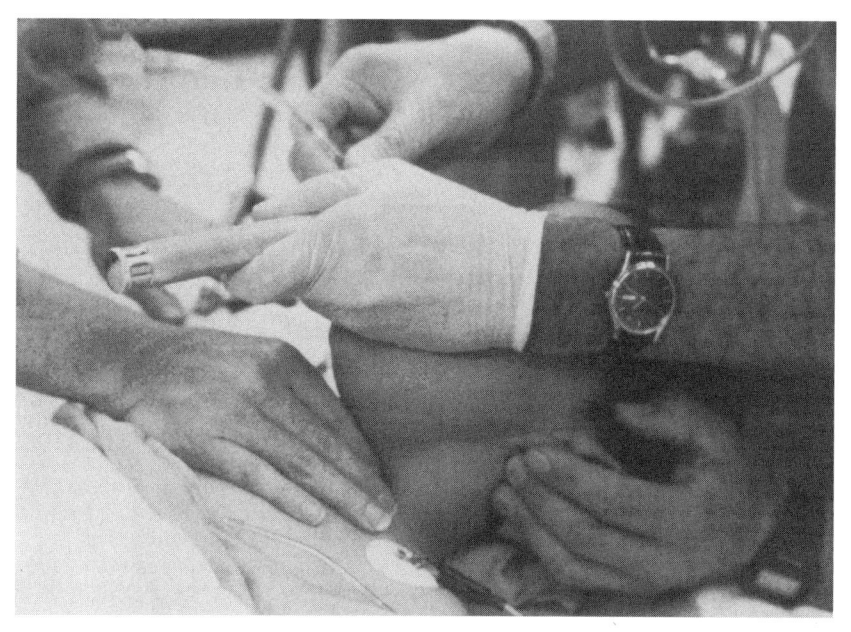

FIG. 34. Direct oral laryngoscopy and endotracheal intubation in a child with suspected cervical injury. Cricoid pressure and in-line stabilization are applied by assistants. In-line stabilization prevents flexion or extension of the child's neck, but does not provide axial traction (see text).

relatively large occiput causes undue neck flexion that prevents adequate laryngoscopy, it is safe to cautiously place a small towel under the shoulders (while maintaining in-line stabilization).

Steward's Algorithm for the Pediatric Difficult Airway

No single approach to the management of the difficult airway will succeed every time. With the addition of the laryngeal mask airway, the infant light wand, and small bronchoscopes, clinicians have additional options that augment previously available tools. When these tools and techniques are used effectively, the truly impossible pediatric intubation becomes exceedingly rare. Effective use of these tools and techniques should follow a logical sequence of action. An excellent example of such a logical sequence of action can be found in David Steward's algorithm for the pediatric difficult airway (Fig. 35).

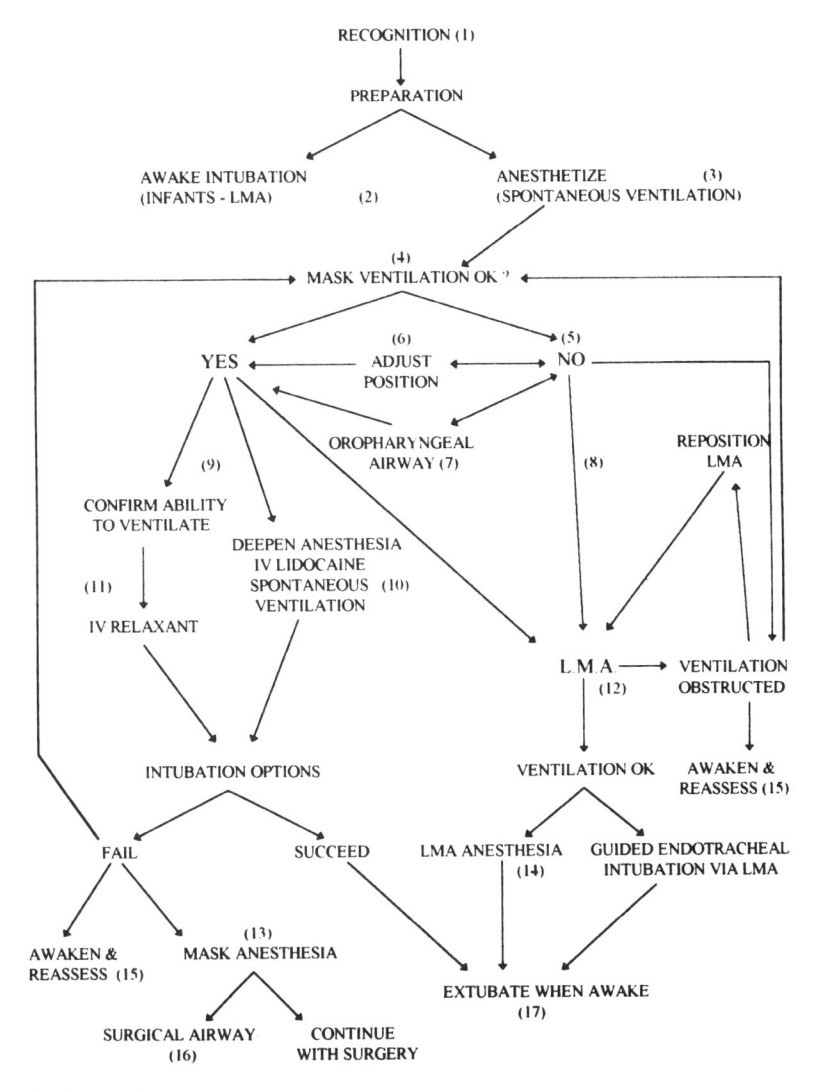

FIG. 35. David Steward's algorithm for the pediatric difficult airway. (Reproduced with permission, from David Steward, M.D.)

A brief description of the use of Steward's algorithm is provided. The numbers in parentheses refer to numbers on the algorithm in Figure 35.

- *Recognition of the potentially difficult intubation before induction of anesthesia is highly desirable (1)*. Unexpected cases of difficult intubation should be handled using the principles outlined in the algorithm.
- *Assess whether to use anesthetized or awake intubation (2)*. Most pediatric patients are managed anesthetized; children are very easily upset and do not usually cooperate during attempts at awake intubation. Small infants may be severely stressed by attempts at awake intubation and are more readily intubated when they are anesthetized. Some small infants may be managed by initial insertion of a well-lubricated laryngeal mask airway while awake; this can then be used as a route to induce anesthesia and complete endotracheal intubation, if indicated.
- *Initial induction of anesthesia is best performed by inhalation (3)*. Intravenous hypnotic agents or relaxants are used with extreme caution in the patient with a potential difficult airway. [see (11)].
- *Assess whether mask ventilation is adequate.*
  - If ventilation is adequate *(4)*, deepen anesthesia using halothane in oxygen and proceed to direct laryngoscopy. (Halothane is preferred to sevoflurane because emergence is less rapid and allows more time for endoscopy).
  - If ventilation is not adequate *(5)*:
    - Adjust the position of the head *(6)* with increased jaw thrust to lift the tongue from the posterior pharyngeal wall and open up the airway (e.g., the survival position—**see Chapter 2**).
  - Insert an oropharyngeal airway *(7)*; be aware that if the patient is very lightly anesthetized, this may result in coughing and laryngospasm.
  - Insert a laryngeal mask airway *(8)*. This may then be used as a route to deepen the anesthesia with inhalation agents, maintaining spontaneous ventilation. It may also be used as a route for fiberoptic or other guided intubation.
- *Once deep anesthesia with halothane and oxygen has been achieved, direct laryngoscopy may be attempted to assess the airway and perform intubation (9)*. The anatomy of the airway and the ease or difficulty of intubation, together with details of laryngoscope blades used, should be carefully recorded for use during any subsequent anesthesia. There are two possible methods to achieve this laryngoscopy:
  - During deep anesthesia, with spontaneous ventilation, give 1 to 2 mg/kg of intravenous lidocaine (to reduce incidence of breath-holding or coughing) *(10)*. The use of an oxyscope will provide for oxygenation during endoscopy.
  - After confirming the ability to ventilate the patient with bag and mask *(11)*, a short-acting muscle relaxant (e.g., succinylcholine or mivacurium) may be administered. Laryngoscopy may now be attempted during apnea with complete relaxation. This may make intubation slightly easier, but does limit the time available for each intubation attempt. Keep in mind that small children desaturate more rapidly during apnea than do older children or adults.
  - Note: Whichever method is used, once the laryngoscope is inserted it may be possible to push the larynx into view by external pressure on the neck. A two-man approach to intubation may be needed—one to hold the larynx in view and the other to insert the tube **(see Creighton's Two-Person Technique)**.

- If laryngoscopy is impossible by direct vision, other options must be considered:
  - Insertion of a laryngeal mask airway to continue anesthesia *(12)*, and, if necessary, to use as a route for endotracheal intubation. If the airway is not clear after insertion of the laryngeal mask airway, the mask must be removed and repositioned.
  - Direct fiberoptic intubation via the oral or nasal route.
    - Bullard laryngoscopy
    - Light wand intubation
- If intubation options are failing, consider the following:
  - Can this case be done with mask anesthesia *(13)*?
  - Can this case be done with laryngeal mask airway anesthesia *(14)*?
  - Should the patient be reawakened *(15)*?
  - Is a surgical airway needed *(16)*?
- Extubation *(17)*. Every patient with a difficult airway should be extubated or have the laryngeal mask airway removed *only* when fully awake and when all danger of swelling in the region of the airway has passed.

SUMMARY

In this chapter, I have described techniques for successful airway management. The information is aimed at helping to provide safe and pleasant experiences for you and the children you anesthetize. Remember John Relton's sage advice, "...a complication-free anesthetic begins with a first-rate IV and a first-rate airway" (15).

REFERENCES

1. Creighton RE: The infant airway. *Can J Anaesth* 1994; 41:174–176.
2. Brain AI: Three cases of difficult intubation overcome by the laryngeal mask airway. *Anaesthesia* 1985;40: 353–355.
3. Fisher JA, Ananthanarayan C, Edelist G: Role of the laryngeal mask in airway management. *Can J Anaesth* 1992;39:1–3.
4. Nanji GM, Maltby JR: Vomiting and aspiration pneumonitis with the laryngeal mask airway. *Can J Anaesth* 1992;39:69–70.
5. Asai T, Fujise K, Uchida M: Use of the laryngeal mask in a child with tracheal stenosis. *Anesthesiology* 1991; 75:903–904.
6. Hasan MA, Black AE: A new technique for fibreoptic intubation in children. *Anaesthesia* 1994;49: 1031–1033.
7. Heath ML, Allagain J: Intubation through the laryngeal mask. A technique for unexpected difficult intubation. *Anesthesia* 1991;46:545–548.
8. Ellis DG, Jakymec A, Kaplan RM, et al: Guided orotracheal intubation in the operating room using a lighted stylet: a comparison with direct laryngoscopic technique. *Anesthesiology* 1986;64:823–826.
9. DeLisser EA, Muravchick S: Emergency transtracheal ventilation. *Anesthesiology* 1981;55:606–607.
10. Miyasaka K, Sloan IA, Froese AB: An evaluation of the jet injector (Sanders) technique for bronchoscopy in paediatric patients. *Can Anaesth Soc J* 1980;27: 117–124.
11. Tate N: Excessive airway pressure during anaesthesia. (Letter). *Anaesthesia* 1979;34:212.
12. Oliverio R Jr, Ruder CB, Fermon C, Cura A: Pneumothorax secondary to ball-valve obstruction during jet ventilation. *Anesthesiology* 1979;51:255–256.
13. Vivori E: Anaesthesia for laryngoscopy. *Br J Anaesth* 1980;52:638.
14. Harris JH, Harris WH: *The radiology of emergency medicine,* ed 2. Baltimore: Williams & Wilkins, 1981: 108–111.
15. Personal communication.

Clinical Pediatric Anesthesia, edited by
J.M. Badgwell. Lippincott–Raven Publishers,
Philadelphia © 1997.

5

Delivery and Monitoring of Alveolar Ventilation

J. Michael Badgwell

"The wind that gave our grandfather his first breath also receives his last sigh."
—Chief Seattle

Modifications for pediatric ventilation equipment and monitors have traditionally relied on adaptations and innovations of standard adult equipment applied to pediatric use. No small amount of inventiveness, energy, and expense has gone into the design and application of special equipment and techniques for the administration of alveolar ventilation to pediatric patients.

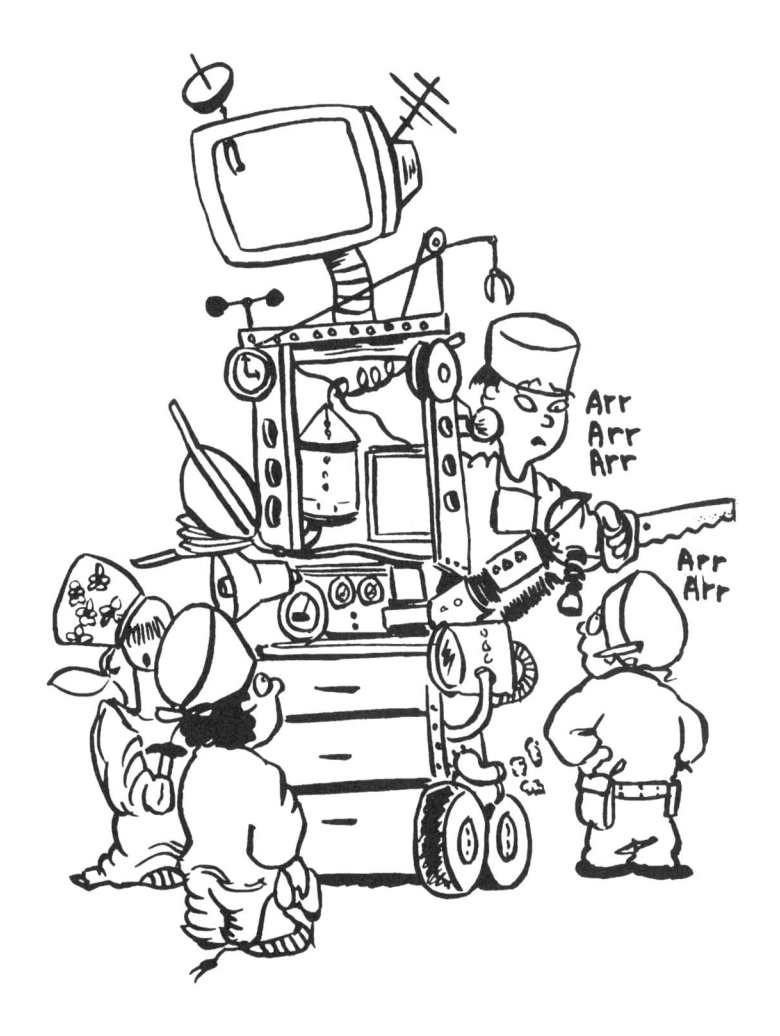

This effort has been for good reason. Poor equipment design and lack of clinician familiarity may contribute to compromised anesthetic care. The American Society of Anesthesiologists' closed claims study found a greater incidence of equipment-related problems in children compared with that found in adult patients. Almost 50% of problems occur in children less than 2 years of age (1). In an effort to reduce unfamiliarity with existing equipment, this chapter attempts to explain and simplify currently available techniques to provide and monitor alveolar ventilation in infants and children.

DELIVERY OF VENTILATION

The Anesthesia Machine

Most pediatric patients can be anesthetized with any standard anesthesia machine. No specific differences exist between a pediatric and an adult anesthesia machine. Insofar as an anesthesia machine's purpose is to deliver known and precise quantities and concentrations of oxygen and anesthetic gases, its design and checkout are identical for adult and pediatric use. Anesthesia machines are generally equipped with a flow meter and cylinder yoke for air, providing the capability to dilute oxygen with air and thus avoid the use of nitrous oxide. This capability may be of particular value when nitrous oxide is contraindicated, as in premature infants in whom a high inspired oxygen concentration as well as nitrous oxide is potentially disadvantageous.

As with adults, an in-line oxygen analyzer is necessary to quantitate the inspired oxygen concentration. This is especially critical when air is used, because there is no interlock between air and oxygen as there is between nitrous oxide and oxygen and because a lower-than-expected inspired oxygen concentration could therefore be delivered unintentionally.

Controlled Ventilation: Breathing Circuits

Controlled ventilation of infants and children using volume-limited (volume preset, time cycled) ventilators and circle breathing systems is commonplace in modern practice. At first glance, it appears that two methods of mechanically controlled ventilation are available to the clinician:

- Conversion of an adult volume ventilator to a pressure ventilator
- Using a volume ventilator with preset tidal volumes and compliant breathing circuits

In practice, usually a volume-limited ventilator with pressure limitations is used **(see Volume-Controlled Ventilation by Means of Compliant Breathing Circuits and a Preset Tidal Volume)**. Therefore, this whole issue may be one of semantics.

Conversion of Adult to Pediatric Ventilators

When beginning controlled ventilation of infants, clinicians can start with low-set tidal volumes and progressively increase the delivered tidal volume until chest expansion is appropriate and peak inspiratory pressure (PIP), end-tidal CO_2, and oxygen saturations are adequate. In effect, this practice is for clinicians to convert an adult ventilator to a pressure ventilator.

Volume-Controlled Ventilation by Means of Compliant Breathing Circuits and a Preset Tidal Volume

"The wind goeth toward the south, and turneth about unto the north; it whirleth about continually, and the wind returneth again according to His circuits."
—Ecclesiastes 1:6

Volume-controlled ventilation and circle breathing systems may be used safely and effectively in neonates, infants, and children (2). Volume-controlled ventilation is made possible in even very small infants because of the large compression volume (volume lost through compression of gases and expansion of the breathing circuit) in the circle breathing system and CO_2 cannister. Whereas circle breathing systems work well in most infants and children, using a relatively compliant breathing system with large compression volume may do little to ventilate the stiff lungs in an infant with very poor pulmonary compliance. With the caveat that some infants' lungs (e.g., those with extremely poor compliance) may not be adequately ventilated, appropriate preset tidal volume ($V_t$set) may be delivered to small patients and is dependent on patient weight. Table 1 contains approximate formulas according to weight.

Relatively larger $V_t$set/kg is needed in small infants because proportionally more of the $V_t$set becomes compression volume. Nevertheless, volume-controlled ventilation in small infants is not without potential hazard, most notably barotrauma. Excessive delivered tidal volume and subsequent barotrauma may be prevented by the practice of beginning with a very low $V_t$set and then adjusting inspiratory pressure to desired parameters (e.g. chest movement and measured PIP). Furthermore, modern ventilators, including the Ohmeda 7800, have a pressure-limiting valve that can be set to prevent excessive PIP and barotrauma. Finally, an endotracheal tube that allows a leak at approximately 30 cm H_2O will help to prevent barotrauma.

Perhaps it is most important to recognize that if a noncompliant breathing circuit (e.g., a Jackson-Rees modification of the Ayre's T-piece) is used in conjunction with a volume-controlled ventilator, the risk for barotrauma is increased because less of the delivered tidal volume is lost as compression of gases or expansion of the circuit. Although the Bain circuit is a Mapleson circuit (type D) in the Ohmeda gas management system (GMS), large compression volume is created because gas is routed through the CO_2 canister. The relatively low compliance of Mapleson D circuits lacking a GMS may preclude them from being used with volume-controlled ventilation if the tidal volume cannot be set sufficiently low.

Some clinicians may not have developed a trust that mechanical ventilation is reliable in infants. Indeed, manual ventilation of the lungs may be required during changing clinical and surgical conditions, including loss of compliance, or when timing of chest expansion must be coordinated with surgical considerations. For the most part, however, using mechanically controlled ventilation leaves the clinician's hands free for the many other tasks required for the care of infants and children.

Alternate Systems for Use When a Circle System Is Not Appropriate

Despite evidence suggesting that changes in pulmonary compliance can be detected equally when using either a circle or Bain system (3,4), many experienced clinicians probably have a better feel for compliance changes when using a low-compliance Mapleson D circuit (Fig. 1). Attempts to achieve this better feel as well as to eliminate dead space[b] and reduce the work of

TABLE 1. *Tidal volume delivery according to body weight*

Preset tidal volume (ml/kg)[a]	Body weight (kg)
200–250	1
50	5
25	10

[a]Ed. Note (JMB): Therefore, for the starting preset tidal volume in infants weighing 1 to 10 kg, one size fits all (i.e., 250 mls will work for all). This holds true for circle breathing circuits because compression volume loss is large in comparison to the amount of gas reaching the infant's lungs. One must use, however, other measures to further avoid barotrauma, (e.g., fresh gas flow should be kept low [~2 to 3 L/min] and a pressure-limiting valve should be set to limit PIP to ~20 to 30 cm H_2O.)

[b]Ed. Note (JMB): Based on answers the editors hear when questioning trainees, there is much room for clarification of the dead-space issue in pediatric anesthesia breathing circuits. Dead space in any breathing circuit only extends to where fresh and exhaled gases are mixed. Once gas is separated, dead space no longer exists; gas then becomes a portion of compressible circuit volume. The dead space of the Y-connector in a circle system extends to the crotch of the Y down to the tip of the endotracheal tube. This dead space can be decreased by the addition of a median septum into the Y. I don't, however, know of anyone who does this. Likewise, the dead space of an elbow in a Mapleson D system can be decreased by decreasing the functional circumference of the elbow ("Norman elbow"). We don't know anyone who still uses a Norman elbow either. In short, dead space may be a dead issue. As long as fresh gas flow (FGF) is adequate and ventilation controlled when using either a circle or Mapleson D breathing system, and as long as end tidal CO_2 is monitored to ensure adequate ventilation, dead space is a relatively moot issue. On the other hand, if you stick other things in the breathing system of a small spontaneously breathing infant (e.g., an adult-sized heat and moisture exchanger with 10 ml added dead space), you may bring this dead issue to life. (The Humid-vent Micro and Humid-vent Mini are less troublesome in this regard, adding only 1.1 and 2.4 ml dead space, respectively).

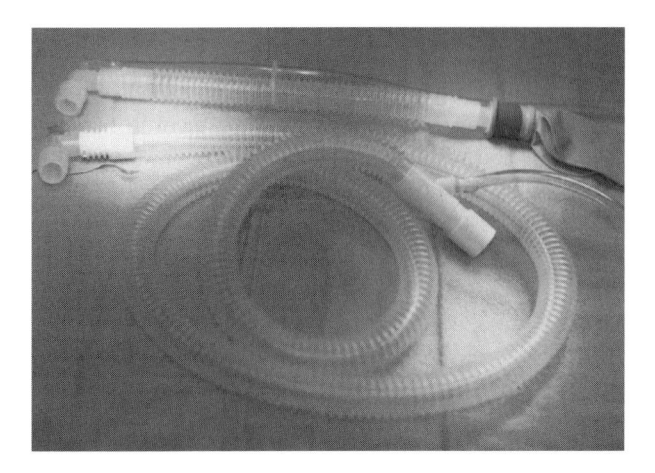

FIG. 1. The Jackson-Rees modification of the Ayre's T-piece **(top)** and the Bain circuit **(bottom)** are examples of Mapleson D circuits. Mapleson E and F systems are really modifications of the D system—take off both the exhalation valve and the reservoir bag from a D and you've got an E; take the valve off a D and you've got an F (Fig. 2). Add a ventilator with an exhalation valve to the E or F and you've got a D. There is no real functional difference between the D, E, and F as they are used in modern practice.

breathing for the child have inspired many of the modifications made in circuits used in infants and young children. The classic example of such a modification is Ayre's T-piece, which contains no valves and no reservoir bag (5,6). Ayre's T-piece was further modified by Jackson-Rees to include addition of a respiratory reservoir (an anesthesia bag) to the expiratory limb (7). Each of the Mapleson circuits (A to E) are similar in configuration—consisting of a source of FGF, a reservoir bag, a pop-off (pressure-release) valve, and an adaptor for the mask or endotracheal tube (Fig. 2) (8). The position of the reservoir bag and pop-off valve determines the name of the configuration, A through E.

Modern anesthesia practice in the United States has virtually eliminated variations except the Mapleson D, which includes the Bain circuit and the Jackson-Rees modified Ayre's T-piece. In Mapleson D circuits, fresh gas is introduced just proximal to the connection for the anesthesia mask or endotracheal tube and thus washes alveolar gas out of the expiratory limb during expiration. Although other factors are involved, the extent to which these circuits prevent rebreathing primarily depends on the FGF, the size of the patient, and whether ventilation is controlled or spontaneous. The heavier the patient, the greater the CO_2 production and the greater the FGF required to prevent hypercapnia (9). Although many for-

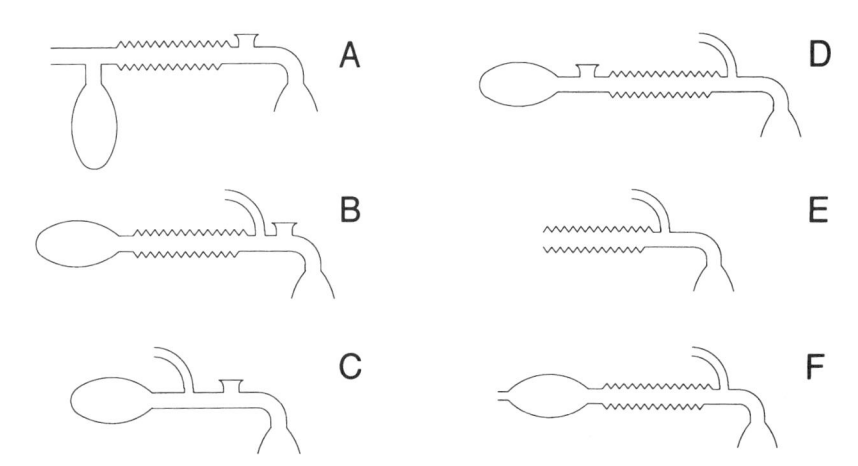

FIG. 2. Mapleson classification of breathing systems.

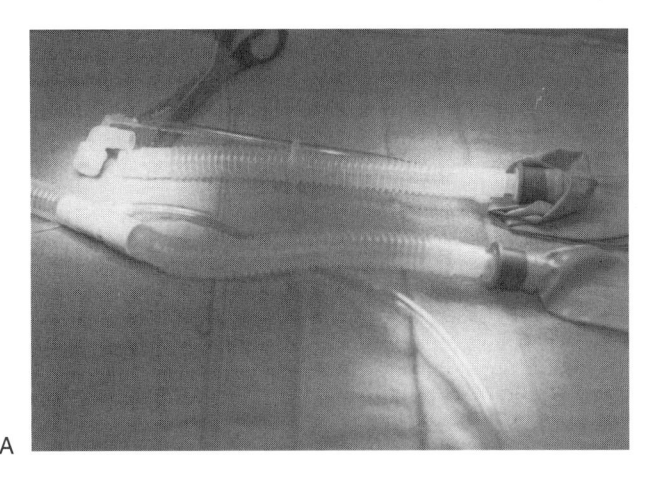

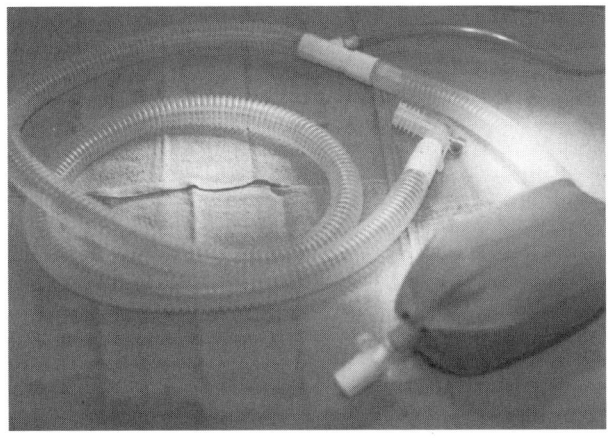

FIG. 3. How to make an extra long breathing circuit for use in magnetic resonance imaging (MRI). **(A)** A Jackson-Rees circuit is disassembled and attached to the back end of a Bain circuit. **(B)** The finished product is an extra long circuit that will reach the patient in the MRI tunnel. For manual-controlled or spontaneous ventilation, a reservoir bag is attached; for mechanical-controlled ventilation, a ventilator may be attached.

mulas for the ideal FGF exist (9,10), most are clinically impractical because their use requires calculation of minute ventilation, which in turn requires an accurate measurement of tidal volume.[c] These formulas may serve as approximate starting flows. In the final analysis, monitoring the end-tidal CO_2 (see **Monitoring the Adequacy of Ventilation**) stands as the most precise way of adjusting FGF when using Mapleson D systems (10).

Adaptation of the Mapleson D for Use in Magnetic Resonance Imaging

An extra long breathing circuit is often needed in the magnetic resonance imaging (MRI) suite as patients are some distance away from the anesthesia machine. A long circuit may be created by combining Bain and Jackson-Rees circuits (Fig. 3). This long circuit will allow spontaneous or controlled ventilation.

---

[c] Ed. Note (JMB): If you really must have a FGF formula, here is a simple one, accurately derived (10).
For controlled ventilation:
FGF = 250 ml/kg/min (for $ETCO_2$ = 38 mmHg)
FGF = 500 ml/kg/min (for $ETCO_2$ = 30 mmHg)
where FGF = fresh gas flow and $ETCO_2$ = end-tidal CO_2. These formulas work as long as $FGF \geq \dot{V}_e$, but you really don't need to remember that because $\dot{V}_e$ is almost always ≤ FGF at normal clinical ventilation settings (e.g., PIP = 20 to 30 cm H_2O and respiratory rate ~20 to 30 breaths per minute).

Anesthesia Ventilators

"Man will never be enslaved by machinery if the man tending the machine be paid enough."
—Karel Capek

Current anesthesia machine ventilators are typically pneumatically and electronically powered and controlled, have ascending bellows and constant flow, and are time-cycled. Most infants and children (even those very small and critically ill) can be ventilated well with currently available ventilators, notwithstanding differences in compressible volume of the ventilator bellows and breathing circuit. Although ventilators may be classified according to any number of things (e.g., power source, method of control, bellows type, waveform-generated, and alarm systems), they are typically referred to by the variable that limits or ends the inspiratory cycle (e.g., volume- or pressure-limited). The following pressure- and volume-limited ventilators are useful in pediatric patients:

- Sechrist Infant Ventilator, Models IV-100B and IV-200 (pressure-limited)
- Siemens-Elema 900C Servo Ventilator and 900D Anesthesia Machine (volume- or pressure-limited)
- North American Drager Narkomed (volume-limited)
- Ohmeda 7800, 7810 (volume-limited), and 7900 (volume- and pressure-limited)

Sechrist Infant Ventilators

The Sechrist infant ventilators are described as "time-cycled, flow-controllers" (a fancy term for a "mechanical thumb") but are basically pressure-limiting ventilators. Closure of the expiratory valve (the mechanical thumb) creates positive pressure in the breathing circuit and inflates the lungs. When pressure in the breathing circuit reaches the set pressure limit, an expiratory valve opens and gas within the breathing circuit is removed. Therefore, the Sechrist ventilators are pressure ventilators. Both of these ventilators allow the user to set the PIP, positive end-expiratory pressure (PEEP), respiratory rate, and inspiration-expiration (I:E) ratio.

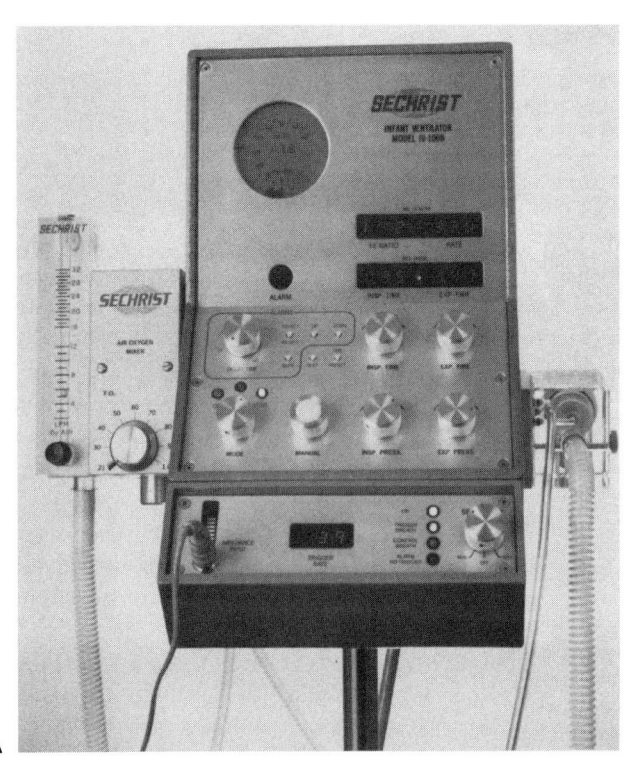

FIG. 4. The Sechrist IV-100B ventilator **(A)**

IV-100B

The IV-100B ventilator may be applied to a Mapleson D breathing circuit simply by connecting the Y-connector of the ventilator breathing circuit to the end of either a Jackson-Rees circuit or a Bain circuit (Fig. 4). Therefore, the FGF from the anesthetic machine enters the breathing circuit at the place it usually enters. Alternatively, this ventilator may be configured so that gas from the anesthesia machine is delivered through the inspi-

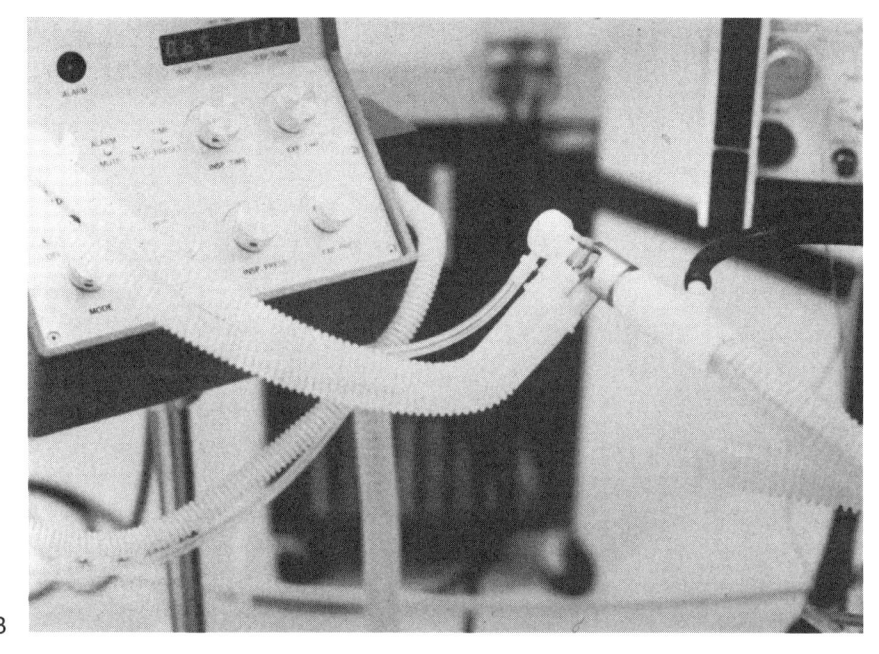

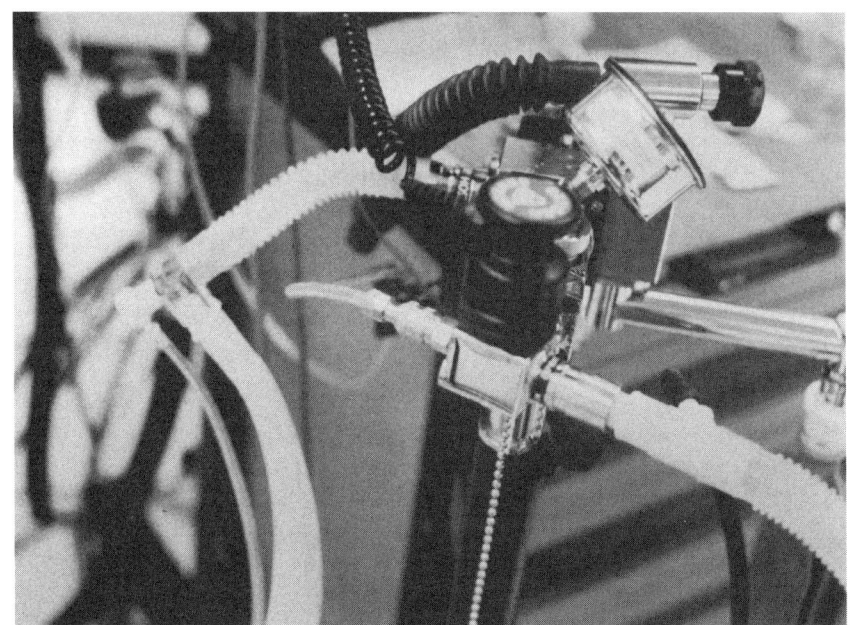

B

C

may be connected directly into a Bain circuit **(B)** or to the Bain circuit adaptor on the anesthesia machine **(C)**.

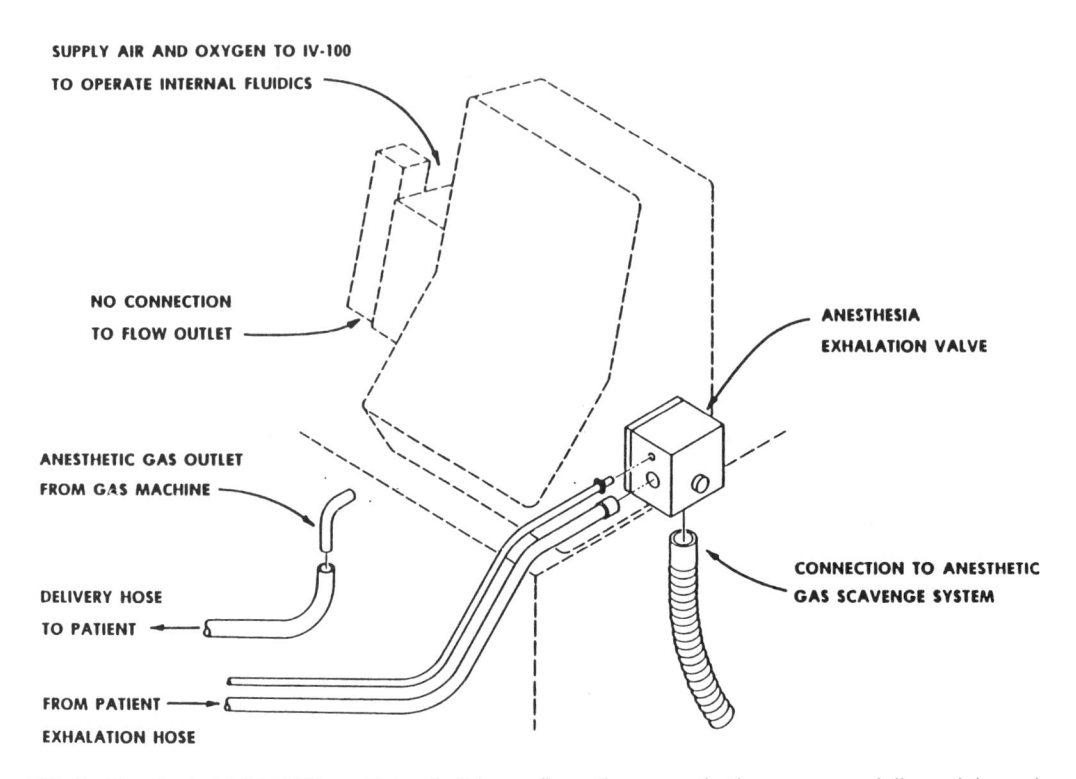

FIG. 5. The Sechrist IV-100B ventilator. In this configuration, anesthetic gases are delivered through the inspiratory limb of the ventilator breathing circuit. The anesthesia exhalation valve acts as a mechanical thumb that is released when the desired inflating pressures are reached. (Diagram provided courtesy of Sechrist Industries, Inc.)

ratory limb of the ventilator's breathing circuit (Fig. 5). Ventilator variables (e.g., respiratory rate, I:E ratio) and inflating pressures are adjusted by dials on the control panel (Fig. 4A).

IV-200

The IV-200 ventilator was designed to be used primarily for newborn intensive care. With the use of a metal exhalation valve (P/N 20084), however, it can be used as an infant anesthesia ventilator. To accomplish this, the IV-200 must be used in conjunction with a conventional anesthesia machine. The total system should be configured so that continuous gas flow of the desired anesthetic agent is generated by the anesthesia machine, routed to the patient connection and then to the IV-200 exhalation valve (Fig. 6). It is necessary to locate a safety pressure relief valve near the origin of the gas from the anesthesia machine. This safety pressure relief valve should be capable of being adjusted within a range of 15 to 75 cm H_2O. Supply gases of air and oxygen at 50 psi are required for ventilator operation. In this application, however, the internal air-oxygen mixer will not be used to control the gas concentrations being delivered to the patient, and the flow meter may be turned off.

Mechanical ventilation is accomplished with the IV-200 in a conventional manner. All anesthetic gases venting from the system may be collected with a gas scavenging system connected to the outlet port of the metal exhalation valve (30-mm taper fitting). This ventilator allows for precise adjustment of ventilator variables useful when pressure-limited ventilation is required in critically ill infants (Fig. 7).

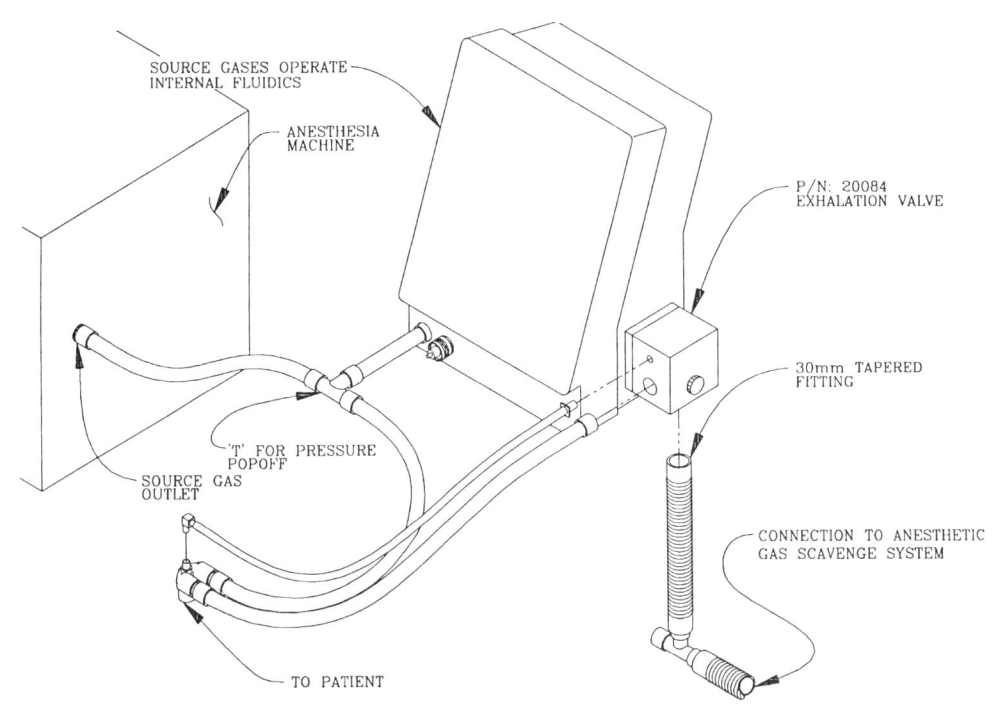

FIG. 6. Application of the Sechrist IV-200 for anesthesia (anesthesia exhalation valve). (Diagram provided courtesy of Sechrist Industries, Inc.)

Seimens-Elema 900C Servo Ventilator and 900D Anesthesia Machine/Ventilator

These complex but useful ventilators allow for precise control of volume or pressure as well as PEEP and provide for a variety of ventilator modes (e.g., continuous positive airway pressure, pressure support). Therefore, they may be particularly useful in critically ill patients, especially those already on mechanical ventilation in the intensive care unit. The Seimens 900C ventilator is used by attaching the FGF from the machine to the low-pressure gas inlet. The Seimens 900D is an anesthesia machine complete with vaporizers as well as a ventilator. As a practical point, it should be noted that the 900D system has two ventilator bellows, interior and exterior. For infants < 10 kg in body weight, the exterior concertina bellows may provide excessive tidal volumes. Therefore, the external bellows is inactivated when ventilating these smaller infants by turning off a rebreathing knob found on the left front of the machine. Appropriate ventilation is then provided by the interior bellows. In both 900C and 900D systems, when FGF ≥ the set minute ventilation adequate working pressure (as indicated by a gauge on the ventilator) will be provided.

North American Drager Narkomed

The North American Drager Narkomed series of anesthesia machine/ventilators include models 2A, 2B, 2C, 3, and 4. Ventilators on all Narkomed anesthesia machines may be used with either adult or pediatric bellows. When using the adult bellows (which, as previously mentioned, is usually appropriate even for pediatric patients), tidal volume is adjusted according to markings on the bellows cannister (the preadjusted bellows height) (Fig. 8). By contrast, when using the pediatric bellows, tidal volume is independent of the bellows markings, but is dependent on inspiratory flow adjusted using the inspiratory flow dial. An adjustable inspiratory pressure-limiting valve (PLV) is present on Narkomed models 2C, 3, and 4 (Fig. 8), but this important PLV is absent on models 2A and 2B (Fig. 9). The absence of a pressure-limiting device may lead to barotrauma in small infants if excessive pressure or tidal volume is delivered inadvertently. This PLV may be retrofitted onto the earlier models. This valve is recommended when infants are to be ventilated with Narkomed anesthesia machines.

Although the Narkomed delivers small tidal volumes, it is capable of measuring exhaled tidal volumes of only 100 ml or greater—a slight drawback (because the volume monitor continuously alarms) when used in small infants whose tidal volumes are less than 100 ml, especially if there is a large leak around the tracheal tube. Ventilation of the infant lungs could well be adequate despite a low volume monitor that continues to alarm.

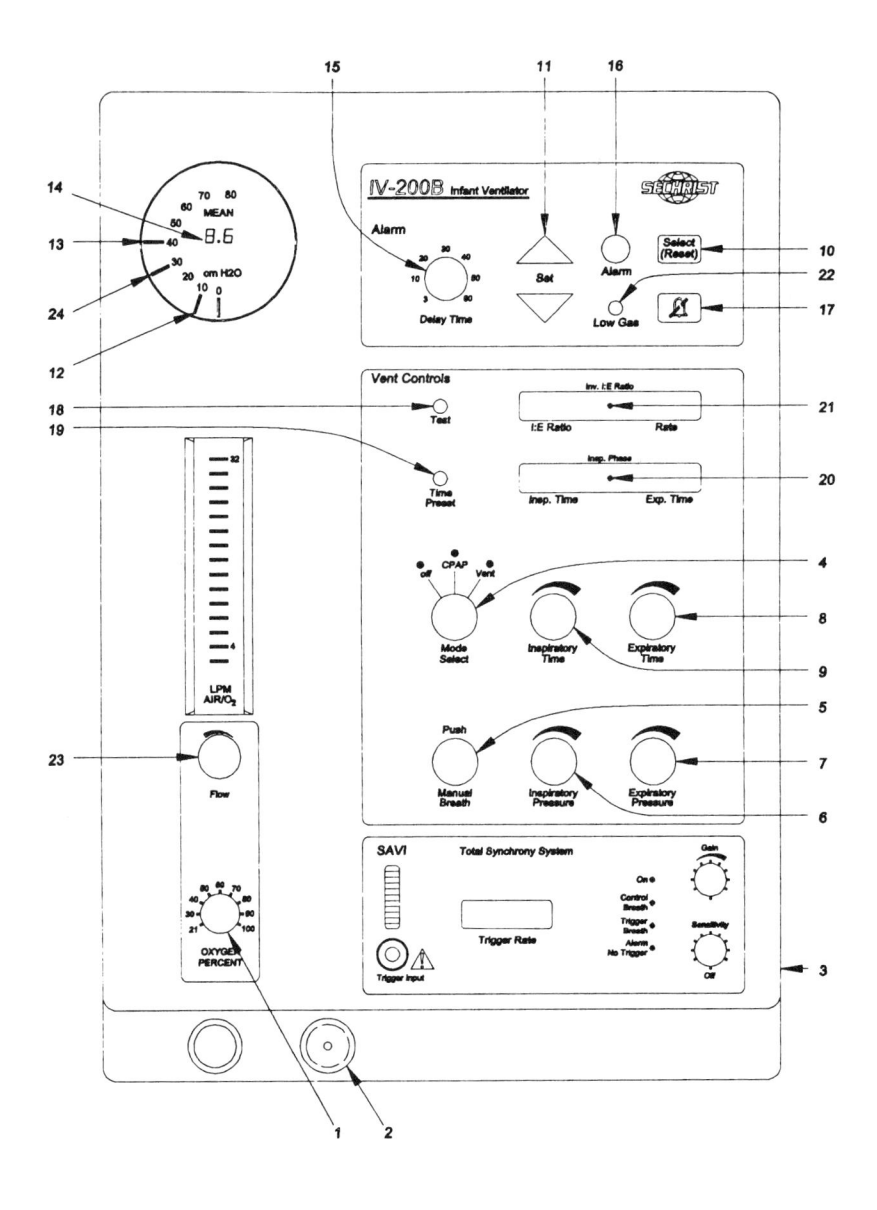

A Bain system may be used with the Narkomed series of anesthesia machine by using a special adaptor (Fig. 10).

Ohmeda Anesthesia Ventilator

Ohmeda 7800 (7810)

The Ohmeda 7800 ventilator is a volume controller with adult and pediatric bellows (300 ml maximum tidal volume) (Fig. 11). This ventilator may be connected to a circle system or a Bain circuit, both of which channel gas through a CO_2 absorber in the Ohmeda GMS system. This ventilator may be used in pediatric patients of all sizes including premature infants, neonates, and ex-prematures if the previously mentioned precautions are considered (2). The 7800 (7810) is capable of measuring exhaled tidal volumes as small as 30 ml,[d] a slight advantage for this ventilator over other volume ventilators. Excessive inflating pressures and subsequent barotrauma are prevented by a pressure-limiting pop-off valve controlled by a preadjustment dial found on the external control panel of the 7800 (7810). By setting this dial to a maximum pressure, the inspiratory cycle ends before barotrauma can result. In essence, one is using this volume ventilator in the pressure mode.

---

[d]Ed. Note (JMB): This statement regarding the lowest measurable tidal volume (Ohmeda [30 ml] and Narkomed [100 ml]) is true when the peritracheal gas leak is small (i.e., the exhaled tidal volume is returned to the volume monitor). In the presence of a large peritracheal gas leak (as many well-intended anesthesiologists prefer), much of the exhaled tidal volume is lost and the volume monitor will continuously sound the low-volume alarm despite what is adequate alveolar ventilation.

FIG. 7. The Sechrist IV-200 control panel (1). Air-oxygen mixer: controls F_iO_2. (2) Safety pressure relief valve: relief pressures between 15 and 85 cm H_2O can be obtained. (3) Power switch: AC power must be on for the ventilator to operate. (4) Mode select: off, continuous positive airway pressure (CPAP), or ventilator. (5) Manual breath: inspiration will occur as long as the button is pushed. (6) Inspiratory pressure adjusts the pressure to the exhalation valve ("mechanical thumb"). Range is from 5 to 70 cm H_2O. (7) Expiratory pressure: selects desired CPAP or positive end-expiratory pressure (PEEP). (8) Expiratory time. (9) Inspiratory time. Dials 8 and 9 determine the I:E ratio. (10) Select (reset) button: this button allows the operator to select the multiple options of the electronic manometer. The selectable options are: mean airway pressure, respiratory rate, inspiratory time, peak airway pressure, high limit alarm pressure, low limit alarm pressure and high breath rate alarm. (11) Set Arrows (up and down): these buttons adjust the alarm limit value for the parameter that has been selected by the SELECT button. (12) Low inspiratory pressure alarm setting ("L LIM SET"): this setting establishes the set point for the low inspiratory alarm for the range −5 to 75 cm H_2O, (−0.5 to 7.5 Kpa). (13) High inspiratory pressure alarm setting ("H LMT SET"): this setting establishes the set point for the high inspiratory pressure alarm for the range 0 to 80 cm H_2O (0.0 to 8.0 Kpa). (14) Mean airway pressure display: this three-digit numeric display shows the mean airway pressure as measured in the patient circuit. (15) Delay time ("Low Delay"): this control sets the time delay before the low inspiratory pressure audible and visible alarms are activated. (16) Alarm visible indicator: this light flashes red during an alarm situation. Simultaneously, an audible beep can be heard. (17) Alarm silence: pushing the button silences the audible alarm indicator for approximately 30 seconds under some alarm conditions. (18) Test: pushing this button when the ventilator is operating in the VENT mode initiates a self-test sequence. (19) Time preset: pushing this button when the mode selector is in the CPAP position allows the operator to observe the settings of the inspiratory and expiratory times before switching to the VENT mode and to make adjustments to the controls if desired. (20) Inspiratory phase light: this light (red LED) is illuminated for the duration of the inspiratory phase when the ventilator is used in the VENT mode. (21) Inverse I:E ratio light: this light (red LED) indicates an inverse I:E ratio (inspiratory time greater than expiratory times). (22) Low inlet gas pressure alarm indicator: if air, oxygen, or both of the inlet gas supplies drop below 30 psi, this visual alarm activates as well as an audible alarm tone. (23) Flow control valve: this control allows the clinician to adjust delivered peak inspiratory flow (continuous flow). (24) PIP indicator: highest inspiratory pressure activated with last inspiration is indicated by a cursor mark. (25) Low pressure alarm delay time indicator: displays the set alarm delay time for the low pressure alarm. (Diagram provided courtesy of Sechrist Industries, Inc.)

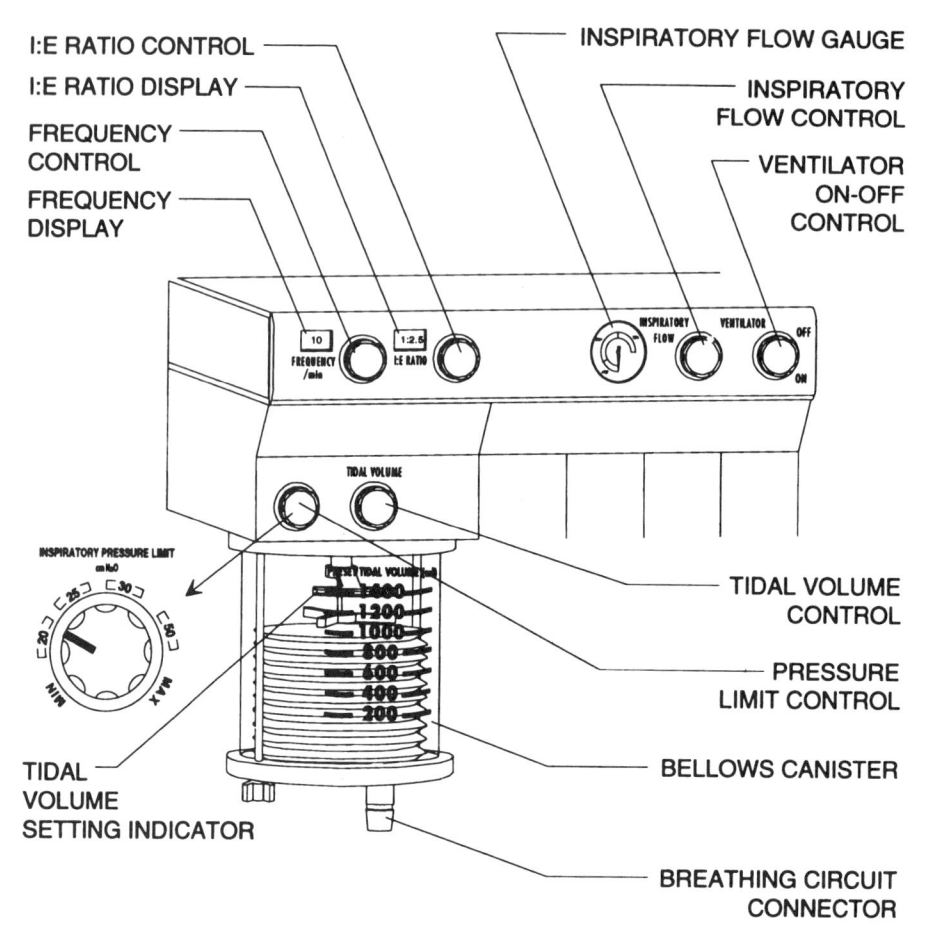

FIG. 8. The control panel and bellows of a North American Drager Narkomed 2C. Using the adult bellows, tidal volume is adjusted by setting the tidal volume control dial. Using the pediatric bellows, tidal volume is adjusted by setting the inspiratory flow control dial. Note the presence on this model of the all-important inspiratory pressure limit dial. (Reprinted from Narkomed 2B Users Manual, courtesy of North American Drager Co.)

Ohmeda 7900

The Ohmeda 7900 ventilator is a microprocessor-controlled ventilator with internal monitors for inspired oxygen, airway pressure, and exhaled volume (Fig. 12). It provides two ventilation modes: volume control and pressure control. By providing both volume control and pressure modes, the 7900 is a very useful ventilator in pediatric anesthesia. In a sense, it is much like an intensive care type of ventilator. Although untested in a large series of clinical pediatric patients, there is reason to believe (based on design characteristics) that this ventilator will be useful in very small critically ill infants, even those with poor pulmonary compliance. The 7900 ventilator has a tidal volume compensation system that allows for automatic compensation of compression losses, changes in fresh gas concentration, and leakages within the absorber and bellows. An electronic PEEP mechanism is a standard feature of the Ohmeda 7900. An autoclavable, latex-free bellows and expiratory valve manifold and an easily accessible absorber are also present in this system. This ventilator can be included on Ohmeda Excel SE and Modulus SE Anesthesia Delivery Systems.

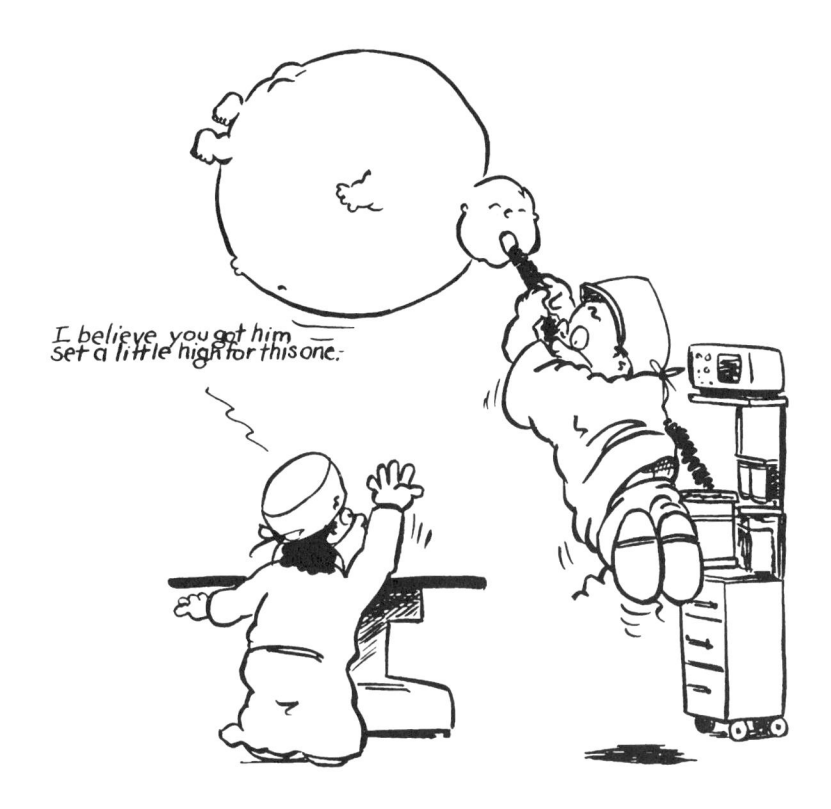

THE EFFECT OF FRESH GAS FLOW ON CONTROLLED VENTILATION

It is important to understand the effect on ventilation of alterations in FGF. Most ventilators used in the operating room combine output from the ventilator bellows with the FGF coming into the anesthesia circuit. Thus, increases or decreases in FGF change the delivered tidal volume even though no change has been made to other ventilator settings (11,12). Such increases or decreases in ventilation are of minimal consequence for adults or older pediatric patients but may have serious consequences for smaller pediatric patients. For example, in infants who weigh approximately 10 kg, increasing FGF from 1.5 to 6 L/min without making any adjustment to the ventilator may result in up to a 40% increase in delivered minute ventilation and PIP (12). Obviously, this consideration may have important implications for pediatric patients, in whom prevention of barotrauma is a major concern (e.g., an ex-premature infant with bronchopulmonary dysplasia). In the final analysis, this information underscores the importance of careful clinical observations: auscultation of breath sounds and chest expansion, monitoring of peak inflation pressure, and accurate determination of expired CO_2.

POSITIVE-PRESSURE VENTILATION THROUGH A LARYNGEAL MASK AIRWAY

The laryngeal mask airway (LMA) provides an effective airway for positive-pressure ventilation (PPV) in infants and children (13). In a recent study, a size 2 LMA was used in patients weighing 6.5 to 25 kg (38 ± 21 months of age), and PPV was adequately performed. If one chooses to use this technique, I recommend using the appropriate-sized LMA **(see Chapter 4)** and monitoring the patient for gastric distention. An increase in the patient's abdominal circumference, especially if ventilation is compromised, would be an indication

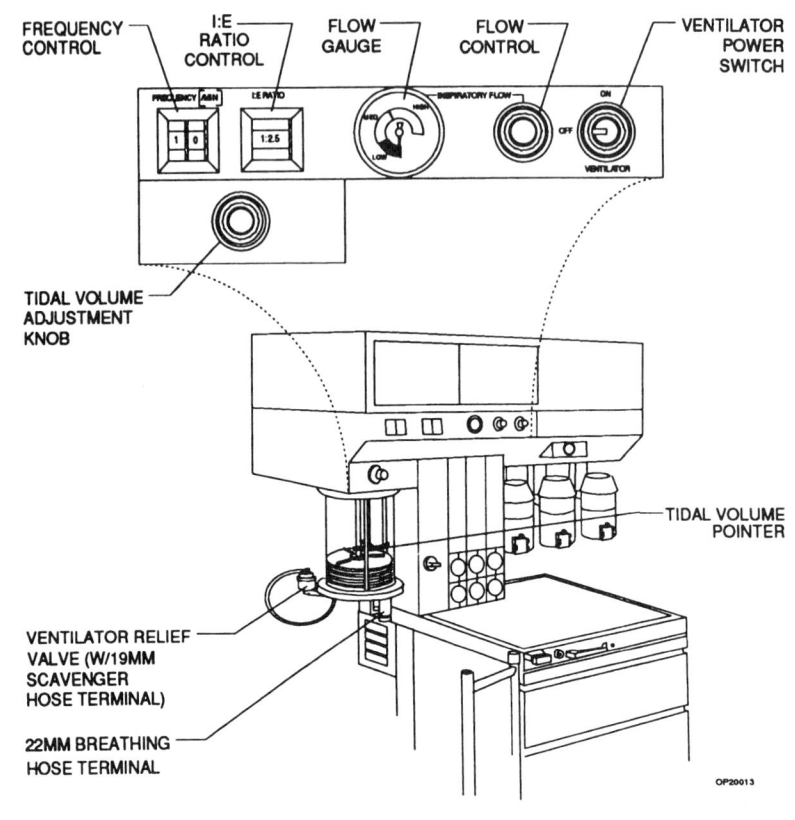

FIG. 9. (A) A diagram of the North American Drager Narkomed 2B anesthesia machine. Using the adult bellows, tidal volume is adjusted by setting the tidal volume adjustment dial. (Reprinted from Narkomed 2B Users Manual, courtesy of North American Drager Co.)

to suction the stomach and manage the airway with another technique (e.g., endotracheal intubation). In addition, leak pressure around the LMA cuff varies from patient to patient depending on (a) size of the cuff in relationship to the patient's anatomy and (b) the amount of air in the cuff. An excessive cuff leak (e.g., at ~10 to 15 mm Hg) may contribute to gastric distention and fail to provide adequate ventilation. Therefore, if measures to decrease a large leak fail, an alternative airway management technique may have to be used.

CONTROLLED VENTILATION: CONCLUSIONS

In conclusion, proper use of equipment may lead to improved safety in pediatric anesthesia. For instance, if done properly, mechanical ventilation with either an adult or pediatric circle breathing system is appropriate even for very small infants. In addition, in a large service in which anesthesia is administered to all age groups and by varied personnel, there may be an advantage in using basic equipment (i.e., volume ventilators and circle systems) serviceable for patients of any size. Using the same equipment for adults and pediatric patients provides a lesser chance for misconnection or otherwise faulty setup between cases. For small infants, when there is reduced compliance, it may be necessary to provide low-compliance breathing circuits and manual or pressure-limited ventilation. In the final analysis, one must rely on clinical skills and judgment. For example, if any ad-

(B) Using the pediatric bellows, tidal volume is adjusted by setting the flow control dial. Note the absence of an inspiratory pressure limit dial.

BAIN SYSTEM - BASED ON MAPLESON "D"

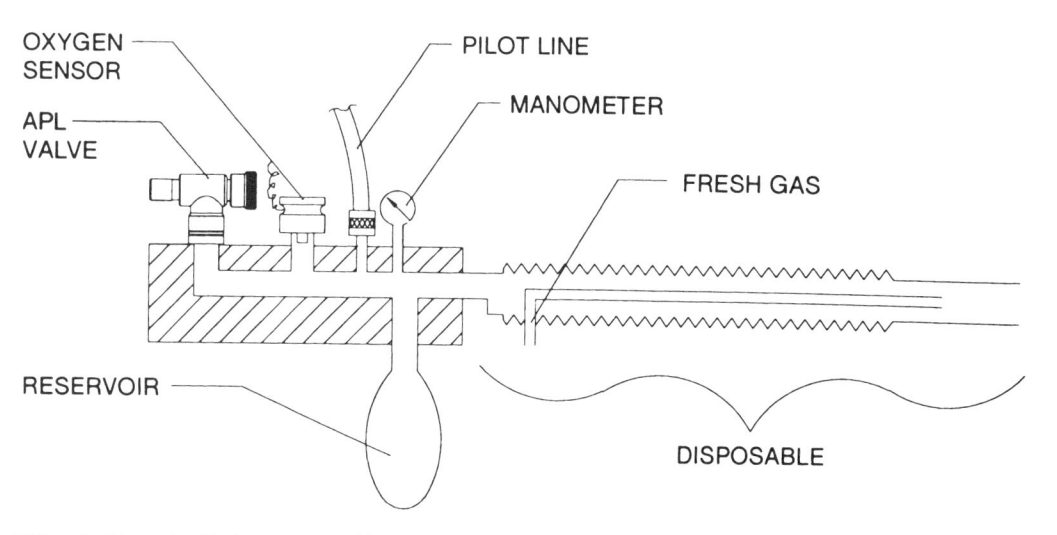

FIG. 10. Use of a Bain system with the Narkomed anesthesia machine. (Reprinted from Narkomed 2B Users Manual, courtesy of North American Drager Co.)

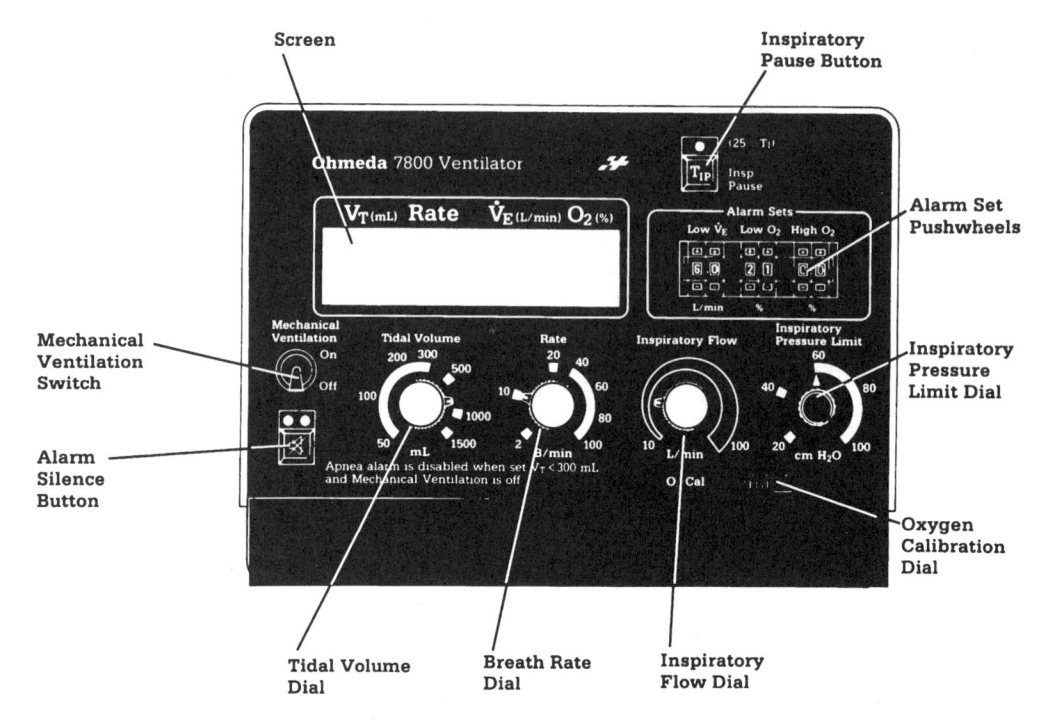

FIG. 11. The Ohmeda 7800 Ventilator. The display screen provides numeric readouts for expired tidal volume, breath rate, expired minute volume and inspired oxygen concentration and displays messages such as alarms and control settings. The tidal volume dial sets the tidal volume from 50 to 1500 ml. The rate dial changes the breath rate used for mechanical ventilation. The inspiratory flow dial sets the inspiratory flow rate from 10 to 100 L/min. Whenever you adjust or just touch the inspiratory flow dial, the ventilator will display the current I:E ratio, which it calculates based on the set inspiratory flow, tidal volume, breath rate, and the inspiratory-pause variables. Thus, a change in any of these variables changes the I:E ratio. To maintain a constant I:E ratio when rate or tidal volume is changed requires an adjustment of the inspiratory flow. Both the maximum-inspiratory-pressure and sustained-pressure alarm limits are set by the inspiratory pressure limit dial, which must be pushed in while turning to change the settings. The ventilator sets the sustained pressure limit to correspond to the inspiratory pressure limit dial setting. For inspiratory pressure limits of 20 cm H_2O to 60 cm H_2O, the ventilator sets the sustained pressure limit to one half the inspiratory pressure limit. Pressing the inspiratory pause button adds an inspiratory pause—an inflation hold—to the inspiratory cycle. (Reprinted with permission of Ohmeda Inc.)

verse change in pulmonary function or adequacy of ventilation is detected, the clinician should probably revert to manual ventilation while observing the patient clinically.

MONITORING THE ADEQUACY OF VENTILATION

"What business has science and capitalism got, bringing all these inventions into the works, before society has produced a generation educated up to using them!"
—Henrik Ibsen

Developments in monitoring of oxygenation and alveolar ventilation have improved the anesthetic care of infants and children. Pulse oximetry (SpO_2) and capnometry are now essential monitors in pediatric anesthesiology (14). Whereas SpO_2 gained almost immediate acceptance and widespread use in pediatric anesthesia, capnography in young patients was at first viewed skeptically because of limitations in obtaining accurate measurements (15). In 1986, the editors of *Health Devices* (a medical consumer's guide

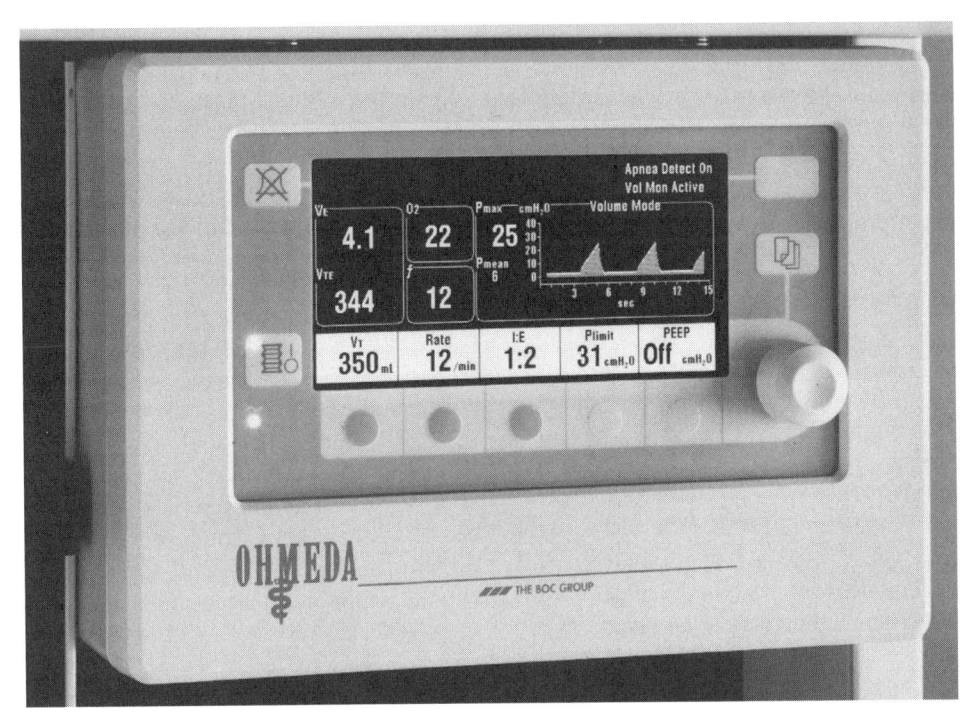

FIG. 12. The Ohmeda 7900 Ventilator. (Reprinted with permission of Ohmeda Inc.)

produced by the Emergency Care Research Institute) did not bother to rate the performance of capnometers in neonates and infants because it was unclear whether a valid end-tidal CO_2 measurement could be obtained in these patients (16).

Following is a review of the technology and clinical application of SpO_2 and capnography, as well as their effectiveness and limitations in the pediatric age group. We will explore how pediatric capnography has become increasingly accurate and how the two monitors, SpO_2 and capnography, work together to monitor oxygenation and alveolar ventilation of infants and children.

Pulse Oximetry

Pulse oximetry (SpO_2) provides instantaneous measurements of arterial oxygen saturation by determining the absorbance of two specific wavelengths of light by blood as it flows between a light source and a photodetector. Two wavelengths are emitted by the light source: red light at 660 nm and infrared light at 990 nm. During each cardiac cycle, light absorption varies cyclically. Pulsatile absorption (AC absorption) occurs during systole when arterialized blood pulsates into the tissue bed. Baseline absorption (DC absorption) is determined in the tissue bed during diastole. The pulse oximeter determines the arterial hemoglobin oxygen saturation (SaO_2) as an absorption ratio of red to infrared wavelength during the AC and DC components of the arterial pulse.

Physiologic Factors That Affect Pulse Oximetry

Because pulsatile blood flow is a requisite for accurate pulse oximetry, a measurement of SpO_2 may be absent or erroneous in the presence of inadequate pulsatile flow. SpO_2 may fail when cardiac output decreases. In this sense, SpO$_2$ may be used as a plethysmograph. Likewise, SpO$_2$ may vary according to the site of the SpO$_2$ sensor. The response time for changes in SpO$_2$ is 5 to 10 seconds using ear probes, and it may be up to 30 seconds using finger probes (17).

Factors That May Interfere With Accuracy

Intrinsic

Methemoglobin has the same absorption coefficient at both red and infrared wavelengths (18). This 1:1 absorption ratio leads to a saturation reading of 85%. Therefore, in the presence of high levels of methemoglobin, SpO$_2$ is erroneously low when SaO$_2$ is greater than 85% and erroneously high when SaO$_2$ is less than 85%. Carboxyhemoglobin has the same absorption coefficient as oxyhemoglobin at 660 nm (19). Therefore, if a patient has a 90% oxyhemoglobin and 7% carboxyhemoglobin, the SpO$_2$ will read 97%. The intravenous administration of some dyes (e.g., methylene blue) produce erroneous SpO$_2$ readings because the dyes change the absorption characteristics of the blood (20). Fetal hemoglobin (21) and bilirubin (22) do not affect the accuracy of SpO$_2$.

Extrinsic

Ambient light interferes with the accuracy of SpO$_2$ and may be minimized by covering the sensor with an opaque shield. During low perfusion, the pulse oximeter will amplify a small pulsatile absorbance signal. Unfortunately, when a weak signal is amplified, the background noise (static) is also amplified, and the pulse oximeter may generate an erroneous SpO$_2$ reading. Most pulse oximeters are designed to minimize this problem or to display a plethysmographic waveform for identification of noise. As with all plethysmography, the pulse oximeter will detect a complete loss of peripheral pulse, but is not designed to quantify peripheral blood flow. SpO$_2$ may be used, however, to confirm collateral blood flow to the hand in corroboration with the Allen's test. Many pulse oximeters have a time-averaging mode to help prevent patient motion artifact. These artifact-rejection schemes, however, may also affect the accuracy and response time of the pulse oximeter.

Accuracy during Arterial Hemoglobin Oxygen Desaturation

Most pulse oximeters are accurate to within ±2% (SD) between an SaO$_2$ of 70% to 100%. In many pulse oximeters, however, the accuracy decreases as the SaO$_2$ falls below 70% (23). This may be a moot point in most children, since investigation of the desaturation should begin when SpO$_2$ falls below about 95%. In children with cyanotic congenital heart disease, the accuracy of measurements at low saturations is of great importance.

Clinical Uses

Current standards dictate that SpO$_2$ be used in every instance of general anesthesia and conscious sedation (14). This recommendation is based on studies such as the one by Coté and colleagues (24), who found that the incidence of major desaturation events (SaO$_2$ ≤ 85%) decreased when SpO$_2$ was available. Although SpO$_2$ is required in all cases, there are some pediatric cases for which SpO$_2$ is particularly helpful:

- Titration of F$_I$O$_2$ in infants at risk for retinopathy of prematurity (we recommend SpO$_2$ = 93% to 95%)
- Pulmonary artery banding procedures (desaturation may indicate that the pulmonary artery band is overly restrictive)
- Cases in which return to fetal circulation may occur (e.g., reopening of the ductus arteriosus)

In cases of ductus arteriosus reopening, preductal and postductal sensors may be helpful in determining shunt direction. Furthermore, recent evidence indicates that arterial hemoglobin oxygen desaturation may occur during transfer from the operating room to the postanesthesia care unit (25) or while in the postanesthesia care unit despite a wakeful clinical appearance (26).

Complications

As with any device that contacts patients directly, injury can occur when a pulse oximeter probe is applied. However, few complications have been reported despite its almost universal use. Reported complications included overheating of a damaged light-emitting diode probe, which resulted in skin blistering in three adults (27). Additional injuries in adults include digital ischemia resulting from mechanical pressure by a probe on a finger. One such episode occurred in an elderly woman after prolonged application of a spring-tipped probe in the intensive care unit (28), and one occurred in a 16-year-old patient during anesthesia with controlled hypotension for an 11-hour maxillofacial reconstruction (29). Complications have also been reported in infants. These include a blister from a probe that overheated, an area of mild skin erosion after an ear probe was applied for over 48 hours, and a localized tanned area caused by the continuous application of fiberoptic finger probe for 5 days (30). A third-degree skin burn has also been reported during an MRI scan. This may have been caused by an electromagnetic field induced in the cable that led from the pulse oximeter to the finger probe (31).

These injury reports remind us of the precautions necessary when using SpO_2. All instruments need routine inspection and maintenance. Probes with damaged light-emitting diode components should be discarded. The probe should be positioned such that no pressure or torque is applied to the probe or the finger. After application of the probe, the extremity should be inspected for reduced blood flow. The quality of pulsations should also be monitored and the probe repositioned periodically to prevent prolonged local contact. During MRI procedures, all cables in contact with the patient should be positioned in such a way that conductive loops are not formed.

Pediatric Capnography

As with life in general, kids have a tendency to complicate matters. Respiratory monitoring during anesthesia is no exception (15). In truth, the measurement of respiratory gases is no more complicated or difficult in children than it is in adults. Let's simplify by starting with some simple definitions.

Capnometry is the measurement and numeric display of expired CO_2, whereas *capnography* is the measurement and graphic display of expired CO_2. If the graphic display is calibrated, capnography includes capnometry. Therefore, capnography is often used to indicate both capnometry and capnography. Gas for analysis of CO_2 may be aspirated from the airway (sidestream, or more appropriately, "aspirating capnography") or analyzed as it flows through a sensor inserted into the breathing circuit (mainstream, or more appropriately, "flow-through capnography"). Gas can be measured from any location in the breathing circuit or tracheal tube. If measured from the elbow of the breathing circuit, it is referred to as proximal end-tidal CO_2. Measurement from a distal location in the tracheal tube is referred to as distal end-tidal CO_2. The CO_2 may be measured by infrared analysis, mass spectrometry, acoustic spectroscopy (32), or Raman scattering (33).

Accurate Aspirating Capnography

In capnography, inaccuracy refers to erroneous difference between the measured end-tidal CO_2 ($P_{ET}CO_2$) values and the true and end-tidal values. Although a small physiologic difference may exist between $P_{ET}CO_2$ and $PaCO_2$, the $P_{ET}CO_2$ usually approximates $PaCO_2$ in intubated children in the absence of significant lung disease or congenital cyanotic heart disease (34).

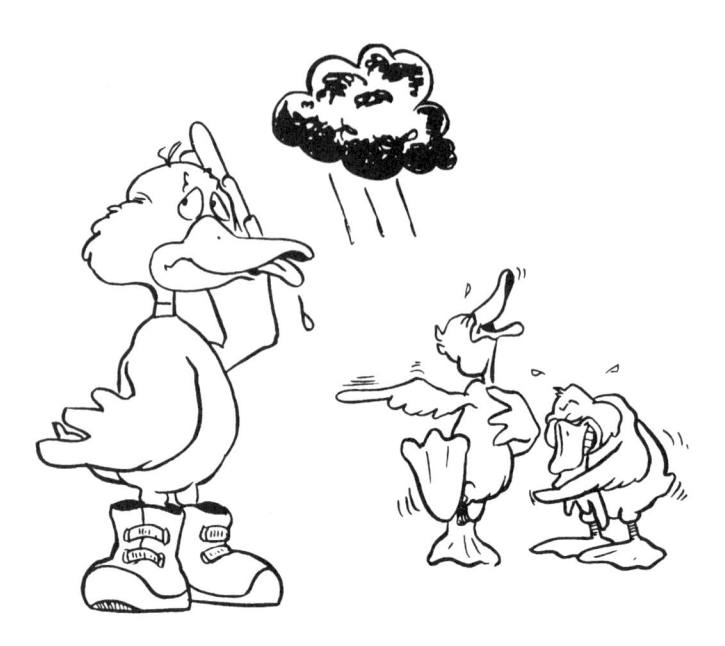

Sampling and the Smoke Line

To understand accurate aspirating capnography in infants and children, it is necessary to first consider the physiologic reasons why the measurement of respiratory gas in these patients is different. Infants and children have smaller tidal volumes (V_t) relative to breathing circuit volume (V_{bc}) and relative to the large amount of FGF entering the circuit. Therefore, exhaled CO_2 becomes diluted, and subsequently CO_2 values have the potential to be inaccurate when measured by capnography sampled from a diluted region of the breathing circuit (Fig. 13) (34).

Are these large V_{bc}:V_t and FGF:V_t ratios a significant impediment to accurate capnography? Not really. When using a circle system, proximal capnography is usually accurate (35). I insert a sampling snorkel, however, into the endotracheal tube of every child anesthetized, whether I am using a Mapleson D or circle system and regardless of the size of the child. This is a lot like putting rubber boots on ducks and

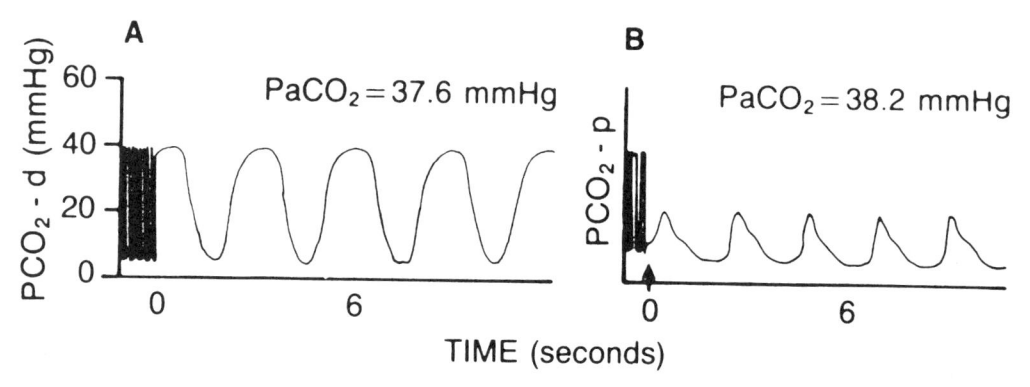

FIG. 13. Capnographic waveforms in a 6.9-kg, 9-month-old infant ventilated through a Mapleson D breathing circuit. **(A)** When gas is sampled from the distal end of the endotracheal tube, end-tidal CO_2 is accurate. **(B)** When gas is sampled from the proximal end (at the elbow of the breathing circuit), end-tidal CO_2 is diluted with fresh gas flow and underestimates the $PaCO_2$. (From Badgwell et al, ref. 34, with permission.)

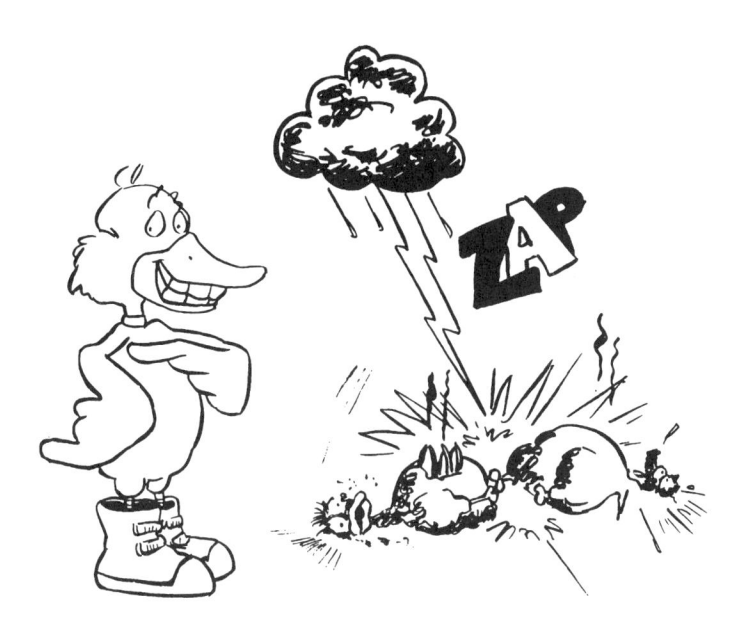

in some instances (e.g., in older children or when a circle system is used) represents overkill but is associated with a very high benefit:cost ratio.

When using a Mapleson D Circuit, it has been shown that one needs only to sample "below the smoke line" for accurate capnography (36). The *smoke line* refers to the leading edge of a column of smoke arising into the endotracheal tube when paraffin is burned in a lung model (36). Basically speaking, this smoke represents the exhaled CO_2 (*capnos* is the Greek work for smoke). Provided that one aspirates from below the smoke line (which is about the middle of the endotracheal tube adaptor, or anywhere in the endotracheal tube), one will get accurate capnography (37). It is easy to sample below the smoke line by using commercially available "snorkels" (sampling catheters) (34) or endotracheal tubes with built-in sampling catheters or adaptor ports (Fig. 14).[e] Distal sampling catheters are particularly helpful in improving accuracy of capnography in the infant or child with a RAE tube (Fig. 15).

Position of the Heat and Moisture Exchanger

The accuracy of proximally aspirated measurements is improved by inserting a small heat and moisture exchanger (e.g., a miniature Humid-Vent, Gibeck Respiration, Upplands Väsby, Sweden) between the fresh gas inlet and the tracheal tube connector. The use of such an exchanger, however, may lead to the accumulation of water within the sampling line, which could block the sampling line or damage the capnograph. The use of water filters, traps, and water-permeable sampling lines (e.g., Nafion) can minimize these effects.

Sample Flow Rate

The sample flow rate for aspirating capnography in infants and children is similar to that used in adults. This has led to apprehension that the sampling flow rate of aspiration capnography may compromise ventilation by extracting large volumes of gas from the tiny lungs of infants. If, however, one works out the mathematics for sampling flow rates as high as 240 ml/min

---

[e]Ed. Note (JMB): Regarding endotracheal tubes with the catheter built into the tube: Although these devices may provide accurate measurements, if the sampling catheter becomes obstructed (such as with secretions), it may be necessary to flush the secretions back into the trachea or, alternatively, change tubes. A new endotracheal tube may be problematic if intubation was difficult or if the airway is inaccessible.

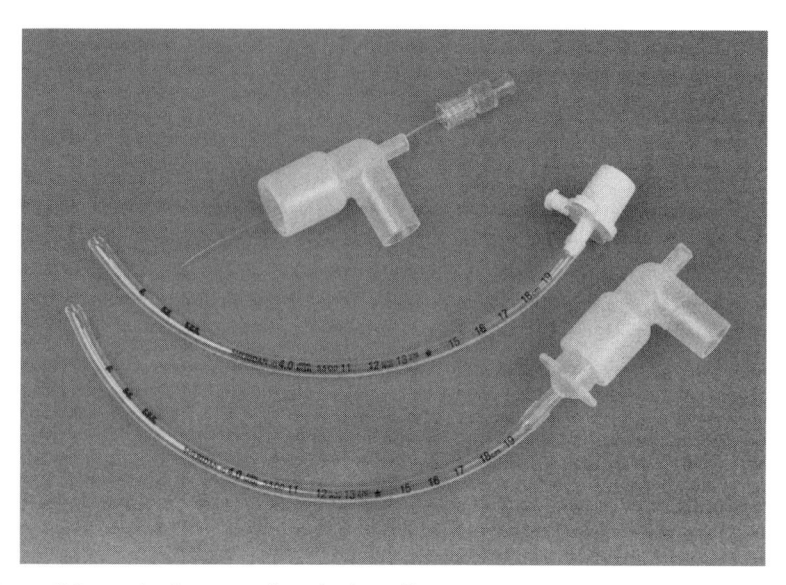

FIG. 14. Airway CO_2 aspiration sampling devices (from top to bottom): *(1)* A small-channel aspiration catheter fitting through an elbow adaptor (with permission of Gibeck-Dryden Corporation, Indianapolis, IN; and Datex Instrumentarium Corporation, Helsinki, Finland). *(2)* A 15-mm endotracheal tube adaptor with side port, originally designed for the administration of surfactant during mechanical ventilation, but used for CO_2 aspiration during anesthesia (with permission of Respiratory Support Products, Irvine, CA). *(3)* A standard elbow adaptor with aspiration channel for capnograph (with permission of Datex Instrumentarium Corporation, Helsinki, Finland).

even in very small infants, one would find that tidal volumes are not compromised (38). For example, in a 3-kg infant ventilated at 30 BPM with an inspiratory-to-expiratory ratio of 1:1, a sample flow rate of 150 ml/min will only aspirate 2.5 ml from the tidal volume (8% if tidal volume is 10 ml/kg) (38). This has been confirmed clinically, since it has been shown that sample flow rates of 150 or 240 ml/min do not affect the adequacy of spontaneous (39) or controlled ventilation (39,40).

Spontaneously Breathing Nonintubated Patients

Spontaneously breathing nonintubated patients may be monitored with aspirating

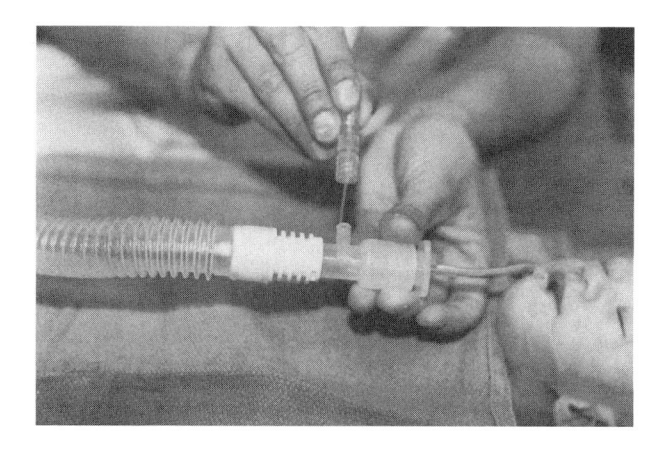

FIG. 15. An aspiration catheter is inserted into a straight connector in the Bain breathing circuit of an infant intubated with an RAE tube.

capnography by taping the sampling catheter adjacent to the external nares. Although a large difference may exist between arterial and end-tidal CO_2 values due to the large dead space of the face mask and high FGFs, this technique may be used to monitor respiratory trends and to detect airway obstruction.

Accurate Flow-Through Capnography

Flow-through capnography has proved to be accurate in infants and children (40–42) even at rapid ventilatory rates (43). There are, however, limitations associated with some models of the flow-through capnometers. The Seimens-Elema 930 CO_2 analyzer comes with a low dead-space pediatric cuvette, but the sensor housing itself is bulky and heavy and requires heating. Therefore, the analyzer may kink or dislodge the tracheal tube, or it may cause a burn injury if it contacts skin for an extended period. Furthermore, since this analyzer recalibrates after each breath and assumes that the inspired PCO_2 is zero, erroneous estimates of the end-tidal CO_2 may result if rebreathing were present (44). The Hewlett-Packard 47201A (Hewlett-Packard Co, Waltham, MA) capnograph has proved to be accurate in very small infants, but even the use of a 2-ml dead-space sensor (14363A) may increase the PCO_2 in small infants (42). The Novametrix 1260 capnograph uses an even smaller dead-space cuvette (0.6 ml). Furthermore, the Novametrix 1260 sensor (Novametrix Medical System, Inc, Wallingford, CT) is lightweight and well insulated to prevent patient injury. This capnograph accurately estimates the end-tidal CO_2 measurement without affecting the adequacy of ventilation (40).

Peritracheal Gas Leak

A large peritracheal gas leak may lead to inaccurate end-tidal CO_2 readings when using flow-through or aspirating capnography (Fig. 16).

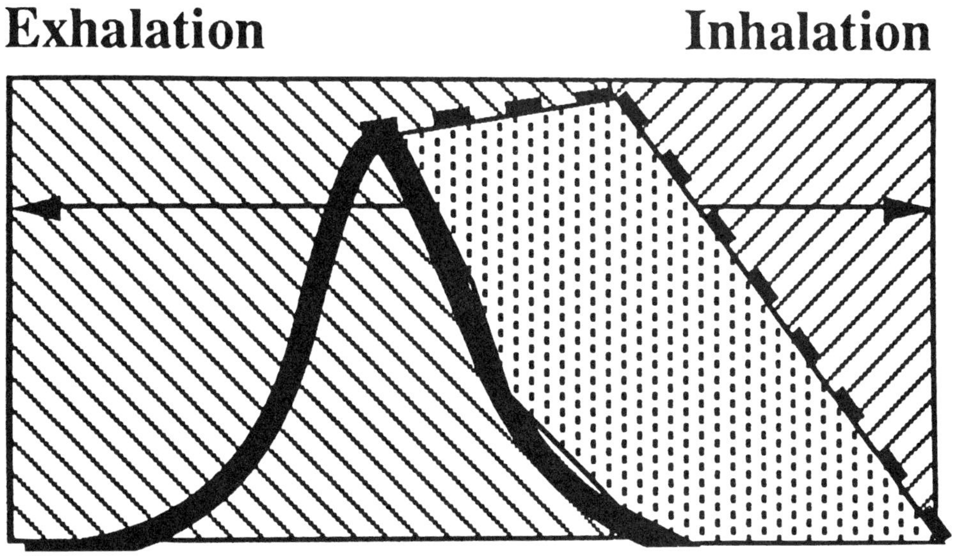

FIG. 16. Gas leak around the endotracheal tube as source of inaccuracy in pediatric capnography. Some alveolar gas, containing CO_2, is exhaled via the endotracheal tube and therefore measured by the capnograph; some escapes around the tube via the trachea and goes undetected *(stippled area)*.

Other Capnographic Considerations Specific to Pediatrics

Capnography at Rapid Respiratory Rates

Other special needs of children relate to their habit of breathing faster than adults. Therefore, one of the perceived problems of respiratory gas measurement has been that these measurements are inaccurate at rapid respiratory rates (45). However, is rate-dependent accuracy really a significant limitation? Probably not. Most capnographs and gas analyzers are very accurate within the physiologic variations of respiratory rates that one would normally encounter in the operating room (20 to 40 BPM). Above 40 BPM, there is a slight decay in end-tidal accuracy and elevation of the capnographic baseline owing to rapid respiratory rate (46).

Capnographic Baseline Elevation

As long as there has been capnography, man has been puzzled to observe the capnographic baseline (the measure of inspired CO_2 or F_iCO_2) ascend to mysterious heights during rapid respiratory rates in children, especially

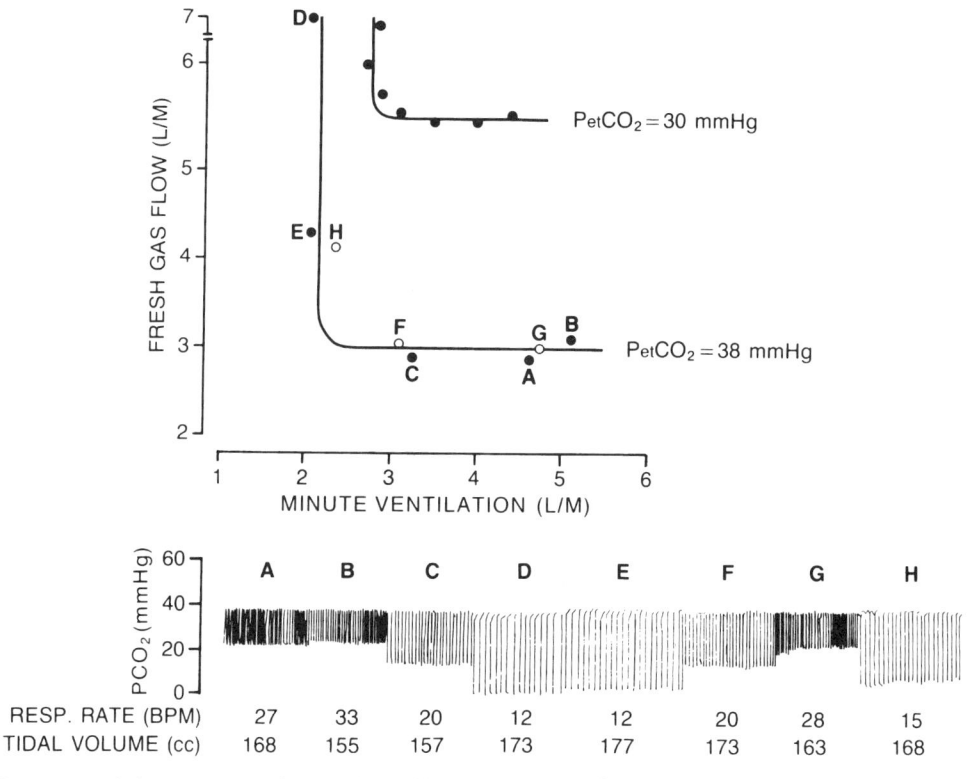

FIG. 17. (Top) Graph shows the relation of fresh gas flow (FGF) and minute ventilation (V_e) in a 12-kg infant with ventilation controlled through a Mapleson D circuit. **(Bottom)** The capnographic waveform at slow paper speed. When V_e FGF and FGF are kept constant, increasing V_e does not change end-tidal CO_2, but inspired CO_2 (rebreathing) increases. An average of many of these isopleths was used as the basis for developing FGF flow formulas (250 ml/kg/min for ETCO$_2$ = 38 mm Hg) (10). These data also help to explain elevation of the capnographic waveform seen at rapid respiratory rates in infants and children. Point B would correspond to ventilatory settings recommended by Rayburn in his CPRAM technique, and Point D would correspond to older recommendations of those who would espouse high FGF and low V_e (e.g., Nightingale et al). These graphs further show that elevation of the capnographic waveform is not particularly bothersome since ETCO$_2$ remains stable and does not increase ("isocapnic ventilation"). (From Badgwell et al, ref. 10, with permission.)

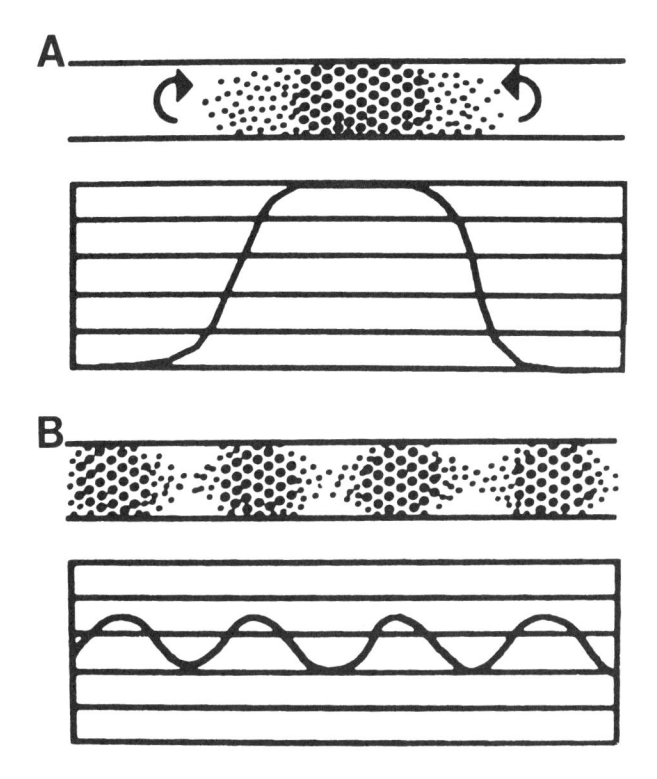

FIG. 18. A plug of CO_2 (stippled area) in a sampling catheter. Below the sampling catheter is the capnogram that would result if this plug reached a CO_2 analyzer. **(A)** As long as the front and back of the plug are well defined, the resultant capnogram will have a sharp upstroke and downstroke and the baseline will return to zero. **(B)** Several CO_2 plugs (as may occur in infants with rapid ventilation measured in a long sampling catheter) follow each other, resulting in a capnographic waveform with poorly defined upstrokes and downstrokes and an elevated baseline. This phenomenon would lead to an artifactual elevation of the baseline of the capnogram. (From Gravenstein JS, Paulus DA, Hayes TJ: *Carbon dioxide and monitoring in capnography in clinical practice.* Boston: Butterworth, 1989:9, with permission.)

when using sidestream (rather than in-line) capnography (Fig. 17). Simply stated, there is nothing too mysterious about baseline elevation of the capnographic waveform. Elevation of the capnographic baseline is attributed to one or both of two factors: true rebreathing and artifact (Fig. 18) (47). Clinically speaking, this phenomenon is of little or no consequence as long as a normal end-tidal CO_2 is maintained.[f]

Other Uses of Capnography in Infants and Children

Waveform Interpretation

In children and adults ventilated through a semiclosed circle system with a CO_2 absorber, the normal capnographic waveform includes a return to zero baseline. The normal pediatric capnogram (like the waveform in adults) includes a sharp upstroke as alveolar gas displaces tracheal gas and a slightly ascending plateau phase. Significant deviations from this morphology suggest an abnormality in the patient, the gas delivery system, or the sampling technique.

Esophageal intubation is diagnosed by the absence of a waveform or a waveform with small rounded humps of decreasing height. Since the stomach could contain some CO_2 after a mask induction, more than one breath should be observed to confirm tracheal tube placement. For instance, when single-use color indicator devices are used to detect CO_2, six breaths are recommended to confirm tracheal placement. Bronchial intubation may initially give normal or slightly lower end-tidal PCO_2 measurements (Fig. 19). If, however, the bronchial placement is allowed to persist for a period of time and the lungs are hypoventilated, end-tidal PCO_2 may increase (Fig. 20) (34). Changes in the capnographic

---

[f]Ed. Note (JMB): For verification of this, one only has to look at Rayburn's CPRAM technique of controlled ventilation in which children are ventilated at rapid respiratory rates (~40 BPM) and low FGFs (1 to 2 L/min) (48). Using Rayburn's technique, rebreathing is maximal (capnographic baseline is elevated [F_ICO_2 is high]), and normal valves for end-tidal and arterial CO_2 are maintained.

138 *CHAPTER 5: ALVEOLAR VENTILATION*

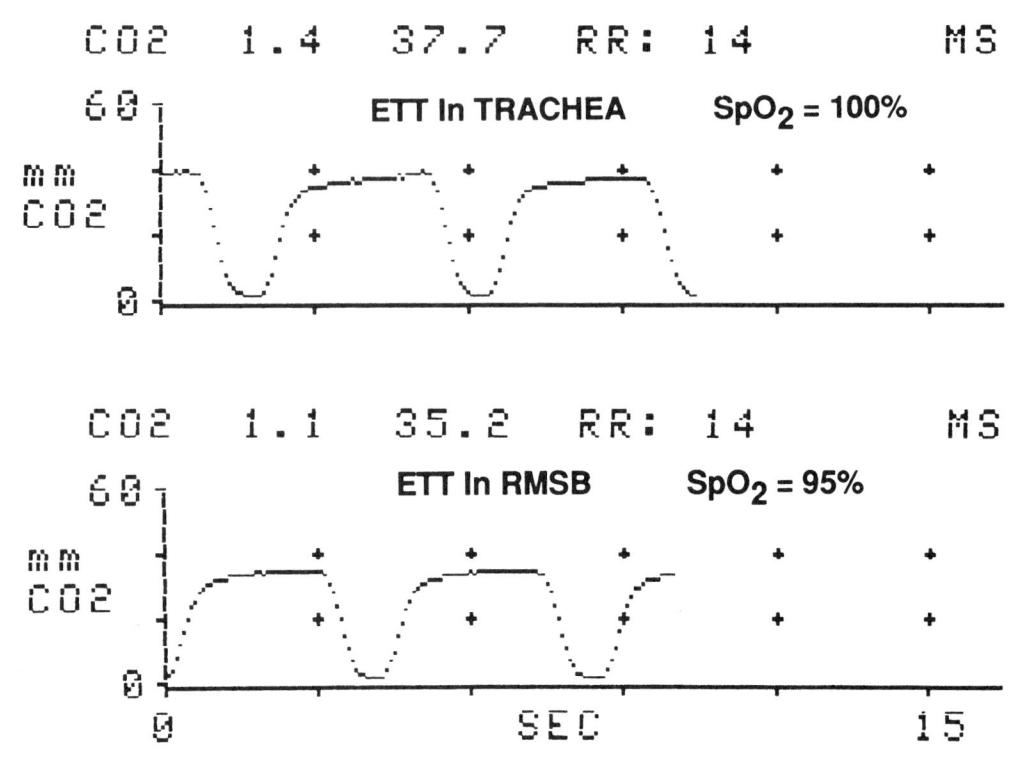

FIG. 19. The capnographic waveform measured by mass spectrometry from a 15-kg 18-month-old child ventilated with an Ohmeda 7810 ventilator and a semiclosed circle breathing system (Ohmeda, Madison, WI). When the endotracheal tube (ETT) was advanced from the trachea into the right main stem bronchus (RMSB) end-tidal PCO_2 decreased from 37.7 to 35.2 mm Hg, and oxygen saturation decreased from 100% to 95%. (Reprinted with permission, from Badgwell JM: Oximery and Capnography Monitoring. In *Anesthesiology Clinics of North America*. Vol 9, No. 4, 1991, p. 830.)

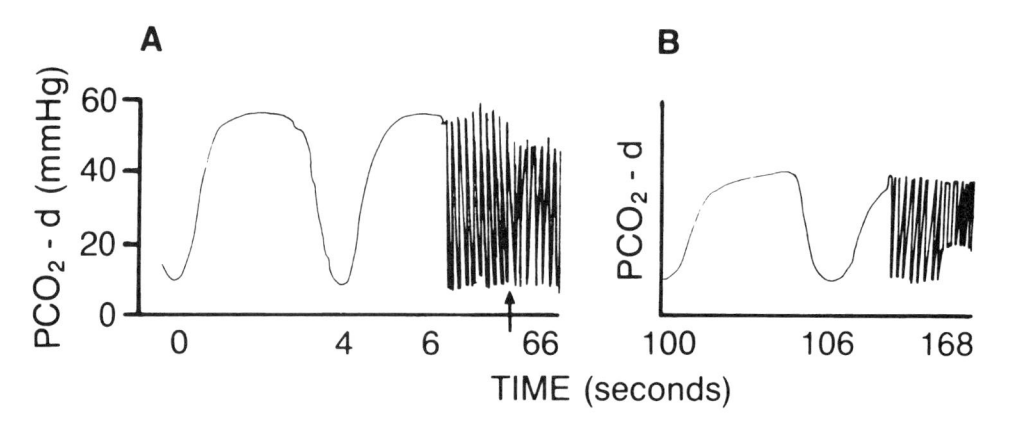

FIG. 20. (A) Capnographic waveform obtained from the distal end of the endotracheal tube and measured by infrared analysis in an 18-kg 4-year-old child ventilated with an Air-Shields Ventimeter. After 20 minutes of controlled ventilation, endobronchial intubation was diagnosed and treated. (B) After correct placement of the endotracheal tube (denoted by *arrow* in **A**) end-tidal PCO_2 returned to normal. (From Badgwell et al, ref. 34, with permission.)

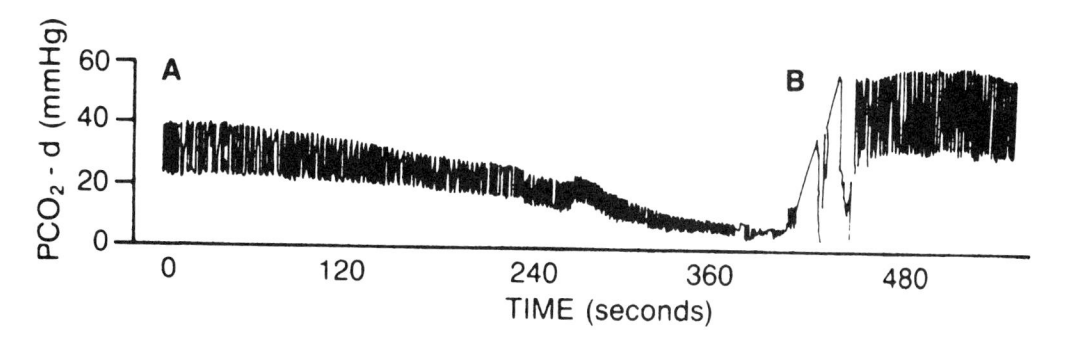

FIG. 21. Capnographic waveform at slow paper speed obtained from the distal end of the endotracheal tube in a 10-kg 1-year-old infant with systemic hypotension that occurred during controlled ventilation with 2% halothane and 70% N_2O/O_2. **(A)** The waveform shows a gradual but profound decrease in $P_{ET}CO_2$, suggesting decreased pulmonary blood flow and CO_2 delivery to the lungs. **(B)** Discontinuation of halothane and the administration of 100% oxygen was associated with a restoration of normal blood pressure and the return of end-tidal PCO_2 to above normal values. (From Badgwell et al, ref. 34, with permission.)

waveform are not diagnostic of a specific disorder. For instance, a sloping expiratory upstroke may indicate a kinked endotracheal tube or airway obstruction (e.g., bronchospasm).

A sudden disappearance of the capnogram indicates complete obstruction, breathing circuit disconnection, or a precipitous increase in dead space (pulmonary embolus or cardiac arrest). A gradual decrease in the end-tidal CO_2 may reflect alveolar hyperventilation of pulmonary hypoperfusion (Fig. 21). In essence, capnography may be used as an estimator of cardiac output. When cardiac output decreases, less CO_2 is delivered to the lungs for elimination and end-tidal CO_2 values will decrease. In fact, the presence of end-tidal CO_2 is often used as an indicator of the success of cardiopulmonary resuscitation. A slowly increasing end-tidal CO_2 may occur with alveolar hypoventilation or in circumstances in which the CO_2 production increases. A very rapid and large increase in the end-tidal CO_2 may suggest malignant hyperthermia. A gradual rise in both inspired and end-tidal CO_2 in a patient ventilated with a circle circuit may indicate faulty inspiratory or expiratory valves. Idiosyncratic inspiratory bumps occur when using the Sechrist Infant Ventilator (Fig. 22). Cardiac oscillations occur in children with slow respiratory rates and can be differentiated from curare clefts by comparing heart rates with the frequency of waveform oscillation (Fig. 23).

Plateaus and Arterial to End-Tidal CO_2 Differences

The presence of a plateau on the capnographic waveform does not always indicate that the end-tidal CO_2 value reflects the arterial CO_2 value. A flat plateau in the presence of a large arterial to end-tidal difference may occur in small infants when proximal sampling is used inappropriately (34) and in patients with large dead-space ventilation (e.g., bronchopulmonary dysplasia) (Fig. 24). By contrast, when accurate sampling is available in healthy infants and children, the arterial to end-tidal PCO_2 differences are small, negligible, or possibly of negative value (34). These data suggest that dead-space ventilation is minimal in these patients.

In infants and children with acyanotic congenital heart disease, end-tidal PCO_2 measurements are a reliable estimate of arterial PCO_2 (49). In infants and children with cyan-

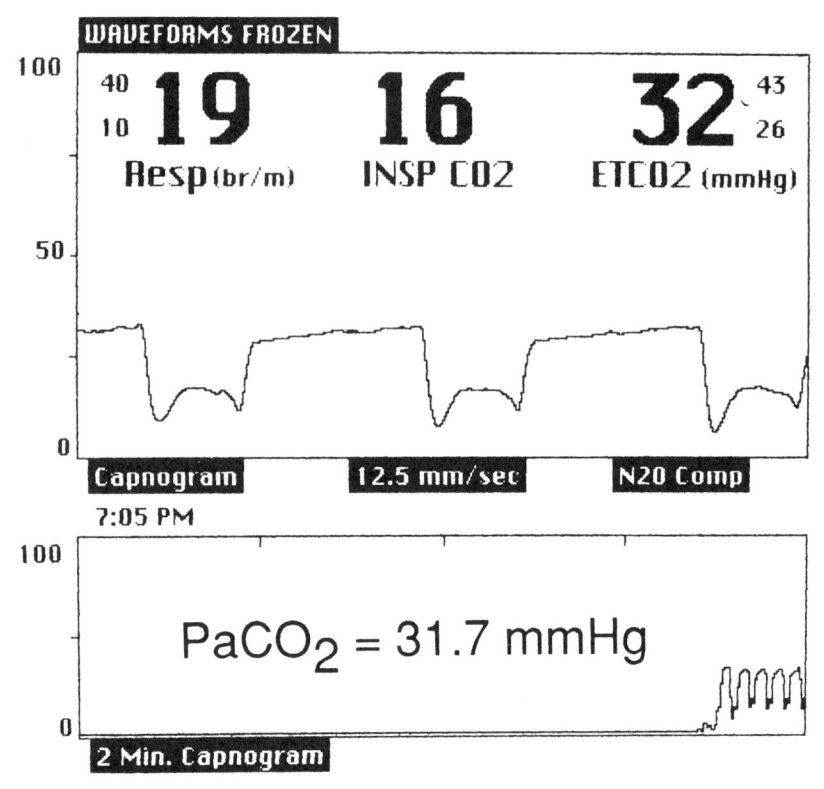

FIG. 22. Capnographic waveform measured by flow-through capnography from an 8.1-kg 10-month-old infant ventilated with a Sechrist Infant Ventilator. The humps that occur during the inspiratory phase are idiosyncratic for the Sechrist Ventilator and do not affect the adequacy of ventilation (unpublished data). Resp (br/m), respiratory breaths per minute; Insp, inspiratory, end-tidal CO2, nitrous oxide compensation. (Reprinted with permission, from Badgwell JM: Oximery and Capnography Monitoring. In *Anesthesiology Clinics of North America*. Vol. 9, No. 4, 1991, p. 832.)

otic congenital heart disease, end-tidal PCO_2 may not reliably estimate arterial PCO_2. In the latter group, both dead-space ventilation and venous admixture (Qs/Qt) increase the difference between arterial and end-tidal PCO_2. Increasing the Qs/Qt ratio increases the PCO_2 difference by shunting venous blood to the left side of the heart with a greater PCO_2 tension than that in the alveoli.

Relation of Capnography and Pulse Oximetry

SpO_2 and capnography together provide continuous monitoring of oxygenation, ventilation, and tissue perfusion. In the child with a decreasing cardiac output, the capnographic waveform may diminish gradually or suddenly, depending on the rate of cardiac collapse, along with the simultaneous failure of SpO_2. The presence or absence of blood pressure and pulses quickly confirms capnographic and oximetric evidence of a decreasing cardiac output.

SpO_2 reduces both the frequency and severity of hypoxemic events during anesthesia in children (24). Compared with capnography, oximetry is more likely to detect episodes of hypoxemia (50). This is not surprising in view of the nature of these monitors. Before the onset of arterial hemoglobin oxygen desaturation, capnography may provide an early warning of ventilation mishaps that may cause significant morbidity (e.g., esophageal intubation and disconnections). In a well-controlled

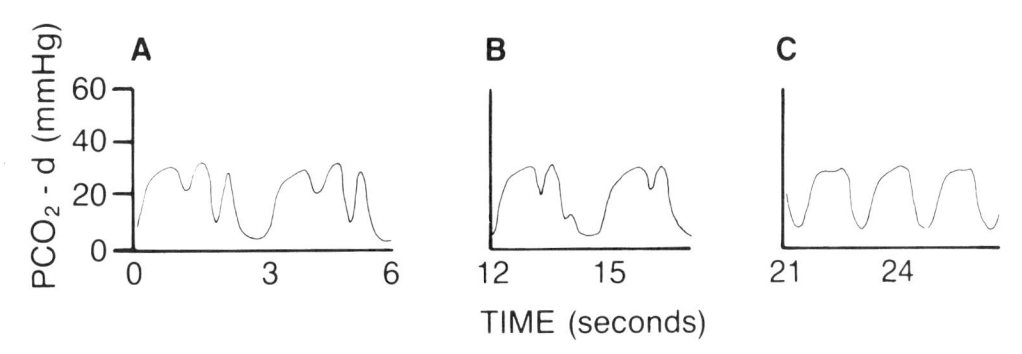

FIG. 23. Curare clefts, or spontaneous respiratory activity, indicating that the muscle relaxant is wearing off. In this case, increasing the rate of controlled ventilation (C) eliminated the curare clefts. (From Badgwell et al, ref. 34, with permission.)

study, anesthesiologists did not respond to changes in the capnograph until arterial hemoglobin oxygen desaturation confirmed the potential ventilation mishap (50). The authors concluded that oximetry is superior to capnography in providing an early warning sign of events that can cause hypoxemia (50). Nevertheless, capnography does have a very important role in preventing ventilation mishaps that could result in hypoxemia.

SUMMARY

Perioperative morbidity and mortality are greatest in childhood. This has been attributed to a large extent to perioperative hypoxic events. The introduction of pulse oximetry and capnography into pediatric anesthetic practice has dramatically decreased the frequency of hypoxic events and airway mishaps. Indeed, these monitors may be more sensitive at detecting adverse events than has the clinician's acumen. Since oximetry and capnography have become minimum standards for anesthetic care, it is our belief that perioperative morbidity and mortality will decrease. The inclusion of these two monitors in pediatric care may be the most important contributions to monitoring since the precordial stethoscope.

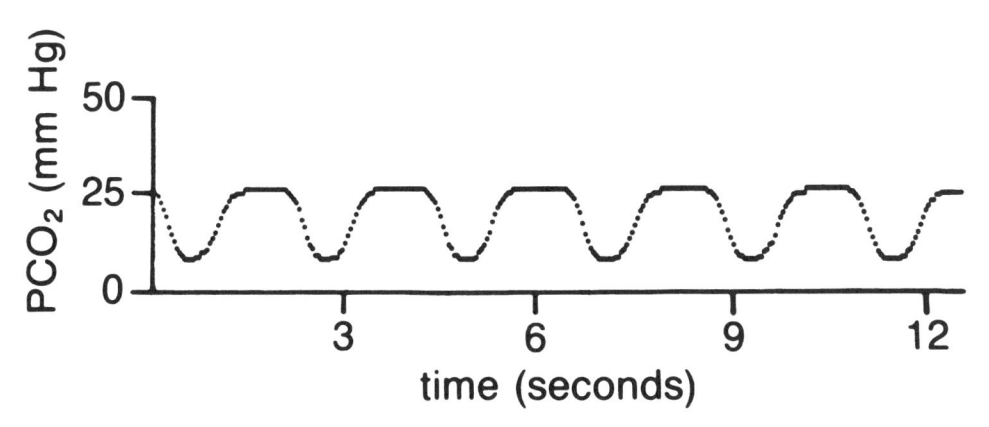

FIG. 24. Capnographic waveform showing the plateau phase in a 4.1-kg 2-month-old infant with bronchopulmonary dysplasia. PaCO$_2$ = 40.3 mm Hg, P$_{ET}$CO$_2$ = 26.4 mm Hg, and the difference between PaCO$_2$ and P$_{ET}$CO$_2$ = 13.9 mm Hg. The large difference between CO$_2$ valve is due to dead-space ventilation in this infant with chronic lung disease. (From Badgwell et al, ref. 34, with permission.)

REFERENCES

1. Morray JP, Geiduschek JM, Caplan RA, et al: A comparison of pediatric and adult anesthesia closed malpractice claims. *Anesthesiology* 1993;78:461–467.
2. Badgwell JM, Swan J, Foster AC: Volume-controlled ventilation is made possible in infants by using compliant breathing circuits with large compression volume. *Anesth Analg* 1996;82:719–723.
3. Spears RS Jr, Yeh A, Fisher DM, Zwass MS: The educated hand: can anesthesiologists assess changes in neonatal pulmonary compliance manually? *Anesthesiology* 1991;75:693–696.
4. Steward DJ: The not-so-educated hand of the pediatric anesthesiologist. *Anesthesiology* 1991;75:555–556.
5. Ayre P: Anaesthesia for hare lip and cleft palate operations on babies. *Br J Surg* 1937;25:313.
6. Ayre P: Endotracheal anesthesia for babies, with special references to hare-lip and cleft palate operations. *Anesth Analg* 1937;16:330.
7. Jackson-Rees GJ: Anesthesia in the newborn. *Br Med J* 1950;2:1419–1422.
8. Mapleson WW: The elimination of rebreathing in various semiclosed anesthetic systems. *Br J Anaesth* 1954;26:323.
9. Bain JA, Spoerel WE: Carbon dioxide output and elimination in children under anaesthesia. *Can Anaesth Soc J* 1977;24:533–539.
10. Badgwell JM, Wolf AR, McEvedy BA, et al: Fresh gas formulae do not accurately predict end-tidal PCO_2 in paediatric patients. *Can J Anaesth* 1988;35:581–586.
11. Ghani GA: Fresh gas flow affects minute volume during mechanical ventilation. *Anesth Analg* 1984;63:619.
12. Moynihan RJ, Cote CJ: Effects of varying ventilatory fresh gas flows on minute ventilation in pediatric patients using a circle system. *Anesthesiology* 1988;69:A270.
13. Gursory F, Algren JT, Skjorsby BS: Positive pressure ventilation with the laryngeal mask airway in children. *Anesth Analg* 1996;82:33–38.
14. American Society of Anesthesiologists: Standards for basic intraoperative monitoring. Anesthesia Patient Safety Foundation, March 3, 1987.
15. Sasse FJ: Can we trust end-tidal carbon dioxide measurements in infants? *J Clin Monit* 1985;1:147–148.
16. Carbon Dioxide Monitors. *Health Devices* 1986;15:225–284.
17. Severinghaus JW, Naifeh KH: Accuracy of response of six pulse oximeters to profound hypoxia. *Anesthesiology* 1987;67:551–558.
18. Eisenkraft JB: Pulse oximeter desaturation due to methemoglobinemia. *Anesthesiology* 1986;68:279–282.
19. Barker SJ, Tremper KK: The effect of carbon monoxide inhalation on pulse oximetry and transcutaneous PO_2. *Anesthesiology* 1987;66:677–679.
20. Scheller MS, Unger RJ, Kelner MJ: Effects of intravenously administered dyes on pulse oximetry readings. *Anesthesiology* 1986;65:550–552.
21. Pologe JS, Raley DM: Effects of fetal hemoglobin on pulse oximetry. *J Perinatol* 1987;VII:324–326.
22. Veyckemans F, Baele P, Guillaume JE, et al: Hyperbilirubinemia does not interfere with hemoglobin saturation measured by pulse oximetry. *Anesthesiology* 1989;70:118–122.
23. Severinghaus JW, Naifeh KH, Koh SO: Errors in 14 pulse oximeters during profound hypoxia. *J Clin Monit* 1989;5:72–81.
24. Coté CJ, Goldstein EA, Coté MA, et al: A single-blind study of pulse oximetry in children. *Anesthesiology* 1988;68:184–188.
25. Pullerits J, Burrows FA, Roy WL: Arterial desaturation in healthy children during transfer to the recover room. *Can J Anaesth* 1987;34:470–473.
26. Soliman IE, Patel RI, Ehrenpreis MB, Hannallah RS: Recovery scores do not correlate with postoperative hypoxemia in children. *Anesth Analg* 1988;67:53–56.
27. Sloan TB: Finger injury by an oxygen saturation monitor probe. *Anesthesiology* 1988;68:936–938.
28. Berge KH, Lanier WL, Scanlon PD: Ischemic digital skin necrosis: a complication of the reusable Nelcor probe oximeter probe [letter]. *Anesth Analg* 1988;67:712–713.
29. Chemello PD, Nelson SR, Wolford LM: Finger injury resulting from pulse oximeter probe during orthognathic surgery. *Oral Surg Oral Med Oral Pathol* 1990;69:161–163.
30. Miyasaka K, Ohata J: Burn, erosion, and "sun" tan with the use of pulse oximetry in infants. *Anesthesiology* 1987;67:1008–1009.
31. Shellock FG, Slimp GL: Severe burns on the finger caused by using a pulse oximeter during MR imaging. (Letter). *AJR* 1989;153:1105.
32. Nielsen J, Kann T, Moller JT: Evaluation of two newly developed anesthetic agent monitors: Bruel and Kjaer anesthetic agent monitor 1304 and Datex Ultima. *Anesthesiology* 1990;73:A538.
33. VanWagenen RA, Westenskow DR, Benner RE, et al: Dedicated monitoring of anesthetic and respiratory gases by Raman scattering. *J Clin Monit* 1986;2:215–222.
34. Badgwell JM, McLeod ME, Lerman J, Creighton RE: End-tidal PCO_2 measurements sampled at the distal and proximal ends of the endotracheal tube in infants and children. *Anesth Analg* 1987;66:959–964.
35. Badgwell JM, Heavner JE, May WS, et al: End-tidal PCO_2 monitoring in infants and children ventilated with either a partial rebreathing or a non-rebreathing circuit. *Anesthesiology* 1987;66:405–410.
36. Halpern L, Bissonnette B: Visualizing the mixing of fresh gas and expired gas in the Mapleson D circuit: a laboratory model. *Anesthesiology* 1991;75:A421.
37. Rich GF, Sullivan MP, Adams JM: Is distal sampling of end-tidal CO_2 necessary in small subjects? *Anesthesiology* 1990;73:265–268.
38. Gravenstein N: Capnometry in infants should not be done at lower sampling flow rates. (Letter). *J Clin Monit* 1989;5:63–64.
39. McEvedy BA, McLeod ME, Mulera M, et al: End-tidal, transcutaneous, and arterial PCO_2 measurements in critically ill neonates: a comparative study. *Anesthesiology* 1988;69:112–116.
40. Badgwell JM, Heavner JE: End-tidal carbon dioxide pressure in neonates and infants measured by aspiration and flow-through capnography. *J Clin Monit* 1991;7:285–288.
41. Hillier SC, Lerman J: Mainstream vs. sidestream capnography in anesthetized infants and children [abstract]. *Anesthesiology* 1989;71:318–321.

42. McEvedy BA, McLeod ME, Kirpalani H, et al: End-tidal carbon dioxide measurements in critically ill neonates: a comparison of side-stream and mainstream capnometers. *Can J Anaesth* 1990;37:322–326.
43. From RP, Scammon FL: Ventilatory frequency influences accuracy of end-tidal CO_2 measurements: analysis of seven capnometers. *Anesth Analg* 1988;67:884–886.
44. Badgwell JM, Heavner JE: Rebreathing affects deadspace in the Siemans-Elema 930 CO_2 analyzer. (Letter). *Anesth Analg* 1989;68:698–699.
45. Jameson LC, Popic PM: Adverse effect of respiratory rate on volatile anesthetic reporting in three infrared anesthetic monitors. *Anesthesiology* 1991;75:A418.
46. From RP, Scammon FL: Ventilatory frequency influences accuracy of end-tidal PCO_2 measurements. *Anesth Analg* 1988;67:884–886.
47. Badgwell JM, Kleinman SE, Heavner JE: Respiratory frequency and artifact affect the capnographic baseline in infants. *Anesth Analg* 1993;77:708–712.
48. Rayburn RL, Graves SA: A new concept of controlled ventilation in children with the Bain anesthetic circuit. *Anesthesiology* 1978;48:250–253.
49. Burrows FA: Physiologic deadspace, venous admixture, and the arterial to end-tidal carbon dioxide difference in infants and children undergoing cardiac surgery. *Anesthesiology* 1989;70:219–225.
50. Coté CJ, Rolf N, Liu LM, et al: A single blind study of combined pulse oximetry and capnography in children. *Anesthesiology* 1991;74:980–987.

6

General Anesthesia Maintenance, Emergence, and Tracheal Extubation

Ira S. Landsman, Peter J. Davis, and J. Michael Badgwell

"Sleep opens within us an inn for phantoms. In the morning we must sweep out the shadows."
—Gaston Bachelard

The administration of both intravenous and inhalational anesthetic agents to children presents significant challenges to the pediatric anesthesiologist. With growth and development, infants and small children undergo marked changes with respect to body composition and protein binding. In addition, changes occur with hepatic and renal blood flow and function. For the anesthesiologist, these physiologic perturbations can result in significant variability in patient-to-patient response to anesthetic agents. This chapter reviews the pharmacology of both volatile and intravenous anesthetic agents administered to children during maintenance of anesthesia. Included are tables that contain age-appropriate minimum alveolar concentrations for inhalation agents and dosing for opioid-based anesthesia. This chapter ends with a discussion of emergence from anesthesia and tracheal extubation.

MAINTENANCE OF ANESTHESIA WITH VOLATILE AND INTRAVENOUS AGENTS

There is no perfect maintenance anesthetic agent for infants and children, nor is one route of administration (e.g., vapor or intravenous) generally better than the other for all patients. Instead, most anesthetics in infants and children consist of a combination of volatile and intravenous agents and take into consideration the variability of children.

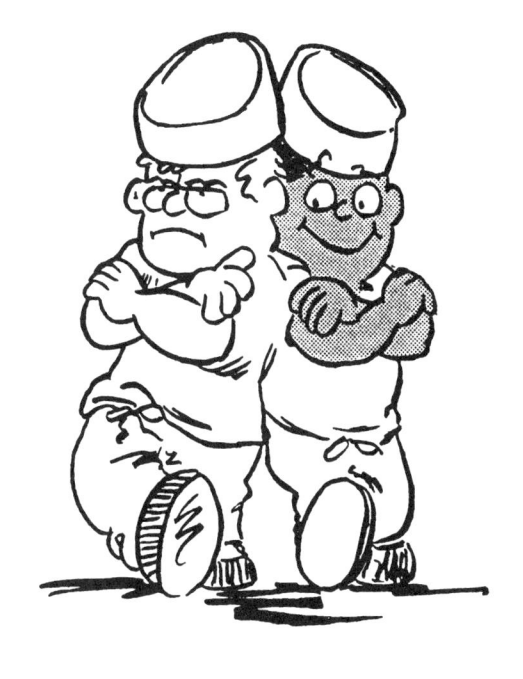

Volatile Anesthetic Agents

Minimum Alveolar Concentration

Age modifies the minimum alveolar concentration (MAC) of inhalation agents. In humans, the MACs for all anesthetic agents are highest between 6 and 12 months of age (Table 1). Inhalation agents have a lower MAC in neonates than in infants older than 1 month. Nevertheless, the MAC of all inhalation agents administered to the full-term newborn infant is equal to that of healthy adult patients. Premature neonates are more sensitive to inhalation agents than full-term babies.

TABLE 1. Age versus mean minimum alveolar concentration in children

Age (months)	Halothane[a]	Isoflurane[b]	Desflurane[c]	Sevoflurane[d]
1	0.87	1.6	9.16	3.2–3.3
2	1.08	1.9	9.4	3.2–3.3
14	0.97	1.8	8.72	2.5
44	0.91	1.6	8.54	2.5
480	0.76	1.2	7.5	2.5

[a]Cook DR, Marcy JH: Pediatric anesthetic pharmacology. In Cook DR, Marcy JH (eds): *Neonatal anesthesia.* Pasadena: Appleton-Davies, 1988:102.
[b]Cameron CB, Robinson S, Gregory GA: The minimum anesthetic concentration of isoflurane in children. *Anesth Analg* 1984;63:418–420.
[c]Taylor RH, Lerman J: Minimum alveolar concentration of desflurane and hemodynamic responses in neonates, infants, and children. *Anesthesiology* 1991;75:975–979.
[d]Lerman J, Sikich N, Kleinman S, Yentis S: The pharmacology of sevoflurane in infants and children. *Anesthesiology* 1994;80:814–824.

Premature infants of less than 32 weeks' gestation have a lower MAC for isoflurane than neonates of longer gestation (1).

Children under 1 year of age anesthetized with inhalation agents are at risk for cardiac toxicity despite their higher MAC requirements. Thus, there is a balance between the infant's need for higher inhalation agent concentrations and the risk of cardiovascular collapse (2–7).

Halothane

Halothane is an inhalation agent commonly administered to pediatric patients. If carefully monitored for bradycardia and hypotension, infants and children tolerate halothane for maintenance of general anesthesia. Halothane is not an ideal inhalation agent, however, because it can cause myocardial depression. The separation between MAC and the lethal concentration of a potent inhalation anesthetic agent defines the safety margin or the drug's therapeutic ratio. During the neonatal period, the therapeutic ratio for halothane is lower than at any other time during childhood. The concentration of halothane in the heart increases more rapidly in infants compared with adults anesthetized with the same inspired concentration of halothane. The short time constant of the infant's heart compared with the adult's heart allows halothane to quickly concentrate in the neonate's myocardium.

Therefore, when multiples of MAC are administered to infants and children (e.g., during induction or when inspired concentrations are changed rapidly), the risk of developing cardiac toxicity is high.

In the pediatric patient, it is not surprising that episodes of anesthetic-related bradycardia and cardiac arrest occur during these periods (8). Halothane may also induce hypotension and bradycardia by attenuation of baroreceptor reflexes. Although atropine reverses halothane-induced bradycardia, it cannot reverse halothane-induced myocardial depression (9,10).

All volatile agents, especially halothane, sensitize the myocardium to the dysrhythmogenic properties of epinephrine (11). Such dysrhythmias are more common in adults than children (12,13). Children rarely develop ventricular irritability despite receiving intravenous doses of epinephrine exceeding 1.7 µg/kg. In fact, if $PaCO_2$ is normal, children anesthetized with halothane who are undergoing cleft palate repair can tolerate 7 to 10 µg/kg of epinephrine combined with 1% lidocaine without ventricular irritability (13,14).

Administration of nitrous oxide or opioids or the use of regional anesthesia techniques as a supplement to general inhalation anesthesia reduces the risk for cardiac toxicity by lowering the MAC of halothane necessary to maintain general anesthesia. With the addition of regional anesthetic techniques, the inhalation requirements for halothane and other potent inhalation agents can be reduced almost to MAC awake levels, making rapid emergence from general anesthesia possible.

Although halothane hepatitis is a concern in adults, it rarely occurs in prepubertal children, even after repeated exposure (15,16).

Isoflurane

Whereas isoflurane causes vasodilation without myocardial depression or bradycardia in adult patients, infants age 5 to 26 weeks, anesthetized with isoflurane (not premedicated with atropine) may exhibit bradycardia, vasodilation, and myocardial depression (17). In older children, isoflurane causes less myocardial depression than halothane. Both isoflurane and halothane decrease blood pressure with a minimal effect on heart rate in unpremedicated children aged 2 to 7 years (18). In these children, however, left ventricular function may be impaired in children receiving halothane compared with those receiving isoflurane (18).

On emergence from anesthesia, pediatric ambulatory surgical patients receiving isoflurane show a more rapid decrease in end-expired concentration than those receiving halothane (19). The times required for response to pharyngeal suction and tracheal extubation, however, are similar for both isoflurane and halothane.

Desflurane

Desflurane is a potent inhalation agent with a blood gas solubility of 0.42 that is similar to nitrous oxide (0.46). As with other inhalation anesthetics, age modifies the MAC of desflurane (see Table 1). Desflurane is an airway irritant. If used as an induction agent, desflurane causes an unacceptably high incidence of laryngospasm, coughing, and hypoxia (20, 21). Emergence from desflurane anesthesia, however, does not seem to cause airway irritability (21).

Compared with those maintained with halothane, children maintained with desflurane have shorter emergence times but similar duration in the postanesthesia care unit (PACU) (22). One can expect to see a higher incidence of postanesthesia agitation and excitement in children receiving desflurane compared with those receiving halothane or sevoflurane anesthesia (22). Therefore, children anesthetized with desflurane may require low doses of intraoperative opioids (1 to 2 μ/kg of fentanyl) to reduce this reaction to emergence. The addition of fentanyl may slow the emergence time, but decrease the intensity of this excitement phase.

The cardiovascular profile of desflurane is similar to isoflurane. At 1 MAC, desflurane, like isoflurane and halothane, appears to attenuate the baroresponse in young children. Thus, hypotension may occur without compensatory tachycardia. However, older children compensate for desflurane-induced vasodilation by reflex tachycardia. In both adults and children, rapid increases in desflurane from 0.55 to 1.66 MAC cause sympathetic stimulation, which in turn causes transient increase in arterial blood pressure and heart rate (23).

Anesthetic doses of desflurane depend on the surgical procedure and associated degree of stimulation. In children, 60% nitrous oxide only decreases MAC by 25% (24). Using regional anesthesia or opioids to supplement desflurane, general anesthesia markedly decreases the MAC of desflurane (25).

Sevoflurane

Sevoflurane is a fluoromethyl propylether with a blood-gas solubility coefficient of 0.68. In children, combining nitrous oxide with sevoflurane greatly increases the uptake of sevoflurane during anesthesia induction (26). In children, the addition of 60% nitrous oxide decreases the MAC by only 25% (27,28). As with other potent inhalation agents, intraoperative regional anesthesia and treatment with intraoperative opioids markedly decreases MAC requirements.

Emergence from sevoflurane anesthesia occurs faster than from halothane (29) but probably slower than from desflurane (26). The rate of emergence delirium and excitement seen in children anesthetized with sevoflurane is higher than halothane (29) or isoflurane, and in our clinical observations, similar to desflurane.

The cardiovascular effects of sevoflurane in children at 1 MAC are similar to those of desflurane. Heart rate at 1 MAC for infants and children under 3 years is preserved. In older children, heart rate increases by 10%. At 1 MAC, systolic blood pressure decreases 20% to 30% from awake values in all children, regardless of age (28). Sevoflurane, like isoflurane and desflurane, minimally sensitizes the myocardium to the dysrhythmogenic properties of epinephrine (30).

The metabolism and degradation of sevoflurane are two potential concerns regarding sevoflurane use in children (31). The metabolism of sevoflurane occurs primarily in the liver by the cytochrome P450 system. Sevoflurane is metabolized to organic and inorganic fluoride. Elevated serum fluoride levels (>50 micromolar [μM]) may cause nephrogenic diabetes insipidus. However, in both adult and pediatric studies there are no reports of nephrogenic diabetes insipidus in patients receiving sevoflurane whose serum fluoride levels were greater than 50 μM. In these patients, desmopressin challenge tests, renal concentrating ability, and creatinine clearance remained normal.

Degradation of sevoflurane occurs in soda lime and barium hydroxide lime and creates two potentially toxic olefins—compound A and compound B. These compounds cause toxicity in animals. However, several studies have demonstrated that adults exposed to anesthetic concentrations of sevoflurane for prolonged times do not produce toxic levels of these olefins and have no clinical evidence of toxicity (32,33).

Opioids

Almost any pediatric patient may be a candidate for opioid therapy. Age-dependent considerations, however, are important to consider. For instance, neonates treated with opioids are at risk for postoperative apnea. There are, however, benefits of opioids in this age group. For example, neonates who receive treatment with high-dose opioids during cardiovascular surgery will have lower levels of stress hormone release than infants anesthetized with only nitrous oxide (34). Attenuation of stress hormone release is good in babies because they have less perioperative protein catabolism and less postoperative instability.

Because infants under 3 months of age metabolize opioids at a slower and more unpredictable rate than older patients, these infants require apnea monitoring for 12 to 24 hours after receiving intraoperative opioids. Furthermore, because neonates may have delayed drug clearance, fentanyl will have a longer duration of action. Therefore, the neonate who receives fentanyl in the intraoperative period may develop apnea in the postoperative period and should be monitored. By 3 months of age, infants develop efficient opioid metabolism. After 9 to 12 months of age, infants actually have faster opioid clearance than adults.

During general anesthesia, opioids may be administered as part of a balanced general anesthetic, reducing the MAC of inhalation agents. For example, in adults, 3 μg/kg of fentanyl reduces the MAC of desflurane by 30% (35). Many clinicians administer 1 to 2 μg/kg of fentanyl and 0.5 MAC isoflurane to infants and children as their bread-and-butter anesthetic. An older child who receives 2 μg/kg of fentanyl during general inhalation anesthesia rarely develops postoperative apnea.

High-dose opioid administration (e.g., an opioid as the sole anesthetic agent) is usually reserved for children with cardiac instability requiring surgical intervention. Since these patients require postoperative mechanical ventilation, opioid-induced apnea is not a concern.

In pediatric ambulatory surgical patients, children less than 6 months of age seldom require opioid therapy. Acetaminophen or ketorolac usually controls pain after insertion of myringotomy tubes or after eye muscle surgery. For patients undergoing lower-extremity procedures or genitourinary surgery, regional anesthesia combined with light general anesthesia provides analgesia during the intraoperative and postoperative periods. Is administration of opioids to infants less than 3 months of age safe in the same-day surgery setting? Although no well-controlled studies have been carried out, infants under 3 months of age who are receiving opioids must have close monitoring for postoperative respiratory depression.

Morphine

Children frequently receive morphine for intraoperative and postoperative analgesia. It has a longer elimination half-life (6.8 compared with 3.9 hours) and clearance (6.3 compared with 23.8 ml/min/kg) in infants 1 to 7 days old than in those over 17 days (35,36). In neonates, interindividual variability in the pharmacokinetics of morphine is large. Therefore, the neonate's clinical response to morphine may be unpredictable. By 30 days of life, the half-life of morphine approaches the 2-hour half-life seen in healthy adult patients (35). After an infant is 3 months of age, morphine clearance is equal to or better than that in the adult patient.

In neonates and infants 2 to 570 days old, morphine serum levels directly correlate with respiratory depression (37). Serum concentrations higher than 20 ng/ml during a morphine infusion are associated with respiratory depression in these patients, regardless of age. After discontinuation of the morphine infusion, adequate breathing resumes when concentrations reach 15 ng/ml or less. Thus, at equal blood levels, age is not a factor in morphine-induced respiratory depression.

When accompanied by potent inhalation anesthesia, a typical intraoperative morphine dose in children over 3 months is 0.1 mg/kg every 2 hours. In either the intraoperative or the postoperative period, treatment of neonates with morphine should proceed at lower bolus doses and wider dose intervals than those recommended for older children.

For surgeries lasting longer than 2 hours, a bolus dose of 0.1 mg/kg per 2 hours of surgical time injected after induction of anesthesia produces excellent intraoperative analgesia and several hours of postoperative analgesia. High-morphine bolus doses stimulate histamine release. Histamine-induced flushing and hypotension are usually minor. However, intravenous injection of morphine with muscle relaxants known to stimulate histamine release can on the rare occasion result in hypotension. Treatment of histamine-induced hypotension, should it occur, includes fluid resuscitation, α_1-agonists, or both.

Fentanyl

Fentanyl, a synthetic, lipid-soluble opioid agonist, is 50 to 100 times more potent than morphine. Because of its lipid solubility, a single dose of fentanyl has a more rapid onset and shorter duration of action than morphine. Multiple doses or continuous infusion of fentanyl eventually saturate inactive tissue sites, leading to prolongation of fentanyl's duration of action (38). Thus, patients receiving high-dose fentanyl or multiple doses of fentanyl have a greater risk of developing late postoperative respiratory depression than those receiving low-dose fentanyl.

Neonates show variable pharmacokinetics, depending on the type and site of surgery. Increased intra-abdominal pressure can diminish hepatic blood flow, increasing the terminal elimination half-life of fentanyl (39). Therefore, duration of action of fentanyl may be prolonged in infants and children after major surgery (e.g., gastroschisis).

As in adults, postoperative fentanyl concentrations are associated with respiratory depression in infants and children receiving fentanyl anesthesia (40). Infants and children over 3 months of age may experience respiratory depression at similar blood concentrations as adults. Infants older than 3 months of age may actually have less hypoventilation than adults. Nevertheless, infants may develop hypoventilation at lower than expected plasma fentanyl concentrations. Thus, infants less than 3 months of age receiving intraoperative fentanyl require monitoring of ventilation and oxygenation postoperatively.

Chest Wall Rigidity

An important complication from fentanyl therapy is chest wall rigidity, severe enough to impede ventilation. Although the mechanism of chest wall rigidity is uncertain, the origin of rigidity is probably outside the stretch reflex arc and originates either in another area of the spinal cord or in higher centers of the brain (41). Glottic rigidity, causing glottic closure and upper airway obstruction, may also occur. Because children are usually anesthetized and paralyzed before opioid administration, chest wall rigidity is an infrequent complication.

Cardiovascular Stability and Respiratory Depression

Cardiovascular stability appears well preserved with opioid anesthesia. In preterm infants 1 day to 6 weeks old undergoing patent ductus arteriosus ligation, the administration of 30 to 50 µg/kg of fentanyl can be expected to maintain "railroad track" hemodynamic stability (42). Even at doses approaching 100 µg/kg, fentanyl will cause bradycardia but not myocardial depression (43). Atropine and pancuronium attenuate fentanyl-induced bradycardia. When using fentanyl as a supplement to balanced general anesthesia, an initial bolus dose of 2 to 5 µg/kg followed by 1 to 2 µg/kg every 1 to 2 hours provides effective analgesia. At these doses, postoperative respiratory depression is usually not a problem. Doses used in high-dose fentanyl anesthesia and fentanyl infusions appear below. **(see Narcotic-Based Anesthetics).**

Alfentanil

Alfentanil is a rapid-acting opioid with short duration of action and 10% of the potency of fentanyl. Because the pKa of alfentanil is 6.8, approximately 90% of alfentanil is in the unionized form at physiologic pH. Because the unionized form quickly crosses the blood-brain barrier, alfentanil has a quick onset time. Its volume of distribution is smaller than that of fentanyl. Alfentanil's brief duration of action is the result of redistribution to inactive tissue sites and hepatic metabolism. Alfentanil is dependent on intact hepatic function for clearance. In adult patients but not children with end-stage liver disease, alfentanil has a prolonged elimination half-life and thus a prolonged clinical effect (44,45). As with fentanyl, bolus doses of alfentanil can cause bradycardia (46). Chest wall rigidity has been observed in all age groups including neonates (47).

Pharmacokinetic studies of alfentanil in pediatric and adult patients demonstrate wide interpatient variability (48–51). The pharmacokinetics of alfentanil is similar in children 3 months to 14 years of age and in adults (50). Prolongation of alfentanil's half-life during the first few days of life is due to immature hepatic metabolism. Neonates in the first 3 days of life have lower clearance and longer elimination half-life than do older children (51).

Alfentanil infusion, delivered with 60% inhaled nitrous oxide, provides adequate general anesthesia. In adults receiving 60% nitrous oxide, different plasma concentrations of alfentanil are required for different levels of surgical stimulation (52). The same may be true for children. Knowing the drug's pharmacokinetics (volume of distribution and clearance) combined with the desired targeted plasma concentrations, simple formulas can be used to calculate a bolus dose and a continuous infusion rate (see equations in following text).

In general, 10 to 15 minutes after termination of alfentanil infusion, children over 3 months of age are alert and ready for extubation. However, wide variability in alfentanil's emergence times may reflect its large variability in clearance. Although postoperative respiratory depression can occur after alfentanil administration, the more common side effects observed with alfentanil are postoperative nausea and vomiting. Because of the increased incidence of nausea and vomiting, patients anesthetized with alfentanil may require longer PACU observation than children undergoing general inhalation anesthesia (22). In children, a bolus dose of 100 to 150 μg/kg of alfentanil followed by a continuous infusion of 2 to 5 μg/kg/min supplemented with 60% inhaled nitrous oxide will provide adequate anesthesia for most pediatric surgical procedures.

Sufentanil

Sufentanil is a synthetic opioid chemically related to fentanyl but 5 to 10 times more potent. Sufentanil's half-life is between that of fentanyl and alfentanil. Like fentanyl, sufentanil maintains cardiovascular stability without stimulating the release of histamine.

During the neonatal period, immature mechanisms for drug metabolism are responsible for sufentanil's longer duration of action (53). In healthy children between 2 and 10 years, sufentanil has a shorter half-life than in adolescents and adults (54). When comparing the sufentanil dose requirements to maintain analgesia or anesthesia in adults and children, neonates require less sufentanil at longer intervals, whereas older children require higher doses at shorter intervals.

As with other opioids, sufentanil can cause bradycardia. In younger children with heart rate–dependent cardiac output, atropine or pancuronium may attenuate hypotension secondary to opioid-induced bradycardia. Like fentanyl and alfentanil, sufentanil causes chest wall rigidity and delayed respiratory depression.

Narcotic-Based Anesthetics

Narcotic-based anesthesia is a method for maintaining general anesthesia primarily with opioids. When using this method, other agents may be necessary to maintain amnesia and ensure hemodynamic stability. Commonly used amnestic agents include nitrous oxide, low-dose potent inhalation agent, benzodiazepines, or scopolamine. Because narcotic-based anesthesia may not completely attenuate stress hormone release, stress-induced hypertension and tachycardia may require treatment with low-dose inhalation agents or antihypertensive agents. High-dose synthetic opioids maintain cardiovascular stability in patients with heart disease. Usual doses for cardiac surgery include fentanyl, 50 to 100 μg/kg, or sufentanil, 8 to 15 μg/kg.

Continuous opioid infusions are popular for providing general anesthesia during major orthopedic and neurosurgical procedures. Many anesthetic agents diminish normal signals measured by somatosensory-evoked response. Opioid infusion with inhaled nitrous oxide, unlike potent inhalation agents and propofol, will not diminish these signals. In patients with intracranial hypertension undergoing neurosurgical procedures, opioid-based anesthesia will not increase cerebral vascular flow.

Doses for opioid infusions are derived from simple general formulas used for calculating continuous infusions of any drug (Table 2).

TABLE 2. *Suggested doses for opioids in children over 3 months old after inhalation induction or intravenous induction with nonopioid agents*

Opioid	Bolus Dose in g/kg[a]	Infusion rate[b]	Time to end infusion (min)[c]	Elimination half-life in minutes
Alfentanil	50–100	2.5–5 μg/kg/min	20	70–90
Fentanyl	5–10	2–4 μg/kg/min	45	185–219
Sufentanil	0.5–1	0.2–0.5 μg/kg/min[d]	30	148–164

[a] Not an induction dose for general anesthesia.
[b] Note infusions are either μg/kg/min or μg/kg/h.
[c] Time required for the patient to regain consciousness after ending the opioid infusion.
[d] Total dose of sufentanil should be less than or equal to 1 μg/kg/h.

TABLE 3. *Target opioid concentrations (ng/ml)*

	Fentanyl	Alfentanil	Sufentanil
Induction and intubation			
Thiopental	3–5	250–400	0.4–0.6
O_2/N_2O only	8–10	400–750	0.8–1.2
Maintenance			
N_2O/potent vapor	1.5–4	100–300	0.25–0.5
O_2/N_2O only	1.5–10	100–750	0.25–1.0
O_2 only	15–60	1000–4000	10–60
Adequate ventilation on emergence	1.5	125	0.25

These formulas require knowledge of the drug's volume of distribution, clearance, and targeted plasma concentration (Table 3). The bolus dose is calculated as the product of the volume of distribution (VD) and the desired plasma concentration (Cp):

$$\text{Bolus dose} = VD \times Cp$$

The maintenance infusion rate (MIR) is calculated as the product of the desired plasma concentration (Cp) and the clearance (Cl):

$$MIR = Cl \times Cp$$

Although these formulas work well at estimating plasma target concentrations, they are not always precise. Consequently, the concept of context-sensitive half-time may better describe how to administer drugs by continuous infusion. The context-sensitive half-life describes the time required for the central compartment drug concentration to decline by 50% after ending an infusion (55). Using complex pharmacokinetic modeling, context-sensitive half-times can predict differences in drug effect in relation to the duration of the drug's infusion. An increase in drug infusion duration generally increases the drug's context-sensitive half-time. This increase in context-sensitive half-time will increase the time required between discontinuation of a drug infusion and the patient awakening from anesthesia (55,56).

After emerging from opioid-based anesthesia, removal of the endotracheal tube should take place only after the patient demonstrates a regular respiratory rate and a normal gag reflex. For 4 hours after discontinuing fentanyl or sufentanil infusions, patients are at risk for developing delayed apnea. These patients require frequent monitoring of depth and rate of respiration. Patients receiving narcotic-based anesthesia rarely develop emergence delirium, but may suffer from nausea and vomiting.

EMERGENCE FROM ANESTHESIA

"No matter what time it is, wake me up, even if it's in the middle of a Cabinet meeting."
—Ronald Reagan

Sooner or later, the infant or child will be allowed to wake up from a general anesthetic. Whether these patients are extubated before or after they wake up is addressed in the following text. Plans for emergence are designed well before the child wakes up (Fig. 1). There are two clinical tips that are important. These tips concern the "sundown sign of imminent awakening" and the "blue-but-well-ventilated-child" with a probe patent foramen ovale.

Sundown Sign of Imminent Awakening

The sundown sign refers to contraction of the inferior rectus muscle of the eye causing the eyeball to look downward toward the toes. This sign is an indication of light anesthesia and occurs just before the patient starts moving and trying to get off the table. The sign is especially helpful to watch for during strabismus surgery. If the ophthalmologist tells you the patient is looking down (instead of the normal straight-ahead gaze associated with deep anesthesia), it may be advantageous to deepen the anesthetic or give a muscle relaxant, depending on where you are in the case.

The Blue-But-Well-Ventilated-Child During Emergence

Approximately 34% of infants and children have a probe patent foramen ovale (PPFO) in the first decade of life (57). If, during emergence (or induction, for that matter), one of these patients with PPFO develops increased pulmonary vascular resistance (e.g., by bucking on the tracheal tube during awakening), a right-to-left (R → L) cardiac shunt may occur across the now patent foramen ovale, and the child will be cyanotic (58). The diagnosis is made only after the child's bucking is overcome and alveolar ventilation through a patent tracheal tube is ensured. Remember that a blue patient during emergence may be cyanotic from other causes, most notably alveolar hypoventilation (e.g., obstructed tracheal tube, esophageal intubation, inadequate ventilation due to chest wall rigidity). These causes must be ruled out before R → L shunt via a PPFO is diagnosed. If PPFO is the diagnosis, it will resolve within a few seconds and the patient will be none the worse. While the child is cyanotic (and other causes of cyanosis are ruled out), the child's lungs should be maintained by ventilation with 100% oxygen and the child should be helped to awaken peacefully while being monitored for adequacy of ventilation (e.g., capnography, observation of chest wall movement) and waiting for the cyanosis to resolve.

Therefore, it is recommended that the lungs be ventilated with 100% oxygen throughout the period of emergence from anesthesia to reduce the incidence and severity of hypoxemia. Failure to ventilate the patient's lungs with 100% oxygen may permit alveolar hypoxia to occur, which, in combination with hemodynamic effects of coughing and straining, can result in pulmonary vasoconstriction, increased right atrial pressure, and as mentioned above, a R → L shunt with profound hypoxemia in children who have a persistent patent foramen ovale.

TRACHEAL EXTUBATION

In most pediatric surgical cases, the tracheal tube is removed at the end of surgery. Clinical practice varies regarding tracheal extubation when the patient is "deep" or "awake." This area is somewhat controversial; emotional advocates can be found on both sides of the issue. For example, devotees of the "deep" school of thought are proud of the "little angels" they deliver to the PACU.

The anesthetic plan determines the manner of extubation. The choice of deep versus awake extubation is made before initiation of anesthesia (Fig. 1). For example, if one plans to administer muscle relaxants and controlled ventilation in an infant for abdominal surgery, then awake is the logical choice for

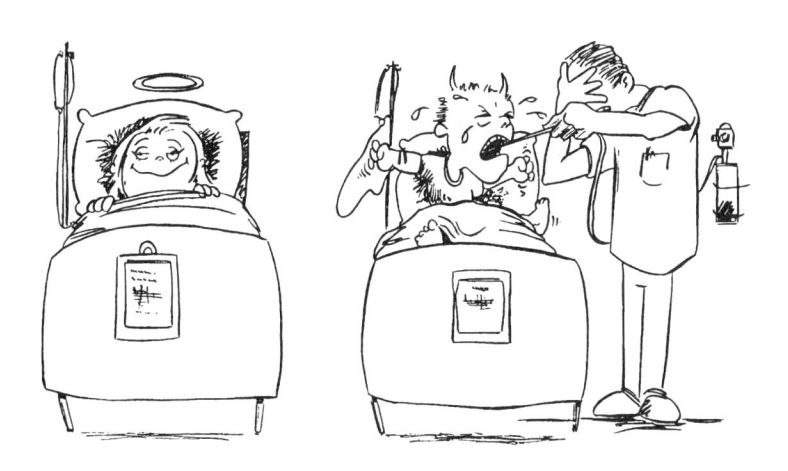

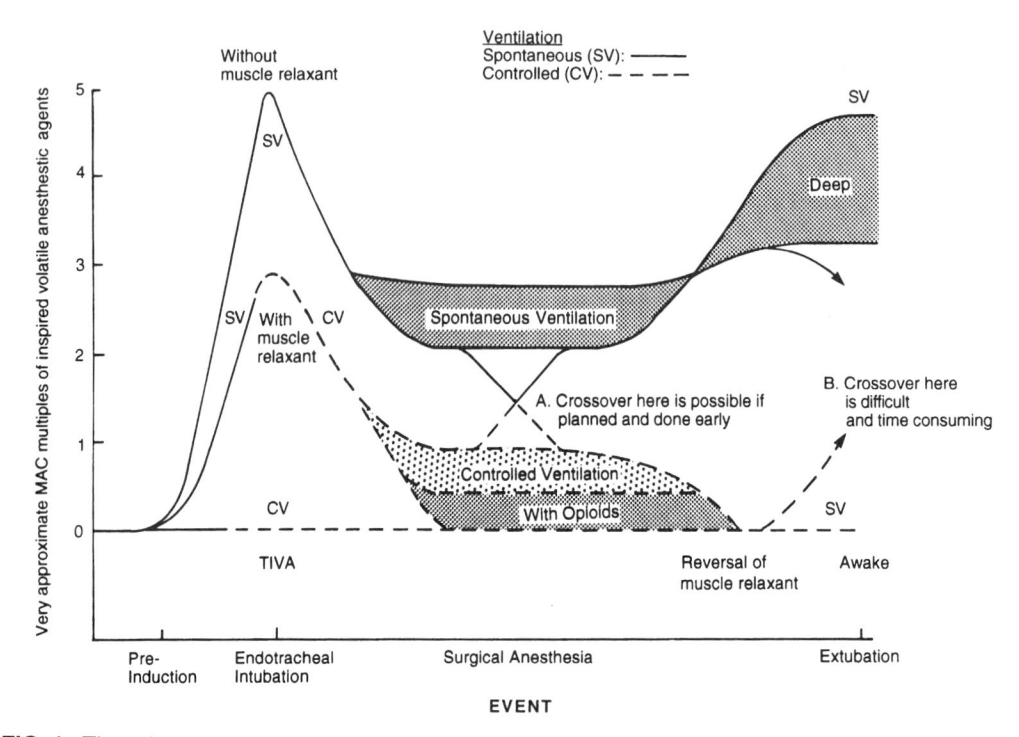

FIG. 1. The relationship of very approximate minimum alveolar concentration (MAC) multiples of inspired volatile anesthetic agents and surgical events. At induction and beginning with a baseline of 0 MAC, the inspired concentration of inhaled agent is increased until the patient is deep enough to tolerate endotracheal intubation. Insertion of an intravenous line and administration of a muscle relaxant and/or an IV agent allow endotracheal intubation at a lower inspired concentration of volatile agent. Of course, an intravenous induction would require no volatile agent, nor would total intravenous anesthesia (TIVA). After endotracheal intubation, the child is allowed to breath spontaneously (SV), or ventilation is controlled (CV). Crossover from controlled to spontaneous ventilation is feasible if planned and done early. Likewise, crossover from spontaneous to controlled ventilation is feasible after careful planning and early institution. By contrast, late crossover—either way—is difficult and time-consuming. Therefore, the method of extubation (e.g., awake versus deep) is decided on early, usually before the induction of anesthesia.

extubation. By contrast, if an older child for dental restoration under inhalational anesthesia is allowed to breath spontaneously, deep extubation is appropriate. As a general rule, spontaneously breathing patients do well with deep extubation and patients with controlled ventilation do well with awake extubation. One technique is to maintain adequate muscle paralysis (e.g., one of four in train-of-four) during the latter portion of the procedure and to incrementally lower the inspired concentration of volatile anesthetic agent. The goal of this technique is to time the wake-up with the last stitch (or last strip of bandage). Gradually, the inhaled agent is discontinued so that it may be eliminated by the child's lungs to amnestic expired concentrations. As the bandage goes on, muscle relaxant reversal is given and the child awakens promptly.

Extubation in Deeply Anesthetized Children

Deep extubation is a colloquial expression describing tracheal extubation while a patient is deeply anesthetized but spontaneously breathing. If done correctly, this method of tracheal extubation decreases the likelihood that tracheal stimulation by the endotracheal tube will cause coughing. This method of tracheal extubation should be done in healthy children who are properly fasted and without airway difficulties.[a] Some clinicians advocate tracheal extubation in deeply anesthetized patients with asthma. By extubating the trachea under a deep plane of anesthesia, bronchospasm in response to tracheal stimulation is attenuated. Removing the endotracheal tube in the deeply anesthetized patient undergoing eye surgery may prevent increased intraocular pressure caused by coughing. Obviously, this technique for extubation does not eliminate the risks of coughing, aspiration, or laryngospasm during the recovery period. In fact, during emergence, blood or mucus draining from the nose or mouth can stimulate the unprotected airway.

The Badgwell Technique of Deep Extubation

The patient is allowed to breathe spontaneously during surgery. For the sake of discussion, isoflurane is our inhalation agent. Inhalation anesthesia is maintained at inspired concentrations necessary to ensure spontaneous breathing without movement to surgical stimulation. When surgery is completed, N_2O is discontinued and the patient allowed to breathe 95% to 97% oxygen. The inspired concentration of isoflurane is increased to 3% to 5%. Before extubation, the patient should exhibit diaphragmatic breathing without the use of intercostal or accessory muscles. While the child is deep, the stomach and posterior pharynx are suctioned to clear secretions. An increase in heart rate, a change in respiratory pattern, or movement suggests the child is at too light a plane of anesthesia to tolerate deep extubation. If the patient shows these signs of being too light for deep extubation, there are two options: (a) deepen the plane of anesthesia or (b) make plans to extubate the child when fully awake.

Both options take time, especially when going from deep to light anesthesia, depending on the depth of anesthesia and the presence or absence of apnea or breath-holding (Fig. 1). Therefore, for many experienced clinicians, deep is deep (e.g., 5% isoflurane). Although studies have defined a MAC for extubation (57,58), a fair number of patients extubated at MAC for extubation experienced airway complications (57,58). "Deep enough" is when the child has only a diaphragmatic flicker remaining and is deep enough to be almost apneic.

Of course, one should avoid pushing the child to the brink of cardiovascular collapse with this technique. Therefore, deep extubation is done only in children who are hemodynamically stable. As a built-in safety factor, children who are allowed to spontaneously breathe volatile agents (even relatively high concentrations) are somewhat protected against myocardial depression because they will stop breathing (i.e., the respiratory control center will be depressed) before myocardial contractility is significantly depressed. By contrast, controlled ventilation with high concentrations of volatile agents will override the respiratory control center and poison the heart. In short, a spontaneously breathing child with stable hemodynamics and stable volume status will not necessarily experience cardiovascular depression during a brief period of inhaling 5% isoflurane for a deep extubation. Nevertheless, hemodynamic monitoring is required and adjustments made to inspired concentrations, if hypotension or bradycardia occurs. The risk of cardiac depression must be measured against the advantage of a deep extubation. Getting the child deep ensures that the airway reflexes are truly attenuated and the risk of coughing, bucking, breath-holding, and laryngospasm are minimized (Table 4).

There are other reasons why appropriately deep (provided the heart is stable) is better than too light. For example, in terms of what

---

[a] Ed. Note (JMB): I do not do deep extubations in infants and children less than 2 years of age. In my experience, these patients almost always develop airway obstruction after deep extubation. Anatomic airway differences (e.g., large tongue, small airways) may explain why these infants develop airway obstruction during light anesthesia and during emergence. This explains why I am much more comfortable with awake extubation in the very young.

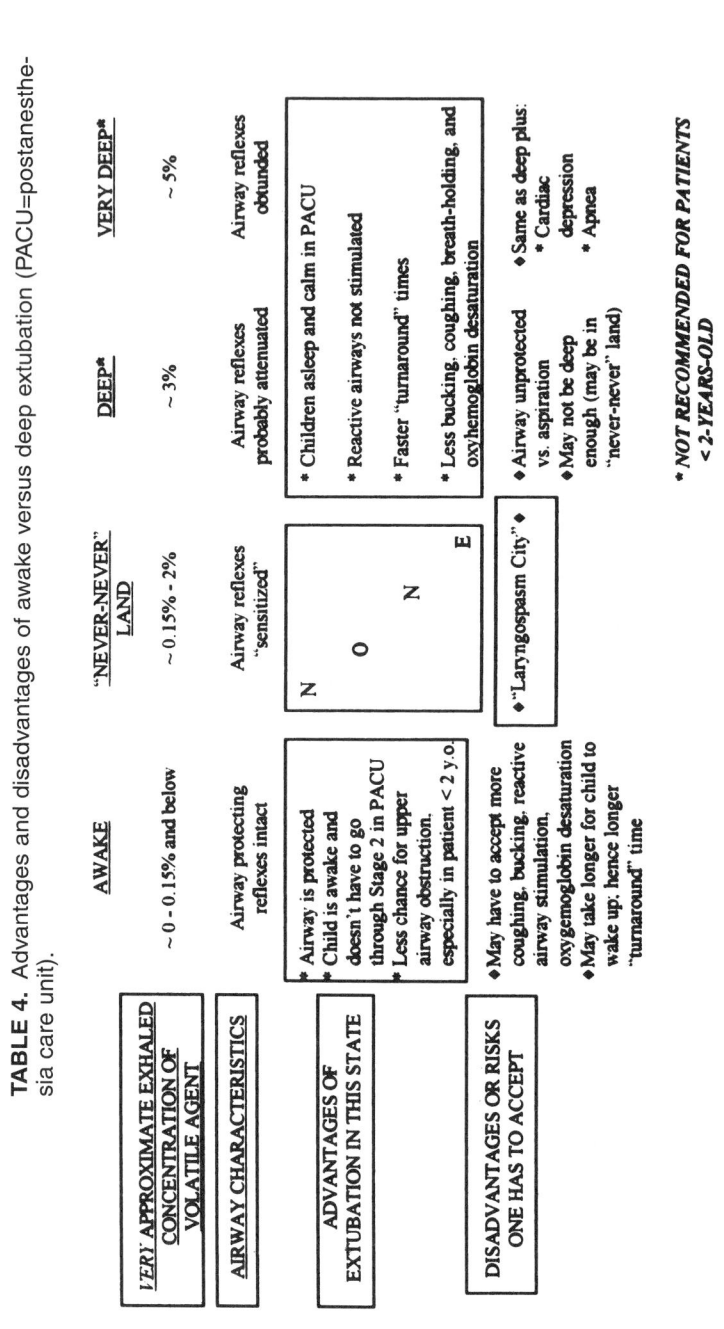

TABLE 4. Advantages and disadvantages of awake versus deep extubation (PACU=postanesthesia care unit).

	AWAKE	"NEVER-NEVER" LAND	DEEP*	VERY DEEP*
VERY APPROXIMATE EXHALED CONCENTRATION OF VOLATILE AGENT	~ 0 - 0.15% and below	~ 0.15% - 2%	~ 3%	~ 5%
AIRWAY CHARACTERISTICS	Airway protecting reflexes intact	Airway reflexes "sensitized"	Airway reflexes probably attenuated	Airway reflexes obtunded
ADVANTAGES OF EXTUBATION IN THIS STATE	* Airway is protected * Child is awake and doesn't have to go through Stage 2 in PACU * Less chance for upper airway obstruction, especially in patient < 2 y.o.	N O N E "Laryngospasm City" ♦	* Children asleep and calm in PACU * Reactive airways not stimulated * Faster "turnaround" times * Less bucking, coughing, breath-holding, and oxyhemoglobin desaturation	
DISADVANTAGES OR RISKS ONE HAS TO ACCEPT	♦ May have to accept more coughing, bucking, reactive airway stimulation, oxygemoglobin desaturation ♦ May take longer for child to wake up; hence longer "turnaround" time		♦ Airway unprotected vs. aspiration ♦ May not be deep enough (may be in "never-never" land)	♦ Same as deep plus: * Cardiac depression * Apnea

NOT RECOMMENDED FOR PATIENTS <2-YEARS-OLD

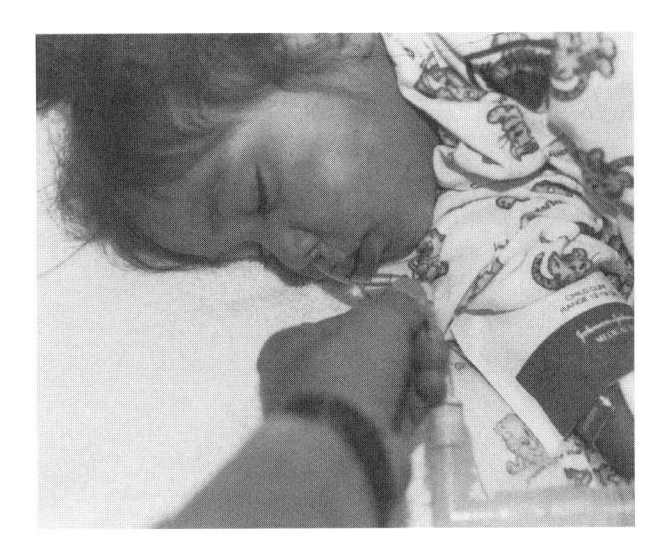

FIG. 2. Tracheal extubation in a deeply anesthetized 3-year-old girl in lateral position after dental restoration. The child had been spontaneously breathing 5.0% inspired isoflurane (see text) and was moved to the transport gurney before extubation. The tube is removed during inspiration in a gentle flowing motion in a pathway following the arc of the tube.

may happen next, the brink of apnea is better than the brink of breath-holding. When apneic from deep anesthesia, spontaneous breathing resumes fairly promptly. Breath-holding due to light anesthesia is a different story (it takes longer to resolve) and may be a harbinger of other untoward events that may occur during light anesthesia (e.g., laryngospasm).

Finally, in the Badgwell technique, the endotracheal tube is not jiggled to see if the child is deep enough. If jiggling the tube discloses that the child is too light, you are faced with one of the two undesirable options—to deepen or to lighten the anesthetic. Why ask for trouble? Better simply to get the child deep and take out the tube.

After ensuring that the child is deeply anesthetized, the child's trachea may be extubated. Immediately after extubation, 100% oxygen by face mask is delivered, and airway patency is verified. Children may be extubated on their side (e.g., in the "tonsil position"), on the operating table, or on the transport bed (Fig. 2). Either way will work fine as long as the child is minimally stimulated after extubation. After extubation, a face mask is gently

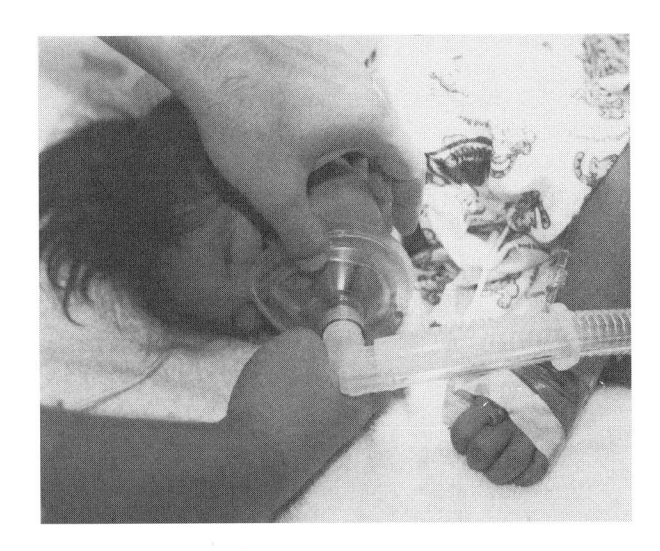

FIG. 3. Immediately after tracheal extubation in the child in Figure 2, oxygen by face mask is applied using a modification of the survival position. After assurance that the child has an unobstructed airway and is breathing spontaneously, the child is transported to the postanesthesia care unit (PACU) with continuous supplemental oxygen delivered through a Jackson-Rees transport circuit. (Note that the intravenous catheter is poorly secured, at least by the editor's standards. More tape and an armboard were applied in the PACU.)

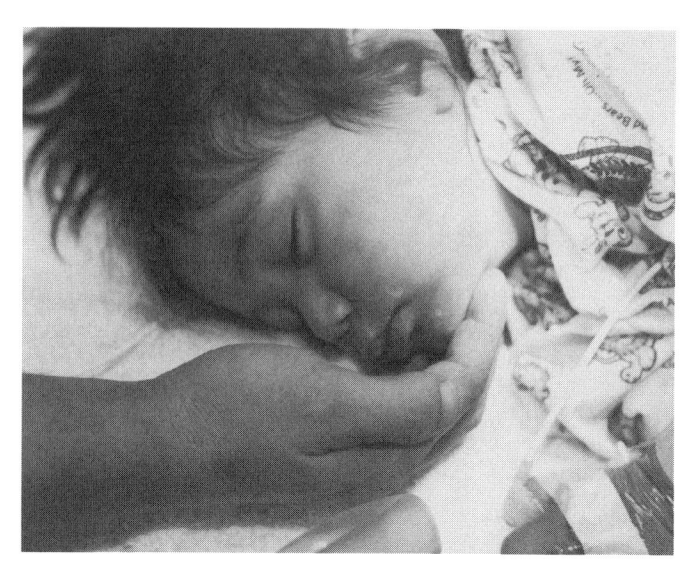

FIG. 4. The 3-year-old child from Figures 2 and 3 is being transported to the postanesthesia care unit. The cupped palm of the clinician is serving as both a human capnograph (the child's breath can be felt on the palm and fingertips) and as a jaw-thrust/chin-lifter to ensure airway patency. Note that oxygen delivery by face mask is close at hand. Alternatively, the elbow of the breathing circuit may be placed between the clinician's fingers to provide oxygen wafting during transport.

applied, using a modified survival position **(see Chapter 2)**, as needed (Fig. 3). When airway patency and spontaneous ventilation are ensured, the face mask is removed, and the patient is observed for ability to ventilate and oxygenate with casual airway support (Fig. 4). Chin lift and respiratory monitoring are provided by placing the clinician's fingertips on the child's chin with the palm over the child's nose and mouth. If the child has been extubated on the operating table, it is important to gently move the patient from the table to the transport bed and then to the PACU.

Emergence from deep planes of anesthesia usually takes place while the patient is being transported. During this period, laryngospasm is easily induced. Emergence from anesthesia then continues in the PACU. During this time, the child requires close observation with minimal stimulation and the immediate availability of qualified personnel to manage the airway.

Children 1 to 8 years of age with normal airway anatomy, who have undergone surgery not involving the pharynx, larynx, or trachea, may tolerate either awake or deep tracheal extubation technique without significant morbidity (59–63). After adenotonsillectomy, tracheal extubation under a deep plane of anesthesia remains controversial (although often practiced) **(see Chapter 11)**.

Extubation in Children Who Are Awake

"Technique is communication. The two words are synonymous in conductors."
—Leonard Bernstein

Awake tracheal extubation refers to the technique of extracting the tracheal tube when the child is fully awake. A fully awake child communicates with you in many ways. The following are signs of a fully awake child:

- Lifts legs with oropharyngeal suction (provided no regional anesthetic administered)
- Opens mouth with oral suction
- Grimaces when stimulated (wrinkles forehead)
- Breathes rhythmically

- Opens eyes
- Tries to take out his or her own tube
- Moves all extremities
- Has complete reversal of muscle relaxant (e.g., four of four in train-of-four and sustained tetanus)
- Has an expired concentration of volatile anesthetic agent of 0.15% or less.

Awake extubation is particularly suitable for those infants and children who:

- Are under 2 years of age
- With full stomachs
- Had muscle paralysis and controlled ventilation for the duration of the procedure
- Are obese
- Have difficult airways
- Have obstructive sleep apnea

The primary concern during extubation is the prevention of laryngospasm. Laryngospasm is a reflex closure of the glottis brought about by stimulation of the vocal cords during light anesthesia. The first stage of laryngospasm is the collapse of supraglottic tissue onto itself. Therefore, to prevent laryngospasm after extubation, one needs to follow a few simple rules:

- Extubate when the patient is deeply anesthetized or fully awake (never in a stage of "light anesthesia").
- Suction secretions before extubation (preferably while the child is "deep")
- Immediately after extubation, stretch the larynx to lengthen the supraglottic structures (Fig. 5).

After awake extubation, immediate concerns for ventilation and patency of the airway are the same as for deep extubation (Figs. 3 and 4). Compared with children extubated deep, children who are extubated awake usually are a little more rambunctious in the PACU, and many require prompt attention to analgesia or sedation needs, especially if regional anesthesia has not been used.

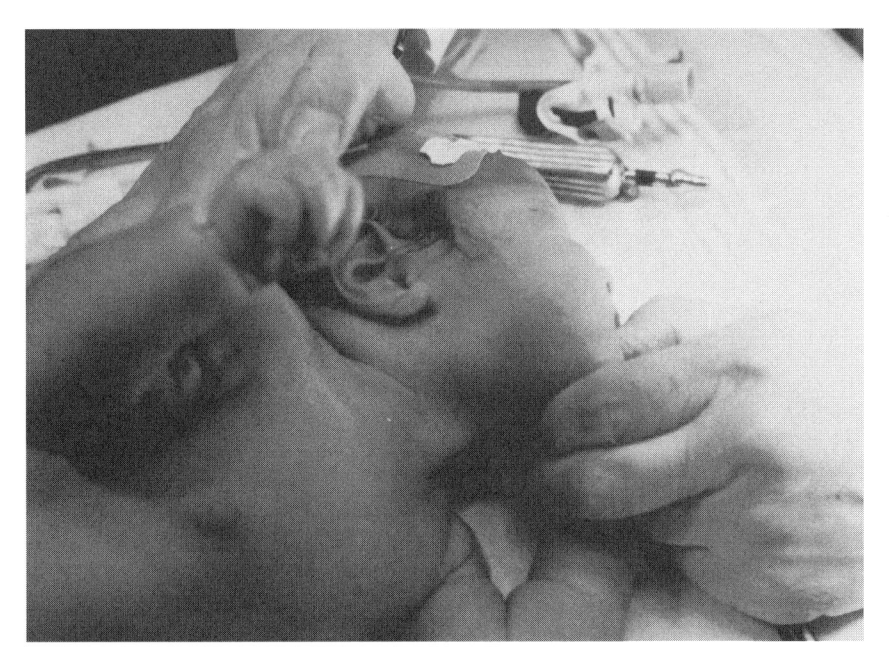

FIG. 5. The hands of Robert Creighton, MD, immediately after extubation, stretching the infant's larynx to prevent laryngospasm. Bass fishermen will appreciate this technique.

SUMMARY

Different modalities are available to the clinician to conduct general anesthesia. Knowledge of the age-related changes in the pharmacokinetics and pharmacodynamics of anesthetic drugs is important to maintain anesthesia safely and allow for a timely emergence from anesthesia. Care must be taken to avoid "cookbook" decisions based on generalizations about the developmental pharmacology of anesthetic drugs. Clinicians providing anesthesia to pediatric patients should use the concepts presented in this chapter to create a rational anesthetic plan that can be modified to meet the needs of the individual patient.

REFERENCES

1. LeDez KM, Lerman J: The minimum alveolar concentration (MAC) of isoflurane in preterm neonates. *Anesthesiology* 1987;67:301–307.
2. Nicodemus HF, Nassiri-Rahimi C, Bachman L, Smith TC: Median effective doses (ED50) of halothane in adults and children. *Anesthesiology* 1969;31:344–348.
3. Gregory GA, Eger EI II, Munson ES: The relationship between age and halothane requirement in man. *Anesthesiology* 1969;30:488–491.
4. Gregory GA, Wade JG, Beihl DR, et al: Fetal anesthetic requirement (MAC) for halothane. *Anesth Analg* 1983;62:9–14.
5. Cameron CB, Robinson S, Gregory GA: The minimum anesthetic concentration of isoflurane in children. *Anesth Analg* 1984;63:418–420.
6. Cook DR, Marcy JH: Pediatric anesthetic pharmacology. In Cook DR, Marcy JH (eds). *Neonatal anesthesia.* Pasadena: Appleton-Davies, 1988:87–125.
7. Taylor RH, Lerman J: Minimum alveolar concentration of desflurane and hemodynamic responses in neonates, infants, and children. *Anesthesiology* 1991;75:975–979.
8. Keenan RL, Shapiro JH, Kane FR, Simpson PM: Bradycardia during anesthesia in infants: an epidemiologic study. *Anesthesiology* 1994;80:979–982.
9. Barash PG, Glanz S, Katz JD, et al: Ventricular function during halothane anesthesia: an echocardiographic evaluation. *Anesthesiology* 1978;49:79–85.
10. Murray D, Vandewalker G, Matherne GP, Mahoney LT: Pulsed Doppler and two-dimensional echocardiography: comparison of halothane and isoflurane on cardiac function in infants and small children. *Anesthesiology* 1987;67:211–217.
11. Katz RL, Epstein RA: The interaction of anesthetic agents and adrenergic drugs to produce cardiac arrhythmias. *Anesthesiology* 1968;29:763–784.
12. Johnston RR, Eger EI II, Wilson C: A comparative interaction of epinephrine with enflurane, isoflurane, and halothane in man. *Anesth Analg* 1976;55:709–712.
13. Karl HW, Swedlow DB, Lee KW, Downes JJ: Epinephrine-halothane interactions in children. *Anesthesiology* 1983;58:142–145.
14. Ueda W, Hirakawa M, Mae O: Appraisal of epinephrine administration to patients under halothane anesthesia for closure of cleft palate. *Anesthesiology* 1983;58:574–576.
15. Carney FM, Van Dyke RA: Halothane hepatitis: a critical review. *Anesth Analg* 1972;51:135–160.
16. Wark H, O Halloran M, Overton J: Prospective study of liver function in children following multiple halothane anaesthetics at short intervals. *Br J Anaesth* 1986;58:1224–1228.
17. Friesen RH, Lichtor JL: Cardiovascular effects of inhalation induction with isoflurane in infants. *Anesth Analg* 1983;62:411–414.
18. Wolf WJ, Neal MB, Peterson MD: The hemodynamic and cardiovascular effects of isoflurane and halothane anesthesia in children. *Anesthesiology* 1986;64:328–333.
19. Kingston HG: Halothane and isoflurane anesthesia in pediatric outpatients. *Anesth Analg* 1986;65:181–184.
20. Taylor RH, Lerman J: Induction, maintenance and recovery characteristics of desflurane in infants and children. *Can J Anaesth* 1992;39:6–13.
21. Zwass MS, Fisher DM, Welborn LG, et al: Induction and maintenance characteristics of anesthesia with desflurane and nitrous oxide in infants and children. *Anesthesiology* 1992;76:373–378.
22. Welborn LG, Hannallah RS, Norden JM, et al: Comparison of emergence and recovery characteristics of sevoflurane, desflurane, and halothane in pediatric ambulatory patients. *Anesth Analg* 1996;83:917–920.
23. Ebert TJ, Muzi M: Sympathetic hyperactivity during desflurane anesthesia in healthy volunteers: a comparison with isoflurane. *Anesthesiology* 1993;79:444–453.
24. Fisher DM, Zwass MS: MAC of desflurane in 60% nitrous oxide in infants and children. *Anesthesiology* 1992;76:354–356.
25. Ghouri AF, White PF: Effect of fentanyl and nitrous oxide on the desflurane anesthetic requirement. *Anesth Analg* 1991;72:377–381.
26. Sarner JB, Levine M Davis PJ, et al: Clinical characteristics of sevoflurane in children: a comparison with halothane. *Anesthesiology* 1995;82:38–46.
27. Katoh T, Ikeda K: The minimum alveolar concentration (MAC) of sevoflurane in humans. *Anesthesiology* 1987;66:301–303.
28. Lerman J, Sikich N, Kleinman S, Yentis S: The pharmacology of sevoflurane in infants and children. *Anesthesiology* 1994;80:814–824.
29. Lerman J, Davis PJ, Welborn LG, et al: Induction, recovery, and safety characteristics of sevoflurane in children undergoing ambulatory surgery. A comparison with halothane. *Anesthesiology* 1996;84:1332–1340.
30. Navarro R, Weiskopf RB, Moore MA, et al: Humans anesthetized with sevoflurane or isoflurane have similar arrhythmic response to epinephrine. *Anesthesiology* 1994;80:545–549.
31. Frink EJ Jr, Isner RJ, Malan TP Jr, et al: Sevoflurane degradation product concentrations with soda lime during prolonged anesthesia. *J Clin Anesth* 1994;6:239–242.
32. Gonsowski CT, Laster MJ, Eger EI II, et al: Toxicity of compound A in rats: effect of a 3-hour administration. *Anesthesiology* 1994;80:556–565.
33. Bito H, Ikeda K: Closed-circuit anesthesia with sevoflurane in humans: effects on renal and hepatic function

and concentrations of breakdown products with soda lime in the circuit. *Anesthesiology* 1994;80:71–76.
34. Anand KJ, Sippell WG, Aynsley-Green A: Randomized trial of fentanyl anaesthesia in preterm babies undergoing surgery: effects on the stress response. *Lancet* 1987; 1:62–66.
35. Lynn AM, Slattery JT: Morphine pharmacokinetics in early infancy. *Anesthesiology* 1987;66:136–139.
36. Chay PC, Duffy BJ, Walker JS: Pharmacokinetic-pharmacodynamic relationships of morphine in neonates. *Clin Pharmacol Ther* 1992;51:334–342.
37. Lynn AM, Nespeca MK, Opheim KE, Slattery JT: Respiratory effects of intravenous morphine infusions in neonates, infants, and children after cardiac surgery. *Anesth Analg* 1993;77:695–701.
38. Murphy MR, Olson WA, Hug CC Jr: Pharmacokinetics of 3H-fentanyl in the dog anesthetized with enflurane. *Anesthesiology* 1979;50:13–19.
39. Koehntop DE, Rodman JH, Brundage DM, et al: Pharmacokinetics of fentanyl in neonates. *Anesth Analg* 1986; 65:227–232.
40. Hertzka RE, Gauntlett IS, Fisher DM, Spellman MJ: Fentanyl-induced ventilatory depression: effects of age. *Anesthesiology* 1989;70:213–218.
41. Sokoll MD, Hoyt JL, Gergis SD: Studies in muscle rigidity, nitrous oxide, and narcotic analgesic agents. *Anesth Analg* 1972;51:16–20.
42. Robinson S, Gregory GA: Fentanyl-air-oxygen anesthesia for ligation of patent ductus arteriosus in preterm infants. *Anesth Analg* 1981;60:331–334.
43. Hickey PR, Hansen DD, Wessel DL, et al: Pulmonary and systemic hemodynamic responses to fentanyl in infants. *Anesth Analg* 1985;64:483–486.
44. Chauvin M, Bonnet F, Montembault C, et al: The influence of hepatic plasma flow on alfentanil plasma concentration plateaus achieved with an infusion model in humans: measurement of alfentanil hepatic extraction coefficient. *Anesth Analg* 1986;65:999–1003.
45. Shafer A, Sung ML, White PF: Pharmacokinetics and pharmacodynamics of alfentanil infusions during general anesthesia. *Anesth Analg* 1986;65:1021–1028.
46. Mulroy JJ Jr, Davis PJ, Rymer DB, et al: Safety and efficacy of alfentanil and halothane in paediatric surgical patients. *Can J Anaesth* 1991;38:445–449.
47. Pokela ML, Ryhanen PT, Koivisto ME, et al: Alfentanil-induced rigidity in newborn infants. *Anesth Analg* 1992; 75:252–257.
48. Roure P, Jean N, Leclerc AC, et al: Pharmacokinetics of alfentanil in children undergoing surgery. *Br J Anaesth* 1987;59:1437–1440.
49. Meistelman C, Saint-Maurice C, Lepaul M, et al: A comparison of alfentanil pharmacokinetics in children and adults. *Anesthesiology* 1987;66:13–16.
50. Goresky GV, Koren G, Sabourin MA, et al: The pharmacokinetics of alfentanil in children. *Anesthesiology* 1987;67:654–659.
51. Killian A, Davis PJ, Stiller RL, et al: Influence of gestational age on pharmacokinetics of alfentanil in neonates. *Dev Pharmacol Ther* 1990;15:82–85.
52. Ausems ME, Hug CC Jr, de Lang S: Variable rate infusion of alfentanil as a supplement to nitrous oxide anesthesia for general surgery. *Anesth Analg* 19813;62: 982–986.
53. Greeley WJ, de Bruijn NP, Davis DP: Sufentanil pharmacokinetics in pediatric cardiovascular patients. *Anesth Analg* 1987;66:1067–1072.
54. Guay J, Gaudreault P, Tang A, et al: Pharmacokinetics of sufentanil in normal children. *Can J Anaesth* 1992;39: 14–20.
55. Hughes MA, Glass PS, Jacobs JR: Context-sensitive half-time in multicompartment models for intravenous anesthetic drugs. *Anesthesiology* 1992;76:334–341.
56. Shafer SL, Varvel JR: Pharmacokinetics, pharmacodynamics, and rational opioid selection. *Anesthesiology* 1991;74:53–63.
57. Hagen PT, Scholz DG, Edwards WD: Incidence and size of patent foramen ovale during the first 10 decades of life: an autopsy study of 965 normal hearts. *Mayo Clin Proc* 1984;59:17–20.
58. Moorthy SS, Dierdorf SF, Krishna G, et al: Transient hypoxemia from a transient right-to-left shunt in a child during emergence from anesthesia. *Anesthesiology* 1987; 66:234–235.
59. Neelakanta G, Miller J: Minimum alveolar concentration of isoflurane for tracheal extubation in deeply anesthetized children. *Anesthesiology* 1994;80:811–813.
60. Griffiths AG, Cranfield K, Forestner J: Minimum alveolar concentration of desflurane for tracheal extubation in deeply anesthetized children. *Anesthesiology* 1995; 83:A1186.
61. Patel RI, Hannallah RS, Norden J, et al: Emergence airway complications in children: a comparison of tracheal extubation in awake and deeply anesthetized patients. *Anesth Analg* 1991;73:266–270.
62. Pounder DR, Blackstone MB, Steward DJ: Tracheal extubation in children: halothane versus isoflurane, anesthetized versus awake. *Anesthesiology* 1991;74: 653–655.
63. Neelakanta G, Miller J: Minimum alveolar concentration of isoflurane for tracheal extubation in deeply anesthetized children. *Anesthesiology* 1994;80: 811–813.

7
Anesthesia for the Neonate

Steven C. Hall

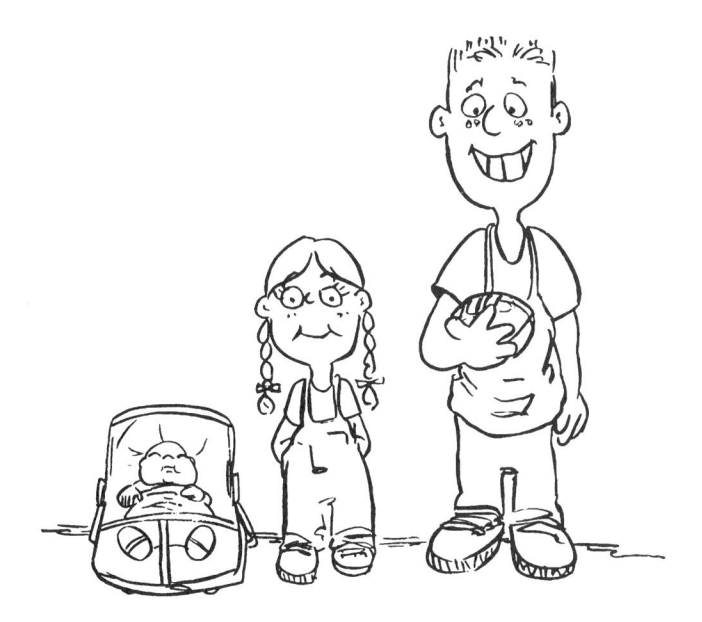

"A baby is a temporarily disabled and stunted version of a larger person...Your job is to help them overcome the disabilities associated with their size and inexperience so that they get on with being that larger person."
—Barbara Ehrenreich

The newborn and infant are widely recognized as having special anatomic, physiologic, and pharmacologic concerns. The anesthesiologist needs to understand the many differences between the newborn[a] and the older child in order to provide safe and timely care. There has been a trend in recent years for surgeons, pediatricians, hospitals, and managed care organizations to insist that infants and newborns undergo surgery in community hospitals rather than regional pediatric medical centers. As a result, anesthesiologists in general practice are increasingly being asked to care for newborns. For this reason, all anesthesiologists should understand the rudiments of neonatal anesthesia, as well as the resources they will need to provide appropriate care.

This chapter discusses not only general topics, such as the evaluation and preparation of the neonatal patient, but also specific surgical conditions and the anesthetic considerations involved in their management. Some of the areas in which new knowledge has changed or expanded our practice are highlighted.

---

[a]Ed. Note (JMB): By definition, newborns are infants in the first day (24 hours) of life, neonates are infants up to 1 month, and infants are infants until age 1 year.

PREOPERATIVE EVALUATION AND PREPARATION FOR SURGERY

"A soiled baby, with a neglected nose, cannot be conscientiously regarded as a thing of beauty."
—Mark Twain

Maternal History

Preanesthetic evaluation follows the form outlined in **Chapter 1**. However, there are specific issues in the newborn that are different from those in the older infant or child. Although there is a tendency to focus only on the newborn, especially when surgery is emergent, there is reason to determine (if possible) whether there are components of either the course of the pregnancy or delivery that can have a material impact on the newborn. Maternal history can provide information about the course of the pregnancy and labor (e.g., toxemia, polyhydramnios, premature labor), maternal medical history (e.g., diabetes, sickle cell disease), and maternal drug history (e.g., narcotics, diazepam, insulin) that may include factors important to the evaluation of the newborn. For instance, it has been determined that newborns of insulin-dependent diabetic mothers have a significant decrease in myocardial contractility for the first few days of life; the cause is unknown (1,2). However, this decrease in cardiac reserve can be significant. Likewise, infants of diabetic mothers may also have a hypertrophic cardiomyopathy that can result in outflow obstruction and heart failure during the first months after birth. Finally, newborns of diabetic mothers are more likely to experience wider swings in blood glucose levels in the neonatal period. The anesthesiologist should not only determine a baseline glucose level before anesthetizing this child, but also be aware that there may be significant alterations in glucose level perioperatively that should be monitored.

Maternal Drug History

Maternal drug history is important. There can be significant depression of a newborn if the mother had received large quantities of narcotics or magnesium sulfate, for instance, during the course of labor and delivery. Chronic medications, such as coumadin, can cross the placenta, causing both fetal and neonatal complications. However, it may difficult to get an accurate history of recreational drug use. Diazepam, opioids, or cocaine may have deleterious effects on the newborn. For example, newborns exposed *in utero* to cocaine have a higher incidence of premature birth (3,4), intrauterine growth retardation (3), patent ductus arteriosus, intracardiac defects (5), conduction and rhythm disturbances (5), seizures, and abnormal respiratory patterns (6,7) including sudden infant death syndrome (3).

Birth History

The anesthesiologist should obtain as complete a neonatal history as possible. Neonatal asphyxia, hypotonia, cyanosis, respiratory distress, or seizures should alert the anesthesiologist to potential underlying lesions or stresses. The lack of crying and vigorous movement after stimulation is disturbing in an otherwise normal newborn. Neonatal asphyxia can limit the cardiac, respiratory, and metabolic responsiveness of the newborn. The asphyxiated newborn can have not only depressed myocardial contractility, with consequent poor cardiac output and metabolic acidosis, but also impaired cerebral autoregulation (8), hypoglycemia, hypocalcemia, hypothermia, and disseminated intravascular coagulation. If medications were given during either neonatal resuscitation or subsequent care, the anesthesiologist must be aware of the drugs used, as well as the dosage and effect. If the patient was intubated after birth, the reason for intubation, need for ventilation, ease of intubation, and evidence of meconium aspiration or other abnormalities should be elicited.

Gestational Age

"I don't dislike babies, though I think very young ones rather disgusting."
—Queen Victoria of Great Britain

Gestational age is another important factor that is estimated from history and physical examination. A newborn is considered full-term if born at 37 weeks' gestation or later and weighs at least 2.5 kg. If the newborn is at least 37 weeks' gestation, but weighs under 2.5 kg, it is considered small-for-gestational age (SGA). The significance of SGA is that intrauterine growth was delayed, often for undefined reasons. SGA newborns appear to have a significantly higher incidence of congenital abnormalities, but also are prone to hypoglycemia, infection, pneumonia, and seizures. In contrast, newborns who are born prematurely (now, more appropriately, called "preterm"[b]), demonstrate physiologic and anatomic abnormalities due to the lack of completion of normal development **(see also Chapter 8)**. Preterm infants are, therefore, at risk for hyaline membrane disease, intraventricular hemorrhage, hypothermia, patent ductus arteriosus, apnea, hypocalcemia, and retinopathy of prematurity. The preanesthetic history should be used to evaluate evidence of these conditions.

RESPIRATORY SYSTEM

The Upper Airway

The newborn is usually an obligate nasal breather; the combination of small nares, relatively large tongue, small mandible, abundant soft tissue, increased anteroposterior diameter of the head, and short neck increases susceptibility to upper airway obstruction. The long, narrow, omega-shaped epiglottis and more cephalad vocal cords make intubation more difficult than in the adult or older child **(see also Chapter 4)**. For these reasons, intubation using a straight blade is usually preferred.

Lungs and Chest

Because of the horizontally placed, flexible ribs and relatively undeveloped intercostal muscles, newborns are diaphragmatic breathers and susceptible to ventilatory embarrassment by gastric or abdominal distention. In contrast to older infants, the diaphragmatic muscle can fatigue under repeated stress, especially in the preterm newborn.

The alveolar bed is incompletely developed at birth. Rapid development occurs through infancy and early childhood, with an adult-type configuration developing by about 8 years of age. The relative size of each of the lung compartments is the same in infancy, childhood, and adulthood. Tidal volumes, on a milliliter per kilogram (ml/kg) basis, are the same in newborns, infants, and children. Although the functional residual capacity of newborns is close to adult levels on a ml/kg basis, the metabolic rate of the newborn is double that of the adult. The minute ventilation/functional residual capacity ratio in adults is about 1.5:1, but approaches 5:1 in the newborn. Therefore, the oxygen reserve provided by the functional residual capacity during apnea is significantly smaller in the newborn compared with that in the adult. This explains why newborns and infants become cyanotic faster during apnea than adults and is the reason why the anesthesiologist must pay meticulous attention to ensuring a clear airway and adequate ventilation at all times.

Apneic Spells

The newborn normally has periodic breathing, but some newborns, especially those who are preterm, will have life-threatening apneic spells. These episodes increase in the presence of stress and after anesthesia and surgery. Also, the newborn responds to hypoxemia by a short period of hyperpnea, followed by hypoventilation. This response is exaggerated in the presence of hypothermia. There is also decreased responsiveness to carbon dioxide. There is evidence that there is a

---

[b]Ed. Note (JMB): Not all of us have switched over to "preterm" for the prematurely born infant **(see Chapter 8)**. And, in fact, we may be unable to change as advancing years set in.

difference in the ventilatory response under anesthesia in newborns (9–11); because of these issues, it has become convention to control ventilation in the anesthetized newborn instead of allowing spontaneous ventilation.

Laboratory Tests

An arterial blood gas or a chest radiograph may be needed if there is a question about the patient's respiratory, cardiac, or metabolic status. Persistent acidosis should alert the anesthesiologist to the possibility of hypovolemia, sepsis, or incomplete recovery from birth asphyxia. Simple correction of the acidosis with bicarbonate is not appropriate; instead, it is crucial to determine the underlying cause and treat this.

CARDIOVASCULAR SYSTEM

Physical Examination

The cardiovascular examination includes the determination of blood pressure, heart rate, rhythm, presence of murmurs, and presence and strength of peripheral pulses. If the patient has cardiac symptoms, consultation with a neonatologist is advisable to help in the assessment of the patient's cardiac status and plan for preoperative therapy to minimize cardiac decompensation. If a murmur is detected, the help of a pediatric cardiologist can be helpful in determining its significance. Weak or absent pulses, cold extremities, diminished urine output, grayish skin color, or lethargy can all be signs of decreased cardiac output.

Laboratory Evaluation

If there is evidence of significant cardiac disease, a chest radiograph, blood gas, and electrocardiogram (ECG) are done. With the help of a cardiologist, noninvasive echocardiography can diagnose the more common congenital cardiac lesions.

Patent Ductus Arteriosus

A patent ductus arteriosus is the most common cardiac lesion detected in the newborn. Blood flow is primarily left to right in these patients, leading to "flooding" of the pulmonary circulation and an increased load on the left ventricle. Medical treatment includes digitalis, diuretics, and mechanical ventilation. The prostaglandin inhibitor, indomethacin, may be used to promote ductal closure.

Newborn Myocardium

The cardiac muscle in newborns has fewer contractile elements than that found in infants or children. The newborn has relatively noncompliant ventricles and a limited ability to increase stroke volume, making cardiac output dependent on heart rate. Bradycardia must be quickly treated to prevent a significant decrease in cardiac output and body perfusion. Although the parasympathetic nervous system is functional at birth, the sympathetic nervous system is not fully developed until about 4 to 6 months of age.

Newborn Pulmonary Vasculature

The neonatal pulmonary vasculature is very reactive; the vessels have a greater muscularis layer than infants and can constrict significantly in the presence of acidosis, hypercarbia, hypoxemia, and other stresses. These responses are heightened in patients with acidosis, congenital hypoplasia of vessels (such as in newborns with congenital diaphragmatic hernia), increased pulmonary blood flow, or prematurity. Sudden increases in pulmonary vascular resistance (PVR) decrease pulmonary blood flow, causing hypoxemia, acidosis, and, potentially, heart failure. Vigorous therapy of the underlying condition, along with hyperventilation, oxygen therapy, and alkalosis may decrease the pulmonary hypertension. The roles of vasodilators, sedation, nitrous oxide, and extracorporeal membrane oxygenation (ECMO) are controversial and subjects of ongoing research.

FLUID AND BLOOD

Total Body Water

Total body water accounts for almost 80% of body weight in the full-term newborn, decreasing to about 60% by the time the child is 2 years of age. Likewise, extracellular water is about 45% at birth and decreases to about 20% at 2 years of age (12). Although the proportion of intracellular fluid stays about the same—35% to 40%—it increases in proportion to total body water and extracellular water in the first 2 years of life. There is a loss of weight in newborns, especially preterms, in the first days of life because of diuresis of some of this interstitial fluid (13). The newborn is especially susceptible to dehydration on the basis of lesser intracellular reserves, high water turnover due to a high metabolic rate, and relative renal immaturity.

Renal Metabolism

Although the neonatal kidney matures (from a functional standpoint) rapidly (usually by the third or fourth day of life), the newborn kidney does not handle extra volumes of salt or water well in the first couple days of life because of a lower glomerular filtration rate and tubular reabsorption. Newborns, especially premature newborns, require low-maintenance fluids for about the first 5 days of life, with the amount gradually increasing over the first month (14,15). A rate of 50 to 70 ml/kg/day is usually enough fluid for the newborn's maintenance during the first 5 days of life. $D_{10}W$ and $D_{10}/0.2$ normal saline are often given because of the newborn's increased metabolic rate and need for glucose. Hypoglycemia (less than 30 mg/dl in full-term infants, 20 mg/dl in preterm infants) is common, especially in the newborn under 2.5 kg, and should be evaluated by using a chemical strip or venous sample.

Anemia

Anemia (hemoglobin [Hgb] < 13.5 mg/dl in the newborn) should be corrected preoperatively. Although relative anemia is decreasingly an indication for transfusion in infants and children, the newborn is unique because lower cardiac, respiratory, and oxygen-carrying reserves make the newborn especially susceptible to tissue hypoxemia. Recent evidence shows that anemia is a risk factor for increased apneic spells in the preterm newborn (16).

Fluid and Blood Requirements

Excess fluid administration correlates with an increased incidence of infant respiratory distress syndrome (IRDS), patent ductus arteriosus, congestive heart failure, and necrotizing enterocolitis. Inadequate fluid administration can cause hypotension and decreased perfusion. Since fluid requirements for any individual surgical procedure can vary widely, it is not reasonable to give absolute guidelines for fluid administration. Clinical experience and close attention to the surgical field, vital signs, acid-base status, and repeat hematocrits are the basis of rational fluid management. A common clinical technique in the newborn is to give crystalloid or, if plasma losses are significant, colloid until the patient demonstrates cardiovascular stability. A hematocrit is then used to guide red blood cell replacement. However, if red cells are being actively lost, replacement is started with red cells.

Maintenance of Normothermia

The newborn is particularly susceptible to cold stress (17). Nonshivering thermogenesis results in acidosis, decreased oxygenation of tissues, hypoventilation, and decreased cardiac output. This should be prevented by maintaining a neutral thermal environment for the baby, using elevated room temperature, heating lights, and blankets,[c] warmed fluids and gases, and protective skin covering (like plas-

---

[c]Ed. Note (JMB): The forced-air warming blankets (e.g., BairHugger by Augustine Medical and WarmTouch by Mallinckrodt Medical) are proving to be the most efficient and cost-efficient way to keep these infants warm **(see Chapter 2)**.

tic wrap). Continual core temperature measurement with either a rectal or esophageal probe is mandatory in newborns. Although it is uncomfortable to work in operating rooms with an elevated temperature, the prevention of heat loss from the newborn is important.[d]

MONITORING

The Precordial Stethoscope

The speed with which things change in the newborn demand that the anesthesiologist be constantly vigilant and anticipate possible problems before they occur. The precordial stethoscope allows constant monitoring of breath sounds, along with the heart sounds, rate, and rhythm during induction and emergence. With just a small amount of experience, the clinician will become adept at assimilating the large amount of information available from the stethoscope. The strength of heart tones, for instance, has been used as an early indicator of a drop in cardiac action and blood pressure. The precordial stethoscope should be the first monitor applied and the last removed at the end of the case—after the patient has been successfully extubated or placed on a ventilator for the postoperative period. An esophageal stethoscope is useful during the middle of a case to monitor heart tones and the presence of breath sounds, but it has the disadvantage of being in a midline position and therefore not helpful if there is a change in breath sounds unilaterally. A precordial stethoscope can be placed over the left hemithorax and is potentially useful in detecting displacement of the tip of the endotracheal tube into the right mainstem bronchus.

Standard Monitors

The standard intraoperative monitors, such as ECG, blood pressure, pulse oximetry, capnography, esophageal stethoscope, and temperature are also used during neonatal procedures. There are some differences in detail because of size and physiology. For instance, because the pressure in newborns is low relative to infants, proper cuff size (one half to three quarters the length of the upper arm) and the additional use of a Doppler probe for accurate readings are useful. Automated blood pressure cuffs (Dinamap) can be used in infancy, but pay special attention to deflation of the cuff to prevent venous stasis. In very small newborns or those with expected wide swings in blood pressure, an alternative to automated blood pressure monitoring is the use of a manual cuff and a Doppler flow probe placed on the brachial or radial artery. This arrangement has the advantage of giving reliable results quickly, even when there is a sharp drop in blood pressure.

Pulse oximetry readings may vary by the site at which the probe is placed. Right arm readings correlate with preductal saturations, while lower extremity readings correlate with postductal saturations. Arterial saturations of 94% to 98% are readily acceptable, and values of 92% to 96% are not uncommon in the normal preterm. With modern equipment, accurate capnograph tracings are available **(see Chapter 5)**.

The most important monitor is the anesthesiologist. Constant observation of the patient and the operation, along with consideration of the trends in vital signs, fluid loss and gain, and anesthetic drugs aid tremendously in the accurate appraisal of the patient's status.

PREMEDICATION AND FASTING

The only premedicant usually given to newborns is atropine or glycopyrrolate. The relatively high parasympathetic tone predisposes the newborn to exhibit bradycardia in response to a variety of stresses. If an intravenous (IV) line is available, administration by IV is the most reliable method. Most newborns come to surgery on an emergency basis, precluding a normal regimen of nothing by

---

[d] Ed. Note (JMB): The use of forced-air warming may allow a cooler room, but each case must be individualized and adjustments in room temperature made based on the patient's core temperature measurements.

mouth. If the case is not emergent, a 2- to 4-hour fast allows adequate emptying of the stomach and avoidance of significant dehydration or hypoglycemia.

Induction

Induction of anesthesia should proceed only after the patient has been properly evaluated and, if needed, resuscitated. The importance of resuscitation cannot be overstressed. Neonates requiring surgery may present with significant volume deficits, ventilatory failure, metabolic acidosis, hypothermia, or sepsis. Although the need for surgical intervention may be emergent, successful survival of the event can depend on the efforts made by the anesthesiologist to resuscitate the newborn before and during the procedure.

Endotracheal Intubation

Awake. Awake endotracheal intubation before induction is recommended by many authors (18). This technique allows protection of the airway before any depressants are given. However, the newborn may struggle enough to make this difficult, even in experienced hands. Specially made *oxyscopes,* blades with a side channel for oxygen administration, allow insufflation during laryngoscopy, decreasing any attendant fall in patient oxygenation. Unless the newborn is extremely ill and weak, thiopental, ketamine, lidocaine, or a narcotic may be used to provide anesthesia and blunt cardiovascular reflexes.

Blades and Tubes. Because of the relatively cephalad (anterior) larynx and long epiglottis, a straight blade (size 0 or 1 Miller) is easiest to use. A size 1 Flagg or 1 Miller blade is most commonly used for a full-term newborn, with the size 0 reserved for the preterm or SGA newborn. A full-term newborn usually needs a 3.0-mm internal diameter endotracheal tube, while the preterm and SGA patient often require a 2.5-mm internal diameter tube.

Maintenance of Anesthesia

Why Pharmacology Is Different in Neonates

The pharmacology of anesthetics in the newborn is distinctly different from that in older children. The newborn has less plasma and tissue protein-binding of drugs, a larger volume of distribution, lesser fat and muscle depots, larger distribution of cardiac output to vessel-rich tissues, and diminished liver and renal function compared with older children. Uptake of inhalation agents is more rapid in the newborn and infant, whereas intramuscular absorption after drug injection is less reliable. Wider distribution of water-soluble drugs, such as neuromuscular blockers, results in higher requirements for succinylcholine in the newborn. Enzymatic metabolism of drugs in blood or liver is diminished in the newborn. Renal elimination is less efficient in the early newborn period, but actually enhanced in the child.

Minimum Alveolar Concentration

The minimum alveolar concentration (MAC) of newborns is lower than that of infants, and that of preterms is lower still. The traditional pediatric volatile agent, halothane, has been shown to have a MAC of 0.87 in newborns and 1.2 in infants (19). The MAC of isoflurane in preterm newborns under 32 weeks' gestational age has been measured as 1.28, whereas newborns between 32 and 37 weeks' gestational age had a MAC of 1.41 (20). In another study, MAC was 1.87 in infants up to 6 months old (21). Although volatile agents are popular for infant and child anesthesia, the drops in blood pressure caused by these agents in newborns can be significant.

Opioids

Opioids have become increasingly popular for neonatal anesthesia, especially because of the relative hemodynamic stability seen with their use. Fentanyl and sufentanil have been used in newborns with little hemodynamic instability (22–24). There are no data available that suggest that one narcotic is superior to another in newborns. An important factor to remember when using narcotics in the newborn is the decreased body clearance and elimination that has been demonstrated for fentanyl (25), sufentanil (24,26), alfentanil (27,28), and morphine (29–31). Fentanyl (5 µg/kg and up) is used extensively in the newborn, along with various nitrous oxide/oxygen/air combinations. There is minimal cardiac depression but there is the disadvantage of an increased need for postoperative ventilation.

Titration of Drugs. Titration of drugs, not dependence on formulas, is appropriate because of tremendous individual variation. However, because drugs like fentanyl may not be "complete" anesthetics, there is always the concern of providing analgesia without anesthesia. For instance, an interesting study by Yaster (32) demonstrated that in newborns, 10 µg/kg of fentanyl blunted hemodynamic responses to surgery, and increasing the dose to 12.5 µg/kg increased the duration of this effect from 75 to 90 minutes. However, we do not understand the consequences of blunting hemodynamic responses with a potent analgesic compared with blunting them with a volatile agent or other drug in which there is greater assurance that the patient is also "asleep."

Hypotension

The newborn's blood pressure may fall dramatically during induction or maintenance. Newborns exhibit different hemodynamic profiles when anesthetized compared with children and adults. For instance, ketamine, fentanyl, halothane, and isoflurane all produce a drop in blood pressure during induction in preterm newborns (33). This hypotension is reversed by surgical stimulation when ketamine or fentanyl are the agents, but significant hypotension can persist with the volatile agents. Changes in blood pressure and heart rate may be significant clinically; therefore, it should be a goal of the anesthetic plan and management to preserve blood pressure and heart rate during induction.

Pain Management

Newborns feel surgical pain, just as children and adults, and should be provided with the benefits of anesthetics, just as are older patients. Our first responsibility in any critically ill patient is to resuscitate first and then administer anesthetics as tolerated. It is unfortunate that some practitioners, in the past, administered only muscle relaxants to newborns, even those who were cardiovascularly stable. This is not an acceptable technique. There is a large literature proving that the newborn not only feels pain, but also mounts significant responses to the stress of pain (34–39). The newborn shows an increase in heart rate, blood pressure, and anterior fontanelle pressure, along with a decrease in transcutaneous oxygen tensions, in response to pain (39). The increase in cardiac output and rise in anterior fontanelle pressure are a particular issue in preterm infants because of the risk of intraventricular hemorrhage. The newborn is also able to mount a dramatic, though short-lived, metabolic response to anesthesia and surgery (35,36,38,40).

The anesthetic management of a newborn undergoing surgery can measurably change the stress response (41,42). The addition of either fentanyl (41) or halothane (42) to a baseline nitrous oxide/relaxant anesthetic will decrease the hormonal stress responses during surgery.

Retinopathy of Prematurity

Both inspired and arterial oxygen concentrations during surgery are important considerations in the newborn. The newborn, especially the preterm infant under 1500 g and 34 weeks' gestation, is at risk for retinopathy of prematurity (ROP). The retinal vasculature is not fully mature at birth and continues its growth toward the periphery, reaching the anterior temporal area somewhere in the first few weeks after birth in the full-term newborn, and later in the preterm. These immature vessels can vasoconstrict, hemorrhage, and vasoproliferate in a random fashion in response to hyperoxia. In severe cases, blindness can result from retinal detachment. Although it has been suggested that 44 weeks' gestation is the time at which vascularization is complete (43, 44), there can be significant individual variability. Two important aspects of ROP should be understood by the anesthesiologist.

First, multiple stresses, such as hypoxemia, acidosis, hypotension, and sepsis, among others, have been implicated in causing ROP (45–47). Although concern has been expressed that enriched oxygen exposure during general anesthesia can precipitate ROP (48), there is not much evidence for this. However, because a sick newborn requiring surgery often is subjected to multiple stresses, it has been stated that the preterm newborn coming to surgery is at no greater risk for the development of ROP than the equivalent infant who does not have anesthesia and surgery (49). Second, the changes in the retina are not immediately observable after a given stress, but take days to weeks to become noticeable. Consequently, examination of the retina just before surgery (and anesthesia) is not a guarantee that ROP will not develop secondary to stresses that occurred before the procedure. Guidelines for administration of oxygen will be discussed in the congenital diaphragmatic hernia discussion that follows and in Chapter 8.

Transfusion Therapy

Transfusion therapy is challenging in the newborn for several reasons. Warming of fluids, either by machine or with your hands, is necessary in these small children to prevent rapid cooling. Second, it is easy to accidentally overload these newborns, causing heart failure, opening of a patent ductus arteriosus, worsening of IRDS, and possibly intraventricular hemorrhage. Calibrated infusion pumps can be used to infuse maintenance fluids at a set rate. Additional fluids are given by syringe or small bolus to avoid overload. Third, the use of non-red blood cell blood components has been guided more by tradition and intuition than scientific study. Platelets and fresh frozen plasma should be given in response to specific needs, not as blanket responses to losses.

Emergence and Postoperative Care

Reversal of neuromuscular blockade and extubation in otherwise healthy newborns is carried out only if several criteria are met. The patient must be awake, normothermic, normotensive, and in good acid-base and electrolyte status, and must be expected to have no significant sequelae either from the operation or from underlying defects. If there is any question about the patient's current or future status, the patient should be left intubated and reevaluated later in the intensive care unit. Transport to the intensive care unit should be in an orderly fashion, with an ECG, Doppler probe, or pulse oximeter monitoring the heart rate continuously. Equipment for intubation and ventilation should be part of the transport equipment, along with a metered oxygen and air source. Wrapping the baby in protective covering such as plastic wrap will keep the patient warm and allows observation of color and perfusion. Once in the intensive care unit, the anesthesiologist gives up responsibility for the patient only after the patient has been stabilized and the care has been assumed by the neonatologist or other physician.

SPECIFIC SURGICAL CONDITIONS

Congenital Diaphragmatic Hernia

Incidence and Etiology

Congenital diaphragmatic hernia (CDH) has been one of the most feared lesions of all of surgery. Despite years of research and trials, the survival rate did not appreciably change. CDH has an incidence of approximately 1 in

2500 live births and is without racial or geographic preference. *In utero,* there is herniation of abdominal contents into the thoracic cavity through the left-sided pleuroperitoneal canal (foramen of Bochdalek), with subsequent compression of growing lung and malrotation of the gut. The hemithorax is filled with stomach and intestines, rarely accompanied by the spleen, liver, or kidneys. Although about 80% of herniations are through the left foramen, there can be herniation through the retrosternal area (Morgagni's foramen) or the right-sided foramen of Bochdalek.

The Pulmonary System

The pulmonary system of the newborn has several unique characteristics that impact anesthetic management. As previously mentioned, newborns are primarily diaphragmatic breathers, with a relatively sparse and undeveloped alveolar bed. In the patient with CDH, herniation of abdominal contents prevents normal development of lung. The earlier in development this occurs (and the larger the herniation), the greater the effect on growth. Not only is there significant impairment of ipsilateral and contralateral lung tissue (50,51), but the pulmonary vasculature is tortuous and decreased in total surface area.

The undeveloped lung may appear compressed at the time of surgery; there is a tendency among inexperienced clinicians to try to expand this lung by overinflation. However, the lung is hypoplastic; increased airway pressures result only in overdistention of more mature (and expandable) lung tissue and subsequent barotrauma. Consequently, sudden deterioration may occur either intraoperatively or postoperatively from a tension pneumothorax, often on the contralateral side where more mature alveoli have been overdistended. Increased airway pressures also have the disadvantage of significantly decreasing venous return to the lungs. Therefore, it is important to ventilate these patients using higher rates and lower peak airway pressures.

Clinical Presentation

Physical Signs

Newborns who present with signs of respiratory distress shortly after birth have a greater degree of lung hypoplasia and a greater mortality rate. The mortality rate approaches 50% in early presenters, whereas those presenting after 24 hours of life have a negligible mortality rate (52,53). The first signs can appear as soon as the umbilical cord is clamped, with cyanosis, tachypnea, retractions, and grunting. Physical examination can reveal a scaphoid abdomen, a barrel-shaped thorax, and decreased chest expansion on the affected side. Although breath sounds on the affected side are usually diminished, this is not always true. Often, bowel sounds can be heard over the chest. With presentation later in life, signs of bowel obstruction may predominate.

Imaging Evaluation

Although intrauterine diagnosis by ultrasonography is increasingly common, the diagnosis in many patients is made after birth. The diagnosis is usually confirmed by chest radiograph, with multiple loops of air-filled bowel in the chest and displacement of the mediastinum toward the unaffected side. Occasionally, it is useful to insert a radiopaque orogastric tube because the repeat radiograph will reveal the catheter in the chest, thus ruling out lesions such as lobar emphysema. Rarely, angiography or computed tomography scans will be used to establish the diagnosis. Arterial blood gases usually demonstrate profound hypoxemia, as well as both a respiratory and metabolic acidosis.

Associated Congenital Anomalies

As is typical of many major congenital syndromes, a significant proportion of newborns with CDH have associated congenital anomalies, primarily cardiovascular (atrial septal defect, ventricular septal defect, tetralogy of Fallot), central nervous system (hydrocephalus, myelomeningocele), or gastrointestinal (duodenal bands, atresia) (54). The presence of other major abnormalities, especially cardiac abnormalities, increases the overall mortality rate. Evaluation for the presence of cardiac abnormalities should be part of the initial evaluation of the patient.

Initial Evaluation and Therapy

Initial evaluation and therapy depends on the severity of presentation. If the newborn is stable, an orogastric tube and venous access are started, and the patient is nursed or transported in a warmed environment with supplemental oxygen by face mask or head hood. If the newborn is acidotic, hypoxemic, and hypercarbic, an awake oral intubation is performed and hyperventilation with rapid, shallow breaths begun. It is helpful, both in the operating room and elsewhere, to have an airway pressure gauge in-line to avoid pressures above 30 cm H_2O. It is important to remember that pneumothorax can produce sudden hypotension and arrest and is more likely to occur on the contralateral side.

If repeat blood gases after ventilation is controlled show significant metabolic acidosis, sodium bicarbonate (1 to 2 meq/kg) is given to temporarily raise the pH. If the patient is hypotensive, inotropic support with dopamine and colloid are added, as needed. Blood samples are sent for hematocrit and for typing and cross-match, although blood transfusion is rarely required for surgical bleeding.

Ventilatory and Cardiac Support

The amount and timing of ventilatory and cardiac support provided before surgically reducing the hernia are controversial. It used to be common to give a short course of aggressive medical management during transport of the newborn, but then proceed quickly to the operating room to reduce the hernia and hopefully improve the cardiopulmonary status. However, there is a strong trend to delay surgery until the patient has been stabilized for a longer period of time (55). ECMO and inhaled nitrous oxide are increasingly used to improve the status of the newborn before surgical repair (56–59). Because of survival of newborns undergoing these treatments that otherwise were not expected to survive, there is growing interest in stabilization using these newer modalities both preoperatively and postoperatively. The end-result has been that fewer patients are presenting emergently to the operating room.

Anesthetic Management

Room Preparation

Despite appropriate medical management, a rapidly deteriorating patient with both respiratory and metabolic acidosis may present to the operating room. All the normal considerations of newborn anesthesia are observed. The room is warmed to 26° to 28° C before arrival of the patient, and heating lamps, monitors, transducers, and infusions are prepared. Depending on the status of the patient, infusions of an inotropic agent such as dopamine or dobutamine (60) and a vasodilator such as sodium nitroprusside are prepared. Finally, drugs for resuscitation are prepared.

When the Patient Arrives

When the newborn arrives, standard monitors are immediately applied. The pulse oximeter probe is placed on the ear or right hand to ensure preductal measurements. Dependable venous access must be established before induction. If the patient is stable, an arterial line is established; otherwise, it is started after induction. The patient may arrive with an umbilical arterial line in place; it is useful to replace this with a right radial arterial line, if possible, for several reasons. A right radial or temporal line gives preductal readings, indicating the status of blood perfusing the eyes, coronaries, and brain, whereas arterial blood from the umbilical artery is a mixture of blood from the left ventricle and any right-to-left shunting across the ductus. Also, umbilical lines are associated with a higher incidence of complications, and, lastly, the umbilical line may be in the way of the abdominal procedure and be at risk for dislodgement.

Endotracheal Intubation

Endotracheal intubation is usually performed awake in the newborn patient with CDH because of the patient's tenuous status, although it is reasonable to use an IV technique. Positive-pressure mask ventilation is avoided because of the potential for gastric distention and increased intrathoracic pressure. After intubation, an esophageal stethoscope and temperature probe are placed. No matter what anesthetic circuit is used, an airway pressure gauge is used to constantly monitor peak pressures, trying to keep peak pressures below 20 to 30 cm H_2O. Although many pediatric anesthesiologists feel that hand ventilation, using rapid rates (70 to 140 breaths/minute) and small tidal volumes, allows detection of small changes in lung compliance and minimizes the danger of pneumothorax, this has been inconclusive when studied *in vitro* (61).

Supplemental Oxygen

Initially, 100% oxygen is administered until blood gases indicate it is safe to lower the F_IO_2. IV agents, such as ketamine (62) and fentanyl, are used instead of inhalation agents because uptake of inhalation agents may be poor, and the cardiovascular depressant effects of the inhalation agents is undesirable. Nitrous oxide is avoided because of possible distention of bowel in the chest.

How much oxygen is too much in the newborn? In these particular patients, it is desirable to keep the PaO_2 above 60 to 80 mm Hg to minimize pulmonary vasoconstriction (63). The newborn, especially the preterm weighing under 1500 g and less than 34 weeks' gestation, however, is at risk for ROP **(see Chapter 8)**. Although the limits of safe levels of administered oxygen in the newborn are not yet completely accepted, it is prudent to keep the preductal (blood obtained from the right radial or superficial temporal arteries) PaO_2 from 50 to 80 mm Hg in the full-term newborn and from 40 to 60 mm Hg in the preterm. These are levels that the normal newborn will demonstrate in room air without supplemental oxygen (64,65).

Considerations during Surgery

The surgical procedure is straightforward, with reduction of the hernia through an abdominal incision and closure of the diaphragmatic defect primarily or with the addition of a plastic patch (52). As the abdominal contents are reduced, ventilating pressures often decrease dramatically, and blood gases improve. Lack of improvement is a poor prognostic sign, often indicating that the ipsilateral lung is exceptionally hypoplastic. Efforts should not be made to expand either the ipsilateral or contralateral lung. A chest tube may be placed prophylactically on the ipsilateral side, both sides, or not at all. Unless the hernia was exceptionally small, the newborn is left intubated and ventilated for transfer to the intensive care unit.

Postoperative Management

Treatment of Pulmonary Hypertension

The ongoing medical care of the newborn with CDH is crucial to long-term survival and is a continuation of intraoperative management. Pulmonary hypertension and lung hypoplasia are the primary determinants of mortality. Immediately after surgery, there is often an improvement in arterial blood gases values and a decrease in ventilating pressures. This "honeymoon period" often lasts for several hours, but the patient then deteriorates because of increased pulmonary artery and airway pressures. This persistent fetal circulation, with right-to-left shunting and occasionally myocardial failure, is responsible for most deaths in the postoperative period. Medical management is directed at preventing and reducing rises in PVR, using some of the same techniques used in the operating room. Hypothermia, metabolic acidosis, and pain all can stimulate a rise in PVR; consequently, general medical care and attention to detail are needed prospectively to avoid unexpected deterioration. Special attention is directed to ventilatory management.

Hyperventilation

Hyperventilation to a $PaCO_2$ of 25 to 30 mm Hg is used to reduce PVR (66). There often is a precipitous decrease in PVR and a rise in PaO_2 when the pH reaches 7.55 to 7.7. As in the operating room, rapid rates and small tidal volumes are used. The use of high-frequency ventilation or oscillation is theoretically attractive because of the potential reduction in barotrauma with lower distending pressures. However, because of the diversity in equipment and rates used, it is not clear which regimen is clearly best. High levels of positive end-expiratory pressure (PEEP) do not improve oxygenation and should be avoided. Throughout the management of these patients, pneumothorax and pneumomediastinum can develop at any time and precipitate rapid deterioration.

Control of F_IO_2

In addition to hyperventilation, oxygen administration is closely managed. Hypoxemia will raise PVR, increasing the right-to-left shunting. Comparing preductal and postductal PaO_2 will indicate the amount of shunting through the ductus arteriosus, foramen ovale and pulmonary circulation (67). The F_IO_2 is adjusted primarily to avoid hypoxemia. As in the operating room, there is concern about oxygen toxicity in susceptible infants, but remember that decreasing the F_IO_2 precipitously can cause sudden decreases in PaO_2, triggering a substantial increase in PVR and rapid deterioration. When the F_IO_2 is lowered, use small increments with the patient observed closely for changes in oxygenation.

Extracorporeal Membrane Oxygenation and Nitric Oxide

Two modalities, extracorporeal membrane oxygenation (ECMO) and inhaled nitric oxide, have been used in newborns with CDH with varying degrees of success and enthusiasm.

ECMO has been used not only in newborns who don't respond to aggressive medical therapy within the first hours of life, but also in those who deteriorate after surgical repair. The goal of ECMO is to ensure adequate cardiopulmonary function for the first few days of life, with the hope that the pulmonary vascular system will stabilize and the persistent fetal circulation will abate. Both arteriovenous and venovenous bypass has been used, with venovenous bypass usually preferred as initial management. Unlike conventional cardiopulmonary bypass, the heart continues to provide some component of cardiac output during ECMO. There is increasing enthusiasm about its effects (68–70), with survival rates of around 50% to 60% being reported in selected patients in whom a 90% mortality rate would otherwise be expected. This has led to a controversial recommendation to consider all newborns with CDH for ECMO therapy if they have failed maximal medical and ventilatory therapy (71,72). Although ECMO is resource- and personnel-intensive, it has been a significant addition to our armamentarium **(see also Chapter 8)**.

Inhaled nitric oxide is the other modality that has been used to decrease PVR in these patients. Nitric oxide is a potent local vasodilator with a very short half-life, making inhalation a method of producing pulmonary vasodilation without systemic vasodilation. This is a true advantage because the general experience with a wide variety of other vasodilators in newborns with CDH has been disheartening. Unfortunately, nitric oxide is difficult to administer and is currently limited to a few centers involved in investigations. This may change in the near future. As with ECMO, there are both supporters and detractors for the effectiveness of nitric oxide. Further research will more clearly delineate the role of each technique.

Prognosis

Newborns requiring surgery in the first hours of life continue to have a high mortality rate (52,53). Significant nonpulmonary congenital anomalies, prematurity, preoperative pH less than 7.0, and preoperative P(A-a)O$_2$ greater than 500 torr all correlate with a high mortality rate. Newborns that do not improve after surgical repair and have a P(A-a)O$_2$ greater than 500 torr after reduction of the hernia generally do not survive (73). On the other hand, children who survive the neonatal period usually do well in childhood and grow normally. Although pulmonary function tests demonstrate some persistent ventilation/perfusion abnormalities (74), the patients usually are functionally asymptomatic.

TRACHEOESOPHAGEAL FISTULA

Tracheoesophageal fistula (TEF) is a test of the anesthesiologist's skill with the airway. TEF occurs in between 1 in 3000 and 1 in 4500 live births, making it one of the more common conditions requiring surgical intervention in the newborn. Both the trachea and the esophagus develop from the median ventral diverticulum of the foregut, and if normal separation does not occur, the child will have a TEF, esophageal atresia without fistula, or, rarely, a laryngoesophageal cleft (75). There are several different potential abnormalities, but the most common form (over 85% of affected patients) is a combination of proximal esophageal atresia ("blind pouch") and a fistula connecting the distal esophagus and distal trachea. The second most common abnormality is esophageal atresia without fistula, present in up to 10% of cases; TEF without esophageal atresia (H-type fistula) accounts for about 2% of the cases, and other combinations occur at less than a 1% rate.

Associated Congenital Anomalies

The most important marker for mortality and morbidity in TEF patients is the presence of other major congenital anomalies. Between 30% and 50% of these newborns have these anomalies (76), with the most important associated problems being cardiac (ventricular septal defect, tetralogy of Fallot, atrial septal defect, and atrioventricular canal). The acronym VATER, for *V*ertebral defects, *A*nal atresia, *T*EF, r*E*nal defects, and *R*adial limb dysplasia, has been used to designate which congenital abnormalities are most commonly associated with TEF. An important part of preanesthetic evaluation is consideration of the presence of associated abnormalities. A second major contributor to morbidity and mortality is prematurity, with up to 30% of newborns with esophageal atresia being preterm. Survival has been linked very closely to birth weight. An immature respiratory system is a particularly important consideration in these patients, because aspiration pneumonitis from the TEF may be complicated by IRDS, making ventilation and oxygenation especially challenging.

Clinical Presentation

The clinical manifestations of patients with TEF usually occur shortly after birth, often with the first feeding. On attempted feeding, the child may demonstrate the "three C's" of esophageal atresia—choking, coughing, and cyanosis—because of inability to swallow beyond the blind pouch and because of aspiration of the food. Paradoxically, the newborn may gasp air that passes through the fistula into the distal esophagus, producing a distended abdomen. The distended stomach, combined with vigorous coughing, can precipitate further aspiration—this time of gastric contents up the distal esophagus into the trachea and lungs. In these patients, aspiration pneumonitis can become life-threatening, with severe hypoxemia and hypercarbia (75,76).

Preoperative Evaluation

Diagnosis

In the past, diagnosis of atresia and fistula was made using radiocontrast dye in the upper pouch. Because of the risk of further aspiration (dye), insertion of a radiopaque orogastric tube is used to demonstrate esophageal obstruction, usually at the 10- to 12-cm depth. A radiograph of the abdomen will demonstrate air in the bowel if there is an associated fistula. Children with an H-type fistula without esophageal atresia usually present later in infancy with recurrent pneumonias and will be detected only on close examination of upper gastrointestinal dye examinations.

Initial Priorities

Initial priorities of management are to prevent further aspiration, treat any pneumonitis, and diagnose existing abnormalities, especially cardiac. An orogastric tube will drain any accumulations in the upper pouch, while nursing in a semi-upright position will discourage passive regurgitation through the TEF. Antibiotic therapy may be started if there is evidence of pneumonitis, whereas supplemental oxygen is administered if there is evidence of hypoxemia. Rarely, the newborn with overwhelming pneumonitis, IRDS, or heart failure will need intubation and ventilation before surgical repair is attempted; in these patients, a gastrostomy is usually done under local anesthesia to drain the stomach, preventing further soiling of the lung (77,78). When the pulmonary status has improved, usually in 3 to 5 days, definitive surgery can proceed. Increasingly, the decision to perform definitive repair versus a staged repair is based on the physiologic status of the patient, not the gestational age, weight, or presence of major anomalies (75,79).

Other Systems

Preoperative evaluation also focuses on nonpulmonary systems. Because the newborn has not been able to effectively swallow, hydration and glucose levels are checked. If there is significant dehydration or hypoglycemia, they should be corrected before proceeding with anesthesia and surgery. Although transfusion is not routinely needed, a type and cross-match should be done because of the proximity of the operative site to major vascular structures.

Surgical Repair

Although repair of a TEF is not usually a true life-threatening emergency, it is useful to proceed expeditiously to minimize further pulmonary aspiration. There is some variation in surgical approach; some pediatric surgeons preferring a primary esophageal repair and fistula closure after gastrostomy local anesthesia, whereas others prefer to omit the gastrostomy (75,76,80). If the distance between the proximal and distal esophageal segments is too long for primary closure, the TEF can be divided and the upper esophagus externalized, delaying primary anastomosis until later.

Anesthetic Management

Monitors

Standard monitoring is used for these patients, with two notable changes. Although an esophageal stethoscope is placed after intubation, it will not be present for the whole operation because it will have to be removed when the esophageal anastomosis is made. Until then, it will be used by the surgeon to define the lower limits of the upper pouch. Because the esophageal stethoscope is only temporary, a precordial stethoscope is placed in the left axilla to keep it out of the surgical field. It is useful in this position because of its ability to detect mainstem intubations during the course of the case. For the same reason, rectal temperature monitoring is used instead of esophageal. Core temperature monitoring is important because of the potential for large heat losses during the thoracotomy.

Pulse Oximetry

Pulse oximetry is especially useful in this surgery because there are often sudden episodes of hypoxemia from compression of the lung, kinking of the tracheobronchial tree, and loss of ventilation through the fistula at the time of division. In these small children, it is useful to place a second probe at the start of the procedure because of the not-infrequent failure of one of the probes as the case proceeds.

Capnography. Capnography is especially useful in this surgery to diagnose any sudden absence in effective ventilation secondary to movement of the endotracheal tube or opening of the fistula.

Blood Pressure Monitoring. Arterial pressure monitoring for blood gas and pressure monitoring is important; pressure monitoring is probably more important because of the possibility of sudden hypotension due to compression of great vessels by the surgeon's hands. A caveat to this is that with pulse oximetry, capnography, and Doppler-assisted blood pressure measurements, it has been possible to safely monitor full-term newborns undergoing TEF closure without arterial lines. The decision to use arterial-line monitoring depends on the anesthesiologist's preference, the underlying medical status of the patient, and the anticipated need for the monitor in both the intra- and postoperative periods.

Endotracheal Intubation of the Newborn with TEF

Technique. Intubation of the newborn can be challenging under the most controlled conditions; in the newborn with TEF, there is the additional problem of the fistula. Consequently, good technique is vital. Several factors—relatively large tongue, small mandible, long, narrow, omega-shaped epiglottis and more cephalad vocal cords (C4 versus C6 in the older child), increased anteroposterior diameter of the head, and short neck—increase the susceptibility to upper airway obstruction and make intubation more difficult **(see also Chapter 4)**. A straight blade is usually preferred to allow displacement of the relatively large tongue to the side.

Proper Placement. In the patient with a TEF, the proper placement of the endotracheal tube is probably the most important contribution of the anesthesiologist in this surgery. By placing the tip of the tube beyond the fistula, the anesthesiologist will be able to ensure adequate ventilation and oxygenation during the thoracotomy; if the tip of the tube is not beyond the fistula, ventilation will preferentially go to the lower-resistance gastrointestinal tract, with subsequent hypoventilation and hypoxemia. Intubation may be done in the awake patient, since it may take more than one attempt to place the endotracheal tube in the optimal position, although some experienced clinicians have preferred to use either IV or inhalation inductions in full-term, healthy patients (81).[e]

The use of adequate preoxygenation and an oxyscope minimizes desaturation during awake endotracheal intubation. If the fistula is intubated using these techniques, the patient will not suffer significant desaturation as long as the tube position is quickly recognized and the tube withdrawn. The key to proper placement is to remember two details about the anatomy in the typical TEF patient:

- The fistula from the distal esophagus enters the posterior surface of the trachea. By turning the tip of the bevel of

---

[e]Ed. Note (JMB): I am one of those clinicians who prefers to use general anesthesia to intubate these patients. As with everything in anesthesia, one has to choose which set of risks one is willing to accept. By anesthetizing the infant, I am accepting the risk that I might be unable to achieve proper tube placement, but this hasn't happened yet. By contrast, in awake intubation, one must accept the potential struggle to intubate the trachea in an otherwise vigorous infant. In addition, awake intubation does carry some risk of causing the infant to become hypertensive, have increased intracranial pressure, and/or have oxygen-hemoglobin desaturation—events not particularly beneficial to newborn infants, particularly those prone to intraventricular hemorrhage (e.g., premature infants).

the endotracheal tube at 90 degrees to normal so that the longest, leading surface rests on the anterior wall of the trachea, one can advance the tube down the trachea and past the fistula without entering the fistula.

- The fistula enters the trachea at various levels, but most commonly just above the carina. Because of this, one should advance the endotracheal tube past the carina into a mainstem bronchus and then withdraw until there are bilateral breath sounds and bilateral chest expansion. If a gastrostomy has been previously placed, it is possible to put the gastrostomy tube under water and look for bubbles, indicating that the tube is above the fistula and needs to be advanced farther. A normal capnographic trace, good bilateral breath sounds, and an absence of breath sounds over the abdomen are useful monitors for correct tube placement.

Unfortunately, there may rarely be a significant leak into the fistula, even when the endotracheal tube is at the carina. The best solution to this problem requires a bit of experimenting by the anesthesiologist. Turning the tube's bevel can sometimes occlude the fistula, and others have suggested right mainstem intubation with reliance on the Murphy eye for left-sided ventilation (82). Another suggestion has been to occlude the lower esophagus by a balloon-tipped catheter inserted through a gastrostomy (80).

Maintenance of Anesthesia

Spontaneous or Controlled Ventilation

Although there are some theoretical advantages to spontaneous ventilation (minimizing flow through the fistula) until the surgeon has quickly opened and clamped the fistula, spontaneous ventilation in the lateral position for a thoracotomy in a newborn is difficult to maintain without significant hypoventilation, hypoxemia, and hypotension. Gentle, assisted ventilation or controlled hand ventilation with faster rates and low peak airway pressures is more commonly used. Several different anesthetic regimens have been successfully used for TEF repairs; there is little to recommend one technique over another. However, there is often significant lung compression during the procedure, necessitating higher than expected levels of oxygen. For this reason, nitrous oxide is usually omitted, and variable combinations of oxygen and air or oxygen and nitrogen are used.

Intraoperative Considerations

A retropleural approach is commonly used to expose the esophagus and trachea, with the child in the left lateral position. During dissection, the lung and the trachea will be compressed, increasing airway pressures and making ventilation more difficult. Many clinicians ventilate manually at this stage of the procedure to judge the changes due to compression and compensate for them. In consultation with the surgeon, it will sometimes be necessary to halt the dissection for a short time and reinflate the lungs, restoring adequate oxygenation and ventilation. Constant communication with the surgeon is crucial for maintaining adequate ventilation. At the time the TEF is divided, there can be significant loss of gases through the open fistula into the wound. If there is a fall in oxygenation, the surgeon should manually occlude the hole to allow restoration of adequate oxygenation before proceeding with the repair. After the fistula closure, the anesthetic technique is straightforward for the rest of the case. However, there may continue to be sudden desaturation or hypotension from surgical compression. A cause of sudden desaturation that should always be considered is inadvertent movement of the endotracheal tube, positioned near the carina, into a mainstem bronchus.

Extubation

At the end of the procedure, it is often possible to extubate the trachea (83). Advantages of extubation include lack of pressure on the tracheal suture line and avoidance of positive pressure at that site. However, patients with significant pneumonitis or IRDS, very low birth weight, symptomatic heart disease, or incomplete recovery from anesthetics or muscle relaxants will benefit from continued ventilation.

Postoperative Considerations

In the postoperative period, there can be several complications related to the pulmonary system. These newborns have tracheomalacia at the site of the fistula and do not have the usual effective ciliary mechanisms to remove secretions (84). Warm, humidified gases, frequent changes in position, and gentle suctioning will control secretions and prevent atelectasis (83). Also, preexisting pneumonitis may worsen, precipitating ventilatory failure. It occasionally becomes necessary to remove secretions by inserting a suction catheter into the trachea under direct laryngoscopic vision at the bedside. Leakage from the esophageal anastomosis site can cause mediastinitis, sepsis, and lung compression from pneumothorax or pneumomediastinum. If there is rapid deterioration in the first few days after surgery, transillumination of the chest may quickly identify pneumothorax as the cause, speeding chest tube drainage of the air. Finally, there is usually some residual esophageal dysfunction from gastroesophageal reflux, decreased esophageal motility, and stricture formation, which can cause recurrent respiratory tract infections secondary to aspiration and poor clearing of secretions during the first few years of life. As these children age, they show good growth, although respiratory reserve does appear somewhat diminished into childhood (85–87).

Prognosis

Prognosis in TEF is primarily dependent on the presence of other congenital anomalies, prematurity (88), and aspiration pneumonitis (89). Because congenital heart disease is the most prominent cause of mortality (76), aggressive treatment of cardiac anomalies may contribute to greater survival (90). For full-term newborns without pneumonitis or major anomalies, a survival rate of almost 100% can be expected with modern techniques, but preterm newborns with severe pneumonitis or major associated anomalies will have a reduced survival rate of about 50% to 75% (75,84).

OMPHALOCELE AND GASTROSCHISIS

One of the best definitions of a pediatric anesthesiologist is someone who can correctly spell both gastroschisis and omphalocele. Omphalocele occurs in between 1 in 3000 and 1 in 10,000 live births and results from herniation of abdominal contents into an avascular sack of peritoneum and amniotic membrane at the base of the umbilical cord. If the sack tears or ruptures before surgery, the newborn may experience significant fluid and temperature losses. The sack may be filled with only a small amount of small intestine or with a very large amount of intestine, spleen, liver, bladder, and stomach. With the larger omphaloceles, both the abdominal and thoracic cavities are smaller than usual for the child's length. Other congenital anomalies occur in about 50% of all patients with omphalocele, contributing significantly to mortality and morbidity (91). These anomalies can include exstrophy of the bladder, malrotation, diaphragmatic hernia, meningocele, cleft palate, and congenital heart disease. Congenital heart disease, such as tetralogy of Fallot, increases reported overall mortality rates from 30% to 80% (92). Beckwith-Wiedemann syndrome occurs in about 6% of omphalocele patients. This syndrome consists of the omphalocele, macroglossia, gigantism, microcephaly, and hypoglycemia, and it can complicate management (93).

Gastroschisis occurs less frequently than omphalocele, 1 in 30,000 live births, although there is some evidence that there is an increased incidence of gastroschisis in Northern Europe and the United States, making it slightly more common than omphalocele in some regions (93). Gastroschisis is a defect in the abdominal wall to the right of the umbilicus that has no sack covering the exposed viscera, possibly because of a vascular accident during development of the abdominal wall. Because the viscera have been exposed to amniotic fluid, the contents are usually edematous and adherent from inflammation. Premature labor and delivery are common with gastroschisis, possibly from irritation of the exposed bowel. Most newborns with gastroschisis are preterm, whereas omphalocele is associated with a slightly increased rate of prematurity (94). Of interest, associated congenital lesions are not particularly increased in patients with gastroschisis.

Preoperative Evaluation

Although the diagnosis of gastroschisis and omphalocele is obvious at birth, proper evaluation focuses not only on associated lesions and problems, but also on the hydration status of the patient. The exposed abdominal area is covered with warm, saline-soaked sponges, and the child nursed in a warm, humidified environment. An orogastric tube is usually placed to decompress the stomach and minimize the risk of aspiration. Patients with large expanses of exposed bowel may develop three early complications, all of which are manifested as hypotension.

Hypotension in the Newborn with Omphalocele or Gastroschisis[f]

Transition from Fetal Circulation

The newborn must adjust quickly from the fetal to the neonatal state in the cardiovascular system to survive. The fetal circulation is designed to allow placental blood to pass through the foramen ovale into the left atrium, bypassing the pulmonary circulation. Blood that does flow into the right ventricle and pulmonary artery primarily flows across the ductus arteriosus into the aorta instead of through the pulmonary circulation because of the high PVR and low systemic vascular resistance. At birth, expansion of the lungs results in a precipitous drop in PVR and an increase in pulmonary blood flow. When venous return to the left atrium increases, the flap-like valve of the foramen ovale closes, eliminating shunting of unoxygenated blood. Because anatomic closure takes months to years to accomplish, there continues to be a risk for reopening and shunting in the presence of elevated PVR, coughing, or crying (95).

The ductus arteriosus closes as the intramural muscle contracts in response to a fall in prostaglandin E_2 levels induced by increased blood oxygen concentrations. As the ductus closes, pulmonary blood flow and oxygen uptake increase. If PVR is low, there may be left-to-right shunting with pulmonary edema and heart failure, but shunting will go right to left, with the potential for hypoxemia and heart failure, if PVR is high. Although small degrees of shunting are usually well tolerated, larger shunts can produce a cycle of progressive ventilation/perfusion mismatching and heart failure.

More about the Neonatal Myocardium

The neonatal myocardium is different from the adult myocardium (96). Neonatal myocytes are smaller and less tightly packed than adult cells (97), resulting in a myocardium that is less compliant than in the older child. Although the atria may dilate in response to preload, the ventricles have a limited ability to respond, producing a fixed stroke volume. Cardiac output becomes heart rate–dependent, although there is some controversy on this point (98). The neonatal myocardium also has a greater dependence on carbohydrates as fuel, compared with the adult myocardium, giving newborns the ability to effectively use not only glycolysis, but also glycogenolysis, for en-

---
[f]Ed. Note (JMB): What follows is a beautiful description of intraoperative hypotension in the newborn in general. Although it occurs frequently in infants with omphalocele and gastroschisis, it is not a phenomenon restricted to these disorders; it can, and does, occur all too frequently in newborn infants anesthetized for any reason. It is presented in the text at this particular point because it is highly common in infants with omphalocele or gastroschisis.

ergy; this may be one of the reasons why the neonatal heart tolerates periods of ischemia or anoxia better than does the adult heart (99).

Sympathetic Innervation of the Heart

Although the parasympathetic nervous system is fully functional at birth, the sympathetic system is not fully developed until the infant is 4 to 6 months of age. Because the neonatal myocardium has decreased sympathetic innervation, there is less response to cardioactive drugs that act indirectly, such as dopamine.

Pulmonary Vascular Resistance

As discussed earlier, the pulmonary vascular bed is very responsive in the neonatal period. PVR may increase in an exaggerated fashion in response to stresses such as hypoxemia, hypercapnia, hypothermia, sepsis, or acidosis. A large increase in PVR causes blood to be shunted away from the pulmonary circulation through the foramen ovale or ductus arteriosus, causing persistent transitional circulation or persistent pulmonary hypertension of the newborn, with a cycle of increased right-to-left shunting, hypoxemia, progressive acidosis, right ventricular failure, and death. The therapy is the same as mentioned for CDH—hyperventilation, oxygen therapy, vasodilators, and, in extreme cases, ECMO. However, no treatment has been shown to be totally reliable (100).

Systemic Vascular Resistance

The systemic vascular bed also undergoes dramatic changes in the newborn. Peripheral vascular resistance increases in the first days and weeks of life, but the relative immaturity of the sympathetic nervous system prevents effective increases in systemic vascular resistance in response to hypovolemia. Because of this, timely volume replacement is especially critical to maintain adequate preload. Other reflexes, such as the baroreceptor reflexes, are present at birth, but not as efficient, and may be blocked by anesthetics in the newborn (101).

Causes and Treatment of Hypotension in the Newborn

Stress Factors. Hypotension in the newborn is not usually caused by intrinsic congenital heart disease, but is a result of other stresses, such as hypoxemia, hypovolemia, or sepsis. In the newborn with gastroschisis or omphalocele, hypovolemia can occur because of losses of both crystalloid and colloid from the exposed surfaces and into indurated bowel. If uncorrected, hemoconcentration, metabolic acidosis, and hypotension develop. Because of this, IV replacement is started immediately with a balanced salt solution at two to three times normal maintenance, or 8 to 12 ml/kg/hour. Additional boluses of balanced salt or colloid, 10 ml/kg, are given if there is evidence of hypovolemia, such as urine output < 1 ml/kg/hour, tachycardia, hypotension, or metabolic acidosis. It is important to remember that the proper treatment of a metabolic acidosis secondary to fluid loss is additional fluid, not sodium bicarbonate. Sodium bicarbonate therapy is only appropriate for the rare case when acidosis is dangerously high (i.e., < 7.2) and is impairing myocardial function. Serum electrolytes, glucose, and acid-base status are followed up during rehydration to guide management. Glucose monitoring is especially important because these patients may develop hypoglycemia or hyperglycemia as a response to stress. Administering glucose, either D_5 or D_{10}, in salt solution at 4 ml/kg/hour is usually appropriate to provide adequate calories as a maintenance. However, repeat measures of glucose levels are necessary to identify either hypoglycemia or hyperglycemia.

Hypothermia. The second cause of hypotension in patients with omphalocele and gastroschisis is hypothermia. The exposed bowel can undergo large losses of heat in both the preoperative and intraoperative period. Preventive measures, such as a warm room or incubator, warmed gases and IV fluids, forced-air warming blankets or clear plastic covering (e.g., Saran Wrap), and warming lights help to minimize heat loss. Thermoregulation is different in the newborn because of a lack of adequate shivering, vasoconstriction, and insulation. The newborn exposed to a cold stress uses increased metabolic activity, especially in the central mitochondria-rich fat deposits ("brown fat"), as the primary component of heat production (102). However, this may be inhibited by certain anesthetics (103). Unfortunately, the use of this nonshivering thermogenesis is associated with increased oxygen consumption, ketone production, acidosis, and osmotic diuresis. Prevention of heat loss by aggressive prospective management is preferable to rewarming a cold, acidotic infant.

Sepsis. The third cause of hypotension in these patients is sepsis. Although antibiotics are usually started early in the course of management, the sudden appearance of unexplained tachycardia and hypotension may be the first signs of sepsis. Symptomatic treatment with fluids and, if needed, inotropic therapy are needed.

Anesthetic Management

Preoperative Preparation

The first step in anesthetic management is to ensure that there has been adequate fluid resuscitation before induction. This may take several hours, with repeated reevaluation and monitoring, before resuscitation has been accomplished. Standard monitoring is applied before induction, with radial artery monitoring particularly useful for blood pressure, hematocrit, blood gas, and glucose measurements, with glucose measurements especially important in the child with Beckwith-Wiedemann syndrome (93). If arterial-line monitoring is problematic, Doppler-assisted blood pressures can be used. Although it has been suggested that central venous pressure monitoring can be useful for evaluation of both intravascular volume and the degree of compromise during abdominal closure (104), it is not widely used for the latter purpose.

The stomach is suctioned before induction. After preoxygenation, a rapid sequence induction is used for intubation in the hemodynamically stable patient. Although awake intubation with an oxyscope is used if the intravascular status is uncertain or if a difficult intubation is anticipated, it is usually not necessary.

Maintenance of Anesthesia

Maintenance of anesthesia can be accomplished with a wide variety of volatile agent or narcotic-based techniques. Air or nitrogen is added to oxygen to maintain acceptable SaO_2 (or PaO_2), but avoiding nitrous oxide because of its potential for bowel distention. A nondepolarizing muscle relaxant is used to provide maximal abdominal muscle relaxation for abdominal closure. A regional block, such as a caudal or epidural block, can provide both intraoperative and postoperative benefit (105–108), although it is rare to use a block as the sole anesthetic.

Intraoperative Fluid Management

Intraoperative fluid management is a tremendous challenge in these patients. Third-space losses are usually initially replaced with lactated Ringer's solution, using approximations such as 6 to 10 ml/kg/hour for abdominal surgery and 4 to 6 ml/kg/hour for intrathoracic surgery. However, these volumes are just starting points and must be adjusted using hemodynamic parameters, skin perfusion, fullness of the fontanelle, and evaluation of the surgical field as monitors. Laboratory studies such as repeat determinations of the hematocrit, electrolytes, glucose, and pH can be useful. Colloid is often added when there is significant third-space loss, using boluses of 5 to 10 ml/kg of 5% albumin. Although fresh frozen plasma has been empirically used to dilute red blood cells and in situations such as gastroschisis with large losses of colloid, there is no evidence that it is superior to albumin.

Blood Components. Red blood cells and platelets are administered in newborns for the same criteria as in older children and adults. Although a normal hematocrit is 45% to 50% in the newborn and anemia is defined as under 40%, this assumes blood that is primarily fetal hemoglobin. Fetal hemoglobin releases oxygen to the tissue at lower tissue saturations than adult hemoglobin. Therefore, when transfusing adult hemoglobin, it is not necessary to attain the higher levels of hematocrit seen with fetal hemoglobin; if the blood volume is largely replaced by transfused red cells, adult hematocrit levels of 35% to 40% are appropriate. When administering red cells to a newborn, remember that irradiated cells are needed to prevent graft-versus-host potential. Also, filtering for white cells is now felt to be more beneficial than washing of cells.

Citrate Toxicity. With rapid infusion of fresh frozen plasma or blood, there may be significant chelation of calcium by the citrate in the preserved blood products. Because newborns have decreased calcium stores, they are more susceptible to transient hypocalcemia and hypotension. Either calcium chloride (10 mg/kg) or calcium gluconate (30 mg/kg) can reverse the hypocalcemia (109), but rapid infusion has been associated with sudden reflex bradycardia and hypotension.

Surgical Considerations

Although it is desirable for both omphalocele and gastroschisis to have a primary closure, a staged repair with a "silo" is used if the abdominal cavity is too small to accept all the viscera. Compressing too much bowel into the abdomen can result in hypotension, decreased preload, decreased cardiac output (110), ventilatory failure (111), decreased renal blood flow (112), and bowel ischemia. Observation of the blood pressure, heart rate, and perfusion of the lower extremities (113) has been suggested as a useful monitor of adequate aortocaval function during closure. Although spontaneous ventilation was used for these cases in the past and return of viscera to the abdomen stopped when ventilation became strained or inadequate because of diaphragmatic compression, this monitoring method has been abandoned and replaced with observation for changes in airway and blood pressures. The anesthesiologist and surgeon monitor these and decide whether primary closure can be done based on the changes. In our institution, a rise in peak airway pressures of up to 50% of baseline are allowed. When the upper limits of this range are used, elective postoperative ventilation for several days are planned to ensure adequate ventilation and oxygenation.

Aortocaval Compression. A dramatic source of hypotension can be aortocaval compression secondary to abdominal contents. This can appear as the last stitches are being tightened or a couple minutes later, just at the end of the case when attention is starting to be directed to the task of transport to the neonatal intensive care unit. The immediate and appropriate treatment of this hypotension is reopening of the surgical wound to release the compression. After the wound is opened and the normal pressure restored, a decision can be made about further management. In some cases, judicious additional hydration or the addition of inotropic support is adequate to allow reclosure. If an abdominal muscle layer had been closed in the repair, closing only skin may be another solution. However, if it is not possible to obtain primary closure without hypotension, an artificial sac of prosthetic material is constructed around the exposed bowel and suspended to prevent excessive pressure on the underlying bowel and aortocaval system. This silo is systematically reduced over the next days or, in extreme cases, weeks.

Extubation

After primary closure, some patients who are awake, normothermic, vigorous, and strong can be extubated. However, if the abdominal closure has resulted in a tight, tense abdominal cavity, the diaphragms are under significant pressure and will not provide adequate ventilation or ability to clear secretions. Most newborns are left intubated and ventilated for at least the first postoperative day. Remember that significant third-space fluid losses continue into the immediate postoperative period and require vigorous fluid and, occasionally, red blood cell replacement. Sepsis is also a concern that demands constant observation.

Prognosis

Prognosis for patients with gastroschisis and omphalocele depends on several factors. Low birth weight and prematurity are predictors of higher mortality and morbidity (91), but associated congenital anomalies appear to be most important (113). With modern therapy, it is reasonable to expect a survival rate of up to 90% if there are no associated major anomalies, and an overall survival rate of over 60% (91).

NECROTIZING ENTEROCOLITIS

Not all surgical procedures in the newborn are based on congenital abnormalities. Necrotizing enterocolitis (NEC) is most commonly a condition seen in preterm newborns who present with life-threatening bowel distention, peritonitis, and sepsis, with mortality in a range as high as 50% and higher. Most of these newborns are under 38 weeks' gestational age, with a reported incidence between 1% to 5% (114,115), although rates as high as 7.3% have been reported (116). NEC can rarely be seen in full-term newborns who have other abnormalities, such as congenital heart disease, which appears to predispose them to NEC.

Although the exact cause of NEC is inconclusive (117,118), the common element in the different explanations for NEC is the loss of integrity of the intestinal mucosal barrier. Many affected patients have significant systemic stresses, including hypoxemia, hypotension, asphyxia, hypothermia, or heart failure, which may cause a common pathway of decreased mesenteric regional blood flow, leading to bowel ischemia, necrosis, and subsequent sepsis (119). However, these identifiable factors are not present in all newborns who develop NEC. There is an increased incidence after early feedings, especially if the liquid is hyperosmolar, leading to the suggestion that feedings are necessary for bacterial colonization to occur and that this is an integral part of NEC (120).

Preoperative Considerations

The first signs of NEC usually occur before the infant is 10 days of age, with abdominal distention, vomiting (occasionally bile-stained), diarrhea (occasionally bloody), and stools positive for blood, along with abdominal erythema and tenderness. Radiographs of the abdomen may show free air, air in the portal venous system, dilated bowel, and pneumotosis intestinalis (bubbles of subserosal gas) (121). With bowel ischemia and necrosis, overwhelming sepsis may rapidly develop. There can be large shifts of fluid into the ischemic bowel, with resulting hypovolemia, hypotension, lethargy, and apnea. With progressive abdominal distention (and sepsis and hypotension), there is progressive hypoventilation, hypercarbia, and hypoxemia. Disseminated intravascular coagulation and hypothermia commonly appear in conjunction with the sepsis. Finally, hyperkalemia may develop as a result of massive bowel necrosis. This last sign is particularly ominous, being associated with fatal dysrhythmias.

The initial therapy for NEC is medical, not surgical (115). Feedings are stopped, gastric decompression started, and vigorous fluid resuscitation started. Colloid and red blood cells are the mainstay of fluid resuscitation because of the large plasma and blood losses into the gut. Fresh frozen plasma and platelets are often given to replace factors lost with the massive third spacing of fluid and disseminated intravascular coagulation. IV antibiotic coverage for both gram-negative and gram-positive organisms is started (122). If hypotension is refractory to fluid replacement, inotropic therapy with dopamine (5 to 10 µg/kg/min) or dobutamine (5 to 10 µg/kg/min) is started. If metabolic acidosis is not controlled by fluid therapy, inotropes, and antibiotics, sodium bicarbonate is usually given to bring the pH above 7. Finally, the patient is closely monitored with repeat arterial blood gases, electrolytes, platelet counts, and prothrombin time and partial thromboplastin time.

Problems Associated With NEC and Prematurity

Necrotizing enterocolitis is usually a disease of preterm newborns who are often stressed from other causes. Preterms are more likely to have IRDS, a patent ductus arteriosus, a fragile choroid plexus, or immature retina compared with a full-term newborn. IRDS, with its atelectasis, hypoxemia, and hypercarbia, can complicate the management of NEC because the abdominal distention makes adequate ventilation of the diseased lungs harder than usual. The vigorous fluid therapy given during NEC resuscitation can reopen or increase the shunting through a patent ductus arteriosus. With left-to-right shunting through a patent ductus, less cardiac output is directed systemically, leading to further bowel ischemia.

The wide swings in cardiac output and blood pressure associated with this disease and its therapy also puts the preterm at risk for intraventricular hemorrhage. Although the stable preterm infant has intact cerebral blood flow autoregulation, some preterms have lost this ability. Hypercarbia, hypoxemia, perinatal ischemia, and other factors can abolish autoregulation in the preterm newborn (123). Systemic hypotension can lead to impaired cerebral blood flow, whereas hypertension can increase blood flow to a degree that causes hemorrhage. It is interesting that recent data have shown that preterm infants who suffer intraventricular hemorrhages tend to have lower mean blood pressures and wider swings in blood pressure compared with preterms who do not suffer hemorrhages, indicating poorer autonomic control of circulation (124).

Finally, the changes in cardiac output and arterial oxygen levels put the preterm's developing retinal vasculature at risk for ROP **(see Retinopathy of Prematurity)**.

More Preoperative Considerations

Newborns who develop free air are explored, but indications for surgery on other patients are less clear and vary from center to center. It is important to review past therapy, especially volume requirements, and current functional status as part of preanesthetic evaluation. Physical examination focuses on an assessment of hydration, adequacy of cardiac output and peripheral perfusion, effect of the abdominal distention and current medical condition on ventilation, and degree of alertness. Laboratory work for the current acid-base, electrolyte, hematologic, coagulation, and glucose values are important. These patients can deteriorate rapidly, so laboratory work or physical examination from several hours earlier may not be accurate for the patient's status at the time of surgery.

History of Controlled Ventilation. If the patient is not already intubated and ventilated, it is prudent to carefully examine the adequacy of ventilation before transporting to the operating room. If the child has signs of hypoxemia or hypercarbia, intubation and ventilation should be instituted before leaving the intensive care unit.

Blood Pressure Monitoring. Although intra-arterial monitoring is important for both blood pressure and laboratory assessment, it may be technically very difficult to institute, especially in newborns under 1500 g (125). The usefulness of the line must be balanced against the time and risk involved in either cutting down on or cannulating a relatively central artery, such as the femoral or brachial. Central venous lines can be useful for volume management; a central venous cannula is often inserted either during previous medical management or at the time of surgery to allow subsequent IV hyperalimentation. Core temperature monitoring is especially important because of the tendency to develop hypothermia from exposed bowel.

Anesthetic Management

Induction of Anesthesia

Induction and maintenance techniques are dependent on the medical status of the patient.

If not intubated before surgery, full stomach precautions are taken. A poorly responsive, weak infant needs to have the airway secured quickly, often with an awake intubation, whereas a rapid-sequence induction is used in the more vigorous patient. Although concern has been expressed about the potential for increased intracranial pressure during awake intubation (126), the initial priority must be expeditious establishment of a secure airway.

Although sick newborns obviously deserve the same level of anesthesia as other critically ill patients, there has been a tendency to avoid the use of anesthetics in sick newborns because of fear of hemodynamic instability and a lack of concern about the effects of not providing anesthesia.

Maintenance of Anesthesia

For maintenance of anesthesia during laparotomy for NEC, narcotics or low-dose isoflurane or halothane are usually used, but nitrous oxide is avoided because of the distended, obstructed bowel. The NEC patient who requires surgery may be hemodynamically very compromised and sensitive to the depressant effects of any anesthetic agent, making titration of the agent crucial. Nondepolarizing neuromuscular blockers are used to provide adequate surgical conditions, with little to recommend one agent over another.

After the abdomen has been opened, the particular surgical procedure will depend on direct findings (127,128). Perforations in otherwise viable bowel are closed, and necrotic segments of intestine are resected, leaving as much viable bowel as possible. To divert stool and put the bowel at rest, an ileostomy is often performed. Unfortunately, some patients will have almost the entire bowel infarcted. These patients usually are closed without further manipulation and succumb within hours.

The anesthesiologist may be extremely busy during the surgical procedure because of ongoing fluid losses, metabolic acidosis and hypotension. The blood pressure can precipitously fall when the abdomen is opened and releases the tamponade of distended bowel on the abdominal vessels, requiring rapid fluid replacement. When administering fluid, it is important not only to decide which colloid is most appropriate, but also to warm the fluids before administration. The fluid replacement may be spectacular in these cases, sometimes well in excess of a total blood volume. Therefore, it is important to periodically monitor not only the blood pressure, but also the hematocrit, blood gas, potassium, and platelet count. Inotropic infusions or, in the presence of severe deterioration, vasoconstrictor infusions, may be needed to maintain adequate cardiac output. Rarely, a metabolic acidosis will have to be corrected with sodium bicarbonate or hypocalcemia treated with calcium to correct hypotension.

Postoperative Considerations

At the end of the case, peak airway pressures often are elevated as the abdomen is closed. Ventilation is adjusted to provide adequate end-tidal CO_2 and arterial oxygen saturations. As with gastroschisis, a fall in blood pressure with closure indicates that there is some aortocaval compression by bowel. However, this usually responds to fluid replacement and does not require reopening of the surgical wound. It is extremely unusual to extubate a patient in the operating room after surgery for this lesion. Continued fluid losses, sepsis, disseminated intravascular coagulation, or problems related to prematurity (IRDS, patent ductus arteriosus) can interfere with postoperative ventilation.

NEC continues to be a source of significant morbidity and mortality in the preterm population (114,129). With aggressive intensive care, timely surgical intervention, and appropriate anesthetic care, the mortality rate remains about 50% in most series (130). The extreme prematurity of many of these patients bring additional challenges to the management of the bowel ischemia, providing a continuing challenge to all the clinicians involved in treatment.

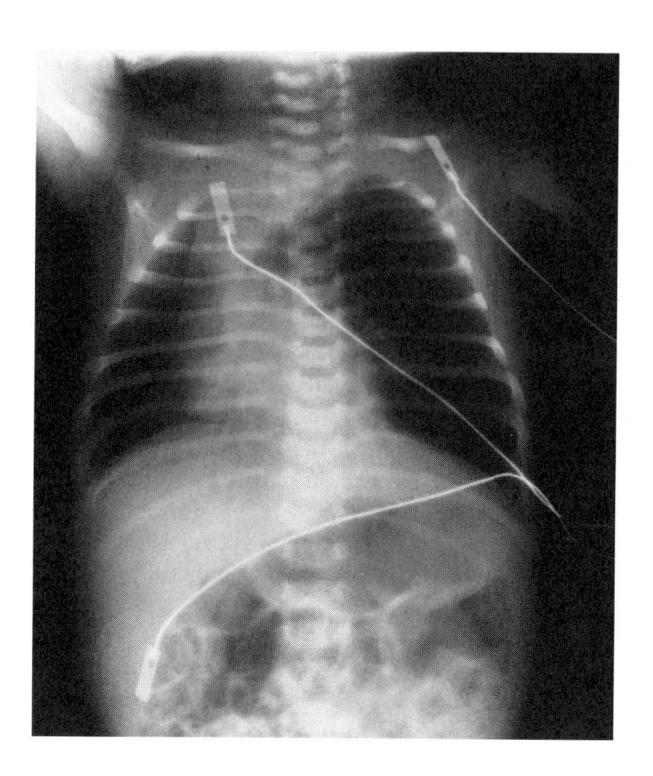

FIG. 1. A 1-month old infant with congenital lobar emphysema. The absence of pulmonary marking in congenital lobar emphysema differentiates it from congenital adenomatous malformation.

CONGENITAL LOBAR EMPHYSEMA

Congenital lobar emphysema (CLE) is a pathologic accumulation of air in one lobe of the lung, usually an upper lobe or the right middle lobe (Fig. 1). Although the clinical presentation of CLE is highly variable, it frequently occurs at birth. The pathophysiology of CLE is similar to that of pneumothorax, and the severity of symptoms (severe dyspnea, cyanosis, wheezing, grunting, and coughing) relate to the degree of cardiopulmonary compromise caused by air accumulation under tension.

Physical examination reveals signs and symptoms similar to hyaline membrane disease (tachypnea, retractions, flaring of the alae nasi, labored breathing, and expiratory wheezing). Lobar distention appears on radiographs as a unilateral radiolucency with marked mediastinal shift away from the affected side and a flattened diaphragm. The presence of bronchial vascular markings differentiate CLE from congenital lung cyst, a disorder that is commonly confused with CLE.

Anesthetic Management

Newborns with CLE and severe cardiorespiratory failure require immediate surgery. An arterial catheter is an essential monitor to allow serial blood gas determinations.

A gentle induction of anesthesia is performed with a volatile anesthetic agent and 100% oxygen. Nitrous oxide and positive-pressure ventilation are contraindicated because of the danger of further expanding the emphysematous lobe. The trachea is intubated without the use of muscle relaxants and spontaneous ventilation is allowed until the chest is opened. If hypotension occurs during the induction or maintenance of anesthesia, the volatile anesthetic agent is decreased or discontinued and supplemental analgesia is provided with ketamine (1 to 2 mg/kg IV). Injection of local anesthetic at the incision site will allow lighter levels of general anesthesia. Hypercarbia in these spontaneously breathing infants may exist. If oxygenation is adequate, as reflected by pulse oximetry and arterial PO_2, the transient hypercarbia that results from relative hypoventilation may be ignored. *One should not be tempted to hyperventilate the patient with positive-pressure ventilation to bring the CO$_2$ down before the chest is opened.* After the chest is opened, the emphysematous lobe permeates through the incision, which eliminates intrathoracic compression. Controlled ventilation can then be started, facilitated by muscle relaxants, if desired.

CONGENITAL HYPERTROPHIC PYLORIC STENOSIS

Congenital hypertrophic pyloric stenosis is a common surgical problem of infancy and may occur in up to 1 in 300 live births in some populations; the incidence has considerable geographic variation. First-born males are more commonly affected.

This lesion consists of hypertrophy of the muscle of the pyloric sphincter causing obstruction and leading to persistent vomiting. Dehydration, hypochloremia, and alkalosis can develop. If the diagnosis of congenital hypertrophic pyloric stenosis is made promptly, severe metabolic derangements may be avoided. In 2% of patients, jaundice is an associated condition. No special treatment is required for this jaundice as it clears after pyloromyotomy.

Special Anesthetic Problems

Special anesthetic problems in the patients with congenital hypertrophic pyloric stenosis include ensuring that dehydration and electrolyte imbalance are fully corrected before surgery. In addition, there is the danger of vomiting and aspiration during the induction of anesthesia. Pyloromyotomy is not an emergency procedure.

Anesthetic Management

Preoperative Considerations

A gastric tube is inserted, and continuous suction is applied. The patient is rehydrated, correcting the electrolyte imbalance. This rehydration and electrolyte correction may take up to 24 to 48 hours. During this preoperative period, the patient is given a intravenous solution as indicated by serum electrolyte values. Potassium chloride (KCl) supplements are added (3 meq/kg/day) when urine flow is established. Surgery is delayed until the infant appears clinically well hydrated and has normal electrolyte levels, acid-base balance, and good urine output.

Immediately preoperatively, the patient is reassessed to ensure that fluid status is satisfactory:

- Clinical signs of hydration (skin turgor, fontanelle, vital signs, activity, moist tongue) are checked.
- Urine output is assessed.
- Biochemistry values are checked. These values should be:
  - pH 7.3 to 7.5
  - Na > 132
  - Cl > 90
  - K > 3.2
  - Bicarbonate < 30 mmol/L

Perioperative Considerations

Atropine may be given intravenously during induction of anesthesia. The infant is placed in either the left lateral or supine position. The stomach is aspirated with a soft catheter, even if the patient has been on continuous gastric suction. 100% oxygen is given by face mask before induction.

Awake intubation or rapid-sequence induction with cricoid pressure is performed to establish an endotracheal tube. Anesthesia is induced and maintained with nitrous oxide and halothane (0.5%), isoflurane (0.75%), or other volatile agents. A muscle relaxant is given and ventilation is controlled. Controlled ventilation permits the use of lower concentrations of anesthetic agents. The choice of relaxant is dictated by the probable duration of surgery (i.e., the speed of the surgeon).

Atracurium, 0.3 mg/kg IV, is useful for short procedures. The infant is well relaxed and maintained in an immobile position while the pyloric muscle is being split. Coughing or movement could result in surgical perforation of the mucosa. At the end of the operation, the patient must be wide awake and in the lateral position for extubation.

Postoperative Considerations

IV infusion of fluids is maintained until oral intake is adequate (usually 25 hours). Oral feeding is started with clear fluids 6 to 12 hours postoperatively. Hypoglycemia has been reported when IV fluids containing glucose are discontinued before oral intake is adequate.

SUMMARY

The newborn presents a series of challenges to the clinician that demands meticulous attention to detail. The anatomic, physiologic, and pharmacologic differences in the newborn require an approach to evaluation, preparation, and perioperative management that is different from that used in older infants and children. Within the newborn population, the preterm infant represents unique problems that must be addressed in addition to the other considerations for all newborns.

"It is a pleasant thing to reflect upon, and furnishes a complete answer to those who contend for the gradual degeneration of the human species, that every baby born into the world is a finer one than the last."

—Charles Dickens

REFERENCES

1. Way GL, Wolfe RR, Eshaghpour E, et al: The natural history of hypertrophic cardiomyopathy in infants of diabetic mothers. *J Pediatr* 1979;95:1020–1025.
2. Weber HS, Copel JA, Reece EA, et al: Cardiac growth in fetuses of diabetic mothers with good metabolic control. *J Pediatr* 1991;118:103–107.
3. Chasnoff IJ, Burns KA, Burns WJ: Cocaine use in pregnancy: perinatal morbidity and mortality. *Neurotoxicol Teratol* 1987;9:291–293.
4. Kain ZN, Rimar S, Barash PG: Cocaine abuse in the parturient and effects on the fetus and neonate. *Anesth Analg* 1993;77:835–845.
5. Lipshultz SE, Frassica JJ, Orav EJ: Cardiovascular abnormalities in infants prenatally exposed to cocaine. *J Pediatr* 1991;118:44–51.
6. Suguihara C, Hehre D, Huang J, et al: Decreased ventilatory response to hypoxia in sedated newborn piglets prenatally exposed to cocaine. *J Pediatr* 1996;128:389–395.
7. Wingkun JG, Knisely JS, Schnoll SH, Gutcher GR: Decreased carbon dioxide sensitivity in infants of substance-abusing mothers. *Pediatrics* 1995;95:864–867.
8. Lou HC, Lassen NA, Friis-Hansen B: Impaired autoregulation cerebral blood flow in the distressed newborn infant. *J Pediatr* 1979;94:118–121.
9. Morray JP, Nobel R, Bennet L, Hanson MA: The effect of halothane on phrenic and chemoreceptor responses to hypoxia in anesthetized kittens. *Anesth Analg* 1996;83:329–335.
10. Brown KA: Pattern of ventilation during halothane anaesthesia in infants less than two months of age. *Can J Anaesth* 1996;43:121–128.
11. Tashiro C, Matsui Y, Nakano S, et al: Respiratory outcome in extremely premature infants following ketamine anaesthesia. *Can J Anaesth* 1991;38:287–291.
12. Friis-Hansen B: Water distribution in the foetus and newborn infant. *Acta Paediatr Scand* 1983;305:7–11.
13. Bauer K, Bovermann G, Roithmaier A, et al: Body composition, nutrition, and fluid balance during the first two weeks of life in preterm neonates weighing less than 1500 grams. *J Pediatr* 1991;118:615–620.
14. Sandstrom K, Nilsson K, Andreasson S, et al: Metabolic consequences of different perioperative fluid therapies in the neonatal period. *Acta Anaesthesiol Scand* 1993;37:170–175.
15. Lorenz JM, Kleinman LI, Ahmed G, Markarian K: Phases of fluid and electrolyte homeostasis in the extremely low birth weight infant. *Pediatrics* 1995;96:484–489.
16. Cote CJ, Zaslavsky A, Downes DJ, et al: Postoperative apnea in former preterm infants after inguinal herniorrhaphy. A combined analysis. *Anesthesiology* 1995;82:809–822.
17. Bach V, Bouferrache B, Kremp O, et al: Regulation of sleep and body temperature in response to exposure to cool and warm environments in neonates. *Pediatrics* 1994;93:789–796.
18. Krishna G, Emhardt JD: Anesthesia for the newborn and ex-preterm infant. *Semin Pediatr Surg* 1992;1:32–44.
19. Cameron CB, Robinson S, Gregory GA: The minimum anesthetic concentration of isoflurane in children. *Anesth Analg* 1984;63:418–420.
20. Lerman J, Robinson S, Willis MM, Gregory GA: Anesthetic requirements for halothane in young children 0–1 month and 1–6 months of age. *Anesthesiology* 1983;59:421–424.
21. LeDez KM, Lerman J: The minimal alveolar concentration (MAC) of isoflurane in preterm neonates. *Anesthesiology* 1987;67:301–307.
22. Robinson S, Gregory GA: Fentanyl-air-oxygen anesthesia for ligation of patent ductus arteriosus in preterm infants. *Anesth Analg* 1981;60:331–334.
23. Hansen DD, Hickey PR: Anesthesia for hypoplastic left heart syndrome: use of high-dose fentanyl in 30 neonates. *Anesth Analg* 1986;65:127–132.
24. Greeley WJ, deBruijn NP, Davis DP: Sufentanil pharmacokinetics in pediatric cardiovascular patients. *Anesth Analg* 1987;66:1067–1072.

25. Koehntop DE, Rodman JH, Brundage DM, et al: Pharmacokinetics of fentanyl in neonates. *Anesth Analg* 1986;65:227–232.
26. Meistelman C, Benhamou D, Barre J, et al: Effects of age on plasma protein binding of sufentanil. *Anesthesiology* 1990;72:470–473.
27. Davis PJ, Killian A, Stiller RL, et al: Pharmacokinetics of alfentanil in newborn premature infants and older children. *Develop Pharmacol Ther* 1989;13:21–27.
28. Marlow N, Weindling AM, Van Peer A, Heykants J: Alfentanil pharmacokinetics in preterm infants. *Arch Dis Child* 1990;65:349–351.
29. Lynn AM, Slattery JT: Morphine pharmacokinetics in early infancy. *Anesthesiology* 1987;66:136–139.
30. Lynn AM, Nespeca MK, Opheim KE, Slattery JT: Respiratory effects of intravenous morphine infusions in neonates, infants, and children after cardiac surgery. *Anesth Analg* 1993;77:695–701.
31. Bhat R, Chari G, Gulati A, Aldana O, et al: Pharmacokinetics of a single dose of morphine in preterm infants during the first week of life. *J Pediatr* 1990;117:477–481.
32. Yaster M: The dose response of fentanyl in neonatal anesthesia. *Anesthesiology* 1987;66:433–435.
33. Friesen RH, Henry DB: Cardiovascular changes in preterm neonates receiving isoflurane, halothane, fentanyl, and ketamine. *Anesthesiology* 1986;64:238–242.
34. Anand KJ, Hickey PR: Pain and its effects in the human neonate and fetus. *N Engl J Med* 1987;317:1321–1329.
35. Greisen G, Frederiksen PS, Hertel J, Christensen NJ: Catecholamine response to chest physiotherapy and endotracheal suctioning in preterm infants. *Acta Paediatr Scand* 1985;74:525–529.
36. Anand KJ, Brown MJ, Bloom SR, Aynsley-Green A: Studies on the hormonal regulation of fuel metabolism in the human newborn infant undergoing anesthesia and surgery. *Hormone Res* 1985;22:1115–1128.
37. Anand KJ, Brown MJ, Causon RC, et al: Can the human neonate mount an endocrine and metabolic response to surgery? *J Pediatr Surg* 1985;20:41–48.
38. Anand KJ, Ward-Platt MP: Neonatal and pediatric stress responses to anesthesia and operation. *Int Anesth Clin* 1988;26:218–225.
39. Emhardt JD, Vasko MR: Do neonates need anesthesia? *Adv Anesth* 1990;7:45–81.
40. Larsson LE, Nilsson K, Niklasson A, et al: Influence of fluid regimens on perioperative blood-glucose concentrations in neonates. *Br J Anaesth* 1990;64:419–424.
41. Anand KJ, Sippell WG, Aynsley-Green A: Randomized trial of fentanyl anaesthesia in preterm babies undergoing surgery: effects on the stress response. *Lancet* 1987;1:262–266.
42. Anand KJ, Sippell WG, Schofield NM, Aynsley-Green A: Does halothane anaesthesia decrease the metabolic and endocrine stress response of newborn infants undergoing operation? *Br Med J* 1988;296:668–672.
43. McGoldrick KE: Anesthesia for ophthalmic surgery. In: Motoyama EK, Davis PJ (eds). *Anesthesia for infants and children,* 6th ed. St. Louis: CV Mosby, 1996:647.
44. Keith CG, Doyle LW: Retinopathy of prematurity in extremely low birth weight infants. *Pediatrics* 1995;95:42–45.
45. Merritt JC, Sprague DN, Merritt WE, Ellis RA. RLF: a multifactorial disease. *Anesth Analg* 1981;60:109–111.
46. Lucey JF, Dangman B: A reexamination of the role of oxygen in retrolental fibroplasia. *Pediatrics* 1984;73:82–96.
47. Flynn JT, Sola A, Good WV, Phibbs RH (eds): Screening for retinopathy of prematurity: a problem solved? *Pediatrics* 1995;95:755–757.
48. Betts EK, Downes JJ, Schaffer DB, Johns R: Retrolental fibroplasia and oxygen administration during general anesthesia. *Anesthesiology* 1977;47:518–520.
49. Flynn JT: Oxygen and retrolental fibroplasia: update and challenge. *Anesthesiology* 1984;60:397–399.
50. Dimitriou G, Greenough A, Chan V, et al: Prognostic indicators in congenital diaphragmatic hernia. *J Pediatr Surg* 1995;30:1694–1697.
51. Nagaya M, Akatsuka H, Kato J, et al: Development in lung function of the affected side after repair of congenital diaphragmatic hernia. *J Pediatr Surg* 1996;31:349–356.
52. Reynolds M, Luck SR, Lappen R: The "critical" neonate with diaphragmatic hernia: a 21-year perspective. *J Pediatr Surg* 1984;19:364–369.
53. Jaffray B, MacKinlay GA: Real and apparent mortality from congenital diaphragmatic hernia. *Br J Surg* 1996;83:79–82.
54. Bollmann R, Kalache K, Mau H, et al: Associated malformations and chromosomal defects in congenital diaphragmatic hernia. *Fetal Diagn Ther* 1995;10:52–59.
55. Davenport M, Rivlin E, D'Souza SW, Bianchi A: Delayed surgery for congenital diaphragmatic hernia: neurodevelopmental outcome in later childhood. *Arch Dis Child* 1992;67:1353–1356.
56. Leveque C, Hamza J, Berg AE, et al: Successful repair of a severe left congenital diaphragmatic hernia during continuous inhalation of nitric oxide. *Anesthesiology* 1994;80:1171–1175.
57. Zayek M, Wild L, Roberts JD, Morin FC III: Effect of nitric oxide on the survival rate and incidence of lung injury in newborn lambs with persistent pulmonary hypertension. *J Pediatr* 1993;123:947–952.
58. Van Meurs KP, Robbins ST, Reed VL, et al: Congenital diaphragmatic hernia: long-term outcome in neonates treated with extracorporeal membrane oxygenation. *J Pediatr* 1993;122:893–899.
59. Fuhrman BP, Dalton HJ: Progress in pediatric extracorporeal membrane oxygenation. *Crit Care Clin* 1992;8:191–202.
60. Klarr JM, Faix RG, Pryce CJ, Bhatt-Mehta V: Randomized, blind trial of dopamine versus dobutamine for treatment of hypotension in preterm infants with respiratory distress syndrome. *J Pediatr* 1994;125:117–122.
61. Spears RS Jr, Yeh A, Fisher DM, Zwass MS: The "educated hand." Can anesthesiologists assess changes in neonatal pulmonary compliance manually? *Anesthesiology* 1991;75:693–696.
62. Friesen RH, Morrison JE: The role of ketamine in the current practice of paediatric anaesthesia. *Paediatr Anaesth* 1994;4:79–82.
63. Hazebroek FW, Tibboel D, Bos AP, et al: Congenital diaphragmatic hernia: impact of preoperative stabilization. A prospective pilot study in 13 patients. *J Pediatr Surg* 1988;23:1139–1146.
64. Richard D, Poets CF, Neale S, et al: Arterial oxygen saturation in preterm neonates without respiratory failure. *J Pediatr* 1993;123:963–968.
65. Stebbens VA, Poets CF, Alexander JR, et al: Oxygen saturation and breathing patterns in infancy. I. Full term infants in the second month of life. 2. Preterm infants at discharge from special care. *Arch Dis Child* 1991;66:569–573, 574–578.
66. Fox WW, Duara S: Persistent pulmonary hypertension

in the neonate: diagnosis and management. *J Pediatr* 1983;103:505–514.
67. O'Rourke PP, Vacanti JP, Crone RK, et al: Use of the postductal PaO₂ as a predictor of pulmonary vascular hypoplasia in infants with congenital diaphragmatic hernia. *J Pediatr Surg* 1988;23:904–907.
68. Kanto WP Jr: A decade of experience with neonatal extracorporeal membrane oxygenation. *J Pediatr* 1994;124:335–347.
69. Clark RH, Yoder BA, Sell MS: Prospective, randomized comparison of high-frequency oscillation and conventional ventilation in candidates for extracorporeal membrane oxygenation. *J Pediatr* 1994;124:447–454.
70. Glass P, Wagner AE, Papero PH, et al: Neurodevelopmental status at age five years of neonates treated with extracorporeal membrane oxygenation. *J Pediatr* 1995;127:447–457.
71. Newman KD, Anderson KD, Van Meurs K, et al: Extracorporeal membrane oxygenation and congenital diaphragmatic hernia: should any infant be excluded? *J Pediatr Surg* 1990;25:1048–1053.
72. Vaucher YE, Dudell GG, Bejar R, Gist K: Predictors of early childhood outcome in candidates for extracorporeal membrane oxygenation. *J Pediatr* 1996;128:109–117.
73. Bohn DJ, James I, Filler RM, et al: The relationship between PaCO₂ and ventilation parameters in predicting survival in congenital diaphragmatic hernia. *J Pediatr Surg* 1984;19:666–671.
74. D'Agostino JA, Bernbaum JC, Gerdes M, et al: Outcome for infants with congenital diaphragmatic hernia requiring extracorporeal membrane oxygenation: the first year. *J Pediatr Surg* 1995;30:10–15.
75. Engum SA, Grosfeld JL, West KW, et al: Analysis of morbidity and mortality in 227 cases of esophageal atresia and/or tracheoesophageal fistula over two decades. *Arch Surg* 1995;130:502–508.
76. Spitz L: Esophageal atresia and tracheoesophageal fistula in children. *Curr Opin Pediatr* 1993;5:347–352.
77. Martin LW, Alexander F: Esophageal atresia. *Surg Clin North Am* 1985;65:1099–1113.
78. Alexander F, Johanningman J, Martin LW: Staged repair improves outcome of high-risk premature infants with esophageal atresia and tracheoesophageal fistula. *J Pediatr Surg* 1993;28:151–154.
79. Randolph JG, Newman KD, Anderson KD: Current results in repair of esophageal atresia with tracheoesophageal fistula using physiologic status as a guide to therapy. *Ann Surg* 1989;209:526–531.
80. Karl HW: Control of life-threatening air leak after gastrostomy in an infant with respiratory distress syndrome and tracheoesophageal fistula. *Anesthesiology* 1985;62:670–672.
81. Reeves ST, Burt N, Smith CD: Is it time to reevaluate the airway management of tracheoesophageal fistula? *Anesth Analg* 1995;81:866–869.
82. Salem MR, Wong AY, Lin YH, et al: Prevention of gastric distention during anesthesia for newborns with tracheoesophageal fistulas. *Anesthesiology* 1973;38:82–83.
83. Hall SC: Neonatal surgical emergencies. *Adv Anesth* 1992;9:27–64.
84. Wailoo MP, Emery JL: The trachea in children with tracheo-oesophageal fistula. *Histopathology* 1979;3:329–338.
85. Chetcuti P, Phelan PD: Respiratory morbidity after repair of oesophageal atresia and tracheo-oesophageal fistula. *Arch Dis Child* 1993;68:167–70.
86. Zaccara A, Felici F, Turchetta A, et al: Physical fitness testing in children operated on for tracheoesophageal fistula. *J Pediatr Surg* 1995;30:1334–1337.
87. Robertson DF, Mobaireek K, Davis GM, Coates AL: Late pulmonary function following repair of tracheoesophageal fistula or esophageal atresia. *Pediatr Pulmonol* 1995;20:21–26.
88. Rickham PP: Infants with esophageal atresia weighing under three pounds. *J Pediatr Surg* 1981;16:595–598.
89. Stothert JC Jr, McBride L, Lewis JE, et al: Esophageal atresia and tracheo-esophageal fistula: pre-operative assessment and reduced mortality. *Ann Thorac Surg* 1979;28:54–59.
90. Louhimo I, Lindahl H: Esophageal atresia: primary result of 500 consecutively treated patients. *J Pediatr Surg* 1983;18:217–229.
91. Yazbeck S, Ndoye M, Khan AH: Omphalocele: a 25-year experience. *J Pediatr Surg* 1986;21:761–763.
92. Greenwood RD, Rosenthal A, Nada AS: Cardiovascular malformations associated with omphalocele. *J Pediatr* 1974;85:818–821.
93. Tobias JD, Lowe S, Holcomb GW III: Anesthetic considerations in an infant with Beckwith-Wiedemann syndrome. *J Clin Anesth* 1992;4:484–486.
94. Moore TC, Nur K: An international survey of gastroschisis and omphalocele (490 cases). II. Relative incidence, pregnancy and environmental factors. *Pediatr Surg Int* 1986;1:105–109.
95. Moorthy SS, Haselby KA, Caldwell RL, et al: Transient right-left interatrial shunt during emergence from anesthesia: demonstration by color flow Doppler mapping. *Anesth Analg* 1989;68:820–822.
96. Teitel DF, Sidi D, Chin T, et al: Developmental changes in myocardial contractile reserve in the lamb. *Pediatr Res* 1985;19:948–955.
97. Stammers AH, Bove EL: The neonatal heart: developmental differences, response to ischemia, and protection during cardiopulmonary bypass. *J Extracorp Technol* 1986;18:208–218.
98. Lindner W, Seidel M, Versmold HT, et al: Stroke volume and left ventricular output in preterm infants with patent ductus arteriosus. *Pediatr Res* 1990;27:278–281.
99. Jarmakani J, Nakanishi T, Jarmakani RN: Effect of hypoxia on calcium exchange in neonatal mammalian myocardium. *Am J Physiol* 1979;237:H612–H619.
100. Kinsella JP, Abman SH: Recent developments in the pathophysiology and treatment of persistent pulmonary hypertension of the newborn. *J Pediatr* 1995;126:853–864.
101. Gregory GA: The baroresponses of preterm infants during halothane anaesthesia. *Can Anaesth Soc J* 1982;29:105–107.
102. Ohlson KB, Mohell N, Cannon B, et al: Thermogenesis in brown adipocytes is inhibited by volatile anesthetic agents. A factor contributing to hypothermia in infants? *Anesthesiology* 1994;81:176–83.
103. Dicker A, Ohlson KB, Johnson L, et al: Halothane selectively inhibits nonshivering thermogenesis. Possible implications for thermoregulation during anesthesia of infants. *Anesthesiology* 1995;82:491–501.
104. Yaster M, Buck JR, Dudgeon DL, et al: Hemodynamic effects of primary closure of omphalocele/gastroschisis in human newborns. *Anesthesiology* 1988;69:84–88.

105. Oberlander TF, Berde CB, Lam KH, et al: Infants tolerate spinal anesthesia with minimal overall autonomic changes: analysis of heart rate variability in former premature infants undergoing hernia repair. *Anesth Analg* 1995;80:20–27.
106. Viscomi CM, Abajian JC, Wald SL, et al: Spinal anesthesia for repair of meningomyelocele in neonates. *Anesth Analg* 1995;81:492–495.
107. Webster AC, McKishnie JD, Kenyon CF, Marshall DG: Spinal anesthesia for inguinal hernia repair in high-risk neonates. *Can J Anaesth* 1991;38:281–286.
108. Tobias JD, Rasmussen GE, Holcomb GW III, et al: Continuous caudal anaesthesia with chloroprocaine as an adjunct to general anaesthesia in neonates. *Can J Anaesth* 1996;43:69–72.
109. Cote CJ, Drop LJ, Daniels AL, Hoaglin DC: Calcium chloride versus calcium gluconate: comparison of ionization and cardiovascular effects in children and dogs. *Anesthesiology* 1987;66:465–470.
110. Masey SA, Koehler RC, Buck JR, et al: Effect on abdominal distension on central and regional hemodynamics in neonatal lambs. *Pediatr Res* 1985;19:1244–1249.
111. Bikhazi GB, Davis PJ: Anesthesia for neonates and premature infants. In: Motoyama EK, Davis PJ (eds). *Anesthesia for infants and children,* 6th ed. St. Louis: CV Mosby, 1996:455–457.
112. Harman PK, Kron IL, McLachlan et al: Elevated intraabdominal pressure and renal function. *Ann Surg* 1982; 196:594–597.
113. Stringel G, Filler RM: Prognostic factors in omphalocele and gastroschisis. *J Pediatr Surg* 1979;14:515–519.
114. Kleinhaus S, Weinberg G, Gregor MB: Necrotizing enterocolitis in infancy. *Surg Clin North Am* 1992;72: 261–276.
115. Kliegman RM, Fanaroff AA: Necrotizing enterocolitis. *N Engl J Med* 1984;310:1093–1103.
116. Frantz ID, L'Heureux P, Engel RR, Hunt CE: Necrotizing enterocolitis. *J Pediatr* 1975;86:259–263.
117. Schober PH, Nassiri J: Risk factors and severity indices in necrotizing enterocolitis. *Acta Paediatr* 1994;396: 49–52.
118. MacKendrick W, Caplan M: Necrotizing enterocolitis. New thoughts about pathogenesis and potential treatments. *Pediatr Clin North Am* 1993;40:1047–1059.
119. Morecroft JA, Spitz L, Hamilton PA, Holmes SJ: Necrotizing enterocolitis: multisystem organ failure of the newborn? *Acta Paediatr* 1994;396:21–23.
120. Engel RR, Virnig NL, Hunt CE, Levitt MD: Origin of mural gas in necrotizing enterocolitis. *Pediatr Res* 1973; 7:292.
121. Miller SF, Seibert JJ, Kinder DL, Wilson AR: Use of ultrasound in the detection of occult bowel perforation in neonates. *J Ultrasound Med* 1993;12:531–535.
122. Saez-Llorens X, McCracken GH Jr: Sepsis syndrome and septic shock in pediatrics: current concepts of terminology, pathophysiology, and management. *J Pediatr* 1993;123:497–508.
123. Bada HS, Korones SB, Perry EH, et al: Mean arterial blood pressure changes in premature infants and those at risk for intraventricular hemorrhage. *J Pediatr* 1990; 117:607–614.
124. Kopelman AE: Blood pressure and cerebral ischemia in very low birth weight infants. *J Pediatr* 1990;116: 1000–1002.
125. Hegyi T, Anwar M, Carbone MT, et al: Blood pressure ranges in premature infants: II. The first week of life. *Pediatrics* 1996;97:336–342.
126. Millar C, Bissonnette B: Awake intubation increases intracranial pressure without affecting cerebral blood flow velocity in infants. *Can J Anaesth* 1994;41:281–287.
127. Walsh MC, Kliegman RM: Necrotizing enterocolitis: treatment based on staging criteria. *Pediatr Clin North Am* 1986;33:179–201.
128. Kosloske AM: Indications for operation in necrotizing enterocolitis revisited. *J Pediatr Surg* 1994;29:663–666.
129. Kurscheid T, Holschneider AM: Necrotizing enterocolitis: mortality and long-term results. *Eur J Pediatr Surg* 1993;3:139–143.
130. Poets CF, Southall DP: Noninvasive monitoring of oxygenation in infants and children: practical considerations and areas of concern. *Pediatrics* 1994;93: 737–746.

8

Anesthesia for the Ex-Premature and Ex-Extracorporeal Membrane Oxygenated Infant

Frederic A. Berry and J. Michael Badgwell

"Does the devil possess you? You're leaping over the hedge before you came at the stile."
—Miguel De Cervantes

About 10% of the 4 million births annually in the United States are premature. This amounts to roughly 400,000 premature births per year. Of this group, about 50,000 to 60,000 weigh <1500 g; these are the infants who have the highest risk for developing the various problems of prematurity, such as respiratory distress syndrome, bronchopulmonary dysplasia, retinopathy of prematurity, and apnea and bradycardia. Because of an increased survival rate in the neonatal intensive care unit, more and more "ex-premies" are presenting to the operating room for surgical procedures. This increased survival rate is due to several factors: more aggressive resuscitation, surfactant, better-trained health care providers, and better drugs and equipment. By definition, the premature infant is less than 37 weeks' gestational age[a] and weighs <2500 g. The definition of *extremely low birth weight* is a premature infant weighing <1000 g. Full-term infants weighing <2500 g are defined as *small for gestational age*. An "ex-premie" has reached greater than 37 weeks' conceptual age.

The anesthesiologist is going to be faced with the issues of anesthetizing premature infants primarily in one of two circumstances: (a) during the initial premature period of birth and survival and (b) for surgery of the premature nursery graduate.

Therefore, although this chapter focuses on ex-premature infants, it necessarily includes material relevant to the infant who, by definition, is still premature. Procedures during the premature period include surgery for hydrocephalus, shunt revision, intestinal obstruction, cryotherapy for retinopathy of prematurity (ROP), treatment of necrotizing enterocolitis, and closure of a patent ductus arteriosus. The anesthesiologist will also become involved when the premature nursery graduate returns for elective or urgent surgery. For example, premature infants have a higher incidence of inguinal hernias and a higher incidence of strangulation and incarceration of these hernias.

TYPICAL EX-PREMATURE PATIENT

A 2-month-old infant is listed on the operative schedule for retinal cryotherapy under monitored anesthesia care (MAC). When you visit the child, you discover that gestational age is 28 weeks and postnatal age is 9 weeks, giving the child a conceptual age of 37 weeks. You further discover that the child had severe respiratory distress syndrome (RDS) and was on a ventilator for 2 weeks in the neonatal intensive care unit. As the clinician caring for this infant, you must first ask yourself, "Can I do this case as a MAC?" Choosing to do deep sedation for these infants means that you must

---
[a]Ed. Note (JMB): *Gestational age* is the time from conception to birth. *Postnatal age* is the time period from birth to the present time. *Conceptual age* is from conception to the present time.

be willing to accept and manage the potential risks to the infant's airway for obstruction or development of apnea.[b] General anesthesia, however, is not without its own set of risks.

PREOPERATIVE ASSESSMENT

"If you desire to drain to the dregs the fullest cup of scorn and hatred that a fellow human can pour out for you, let a young mother hear you call dear baby 'it.' "
—Jerome K. Jerome

The clinician's strategies for the management of the premature infant are primarily based on an assessment of the infant's cardiopulmonary system as well as the impact of the surgical problem on other body systems. As an example, infants who have necrotizing enterocolitis often have the complicating problems of hypovolemia, coagulopathy, and sepsis. The spectrum of pulmonary function ranges from the very low birth weight infant with immature lungs and deficient surfactant to the 1500g premature infant who may have completely normal pulmonary function.

To determine the extent of pulmonary involvement is tantamount to an adequate preoperative assessment. Did the child have RDS at birth? Up until about 1990, the major cause of death in premature infants was RDS. The second leading cause was congenital anomalies, which today constitute the major cause of death. Since the introduction of surfactant in 1990, there has been an enormous drop in infant mortality in the United States and the rest of the world. RDS is no longer the leading cause of death in the premature infant. Not only has there been an increase in survivors of prematurity, but there has also been a considerable reduction in morbidity, specifically the issues of severity of RDS, air leak, and the incidence and severity of bronchopulmonary dysplasia (BPD), as well as an apparent reduction in the incidence of intraventricular hemorrhage.

The major problems facing the anesthesiologist for emergency surgery in the first few days of a neonate's life are those relating to RDS. Newborn infants with RDS exhibit tachypnea, inspiratory retraction, expiratory grunt, and oxygen-hemoglobin desaturation. The use of surfactant has greatly reduced the severity and incidence of RDS. For infants who require emergency surgery in the first several days of life, the use of surfactant to improve pulmonary function is an accepted form of therapy. Usually, these infants are intubated and ventilated and are aggressively cared for by the neonatology staff.

When the premature infant or a premature nursery graduate requires surgery, it is generally after the acute phases of RDS, when the child may have some form of residual lung disease—most frequently BPD. The major contributing factors are those of a very low birth weight infant who develops sepsis and a late episode of a patent ductus arteriosus. Immaturity of the pulmonary structures and lack of surfactant requiring intubation and ventilation resulting in barotrauma, oxygen toxicity, and infection are the etiologic factors that contribute to the development of BPD. It is known that high concentrations of oxygen with its formation of toxic radicals will directly damage the lung. In addition, barotrauma disrupts the airway architecture. After the damage occurs, there is a reparative process that is often associated with an inflammatory reaction in the lungs with an associated increase in pulmonary microvascular permeability. These are some of the secondary factors that are thought to play a role in the development of BPD.

Assessing Bronchopulmonary Disease

At preoperative assessment, one must ask whether the infant has BPD (Fig. 1). BPD represents "chronic lung disease" of the premature and is essentially a radiographic diagnosis with the following findings:

- Streaky fibrosis
- Atelectasis

---

[b]Ed. Note (JMB): It is the editor's experience that premature and ex-premature infants require general anesthesia and endotracheal intubation to protect their airway during surgical immobilization.

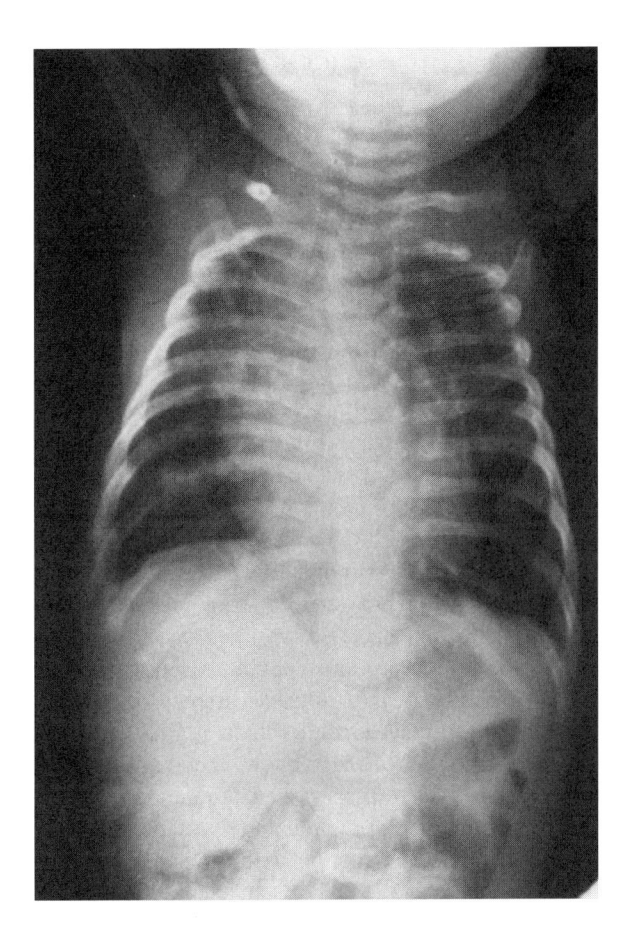

FIG. 1. Characteristic radiographic signs of an infant with chronic lung disease (bronchopulmonary dysplasia): flat diaphragm, streaky infiltration, fibrosis, atelectasis, and patchy overinflation. This film is as good as it gets radiographically for this infant. Therefore, previous films must be compared when deciding whether the infant has an acute process (e.g., superimposed pneumonia).

- Patchy infiltrates
- Hyperinflation

BPD occurs in 10% to 15% of infants who have been intubated and ventilated. *Chronic lung disease* has been defined as a condition during the first 2 months of life in which there is a need for supplemental oxygen for at least 28 days of that time period in association with specific chest radiographic findings. Most infants with chronic lung disease have a history of RDS with varying degrees of BPD. The residual problems of BPD may involve the infant who makes an almost complete recovery as well as the infant who remains oxygen-dependent and may well die of this residual form of lung disease. There has been an increase in the number of infants who develop chronic lung disease and who have very mild or no RDS. Children with known BPD have been diagnosed and are usually being followed up by a pediatrician. However, some premature infants have residual lung disease without parent awareness or a radiographic diagnosis. For the hospitalized patient, the pulmonary status is usually well documented by the neonatologist in charge of the patient.[c] Although the early pathologic changes of BPD may be recognized at the end of the first week of life, it usually takes 3 to 4 weeks before the diagnosis can be made. The current diagnostic tests are clinical signs of persistent respiratory distress requiring oxygen supplementation.

---

[c]Ed. Note (JMB): At our institution, the neonatologists provide each patient with a discharge chest film. These films have proved to be invaluable in differentiating acute from chronic pulmonary processes (e.g., chronic fibrosis from pneumonia).

The chest radiographic changes have also evolved into a broad spectrum of diagnoses. BPD was recognized as a disease only 29 years ago, so that there is little long-term follow-up in affected patients. As a general rule, any infant who has been intubated and ventilated with an increased F_1O_2 should at least be suspected of having the potential for residual lung disease. Children with BPD can be diagnosed by asking the parents whether the infant had the "breathing done for him" and if the infant has had recurrent pulmonary infections. Children with residual pulmonary involvement will have altered pulmonary function tests (Table 1):

Infants with BPD also present with reactive airways. Infants with reactive airways are more sensitive to the noxious effects of inhalation anesthetics. Therefore, with the induction of anesthesia, they may hold their breath, cough, have a low threshold for laryngospasm, and in general can create a headache for the anesthesiologist. In the presence of an intravenous line, there is good reason to treat these infants with an anticholinergic agent such as glycopyrrolate to reduce the secretions and act as a bronchodilator.

Children with BPD often have a large difference between the arterial and end-tidal PCO_2 values owing to loss of adventitial and vascular pulmonary tissue, which results in an increased dead-space ventilation. Small for gestational age infants are prone to aspiration pneumonia and hypoglycemia. Preterm infants, on the other hand, have a high incidence of perioperative apnea **(see Postanesthetic Respiratory Complications)**. Often preterm infants are on corticosteroids and may as well be receiving long-term diuretics, which are thought to improve the outcome of this disease. Therefore, ex-premature infants may be dehydrated when you get them.

INDUCTION OF GENERAL ANESTHESIA

Inhalation Induction

At many institutions, anesthesia is induced using a face mask with spontaneous ventilation and maintained with a volatile agent without endotracheal intubation.[d] This is an acceptable technique if one is able to recognize and treat the potential complications. For example, attempts at preoxygenation often result in an infant who is crying with increased secretions, breath-holding, and coughing; soon what appeared to be a reasonable strategy of preoxygenation may turn into chaos in the control of the airway. For that reason, one approach is to gently blow an increased amount of oxygen over the face of the premature infant and do an intravenous induction with either propofol or thiopental followed by succinylcholine or a short-acting nondepolarizing agent such as atracurium or rocuronium. Rapid intubation and control of the airway then follows.

Lidocaine (4 mg/kg) may be administered topically on the airway at the time of intubation. The lidocaine comes in one of two forms. One form is 4% lidocaine, meaning 40 mg/ml of solution directly sprayed onto the epiglottis and vocal cords with a tuberculin syringe and a no. 23 needle. The dose for even

TABLE 1. *Abnormal pulmonary findings in children with residual pulmonary involvement*

Increased
Functional residual capacity
Airway resistance
Dead-space ventilation
$PaCO_2 - P_{ET}CO_2$ difference

Decreased
Pulmonary compliance

[d]Ed. Note (JMB): If the airway is not a potential problem (e.g., if the infant does not have a difficult airway as in Pierre Robin syndrome), I prefer to induce anesthesia in premature infants by intravenous technique using thiopental (5 mg/kg), atropine (0.02 mg/kg), and a muscle relaxant, followed by endotracheal intubation. If the infant has no preexisting intravenous access, a no. 24 catheter may be placed into a dorsal hand, ventral wrist, or saphenous vein. Alternatively, a butterfly technique using a no. 27 butterfly needle may be used and a "real" intravenous line started later. *Intravenous inductions may be advantageous in premature infants* to avoid potential complications that can occur during mask induction (e.g., breath-holding, apnea, airway obstruction, laryngospasm, vomiting, and hypotension).

a 2-kg child (10 mg), which is 0.25 ml, can be directed onto the appropriate structures. The other possibility is 10% aerosolized lidocaine, which comes in an aerosolized can, with one puff being 10 mg of lidocaine. It is obvious that this solution is useful only in infants who weigh ≥2 kg, since one can easily administer an overdose. The signs of an overdose of topical lidocaine that has become systemically absorbed are primarily those of bradycardia.

The choice of anesthetic technique depends on the nature of the surgery, but the combination of general anesthesia with some form of local or regional block should be considered. The advantages of this combination are a reduction in the amount of volatile anesthetic and a reduction in the need for narcotics and muscle relaxants. A further advantage of this combination is a more rapid awakening at the end of surgery with the return of airway reflexes and the possibility of extubating the infant soon after surgery.

For an infant with hydrocephalus with placement of a shunt, general anesthesia with local infiltration of the skin with dilute solutions of lidocaine or bupivacaine is used. For thoracic or abdominal procedures, various regional techniques are appropriate (e.g., either single-shot caudal or the placement of a caudal catheter). Details of regional anesthesia are discussed in **Chapter 10**. For thoracic procedures, the dose is 1.25 ml/kg of 0.25% bupivacaine or 0.2% ropivacaine with 1 to 200,000 dilution epinephrine. For abdominal procedures, the dose is 1 ml/kg of the same solutions. Various strategies for postoperative pain management include the use of local anesthesia or narcotics or both.

TABLE 2. *Summary of characteristics that justify tracheal intubation in ex-premies*

High incidence of airway obstruction
Poorly developed respiratory control
Biphasic response to hypoxia (tachypnea → apnea)
Circular rib cage, horizontal diaphragm, indicating increased work of breathing
Only 10%–25% type 1 fibers in diaphragm
↑ VO_2, ↓ functional residual capacity, ↑ closing volume

tion, then apnea), and (d) a very compliant, circular rib cage with horizontal placement of the diaphragm (Table 2). The latter factor increases the work of breathing for infants, especially if partial airway obstruction occurs. Furthermore, infants have only about 25% (10% in premature infants) of the type 1 anaerobic-resistant fibers and therefore develop respiratory fatigue more easily than older infants and children. Finally, neonates and ex-prematures have an increased oxygen consumption, decreased functional residual capacity, and an increased closing volume compared with those of older infants and children. For these reasons, *it is usually appropriate to intubate and control ventilation in premature and ex-premature infants.*

The Question of Awake Intubation

Unless the infant is very sick or has a full stomach, general anesthesia before intubation is advised. If awake intubation is performed, it should be done using an oxyscope, which is a laryngoscope blade that allows delivery of supplemental oxygen. Topical lidocaine may be applied to the mucosa of the tongue and posterior pharynx by allowing the infant to suckle lidocaine jelly. The disadvantages of awake intubation in infants are the potential development of bradycardia or hypertension. These factors may in turn lead to increased intracranial pressure or intraventricular hemorrhage. Most infants, unless they are critically ill, can tolerate anesthesia for intubation.

Endotracheal Intubation

It is generally advisable to intubate the trachea of premature and ex-premature infants rather than administer general anesthesia by face mask. The recommendation to intubate is made because these infants have (a) a higher incidence of airway obstruction, (b) poorly developed respiratory control, (c) a biphasic response to hypoxia (initial increase in respira-

Laryngeal Mask Airway

The recent interest in the laryngeal mask airway has extended to the premature infant.

The laryngeal mask airway may be used in infants with BPD to minimize the risk of intubation. This may or may not be an advantage. However, the technique is certainly worth discussion. One technique is to accomplish induction via the intravenous route. Infants may be paralyzed with succinylcholine and then maintained on controlled ventilation with isoflurane and nitrous oxide. The laryngeal mask airway may be left in place at the end of surgery until the infant has recovered airway reflexes as previously described and then extubated. To our knowledge, no airway complications have been reported using this technique. The problem of distention of the stomach may be solved by placing an orogastric tube beside the laryngeal mask airway. This allows any overpressure of the airway that might go into the stomach to be vented through the orogastric tube rather than distending the stomach.

Infants with BPD also often have a history of apnea and bradycardia and need a postoperative period of close postoperative monitoring. Therefore, the guidelines for awake extubation need to be followed. However, in spite of this, the occasional premature infant will go through episodes of breath-holding or bradycardia, and so on, which challenge the most experienced of pediatric anesthesiologists in management of these patients. On occasion, some of these infants ultimately need reintubation and a period of intubation and observation.

DOSAGE CONSIDERATIONS

Volatile Agents

The MAC of isoflurane in preterm neonates of less than 32 weeks' gestational age is $1.28 \pm 0.17\%$, and in neonates of 32 to 37 weeks' gestational age it is $1.41 \pm 0.19\%$ (1). In full-term neonates, the MAC for isoflurane is $1.60 \pm 0.03\%$. The MAC for halothane in premature infants has not been studied.

Fentanyl

There is little information available on the use of fentanyl anesthesia in preterm infants. There is, however, a pharmacokinetic study in preterm infants who received fentanyl (30 µg/kg) at the start of surgery for repair of patent ductus arteriosus (2). In this study, the $T_{1/2}\beta$ was 6 to 32 hours (17.7 ± 9.3), volume of distribution was between 2206 and 3896 ml/kg (2904 ± 517), and clearance was 104.1 ml/kg/min (2.4 ± 1.3). Although blood pressure remained stable throughout surgery, there was a gradual increase in heart rate at the time of skin closure (2). These findings correlate well with the clinical impression that toward the end of this operation, anesthesia becomes lighter after a single dose of fentanyl when no other anesthesia agents are given. Of particular interest was the lack of correlation between the prolonged elimination of fentanyl and the termination of its pharmacodynamic effect (2). At the end of surgery, most infants moved or breathed spontaneously despite high plasma concentrations of fentanyl. This phenomenon is explained by redistribution of fentanyl from the brain into fat and muscle.

In summation, these studies suggest that a bolus of fentanyl (30 µg/kg) as the sole agent provides stable hemodynamics, but may not provide adequate analgesia during skin closure in premature infants. *Therefore, it seems reasonable to use fentanyl (30 µg/kg initially, followed by repeated doses as needed) as the sole agent in premature infants for repair of patent ductus arteriosus.* However, this regimen may delay onset of spontaneous respiration and require mechanical ventilation of infants during the immediate postoperative period. The doses of fentanyl (30 µg/kg) may be appropriate for the preterm infant undergoing patent ductus arteriosus ligation when postoperative ventilation is planned, but this dose may be excessive for the premature or ex-premature infant undergoing minor surgery (e.g., inguinal hernia repair) when early extubation or no endotracheal intubation is planned. In these cases, fentanyl may cause apnea or prolonged respiratory depression requiring continued intubation, especially if the infant has been given other anesthetic agents.

INTRAOPERATIVE PULMONARY CARE

Techniques for ventilation of ex-premature infants depend on the degree of residual disease. If they have little residual disease, gentle ventilation with small amounts of positive end-expiratory pressure (PEEP) are effective. However, in the presence of moderately severe BPD, the usual strategy is that of controlled ventilation with small amounts of PEEP. Therefore, intraoperative pulmonary care typically includes endotracheal intubation, controlled ventilation, and cautious PEEP (2 to 4 cm H_2O) (Table 3). Because of the potential for chronic air trapping in preterm infants with BPD, the intraoperative use of nitrous oxide should be done with caution. Excessive inflation pressures (>35 cm H_2O) should be avoided in infants with BPD. However, because the infants have decreased pulmonary compliance, inflating pressures of ~25 to 30 cm H_2O may be required to adequately inflate the lungs. Intraoperative fluid therapy is monitored carefully to avoid pulmonary edema.

By contrast, underhydration is also poorly tolerated, particularly in infants receiving diuretic therapy. Underhydration would be manifested as unexpected hypotension (especially during induction) and may be corrected by the cautious administration of a balanced salt solution **(see Chapter 9)**.

RETINOPATHY OF PREMATURITY

Retinopathy of prematurity (ROP) is a disease process whereby the retinal vessels constrict, causing ischemia of the retina. Then, a reparative process of neovascularization goes somewhat out of control, resulting in various stages of retinopathy from mild visual impairment to retinal detachment and blindness. The infants most at risk are those that require intervention for survival (e.g., premature infants <1500 g, particularly those requiring intubation and ventilation).

The anesthesiologist plays two roles that may influence ROP: (a) limiting inspired oxygen concentrations during surgery and (b) administering anesthesia for the cryotherapy.

Inspired oxygen is limited to minimize the occurrence of a high PaO_2, which is thought to be one of the etiologic factors in the development of ROP. However, this has never been well documented. The incidence of ROP in premature infants of very low and extremely low birth weights has actually decreased over the last several years. This is thought to be because of the monitoring of oxygen saturation and PaO_2 and attempts at its control, along with the use of surfactant, which decreases the need for respiratory support as well as the administration of vitamin E. At any rate, intraoperatively the anesthesiologist is faced with a problem of how to maintain a saturation that is reasonable for the condition of the infant. This sounds as if it ought to be an easy goal to accomplish, but unfortunately there are no solid data and no compelling literature to help the anesthesiologist with these guidelines. Moreover, the legal profession often takes guidelines such as these and uses them to the detriment of the patient as well as the medical community.

As a general guideline, a saturation of 90% to 95% would result in a PaO_2 in a range of 60 to 80 mm Hg, which is thought to be in the usual range of saturations for premature infants (3). What are the strategies for accomplishing this oxygen-hemoglobin saturation? To begin with, our usual practice is to use two pulse oximeters, for two reasons.

TABLE 3. *Summary of intraoperative pulmonary care in the infant with bronchopulmonary dysplasia*

Endotracheal intubation
Controlled ventilation
Positive end-expiratory pressure (2–4 cm H_2O)
Avoid nitrous oxide
Peak inspiratory pressure ~ 25 to 30 cm H_2O (avoid >35)
Appropriate hydration

- The rule of two pulse oximeters in premature infants : Only one functions at any given time.

- One oximeter is applied to a preductal site (right upper extremity or ear lobes) to look for reopening or shunt reversal in patent ductus arteriosus, and so on.

The brain and retinal arteries are perfused with preductal blood. Varying amounts of either air or nitrous oxide can be added to the inspired oxygen in an attempt to maintain an oxygen-hemoglobin saturation within the above-mentioned guidelines. In the very sick infant, however (or if there are problems maintaining within this guideline) a higher F_IO_2 with saturations between 95% and 100% may have to be used for the survival of the patient. This is obviously a judgment call.

Considerations to Prevent Retinopathy of Prematurity

Whereas preterm infants <44 weeks of gestational age (the age when vascularization of the retina is completed) are at risk for ROP, this is particularly true for infants weighing <1000 g.

As mentioned, PaO_2 is maintained below 80 mm Hg to prevent retinal artery vasoconstriction. Therefore, SpO_2 should be kept between 90% and 95% ($PaO_2 \sim 80$ mm Hg) to prevent excessive oxygenation, retinal artery vasoconstriction, and possibly ROP. Below saturation of 90%, the oxygen-hemoglobin dissociation curve is very steep, and tissue oxygenation may be in jeopardy. *Assessment of PaO_2 in the retina requires measurement of preductal oxygenation.* Therefore, arterial catheters and pulse oximeter probes should be placed in the right upper extremity.

Surgery for Cryotherapy of Retinopathy of Prematurity

There are no special requirements for cryotherapy for ROP except that the infant is motionless. Most infants with ROP still reside in the premature nursery and have varying degrees of BPD and residual lung disease. Some infants come to surgery intubated (with or without a ventilator), and this makes the anesthetic induction rather simple. Induction of anesthesia follows guidelines described in **Chapter 2**.

OTHER INTRAOPERATIVE CONSIDERATIONS

Manual Ventilation

There are times during surgery on neonates (e.g., for tracheoesophageal fistula) when manual ventilation is preferred. For the most part, controlled ventilation with a ventilator is optimal. A recent report refutes the commonly held belief that the "educated hand" permits clinicians to detect subtle changes in pulmonary compliance in neonates during anesthesia (4). Notable authorities agree that "in this day of reliable volume-cycled ventilators...mechanical ventilation provides very predictable and constant gas exchange over long periods of time" (5).

Breathing Circuits

For ex-premature infants, either a Mapleson D breathing circuit (Jackson-Rees modification of the Ayre's T-piece or Bain circuit) or a circle system (pediatric or adult) may be used **(see also Chapter 5)**. Fresh gas flow requirements for Mapleson D circuits are 250 ml/kg/min as a starting point in an attempt to provide an end-tidal PCO_2 of 38 mm Hg (6). When controlled ventilation is used in infants, the resistance and work of breathing added by inspiratory and expiratory valves in circle systems are not issues. Compression volume loss is less in Mapleson D circuits than circle systems unless a CO_2 absorption canister is used with the Bain circuit (e.g., the Ohmeda GMS system).

The Anesthesia Machine

An anesthesia machine may be used in premature and ex-premature infants if the machine has the capability of delivering oxygen and air by means of very low flows.

ENDOTRACHEAL EXTUBATION

"He who hesitates is sometimes saved."
—James Thurber

If the child's condition warrants it or if there is any question about the ability of the infant to be extubated, the conservative approach is to leave the premature infant intubated and return the child to the neonatal intensive care unit for a process of gradual weaning. However, if the infant is doing well at the end of surgery, ventilation is easy, and extubation may well be indicated at the end of surgery or shortly thereafter. The authors avoid the use of narcotics in any neonate and young infant (<6 months) in whom extubation is anticipated at the end of surgery. Regional anesthesia is used intraoperatively as well as for postoperative analgesia. Extubation criteria are very conservative, meaning that the infant needs to demonstrate control of the protective airway reflexes as well as being awake. If the premature infant is crying or opening the eyes and reaching for the endotracheal tube, this is the indication of the time for extubation. If the infant is not ready for extubation but is reacting to the endotracheal tube, then a dose of lidocaine, 1 to 1.25 mg/kg, might well tide the infant over until the tube can be successfully removed. This dose can be repeated once in 5 to 10 minutes.

It is advisable to remove tracheal tubes from ex-premature and premature infants only when the infants are fully awake. If the infant is not fully awake at the end of the operation, the anesthesiologist should delay extubation until the infant meets the awake criteria (Table 4). In small infants, extubation during early awakening and residual light anesthesia often is followed by breath-holding or apnea, which may lead to sudden oxygen-hemoglobin desaturation and hypoxia bradycardia. Therefore, in neonates, it is much safer to delay extubation until they are fully awake. A fully awake infant moves the extremities purposefully and opens the eyes—the true sign of awakening. "Deep extubation" or tracheal extubation while the infant is deeply anesthetized is inadvisable in infants and is reserved for selected older pediatric patients.

During extubation, infants may respond to laryngeal stimulation by breath-holding or laryngospasm. If so, jaw thrust using the survival position (thumbs placed on the mask, fingertips placed behind the ramus of the mandible, anterior traction applied to the temporomandibular joint) and positive-pressure ventilation using a "fluttering" squeezing action on the bag will eventually allow ventilation of the infant's lungs. If this maneuver does not work, reintubation facilitated by succinylcholine may be required.

TABLE 4. *Signs of the fully awake infant ready for extubation of the trachea*

Breathes spontaneously and rhythmically
Opens mouth and brings up legs in response to oropharyngeal suction
Moves extremities purposefully
Opens eyes
Has baseline oxygen-hemoglobin saturation

POSTANESTHETIC RESPIRATORY COMPLICATIONS

Postoperative Apnea

It is well known that premature and ex-premature infants undergoing elective surgery are prone to developing perioperative respiratory complications (7). Preterm infants with a history of idiopathic apnea are more susceptible than full-term babies to develop life-threatening apnea in the postoperative period. Apnea is defined as a cessation of breathing for 20 seconds or more, resulting in cyanosis and bradycardia. This phenomenon occurs in 20% to 30% of preterm infants during the first month of life. Steward (7) reported an 18% incidence of apnea in preterm infants during the first 12 hours after surgery. Liu (8) and others reported an increased incidence of postanesthetic apnea in infants with a conceptual age of <44 weeks. Kurth and associates (9) observed postanesthetic apnea occurring in 61% of infants <42 weeks old, and one case that occurred in an infant of 55 weeks' con-

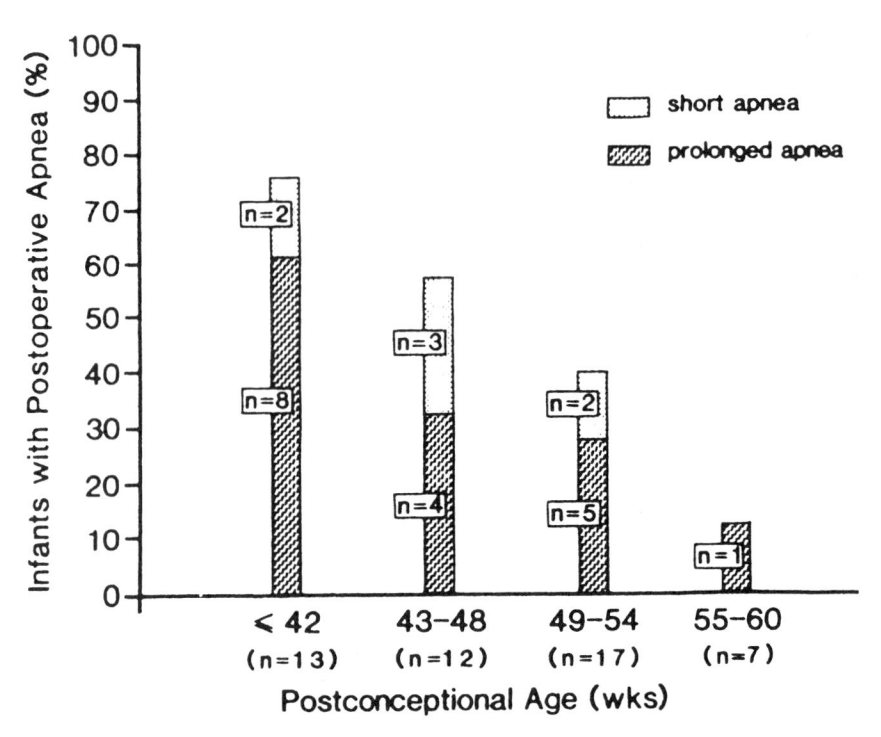

FIG. 2. Incidence of postoperative apnea in babies of different postconceptual ages. The numbers on the bars indicate the number of infants that had either short or prolonged apnea. (Redrawn from Kurth, ref. 9, with permission.)

ceptual age (Fig. 2). These and other studies have led to a controversy regarding recommendations as to when ex-premature infants may be considered as outpatients and when they must be admitted to the hospital for postoperative monitoring.

To summarize all the studies on this issue, the age below which premature infants have been reported to be at risk varies from 40 to 60 weeks' postconceptual age (10). To clear up this issue of when to admit and monitor the ex-premature, Coté and associates (10) did a combined analysis of eight prospective studies in former preterm infants after inguinal herniorrhaphy. These investigators found that the risks of postoperative apnea in nonanemic infants, free of recovery room apnea, is not <5% until postconceptual age is 48 weeks when the gestational age was 35 weeks. This risk is not <1% for that same subset of infants until postconceptual age is 54 (for gestational age = 35 weeks) or 56 weeks (for gestational age = 32 weeks). The authors of this analysis express caution, however, that "... given the limitations of this combined analysis, each physician and institution must decide what is an acceptable risk for postoperative apnea" (10).

How can we help you decide for your institution what is an acceptable risk and how can we best provide you with a rationale for safe guidelines in the care of ex-prematures? We know that in all reported series, no infant suffering postoperative apnea had a first apnea spell more than 12 hours after surgery, with most initial apneic spells occurring within the first 2 postoperative hours. Therefore, we have established an arbitrary set of guidelines (based on the observations just discussed) that will provide acceptable care in most cases:

- Because of the risks of postoperative apnea, elective surgery is postponed until

the premature infant is at least 50 weeks' postconceptual age.
- If surgery is required before this time, the infant is monitored (apnea/heart rate monitor or pulse oximetry) in the hospital for a minimum of 12 hours postoperatively.[e]
- Otherwise healthy preterm infants ≥ 50 weeks' postconceptual age are monitored for a minimum of 2 hours in the postanesthesia care unit and can be discharged home (after minor surgery such as herniorraphy) if they have had no apneic episodes. (The same care is recommended for full-term infants requiring surgery in the first month of life.)

Other Considerations to Prevent Postoperative Apnea

Anesthetic management can affect the incidence of respiratory complications in infants born prematurely. When appropriate, the use of spinal or caudal anesthesia **(see Regional Anesthesia)** rather than general anesthesia will reduce the incidence of desaturation, bradycardia, and postoperative apnea. Spinal anesthesia without sedation is associated with less apnea than is general anesthesia or spinal anesthesia with ketamine sedation (11). Similarly, in former preterm infants given either a spinal or general anesthetic, postoperative arterial desaturation occurred with greater frequency and to greater degrees after general anesthesia (11,12). The incidence of apnea, however, was not significantly different. Caffeine (10 mg/kg) infused at the time of induction may be used to reduce the risk of perioperative apnea (13). Finally, infants with anemia of prematurity, generally a benign condition, are at increased risk of developing postoperative apnea (14). Therefore, if anemia exists, it is preferable to delay elective surgery and give iron supplementation until the hematocrit is above 30%. If surgery cannot be delayed, one should be aware of the increased risk of postoperative apnea.

Management of Apnea

Practically speaking, elective surgery is usually postponed until the premature infant is at least 50 weeks' postconceptual age. If surgery is required before this time, the infant is monitored (apnea/heart rate monitor or pulse oximetry) in the hospital for a minimum of 12 hours postoperatively. Otherwise healthy preterm infants, 50 to 60 weeks' postconceptual age, are monitored for 2 hours in the postanesthesia care unit and can be discharged home if the surgical procedure is relatively minor (e.g., inguinal herniorrhaphy) and the infant has had no apneic episodes. The same 2-hour monitoring period is suggested for full-term infants needing surgery in the first month of life. If apnea occurs, the first step in management is stimulation to initiate spontaneous respirations. Occasionally bag-mask ventilation and even intubation and mechanical ventilation may be required.

REGIONAL ANESTHESIA

Caudal epidural blockade, with or without general anesthesia, may be used for intraoperative and postoperative analgesia after lower abdominal and genitourinary surgery in preterm infants. If general anesthesia is to be used, it is induced using either intravenous or inhalation technique. The trachea may or may not be intubated. Light anesthesia is maintained with nitrous oxide (60% to 70%) and halothane (0.5%). The infant is then turned on the side and given a caudal block with 1.0 ml/kg of 0.25% bupivacaine or 0.2% ropivacaine (maximum dose 3 mg/kg) and epinephrine (1:200,000). If general anesthesia is not used, the block is in-

---

[e]Ed. Note (JMB): To satisfy this 12-hour period, most children need an overnight stay in the hospital. Most hospitals now have a 23-hour stay policy that qualifies as an outpatient stay for insurance billing purposes.

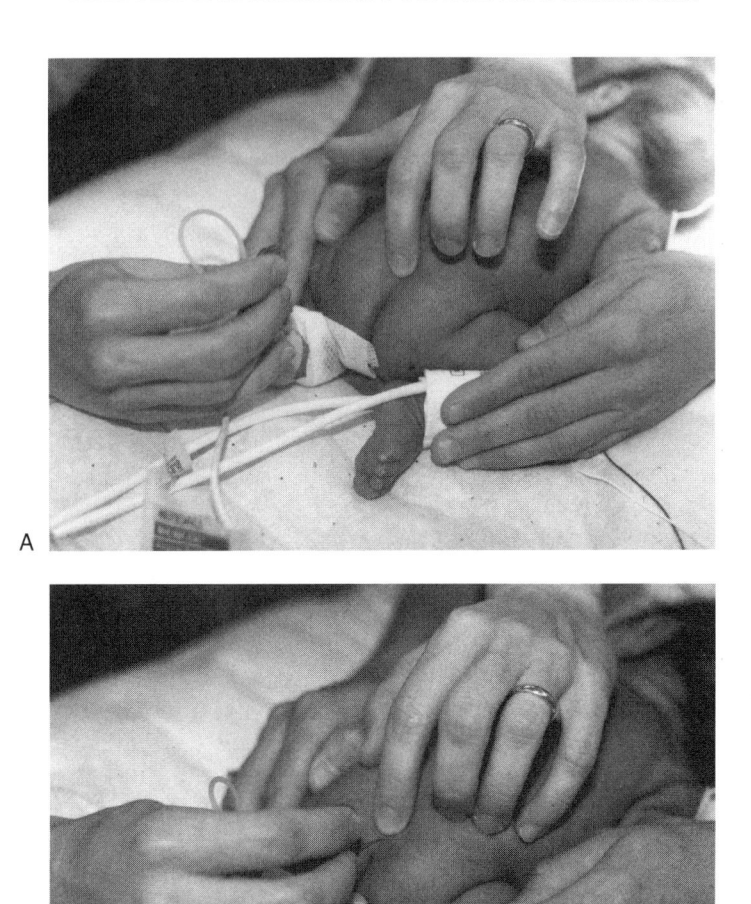

FIG. 3. Caudal anesthesia in an awake ex-premature infant. **(A)** The infant is gently restrained in the prone position. The sacral hiatus is palpated and identified. **(B)** A 25-gauge butterfly short-level needle is inserted at about a 45-degree angle to the skin and advanced until the characteristic pop is felt, indicating that the sacrococcygeal ligament has been pierced and the caudal epidural space entered.

duced using the same technique with the addition of gentle restraint for the infant (Fig. 3). The infant is then given a sugar water nipple to suckle (Fig. 4).

Care must be taken when using a combined general anesthetic with a volatile agent and a regional technique with bupivacaine. It has been shown that the volatile anesthetic agents enhance the toxic effects of bupivacaine when infused intravascularly in small piglets (15). Furthermore, it has been shown that hypoxia (16) and hypercarbia (17), which may occur secondary to airway obstruction, also enhance the toxic effects of bupivacaine. Therefore, meticulous attention must be paid to airway patency when administering a combination anesthetic. For this reason, we prefer to intubate infants during the administration of combined general and regional anesthesia. The first sign of inadvertent intravascular injection of bupivacaine plus epinephrine is elevation of the T-wave on electrocardiogram (18).

The use of spinal anesthesia for hernia repair in premature infants <36 weeks' gesta-

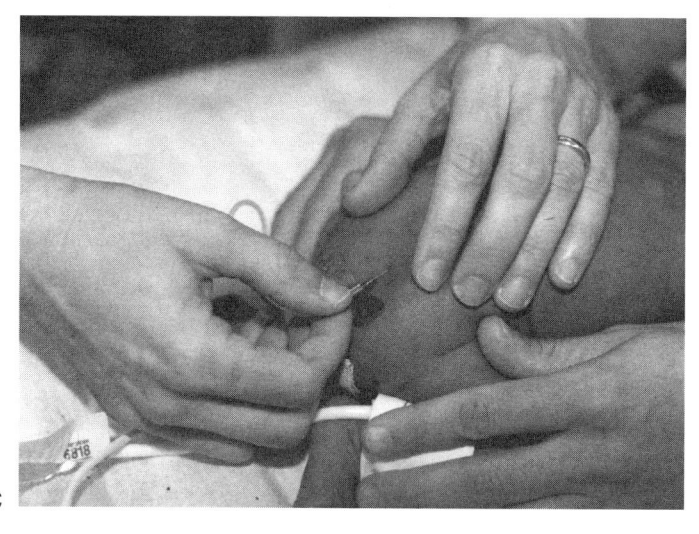

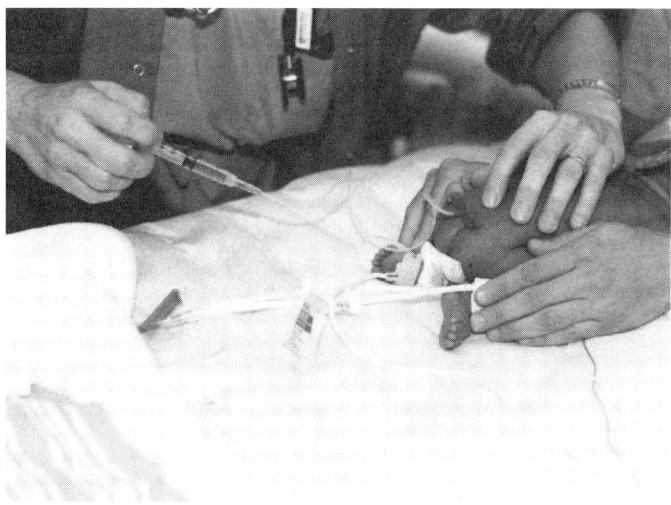

(C) The needle is secured. **(D)** Epinephrine-containing local anesthetic (see text) is injected incrementally (1/3 of the total dose every 20 seconds) feeling for inadvertent subcutaneous injection and watching the electrocardiogram monitor for T-wave elevation (indicating inadvertent intravascular injection, if T-wave changes occur).

tional age recovering from RDS is reportedly a safe and satisfactory alternative to general anesthesia (19). Spinal anesthesia using hyperbaric tetracaine (0.4 to 0.6 mg/kg) inserted at the L_{4-5} level produces good analgesia with minimal cardiovascular instability.

ANESTHETIC CONSIDERATIONS FOR THE ECMO GRADUATE

Extracorporeal membrane oxygenation (ECMO) is widely used to treat infants and children with life-threatening cardiorespiratory failure (20,21). Considerations for the ECMO graduate include (a) the usual concerns of anesthetizing a neonates and premature infants and (b) the following underlying medical disorders that necessitate ECMO:

- Residual pulmonary disease and BPD
- Central nervous system damage from perinatal hypoxemia, including seizures, intraventricular hemorrhage, and hydrocephalus
- Nephrotoxicity from hypoxemia, medications

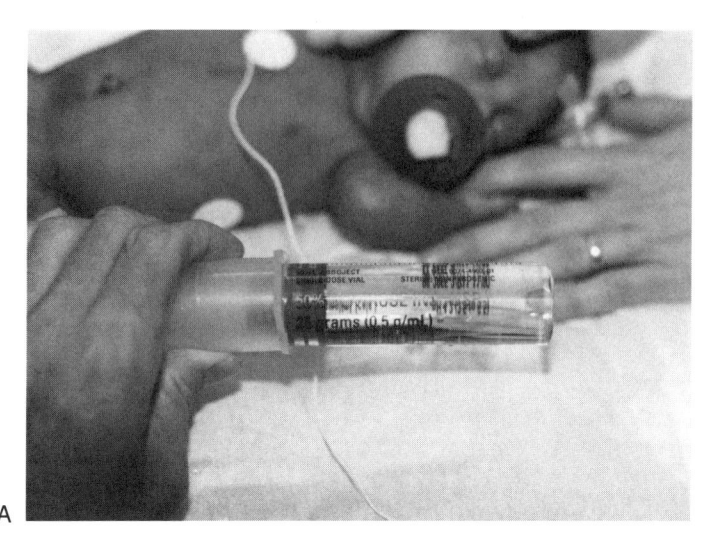

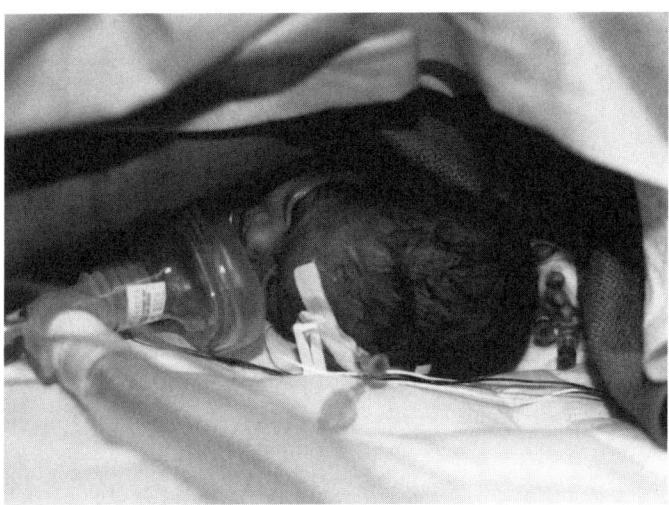

FIG. 4. (A) A sugar water nipple may be prepared by saturating a cotton-stuffed bottle nipple with 50% dextrose in water. **(B)** The sugar water nipple, a little oxygen, and a caudal anesthetic makes for a happy comfortable infant enjoying the herniorraphy.

In addition, there are problems created by ECMO itself, such as the following:

- Ligated carotid artery and internal jugular vein
- Residual coagulopathy from heparin therapy
- Thrombocytopenia from contact with membrane oxygenator
- Anemia from iatrogenic phlebotomy
- Electrolyte imbalances from parenteral hyperalimentation
- Narcotic abstinence syndrome

ECMO Techniques

It is important to consider the techniques currently available for ECMO and to consider how ECMO and its residual effects may make an impact on the anesthetic plan. ECMO was initially introduced in the late 1960s as therapy for infants with what was then known as hyaline membrane disease (RDS) and was later used for respiratory failure in full-term infants (21). Presently, ECMO is indicated for reversible cardiorespiratory failure in full-term neonates who have failed to respond to maximal medical management. The following are some of the more common causes of respiratory failure in the neonate for which ECMO has been used:

- Meconium aspiration syndrome
- Congenital diaphragmatic hernia
- Persistent pulmonary hypertension
- Sepsis
- Older children and adults with cardiorespiratory dysfunction of various origins (22)

Techniques for ECMO include venoarterial, venovenous, and single-catheter venous bypass. Although the latter two techniques offer significant advantages over venoarterial ECMO in that they do not require access to the arterial circulation and carotid ligation, venoarterial ECMO provides the highest level of oxygenation as well as the capability for assisting cardiac output. The single-catheter venous technique is necessary when ECMO is used as a circulatory rather than a respiratory assist device (e.g., cardiac dysfunction after surgery for congenital heart disease, cardiac failure from myocarditis, or a cardiomyopathy) (22). Although venovenous techniques provide excellent carbon dioxide removal, disadvantages include borderline oxygenation due to venous admixture and no capabilities for assisting cardiac output. In venoarterial ECMO, access includes drainage of blood from the right atrium with a catheter placed via surgical cutdown on the right internal jugular with return through a catheter positioned via the carotid artery into the aortic arch with all or part of the cardiac output maintained by the ECMO circuit. Oxygenation and carbon dioxide removal are achieved by using a membrane oxygenator similar to those that are used for cardiopulmonary bypass.

Residual Cardiopulmonary Dysfunction

One of the primary concerns of the clinician in caring for the ECMO graduate is the presence of associated congenital anomalies and residual cardiopulmonary dysfunction. These patients run the gamut from preterm neonates with associated anomalies and respiratory failure to full-term infants with respiratory failure and no other organ system dysfunction. Congenital cardiac lesions are ruled out by echocardiography before the initiation of ECMO. Subtle anomalies missed on echocardiography (e.g., partial anomalous pulmonary venous return) may prevent successful weaning from ECMO. In addition to everything else going on with ECMO graduates, depression of myocardial contractility due to perinatal hypoxemia or sepsis may be present.

Other Concerns

Neurologic. Perinatal hypoxemia and shock may also affect other organ systems (e.g., the central nervous system). Preoperative evaluation of the central nervous system includes a review of birth history, Apgar scores, and subsequent hospital course. These infants may have a preexisting history of severe hypoxemia, central nervous system dysfunction, intraventricular hemorrhage, hydrocephalus, seizures, or apnea and bradycardia.

Renal and Hematologic. Even in the absence of associated renal anomalies, preoperative renal function (e.g., blood urea nitrogen, creatinine, and urinalysis) should be evaluated, since many of these infants will have received potentially nephrotoxic drugs such as antibiotics or diuretics. Evaluation of the hematologic status of these patients is also recommended. Hematologic concerns include a high incidence of iatrogenic anemia due to repeated phlebotomy. Although heparinization is reversed with protamine after ECMO, a residual coagulopathy should be ruled out by measuring the partial thromboplastin time. In addition, these infants have been exposed to several insults that may lead to thrombocytopenia such as the following:

- Heparin therapy
- Contact with the membrane oxygenator
- Sepsis
- Medications

Fluids. Because many of ECMO graduate infants are maintained on total parenteral hyperalimentation, preoperative evaluation should include measurement of electrolytes, calcium, magnesium, phosphorus, and liver enzymes (alanine transaminase, aspartate transaminase) to identify those patients with total parenteral hyperalimentation cholestasis. Maintenance fluid requirements are met by continuing the infant's current hyperalimentation fluid throughout the perioperative period (with monitoring of blood glucose). Intraoperative blood loss and third-space losses are then replaced with an isotonic fluid **(see Chapter 9)**.

Narcotic Dependency. One other issue of concern to the anesthesiologist is the high incidence of narcotic dependency (23). Infants who were on ECMO for longer than 5 days or those who had received total fentanyl doses of greater than 1.6 mg/kg have a high incidence of dependency and often develop neonatal abstinence syndrome after the abrupt withdrawal of opioids. Therefore, the preoperative evaluation should include an assessment of the infant's previous sedation history, the current sedation regimen, and signs and symptoms of neonatal abstinence syndrome (24). Infants requiring large doses of opioids may require higher doses intraoperatively and postoperatively (25).

Difficult Venous Access. Peripheral venous access may be difficult in ECMO graduate infants, and central access may be required. If central venous access is required, catheterization of the left internal jugular vein is avoided. Inadvertent trauma to the left carotid artery may compromise the already marginal cerebral perfusion. Cannulation of the left internal jugular vein may impair cerebral venous drainage, especially if the right internal jugular vein has been ligated. Other appropriate venous access sites include the femoral (26,27) and subclavian veins **(see Chapter 3)**.

SUMMARY

Anesthetic considerations of the ECMO graduate can be summarized into three categories (28): (a) the usual concerns of anesthetizing an infant, (b) associated organ system dysfunction, and (c) sequelae of the ECMO process.

A thorough preoperative review of the history, examination of the infant, and laboratory evaluation will help identify end-organ system dysfunction and allow the provision of a safe anesthetic for these patients. Although ECMO is currently limited to certain centers, its recent success suggests that use of this technique will continue to increase in both the neonatal and nonneonatal populations.

REFERENCES

1. LeDez KM, Lerman J: The minimum alveolar concentration (MAC) of isoflurane in preterm neonates. *Anesthesiology* 1987;67:301–307.
2. Collins C, Koren G, Crean P: The correlation between fentanyl pharmacokinetics and pharmacodynamlcs in preterm infants during PDA ligation. *Anesthesiology* 1984;61:A442.
3. Richard D, Poets CF, Neale S: Arterial oxygen saturation in preterm neonates with respiratory failure. *J Pediatr* 1993;123:963–968.
4. Spears RS Jr, Yeh A, Fisher DM, Zwass MS: The "educated hand." Can anesthesiologists assess changes in neonatal pulmonary compliance manually? *Anesthesiology* 1991;75:693–696.
5. Steward DJ: The "not-so-educated hand" of the pediatric anesthesiologist. *Anesthesiology* 1991;75:555–556.
6. Badgwell JM, Wolf AR, McEvedy BA, et al: Fresh gas flow formulae do not accurately predict end-tidal PCO$_2$ in paediatric patients. *Can J Anesth* 1988;35:581–586.
7. Steward DJ: Preterm infants are more prone to complications following minor surgery than are term infants. *Anesthesiology* 1982;56:304–306.
8. Liu LM, Coté CJ, Goudsouzian NG, et al: Life-threatening apnea in infants recovering from anesthesia. *Anesthesiology* 1983;59:506–510.
9. Kurth CD, Spitzer AR, Broennle AM, Downes JJ: Postoperative apnea in preterm infants. *Anesthesiology* 1987;66:483–488.
10. Coté CJ, Zaslavsky A, Downes JJ, et al: Postoperative apnea in former preterm infants after inguinal herniorrhaphy. A combined analysis. *Anesthesiology* 1995;82:809–822.
11. Welborn LG, Rice LJ, Hannallah RS, et al: Postoperative apnea in former preterm infants: prospective comparison of spinal and general anesthesia. *Anesthesiology* 1990;72:838–842.
12. Krane EJ, Haberkern CM, Jacobsen CE: A comparison of spinal and general anesthesia in the former preterm infant. *Anesth Analg* 1995;80:7–13.
13. Welborn LG, Hannallah RS, Fink R, et al: High-dose caffeine suppresses postoperative apnea in former preterm infants. *Anesthesiology* 1989;71:347–349.
14. Welborn LG, Hannallah RS, Luban NL, et al: Anemia

and postoperative apnea in former preterm infants. *Anesthesiology* 1991;74:1003-1006.
15. Badgwell JM, Heavner JE, Kytta J: Bupivacaine toxicity in young pigs is age-dependent and is affected by volatile anesthetics. *Anesthesiology* 1990;73:297-303.
16. Heavner JE, Dryden CF Jr, Sanghani V, et al: Severe hypoxemia enhances central nervous system and cardiovascular toxicity of bupivacaine in lightly anesthetized pigs. *Anesthesiology* 1992;77:142-147.
17. Heavner JE, Badgwell JM, Dryden CF, Flinders C: Bupivacaine toxicity in lightly anesthetized pigs with respiratory imbalance plus or minus halothane. *Reg Anesth* 1995;20:20-26.
18. Freid EB, Bailey AG, Valley RD: Electrocardiographic and hemodynamic changes associated with unintentional intravascular injection of bupivacaine with epinephrine in infants. *Anesthesiology* 1993;79:394-398.
19. Albajian JC, Mellish RW, Browne AF, et al: Spinal anesthesia for surgery in the high-risk infant. *Anesth Analg* 1984;63:359-362.
20. Bartlett RH, Andrews AF, Toomasian JM, et al: Extracorporeal membrane oxygenation for newborn respiratory failure: forty-five cases. *Surgery* 1982;92:425-433.
21. Kirkpatrick BV, Krummel TM, Mueller DG, et al: Use of extracorporeal membrane oxygenation for respiratory failure in term infants. *Pediatrics* 1983;72:872-876.
22. Bartlett RH, Gazzaniga AB, Toomasian J, et al: Extracorporeal membrane oxygenation (ECMO) in neonatal respiratory failure (100 cases). *Ann Surg* 1986;240:236-245.
23. Arnold JH, Truog RD, Orav EJ, et al: Tolerance and dependence in neonates sedated with fentanyl during extracorporeal membrane oxygenation. *Anesthesiology* 1990;73:1136-1140.
24. Tobias JD, Schleien CL, Haun SE: Methadone as treatment for iatrogenic narcotic dependency in pediatric intensive care unit patients. *Crit Care Med* 1990;18:1292-1293.
25. Anand KJ, Hansen DD, Hickey PR: Hormonal-metabolic stress responses in neonates undergoing cardiac surgery. *Anesthesiology* 1990;73:661-670.
26. Kanter RK, Gorton JM, Palmieri K, et al: Anatomy of femoral vessels in infants and guidelines for venous catheterization. *Pediatrics* 1989;83:1020-1022.
27. Abdulla F, Dietrich KA, Pramanik AK: Percutaneous femoral venous catheterization in preterm neonates. *J Pediatr* 1990;117:788-791.
28. Levy FH, O'Rourke PP, Crone RK: Extracorporeal membrane oxygenation. *Anesth Analg* 1992;75:1053-1062.

9

Perioperative Fluid Management

Eugene B. Freid and J. Michael Badgwell

"So let a man consider of what he was created; he was created of gushing water issuing between the loins and the breast-bones."
—Qur'an. *The Night Star*, 86:5–7.

Despite the watery matrix that bathes all cells, chapters on fluid management are usually "dry" and not particularly interesting to read. This chapter may be no exception. Nevertheless, it is a critical chapter. Even more so than in the adult, improper fluid management in infants and children can cause life-threatening consequences. The inadvertent administration of a seemingly minuscule excess of fluid may cause problems. For example, 100 ml of fluid in a full-term neonate is comparable to a 1- to 2-liter excess in an adult. Likewise, the loss of 3 tablespoons of blood (45 ml) in a 1000-g premature is 50% of the circulating blood volume of the infant. The goal of this chapter is to clarify and simplify and present a practical and "not-so-dry" approach to the perioperative fluid management of infants and children.

TRANSITION AND MATURATION OF THE KIDNEY

In many respects, the newborn kidney is similar to the newborn lung. Both have a high vascular resistance, resulting in a low blood flow. In the kidney, this low blood flow leads to a low glomerular filtration rate. A low glomerular filtration rate results in limited renal function in the first 24 hours of life. Although renal function is incompletely developed at birth, full-term neonates can effectively maintain fluid, electrolyte, and acid-base balance. The kidney of the infant is less able to conserve fluid and has more difficulty than the mature kidney in concentrating urine during periods of fluid restriction. Consequently, fluid restriction may lead to dehydration and hypernatremia.

Shortly after birth, the transition of fetal circulation to that of the neonate results in an increase in systemic pressure and a decrease in renal vascular resistance. These changes lead to improvement in renal blood flow, and by the time the neonate is 4 to 5 days old there is marked improvement in the ability of the neonatal kidney to conserve fluid as well as excrete an overload. On the other hand, fluid turnover in the infant, expressed as a percentage of extracellular fluid volume, is twice that of an adult (1). This rapid turnover makes prompt replacement of fluid deficits and correction for ongoing losses essential.

Newborn infants respond to sudden fluid intake by increasing urine volume and forming dilute urine, but it takes the infant significantly longer to excrete the fluid than it does older children and adults.

BASIC FLUID AND ELECTROLYTE REQUIREMENTS IN INFANTS AND CHILDREN

Maintenance fluids are hypotonic in general and are required for five basic reasons:

- Evaporation from the skin, an essential part of thermoregulation
- Excretion of waste products via the kidney
- Water in the stool
- Water losses from the respiratory tract
- Growth

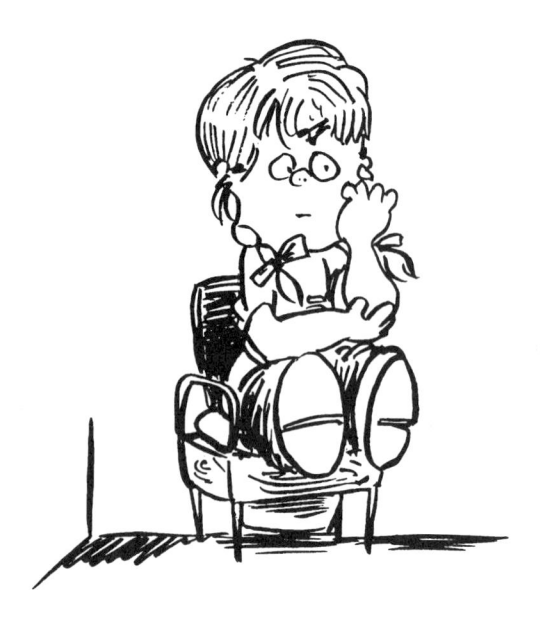

Maintenance fluid requirements vary, depending on the caloric requirements and metabolic rate of the infant or child. For up to 10 kg of body weight, the requirement is 4 ml/kg/hour; 2 ml/kg/hour are required for each kilogram between 10 and 20 kg; and 1 ml/kg/hour for each kilogram over 20 kg. To simplify the calculation of fluid requirements in the intraoperative period, an average amount of maintenance fluid of 4 ml/kg/hour may be used. The electrolyte requirement is for sodium, 2 to 3 meq/kg/day, and potassium, 1 to 2/meq/kg/day. Usually, potassium is omitted in the perioperative period. The combination of maintenance fluid requirements and electrolyte requirements results in a hypotonic electrolyte solution. Therefore, the usual intravenous (IV) maintenance fluid given to children by pediatricians in the hospital is one fourth- to one third-strength saline.

Preoperative Assessment

The preoperative assessment of fluid volume and state of hydration varies from elective surgery patients with no or slowly developing fluid deficit to the severely traumatized patient who is undergoing a dynamic deficit in blood and interstitial volume (rapidly occurring fluid loss) and in whom it is more difficult to evaluate fluid balance. In addition, response to compensatory mechanisms affect the child's clinical picture.

Compensatory Mechanisms for Fluid Loss

The body has a variety of mechanisms to compensate for fluid loss and to maintain the circulation. The compensatory mechanisms to accomplish fluid and electrolyte replacement are either definitive or temporary.

Definitive Compensatory Mechanisms. The definitive mechanism for fluid and electrolyte compensation is through the renal system. Twenty-five percent of the cardiac output goes through the kidneys. Glomerular filtration is the process of ultrafiltration, which is a separation of the plasma water and its constituents from the blood cells and plasma proteins. About 99% of that which is filtered is reabsorbed. Sodium and water deficits result in the almost complete reabsorption of the sodium and water through the distal tubule and collecting duct. A low blood volume or low blood pressure or low sodium in the distal tubule results in activation of the renin-angiotensin-aldosterone system. Renin is released from the kidney, which converts angiotensinogen to angiotensin I. Angiotensin I is converted by the converting enzyme into angiotensin II. Angiotensin II has both definitive and temporary mechanisms for conserving fluid. The definitive mechanism is that angiotensin II will trigger a release of aldosterone from the adrenal gland. Aldosterone circulates back to the kidney, which will result in the reabsorption of sodium from the distal tubule. Along with the sodium, water is reabsorbed, thereby restoring the patient to a normovolemic state with normal electrolytes.

Temporary Compensatory Mechanisms. There are temporary compensatory mechanisms that the body can activate to maintain both normal blood pressure and normal fluid volumes, but each has its own cost. The temporary mechanisms include (a) endogenous vasopressors (antidiuretic hormone, angiotensin II, and catecholamines), (b) transcapillary refill, and (c) antidiuretic hormone. Antidiuretic hormone will result in the reabsorption of free water from the distal tubule and collecting duct, which will in turn result in varying degrees of hyponatremia.

Hypovolemia, hypoperfusion, and hypotension stimulate the release of the endogenous vasopressors, which increase the blood pressure in an attempt to maintain circulation while the blood volume is being augmented through renal mechanisms. Transcapillary refill refers to the process whereby the interstitial fluid volume temporarily refills the plasma volume. The interstitial fluid acts as a volume buffer, but its ability to contract is limited. As the interstitial fluid volume contracts to augment the plasma volume, there will be varying degrees of a decrease in skin turgor. In other words, a loss of skin turgor indicates a loss of interstitial fluid volume, which in turn indicates a loss of sodium from the extracellular fluid volume. Normally, antidiuretic hormone is controlled by the osmoreceptor to maintain normal plasma osmolarity. However, hypotension will stimulate the baroresponse, which will override the osmoreceptor response. The result is a release of antidiuretic hormone, in turn resulting in an increased free water reabsorption and varying degrees of dilutional hyponatremia.

A mild hyponatremia, that is, sodium value of ≥125 is well tolerated. Sodium values lower than this have varying degrees of potential or actual problems. One of the major problem periods for the anesthesiologist is the postoperative period in which there is a potential for the development of postoperative hyponatremia. This issue will be developed later in this chapter.

Loss and Replacement of Fluid in the Perioperative Period

"When the water of a place is bad it is safest to drink none that has not been filtered through either the berry of a grape, or else a tub of malt. These are the most reliable filters yet invented."

—Samuel Butler

Oral Intake in the Child Scheduled to Have Elective Surgery

Maintenance fluids are provided orally to prevent dehydration before elective surgery. In elective procedures, there is almost always time for an appropriate period of fasting from milk, solids, and clear liquids (2) (Table 1).

There is no difference in gastric residual volume or pH in children who have had a standard 8-hour fast (NPO) compared with those allowed to ingest unlimited amounts of clear liquids (apple juice, water, clear gelatin, sugar water) up to 2 hours before anesthetic induction (4–6). The 2-hour NPO interval reduces the likelihood of serious pulmonary aspiration while keeping the child relatively well hydrated. This fasting regimen is also a much more humane treatment for the child and the parents.

As a practical rule of thumb, one may ask the parents or caregivers to withhold all milk and solids after midnight (or after going to sleep for the night) and then offer the child clear liquids 3 hours (rather than 2) before the scheduled procedure. By allowing fluids up to 3 hours in advance of the procedure, if there is a change in the schedule and the procedure takes place up to 1 hour earlier than expected, the child will have been fasting for 2 hours and the physician can feel comfortable in moving the surgery ahead without increasing the risk of pulmonary aspiration (2,3).

Intraoperative Fluid Replacement

Isotonic Replacement Fluid. Isotonic fluid losses are secondary to trauma, burns, peri-

TABLE 1. *Fasting guidelines (hours)*

Age	Milk/solids	Clear liquids
<6 months	4	2
6–36 months	6	2
>36 months	8	2

Note: Most children > 6 months of age can fast from milk and solids after midnight. Any amount of clear liquids (apple juice, water, sugar water) should be offered up to 2 hours before scheduled surgery. Breast milk should be considered as being in the milk and solid group, not as a clear liquid (3).

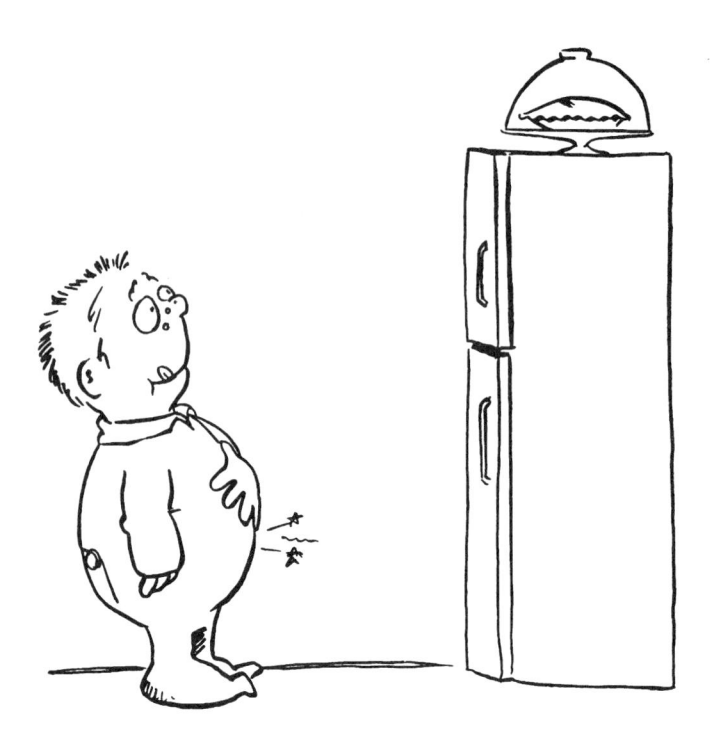

tonitis, bleeding, and losses from the upper gastrointestinal tract.

All of these losses are very high in sodium, that is, 120 to 160 meq/L. As a matter of fact, for purposes of discussion, all of the latter losses can be considered as loss of extracellular fluid. Extracellular fluid is made up of interstitial fluid and plasma volume. The main difference between interstitial fluid and plasma volume is the fact that plasma contains protein. The electrolyte content of the extracellular fluid is basically the same for interstitial fluid and plasma volume. Therefore, any type of injury, surgery, or upper gastrointestinal tract loss should be replaced by a balanced salt solution, that is, one that contains approximately 140 meq/L of sodium, 100 meq/L of chloride, and small amounts of other electrolytes.

One of the major differences in fluid volumes of the body is that in infants, 40% of body weight is extracellular fluid, whereas in children and adults, 20% of body weight is extracellular fluid. The reason for the difference is a larger interstitial fluid volume in the child. The plasma volumes are similar.

Hypotonic Replacement Fluid. Examples of hypotonic fluid loss are sweating and diarrhea. The replacement fluid for these losses is hypotonic (e.g., 0.25 to 0.5 normal saline). However, for practical purposes, balanced salt solution can be used to replace all types of losses—isotonic or hypotonic. The kidney is much better equipped to excrete overloads of sodium than it is to compensate for excess losses of sodium that are not appropriately replaced.

Choice and Quantity of Intraoperative Fluids. In the ideal world, perhaps one would start two IV lines: one with maintenance fluids at a set rate and the other with replacement fluids. However, this is both burdensome and, in most cases, unnecessary. The decision is based on two choices: (a) to give a hypotonic solution such as maintenance fluids and hope that the kidney can excrete the extra water and there will be no further sodium losses (e.g., from vomiting) or (b) to administer a balanced salt solution and rely on the kidney to excrete any extra sodium. The latter is by far the best choice.

TABLE 2. *Guidelines for fluid administration in pediatric patients: balanced salt solution*

1. First hour: hydrating solution, 4 ml/kg for every hour of fluid deprivation prior to surgery
2. Basic hourly fluid = Maintenance + surgical trauma
   Maintenance fluid = 4 ml/kg/h
   Surgical trauma replacement fluids
     Mild trauma (e.g., herniorrhaphy), 2–4 ml/kg/h
     Moderate trauma, 5–7 ml/kg/h
     Severe trauma (e.g., major abdominal tumor resection), 8–12 ml/kg/h
3. Blood replacement with blood or 3:1 volume replacement with crystalloid

Table 2 provides guidelines for fluid administration in pediatric patients. If an IV line is in place and the infant or child is hydrated, then the guidelines start with items 2 and 3. For relatively minor operations or operations in which blood loss of up to 15% to 20% of blood volume is anticipated and assuming that the blood loss will be controllable, either no invasive monitors or urine output is monitored along with routine monitors to determine the adequacy of volume replacement. Remember that in the small infant, blood pressure is an excellent reflection of blood volume. If the blood loss is going to equal or exceed 20% of blood volume or if the blood loss is potentially uncontrollable, then consideration should be given to the use of an arterial line or central venous line for the serial determination of blood pressure, hematocrit, electrolytes, and blood gases.

Glucose

In the last several years, there has been a complete reevaluation of the place of glucose in routine intraoperative solutions. The basic question being: Is glucose necessary in the intraoperative period? It has long been thought that the pediatric patient might be at special risk for developing hypoglycemia. Therefore glucose has been given to prevent that possibility. Whereas it is very difficult to obtain a consensus on the definition of hypoglycemia, in otherwise healthy patients (e.g., those without diabetes mellitus) hypoglycemia is defined as <30 mg/dl in neonates and <40 mg/dl in older infants and children. The neonate tolerates much lower glucose levels than the older child and adult but is more likely to develop hypoglycemia due to its rapid metabolism and limited glucose stores. Welborn and colleagues (7) reported fasting glucose levels on several hundred pediatric outpatients who had been NPO for anywhere between 6 and 17 hours. None of these patients had symptoms of hypoglycemia, and, according to accepted definitions of hypoglycemia, none had hypoglycemia. Therefore, in routine patients, it appears that there is no need for glucose in the intraoperative period, nor is there a need to monitor glucose in these patients. After surgery, when the danger of hypoxia and cerebral ischemia is over, glucose solutions can be started.

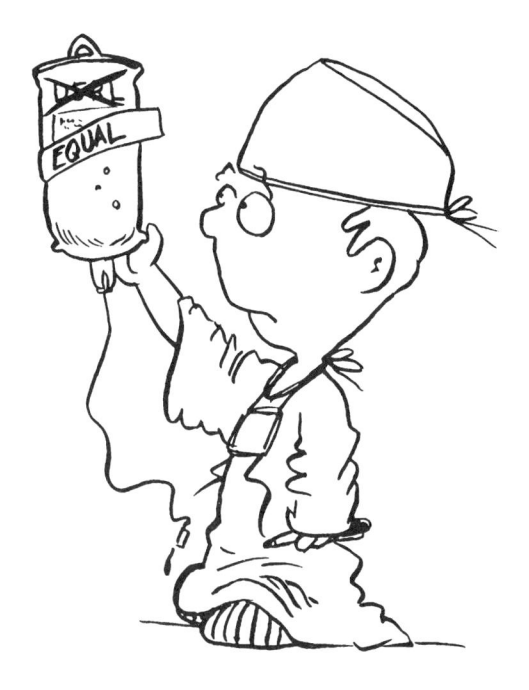

On the other hand, certain high-risk patients do run a danger of hypoglycemia. These patients are those who are receiving glucose-containing or hyperalimentation solutions. Patients who fit into this category should have their hyperalimentation or glucose solution continued in the perioperative period. Certain other patients may be at risk for hypoglycemia, such as infants < 1 month of age, infants of diabetic mothers, neonates, especially those who are small for gestational age, and children who are diabetic. These patients need to have basal glucose infusions or their glucose monitored.

Is Glucose Potentially Harmful in IV Solutions?

There are now a whole host of studies in various animal models which have indicated the potential for the augmentation of ischemic brain injury by glucose infusions. The issue of whether glucose is harmful is directly related to whether our patients have any chance during anesthetic management for hypoxia and cerebral ischemia. The issue is that in the presence of partial cerebral ischemia, the previous administration of a glucose solution will result in an increase in glucose in the brain so that with ischemia, anaerobic metabolism results in the production of large quantities of lactic acid. Lactic acid reduces the pH of the brain cell, which greatly increases the potential for neurologic damage.

Various experimental studies typify a potential clinical situation for anesthesiologists—cardiac arrest occuring during administration of normal amounts of glucose with only modest elevations of blood glucose (8–10). Blood glucose, however, does not necessarily reflect brain glucose. Therefore, hyperglycemia alone does not increase the risk. The increased risk is apparently due to the combination of partial cerebral ischemia and increased glucose "seen" by the brain.

Hyperglycemia or the administration of glucose may be associated with central nervous system injury. In humans, acquired neuropathic lesions have occurred in infants with hypoplastic left heart syndrome who underwent major surgery (11). One of the correlations between acquired neuropathic lesions was with hyperglycemia. In the final analysis, there appears to be no reason to administer glucose in the usual clinical situation. By contrast, there are definite potential hazards.

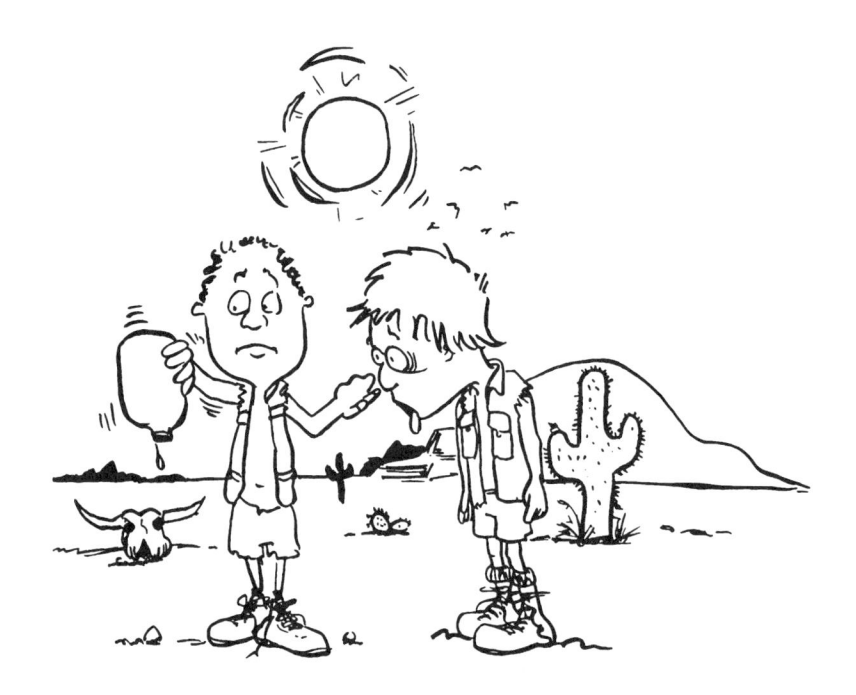

Acute hyperkalemia may be treated with hyperventilation, calcium, sodium bicarbonate, a beta$_2$ agonist (albuterol or terbutaline), and epinephrine. In addition, the administration of glucose has been recommended as part of therapy in hyperkalemia. The clinical efficacy of glucose and insulin to reduce serum potassium occurs on a delayed basis because it takes 15 or 20 minutes for a clinical effect to take place. To administer glucose when the patient is hypotensive or in the situation of arrest might augment cerebral ischemia. Therefore, it would be better to delay glucose and insulin until the patient has a stable circulation.

Changes Related to Volume Status

Slowly Developing Fluid Loss

Slowly developing fluid loss will allow appropriate time for normal definitive mechanisms of the body to compensate for fluid loss if the appropriate electrolyte content is given in sufficient quantity. This means that when the renin-angiotensin-aldosterone system is activated, the first thing that will be noticed is a decrease in urine output. If one were to measure in older children, there would be a markedly decreased amount of sodium in the urine, <5 meq/L. The immaturity of the neonatal distal tubule results in higher amounts of sodium in the urine, 10 to 20 meq/L. If insufficient fluid volume and electrolyte are administered, transcapillary refill is activated whereby interstitial fluid volume will be transferred to the plasma volume. The condition is identified by loss of skin turgor. In the small infant, the fontanelles as well as the eyes may be sunken. The activation of these compensatory mechanisms usually indicates a loss of 5% to 10% of body weight. If the fluid loss continues without appropriate replacement and hypovolemia develops, the baroreceptor will be stimulated by the decreasing blood pressure. Then, the endogenous vasopressors will be activated, resulting in a tachycardia and vasoconstriction in an attempt to maintain normal blood pressure to ensure normal perfusion of vital organs.

Any pediatric patient who has undergone slow progressive volume loss and who has become hypotensive in association with fluid loss can be assumed to have at least 20% loss of blood volume. Therefore, these children need to have at least 20% of their blood volume restored through the use of crystalloid resuscitation. The usual resuscitation fluid for the pediatric patient requiring preoperative fluid resuscitation is balanced salt solution.

Slowly Developing Bradycardia/Hypotension

The causes of slowly developing bradycardia/hypotension are slowly developing fluid loss (see previous text), anesthetic overdose—relative or absolute—hypovolemia, low ionized calcium, and obstruction of major blood vessels with a decrease in venous return. Hypoxia can also cause a slowly developing bradycardia and hypotension; with modern monitors, this would be certainly picked up early. Hypercarbia may cause a vasodilatation, but usually the sympathetic nervous system is stimulated so that there may be an increase rather than a decrease in heart rate.

Rapidly Occurring Fluid Loss

Rapidly occurring fluid loss is the most significant pathophysiologic defect in surgical patients undergoing massive bleeding and in traumatized children with hemorrhagic shock. Shock is manifested in anesthetized and nonanesthetized patients as delayed capillary refill, mottled skin, cool extremities, and tachycardia. In the anesthetized child, diastolic blood pressure is a good indicator of filling pressure and, in the hypovolemic child, may decrease either gradually or rapidly (as in rapid response to anesthetic induction agents). In moderate to severe shock, peripheral pulses may be absent, evidenced by the loss of pulse oximetry. Diminished peripheral pulses, loss of pulse oximetry, and tachycardia should alert the clinician that cardiovascular collapse may be imminent. Arterial pH is a good indicator of circulatory status. If pH is low and carbon dioxide is normal or low, circulating blood volume is probably inadequate. Metabolic acidosis in hypovolemic children is usually corrected by adequate fluid resuscitation. However, if the pH falls below 7.2 in a child with adequate ventilation, sodium bicarbonate may be added to fluid replacement (dose = body weight in kg × 0.15 meq × base deficit, given as an IV bolus, followed by reassessment of the pH) (12).

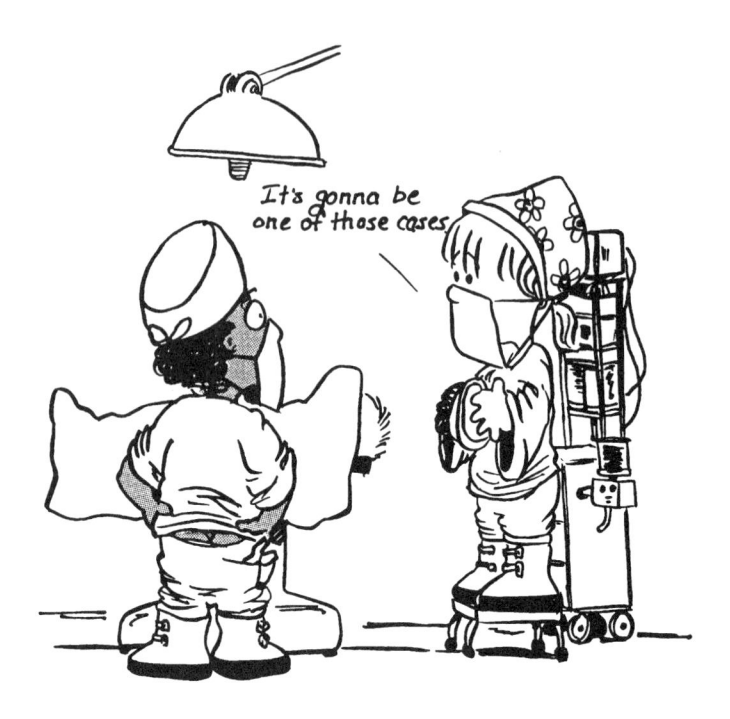

Rapidly Developing Bradycardia/Hypotension

The definition of "sudden" is something that happens over a period of a minute or two. Bradycardia is defined as a pulse rate that drops by at least 40% and hypotension is defined as a blood pressure that drops approximately the same. Because of the differences in pulse rate with age, it is impossible to give a number—hence the percentages.

The major causes of a sudden bradycardia/hypotension are such things as hypoxia, rapidly occurring fluid loss and hypovolemia, anaphylaxis, vagal reflexes, and hyperkalemia. An anesthetic overdose may be responsible for bradycardia and hypotension, but it usually develops over a period of 5 or 10 minutes or longer, depending on the concentration of the inspired agent as well as the rate of ventilation and cardiac output. The following are steps in the treatment of sudden hypotension or bradycardia:

- Notify surgeons.
- Turn off the anesthetics.
- Assure airway and ventilation.
- Ventilate with 100% oxygen.
- Give bolus fluids or blood.
- Have a low threshold to:
  - Apply cardiac compression.
  - Administer IV epinephrine, 5 µg/kg.

If in doubt, cardiac compressions should be done. If the heart goes into total arrest, then the dose of epinephrine may need to be increased up to 50 to 100 µg/kg.

NORMAL (P.D. -90 mV)   **HEMORRHAGIC SHOCK (P.D. -60 mV)**

Normal (mEq/L): $Na^+ = 9.9$, $K^+ = 173$, $Cl^- = 3.9$

Hemorrhagic shock (mEq/L): ↑$Na^+ = 18.4$, ↓$K^+ = 162$, ↑$Cl^- = 11.1$

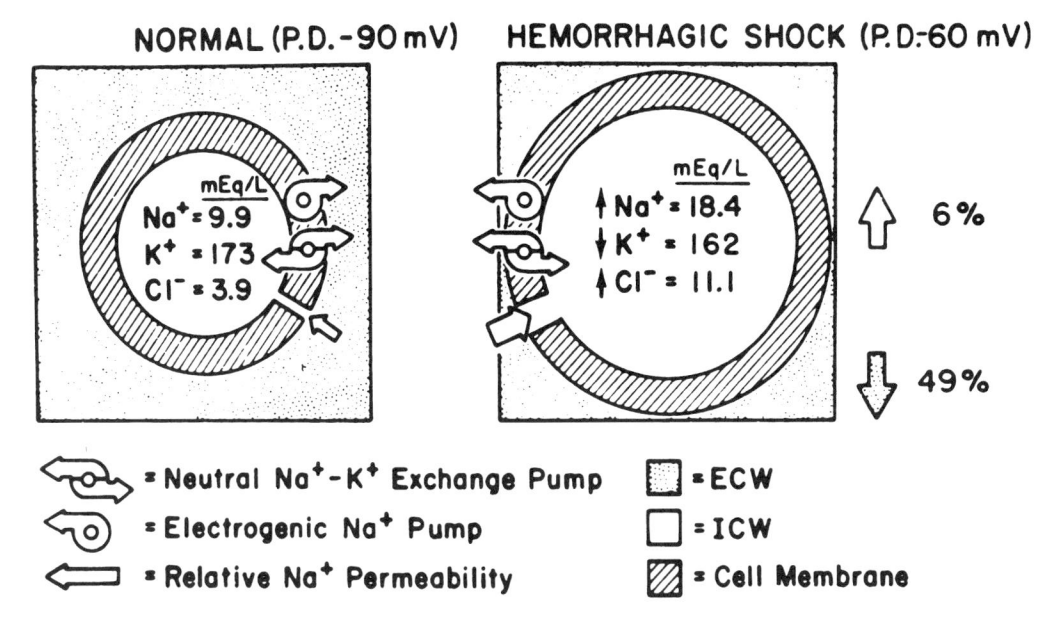

↑ 6% ↓ 49%

- = Neutral Na^+-K^+ Exchange Pump
- = Electrogenic Na^+ Pump
- = Relative Na^+ Permeability
- = ECW
- = ICW
- = Cell Membrane

FIG. 1. The failure of cellular pump mechanisms during hemorrhagic shock causes an increase in intracellular sodium and water and a decrease in extracellular water. Intracellular water excess causes the patient to swell. (Reprinted with permission of the McGraw-Hill Companies. Schwartz S: *Principles of Surgery*. 5th Ed., 1989, p. 121.)

TREATMENT OF HYPOVOLEMIA AND BLOOD LOSS

"In the world there is nothing more submissive and weak than water. Yet, for attacking that which is hard and strong nothing can surpass it.
—Lao-Tzu (6th Century BC)

Crystalloid

The goal of fluid management during maintenance of anesthesia is to replenish vascular and interstitial fluid volumes. Hypovolemic shock is associated with a decrease in functional extracellular fluid volume and an increase in intracellular fluid volume (Fig. 1) (13). Therefore, resuscitative fluid should mimic that of extracellular fluid (sodium concentration 140 to 150 meq/L) (14). Effective resuscitation requires the administration of red cells and crystalloid in excess of the amount of blood that is lost (15).[a] Therefore, effective resuscitation after massive hemorrhage causes edema, swelling, and obligatory weight gain (Fig. 2). The administration of hypotonic solutions (e.g., 5% dextrose in water or 0.2 normal saline) will cause intracellular edema but without the beneficial effects of intravascular and interstitial repletion. Children, like adults, need balanced salt solutions to replace traumatic and surgical losses.

Blood Component Therapy

Measurements of blood loss during massive blood loss are usually unreliable. More reliable are clinical signs, such as capillary refill, temperature gradient (e.g., between rectum and skin), urine output, central venous pressure, or diastolic blood pressure, as a guide for estimating blood loss and volume status. The hematocrit is a reflection only of

---

[a]Ed. Note (JMB): This is the work of G. Thomas Shires, MD (preeminent surgeon and researcher), who is now Director of Surgical Research at the University of Nevada. In 1963, Tom was chief at Parkland Hospital in Dallas, Texas. He was in Galveston presenting an abstract (see ref. 15) on November 22, the day President Kennedy was shot and taken to Parkland Hospital. It is doubtful whether Tom could have done much more than his colleagues to save the President. Nevertheless, the irony of this remarkable situation is not lost on your intrepid editor.

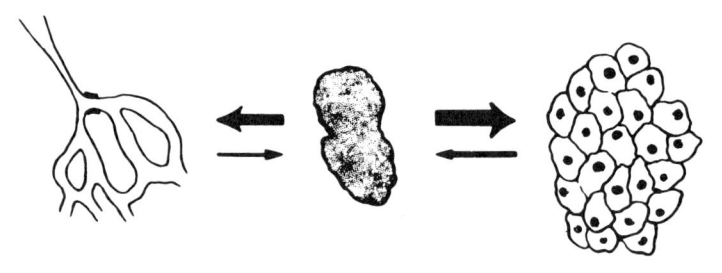

FIG. 2. Interstitial fluid is translocated, intravascularly and intracellularly, after hemorrhagic shock. This translocation of fluid results in a decrease in functional extracellular fluid and an increase in intracellular volume. (Reprinted with permission of the McGraw-Hill Companies. Schwartz S: *Principles of Surgery*. 5th Ed., 1989, p. 121.)

the ratio of red blood cells (RBCs) to crystalloid and colloid. Therefore, hematocrit is not a good reflection of volume status. It may be used, however, to guide further therapy (i.e., more RBCs versus more fluid).

Red Blood Cells

RBCs should be transfused to increase oxygen carrying capacity in children who have lost a significant portion of their RBC mass. The decision to give RBC is less difficult in the traumatized child than in the child undergoing elective surgery. Either O-negative or cross-matched type-specific blood may be used to replace blood that has been previously or continues to be lost by the hypovolemic child. In the equation,

$$\dot{D}O_2 = CO \times CaO_2$$

where $\dot{D}O_2$ = oxygen delivery, CO = cardiac output, and CaO_2 = oxygen content), hemoglobin is the major oxygen "container," and is therefore a major determinant of $\dot{D}O_2$. Anemic children compensate for low hemoglobin by increasing heart rate to increased cardiac output. Although healthy children, or those with chronic anemia may tolerate hemoglobin values of 7 g/dl or less, neonates, children with cardiac disease or chronic pulmonary disease, and children with multisystem trauma, who may have coexisting hypovolemia, hypoxemia, acidemia, and hypothermia, require transfusion to a hematocrit of 33% to 35%.

Although it is necessary to filter (using a 170-μm pore filter), measure, and warm administered blood cells, it is not necessary to filter cells with a very-small-pore filter (e.g., a 20- to 40-μm filter) (16). Children requiring a transfusion should, however, receive blood filtered for white blood cells (when possible) to prevent sensitization to white cell antigens in blood. Leukocyte-depleted blood (blood filtered or irradiated in the blood bank) is especially indicated in certain groups of patients—patients who are immunosuppressed, those with cancer, and those receiving blood from close relatives.

Warm blood may be administered very rapidly to children, by hand or by using a mechanical rapid-infusion system. Although a 7F catheter in an older child will allow blood administration at 750 ml/min, this very rapid flow rate may overload the right heart and rapidly cause pulmonary edema. Because there are no maximum flow formulas that can take into account all of the patient's variables, central venous pressure must be measured and maintained at physiologic values when rapid-infusion systems are used in children.

Guidelines for an Acceptable Hematocrit

An area of fluid management that has undergone the greatest change in both adults and children is in blood replacement. The dangers of blood-borne diseases, such as hepatitis and AIDS along with the experience with the Jehovah's Witness, has resulted in a much more balanced approach to the risk and benefits of blood transfusions. Blood component therapy is largely a judgment issue. As a result, some arbitrary guidelines have been developed to assist the clinician with this sometimes difficult decision. The concept of an acceptable hematocrit and a normal hematocrit will assist the clinician in determining both the adequate preparation of the patient for surgery as well as in recognizing an acceptable hematocrit in the intraoperative and postoperative period.

If an infant has a normal hematocrit, which is within 2 standard deviations for age, then there is no preoperative concern about whether or not the hematocrit is acceptable for surgery. If the hematocrit is <2 standard deviations, attention needs to be directed toward making a diagnosis of why the child is anemic. The degree of anemia may be such that the hematocrit is acceptable for surgery, but still is not considered normal. An acceptable hematocrit is defined as a hematocrit that is tolerated by infants and children without the need for blood transfusion. Table 3 gives a list of normal and arbitrary acceptable hematocrits. These values are subject to change as further clinical experience is gained.

It should be recognized that if the infant or child has an underlying medical condition that involves either the respiratory system or the cardiovascular system and this condition limits either the ability to increase cardiac output or the ability to saturate hemoglobin, then higher guidelines for the hematocrit need to be followed.

Platelets

Platelet deficiency is the usual cause of clinical bleeding after hemorrhage and resuscitation. Although surgical bleeding may occur when the platelet count is 50,000 to 70,000/mm^3, there is no absolute number that relates platelet count to clinical bleeding. Each patient must be individually assessed for signs of bleeding (e.g., oozing in the surgical field). The infusion of 0.1 to 0.3 units of platelets per kg body weight will cause a rise of 20,000 to 70,000/mm^3 in the child's platelet count (17). After massive transfusion, it is not necessary to infuse platelets as a prophylactic measure in the child who is not bleeding. Because hypothermic platelets do not function properly, every effort should be made to keep children warm, especially children who are actively bleeding.

Fresh Frozen Plasma

The prophylactic administration of fresh frozen plasma (FFP) after massive transfusion

TABLE 3. *Normal and acceptable hematocrit in pediatric patients*

	Normal hematocrit		Acceptable hematocrit
	Mean	Range	
Premature	45	40–45	35
Newborn	54	45–65	30–35
3 mo	36	30–42	25
1 y	38	34–42	20–25
6 y	38	35–43	20–25

(>1 blood volume replaced; estimated blood volume = 80 ml/kg) does not prevent clinical bleeding states that are associated with coagulopathy and should not be given merely for volume expansion. FFP is used to increase clotting factors in children with demonstrated deficiencies (e.g., prothrombin time, partial thromboplastin time >150% of normal) (18). Because FFP and platelet concentrates contain a large amount of citrate preservative, rapid administration (>1.5 ml/kg/min) may cause calcium binding and hypotension (19). Hypotension that is secondary to citrate toxicity may be treated with calcium chloride (10 mg/kg) or calcium gluconate (30-60 mg/kg) and the temporary discontinuation of FFP or platelet transfusion.

Postoperative Fluid Problems

Acute Dilutional Hyponatremia

The use of hypotonic IV fluids (e.g., $D_s O.SNS$) in the immediate postoperative period may be appropriate in volume replete pediatric patients. When hypotonic fluids are used in volume depleted patients combined with losses of sodium, however, dilutional hyponatremia may occur. Therefore, acute dilutional hyponatremia is a potential problem in almost every postoperative patient (a) who has undergone any degree of tissue trauma, such as tonsillectomy and adenoidectomy, hernia repair, and other procedures, and (b) who is placed on hypotonic fluids postoperatively.

The most common anesthetic complication is nausea and vomiting. Vomiting results in the loss of fluid that is high in sodium—balanced salt solution. Vomiting together with small losses of blood or third-space tissue trauma fluid can result in the need for postoperative sodium. When hypotonic solutions are used, often the sodium is inadequate to meet the needs of the body. Antidiuretic hormone is released to maintain volume, and acute dilutional hyponatremia occurs. The problem is that when the extracellular fluid becomes hypotonic, the intracellular fluid remains isotonic. Mother Nature cannot stand the osmotic imbalance. Therefore, water is transferred from the extracellular fluid to the intracellular fluid, resulting in cerebral edema. Cerebral edema leads to central nervous system irritability and depression, resulting in a decreasing level of consciousness, disorientation, vomiting, and, in severe cases, seizure activity.

Acute symptomatic hyponatremia is a medical emergency, which fortunately is relatively infrequent, but requires immediate therapy. The drug of choice is sodium bicarbonate, which is a 6% sodium solution (1000 meq/L). The empirical dose is 2 ml/kg of sodium bicarbonate given rapidly (1 to 2 minutes). Sodium bicarbonate, 2 ml/kg, will raise the serum sodium by 6 meq/L. Administration of sodium bicarbonate should be considered for any patient having seizures who is receiving a hypotonic solution postoperatively along with the usual treatment for the seizure (oxygen, ventilatory support, and an antiseizure drug such as lorazepam or midazolam (each in the dose of 0.05 mg/kg initial dose then titrated to response). The hypertonic sodium bicarbonate increases the tonicity of the serum, thereby pulling water from the interstitium of the brain cells. After 2 ml/kg sodium bicarbonate is given, if the seizures have abated, then balanced salt solution can be started as the appropriate fluid. If the sodium concentration is still below 120, consideration should be given to giving 1 ml/kg more of sodium bicarbonate.

Any patient who has a seizure in the postoperative period and who is receiving hypotonic fluids must be considered to have acute dilutional hyponatremia and receive the appropriate therapy. After the sodium is given or while it is being given, a blood sample should be drawn to rule out hypoglycemia or other potential problems. The very simple way to prevent acute symptomatic hyponatremia is to maintain all postoperative patients on balanced salt solution, either until they begin to eat or until they are well through any major period of fluid shifts.

Chronic Hyponatremia

Chronic hyponatremia is exactly what the name implies—hyponatremia that has occurred over a period of time and can be considered chronic. This condition should be managed in a very conservative manner, since too-rapid administration of sodium in chronic hyponatremia has been reported to cause a debilitating neurologic condition referred to as *osmotic demyelination syndrome*. Patients with chronic hyponatremia have usually been on long-term diuretics, have varying degrees of nutritional problems, and need to be managed most conservatively.

SUMMARY

This chapter provides an overview of perioperative fluid concerns in the pediatric surgical patient. An understanding of fluid assessment and the compensatory mechanisms for fluid volume and electrolyte values helps to define the guidelines for appropriate fluid and electrolyte management of the pediatric patient in the perioperative period. In summation, we have described the use of fluids and blood components as well as some of the infrequent but potentially devastating problems associated with the use of intraoperative fluid solutions. We hope that these guidelines will be useful in helping to meet the hydrational and oxygen delivery needs of infants and children and will help the clinician to recognize and prevent potential problems.

REFERENCES

1. Kooh SW, Metcoff J: Physiologic considerations in fluid and electrolyte therapy with particular reference to diarrheal dehydration in children. *J Pediatr* 1963;62:107.
2. Coté CJ: NPO after midnight for children: a reappraisal. *Anesthesiology* 1990;72:589–592.
3. O'Hare B, Lerman J, Endo J, Cutz E: Acute lung injury after instillation of human breast milk or infant formula into rabbits lungs. *Anesthesiology* 1996;84:1386–1391.
4. Schreiner MS, Triebwasser A, Keon TP: Ingestion of liquids compared with preoperative fasting in pediatric outpatients. *Anesthesiology* 1990;72:593–597.
5. Sandhar BK, Goresky GV, Maltby JR, Shaffer EA: Effect of oral liquids and ranitidine on gastric fluid volume and pH in children undergoing outpatient surgery. *Anesthesiology* 1989;71:327–330.
6. Splinter WM, Stewart JA, Muir JG: The effect of preoperative apple juice on gastric contents, thirst and hunger in children. *Can J Anaesth* 1989;36:55–58.
7. Welborn LG, McGill WA, Hannallah RS, et al: Perioperative blood glucose concentrations in pediatric outpatients. *Anesthesiology* 1986;65:543–547.
8. Lundy EF, Kuhn JE: Infusion of five percent dextrose increases mortality and morbidity following six minutes of cardiac arrest in resuscitated dogs. *J Crit Care* 1987; 2:4–14.
9. Nakakimura K, Fleischer JE, Drummond JC, et al: Glucose administration before cardiac arrest worsens neurologic outcome in cats. *Anesthesiology* 1990;72: 1005–1011.
10. Lanier WL, Stangland KJ, Scheithauer BW, et al: The effects of dextrose infusion and head position on neurologic outcome after complete cerebral ischemia in primates: examination of a model. *Anesthesiology* 1987; 66:39–48.
11. Glauser TA, Rorke LB, Weinberg PM, Clancy RR: Acquired neuropathologic lesions associated with the hypoplastic left heart syndrome. *Pediatrics* 1990;85: 991–1000.
12. *Advanced Trauma Life Support Student Manual.* Chicago: American College of Surgeons, 1989:222.
13. Shires GT, Cunningham JN, Backer CR, et al: Alterations in cellular membrane function during hemorrhagic shock in primates. *Ann Surg* 1972;176:288–295.
14. Shires FT, Canizaro PC, Carrico CJ: Shock. In Schwartz SI. ed. *Principles of Surgery,* 3rd ed. New York: McGraw-Hill, 1979:139–144.
15. Shires FT, Coln D, Carrico J, Lightfoot S: Fluid therapy in hemorrhagic shock. *Arch Surg* 1964;88:688–693.
16. *Questions and answers about transfusion practices,* 2nd ed. Dallas: American Society of Anesthesiologists Committee on Transfusion Medicine, 1992:24.
17. Coté CJ, Liu LM, Szyfelbein SK, et al: Changes in serial platelet counts following massive blood transfusion in pediatric patients. *Anesthesiology* 1985;62:197–201.
18. Anonymous: NIH Consensus Conference: fresh-frozen plasma. Indications and risks. *JAMA* 1985;253:551–553.
19. Coté CJ, Drop LJ, Hoaglin DC, et al: Ionized hypocalcemia after fresh frozen plasma administration to thermally injured children: effects of infusion rate, duration, and treatment with calcium chloride. *Anesth Analg* 1988; 67:152–160.

10
Perioperative Pain Management

J. Michael Badgwell, Joseph P. Cravero, Brenda C. McClain, Linda Jo Rice, and Melissa M. McLeod

"So long as little children are allowed to suffer, there is no true love in this world."
—Isadora Duncan

PAIN MANAGEMENT: TIME PERIODS

Preoperative

The control of pain is a continuum that begins in the preoperative period (Fig. 1). Plans to control postoperative pain begins when we first see the patient. For the school-aged child, pain management begins preoperatively by discussing the operative procedure with the child, letting him or her know that there will probably be some pain but that medications can be given to lessen it. Many children are afraid of getting multiple shots, and they should be reassured that this will not happen. Intramuscular (IM) injections should be avoided whenever possible. Preoperatively, many patients have anxiety as well as pain. Will an analgesic agent administered preoperatively carry over and provide pain relief in the postoperative period? There are some instances in which it may. For example, a midazolam and ibuprofen combination may be given to children before many procedures (e.g., dental restoration) to provide postoperative pain relief. There is no reason why this regimen won't work in many areas.

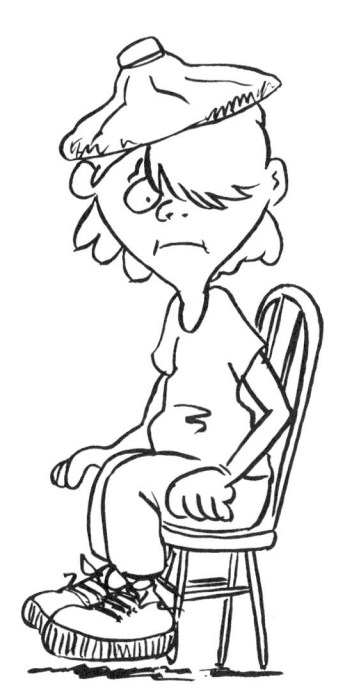

Preemptive Analgesia

"Do not undervalue the headache. While it is at its sharpest, it seems a bad investment; but when relief begins, the unexpired remainder is worth $4 a minute."
—Mark Twain

There is mounting evidence that aggressive analgesia will improve outcome after surgery. Although it is uncertain whether the prevention of pain mediators (preemptive analgesia) affects the level of pain achieved after the analgesic has worn off, anyone who has ever treated his or her own headache knows that it is much easier to control the pain if treatment occurs early than if the headache is allowed to become severe.

Intraoperative

Another window of opportunity to provide postoperative pain relief exists early in the in-

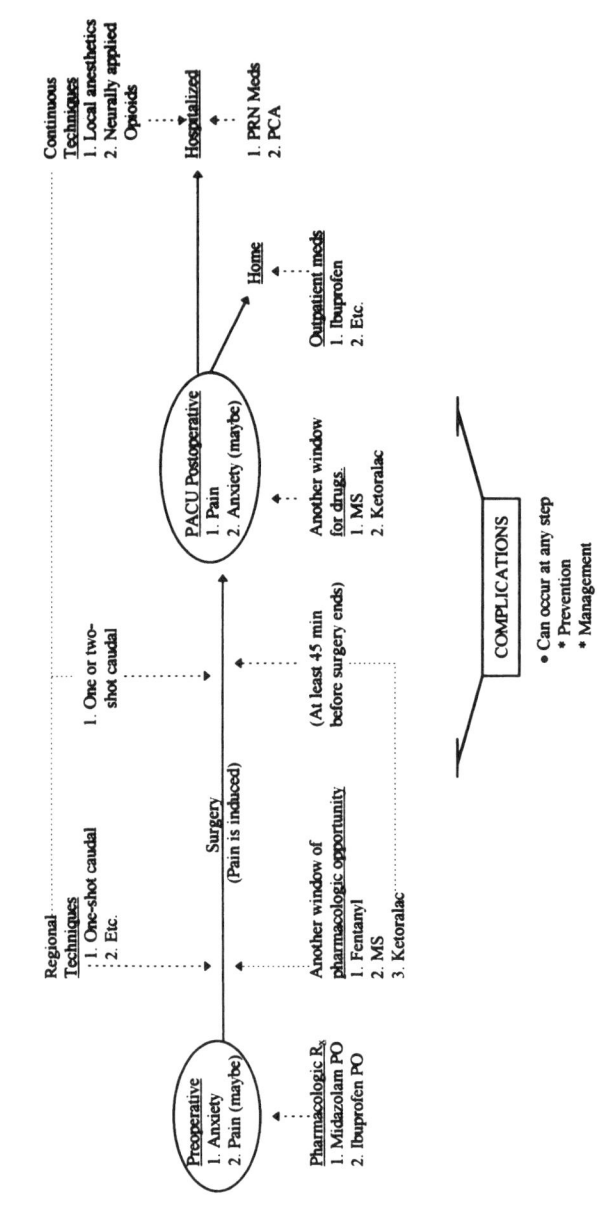

FIG. 1. The management of perioperative pain is a continuum with many windows of opportunity for intervention.

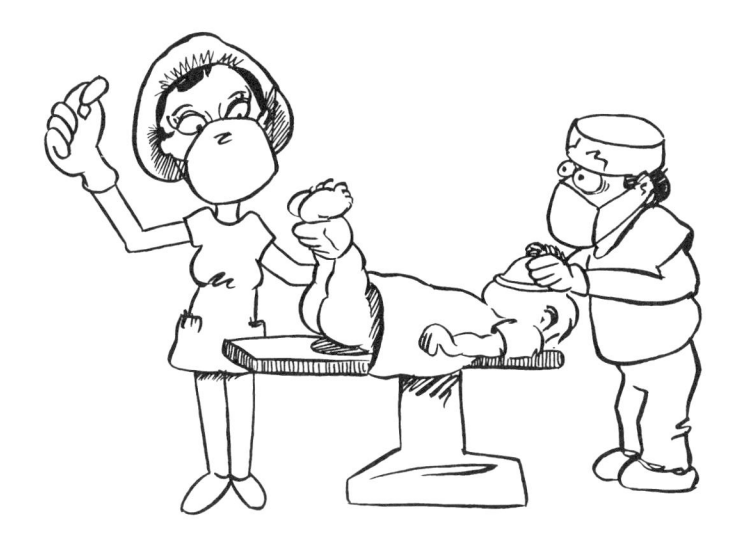

traoperative period with either the use of a regional technique or pharmacologic agents. For example, a one-shot caudal may be given to provide preemptive analgesia to the child with lower abdominal surgery. If this lower abdominal surgery goes longer than 3 hours, a repeat caudal may be done (two-shot caudal) to provide pain relief. Pharmacologic therapy begins early in the intraoperative course with the initiation of a background of narcotic analgesia or nonsteroidal anti-inflammatory drugs (NSAIDs). For example, ketorolac can be given 45 minutes before the end of surgery to provide postoperative pain relief.

Titration of narcotic analgesics, the use of regional techniques, local nerve blocks, intravenous (IV) ketorolac, or rectal administration of acetaminophen all can be accomplished in the operating room with the child asleep.

For high-risk patients (e.g., those with tenuous airway or the neonatal patient), it may be more appropriate to limit the use of narcotics in the operating room, maximize the use of nonnarcotic analgesic techniques, and then titrate additional analgesics in the postanesthesia care unit (PACU) as the child awakes. Failure to administer any analgesic agents before waking a child from a procedure expected to cause postoperative pain will only result in a stormy emergence, a combative patient, and an unhappy PACU staff.

Postoperative Pain

The continuum of pain management continues through to the PACU, the pediatric intensive care unit, the outpatient surgery area, home, or to an inpatient bed. In the PACU, pain and anxiety can be controlled with pharmacologic agents or continuation of the regional technique (e.g., a continuous regional technique). Therefore, the PACU is another window of opportunity to provide either pharmacologic agents or continuation of the regional technique. No child should be discharged from the PACU with uncontrolled pain.

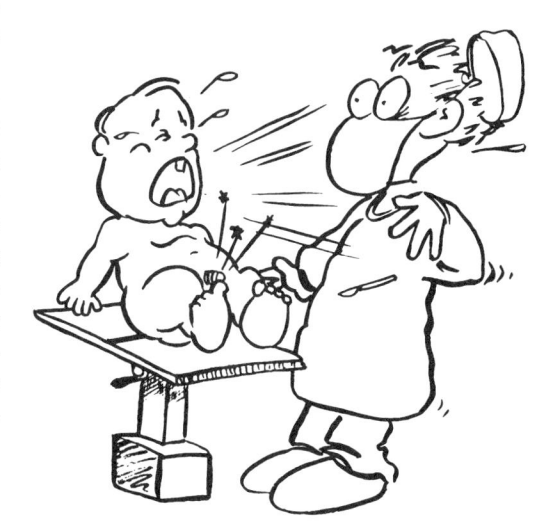

This chapter examines each of these steps along the way, going into practical detail of regional and pharmacologic pain management. In addition, particular attention will be directed toward prevention and management of potential complications of both regional and pharmacologic pain management techniques.

CHILDREN'S PAIN: SAME AS ADULTS' PAIN?

As in adults, surgical procedures in children produce tissue trauma and release potent mediators of inflammation and pain. After pain is produced in children, the severity of pain is influenced by the child's medical condition, the type of procedure performed, and the attitudes of health care professionals and families toward pain management.

The rest of the world has come to realize what mothers (and pediatricians doing circumcisions) have known for years—children feel pain. It is the responsibility of the caregiver to recognize that the child is in pain; it is not up to the child to convince the caregiver that he or she hurts. If it would be painful for a grownup, it will be painful for a baby. In addition, children often have pain for reasons other than surgical pain (e.g., procedures such as lumbar punctures or bone marrow biopsies, or medical problems such as headaches). Furthermore, just as children change in every other aspect of development with age, their response to pain and emotional distress changes over time. Therefore, pain management may be more challenging for children than for adults.

Assessment of Pain in Children

An understanding of children, including their developmental level and their behavior, is necessary to assess pain and distress. Language skills, previous pain experiences, and coping strategies are important. Most of the time, Mom knows best for a preverbal child. Pain questions addressed to a verbal child should be in the child's language—the language of "owies and boo-boos." There are numerous tools for assessing the pain of children of all ages. Because pain is a subjective experience, a self-assessment scale may be preferable to an observer's objective assessment and should be used whenever possible. Younger school-aged children can often use a numeric rating scale, with a score of 10 as "no pain" and 0 as "the worst pain imaginable." Those not able to use numeric

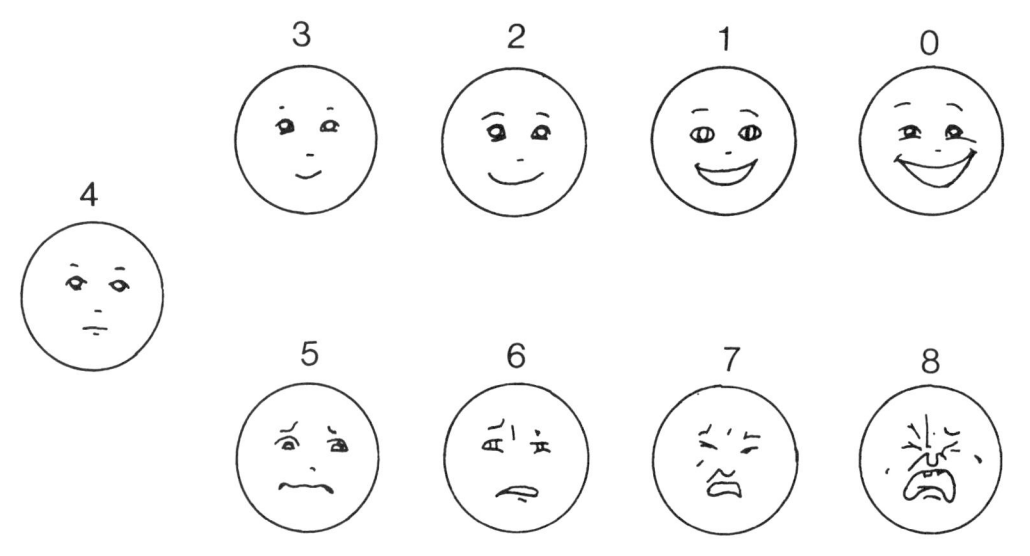

FIG. 2. The Faces Pain Rating Scale: A subjective assessment guide for younger children. The child is asked which face looks like how he or she is feeling.

TABLE 1. Ten-point objective pain-discomfort scale

Points	0	1	2
BP	10%>preop	10% to 20%>preop	20% to 30%>preop
Crying	No crying	Crying, but responds to tender loving care (TLC)	Crying, does not respond to TLC
Movement	None	Restless	Thrashing
Agitation	Patient asleep or calm	Mild	Hysterical
Verbal evaluation or body language	Patient asleep or no pain	Mild pain (cannot localize)	Moderate pain expressed verbally or by pointing

Reproduced with permission, from Broadman LM: 10-Point Objective Pain-Discomfort Scale.

scales may be taught to use one of the visual scales such as the Oucher or Faces Pain Rating Scale (Fig. 2). Presenting these to children in the preoperative period helps to familiarize them with the concept of rating pain and enables them to use the pain scale better after surgery.

By contrast, preverbal children must be assessed by an objective observer. All objective rating systems, such as the Children's Hospital of Eastern Ontario Pain Scale (1), rely on physical signs of sympathetic activity combined with behavioral assessments. Alternatively, one may use a simple 10-point objective pain scale (Table 1).

Using one of the pain assessment techniques, there should be frequent evaluations, an intervention if necessary, and a reassessment to be certain that the pain intervention was effective.

Mechanism of Pain

Stimulation of receptors and sensory neurons lead to pain perception. Nerve fibers of sensory neurons synapse in the superficial layers of the dorsal horn of the brain. The role of the brain cortex in pain perception is controversial, especially in children. It is not controversial, however, that children and even newborn infants perceive pain. Various neurotransmitters secreted at sensory nerve fibers mediate the transmission of pain from the peripheral nerve receptor to the brain. Analgesia is achieved by activation of a powerful inhibitory process that blocks the effect of neurotransmitters at nerve endings. Nonsteroidal anti-inflammatory drugs (NSAIDs; the best known of which are ibuprofen and ketorolac) inhibit the production of cyclooxygenase, a compound that is important in the conversion of precursors to pain neurotransmitters.

PHARMACOLOGIC MANAGEMENT OF POSTOPERATIVE PAIN

As an alternative to regional anesthesia or as an adjunct to regional anesthesia, the pharmacologic approach can be used for the management of pediatric postoperative pain. Pain can be attacked pharmacologically at one or a combination of sites located in the brain or peripheral nerve receptors. Whereas narcotics work primarily in the brain and spinal cord, NSAIDs work at peripheral nerve receptors to provide analgesia.

Intravenous Analgesics

Intermittent Intravenous Injections

Rectal or oral routes of administration have a less predictable onset and longer time to peak effect. They can, however, provide useful supplemental analgesia or primary analgesia if pain is not severe and ample time is given to achieve an effect. Oral medications are not practical for initial pain management in most postoperative patients. For outpatients, it may be useful to provide a dose of the oral analgesic agent planned for home administration before discharge. Acute control of moderate to severe pain in the PACU may be managed with IV narcotics. Longer-acting narcotics may be preferable to short-acting ones, since the pain frequently outlasts practical dosing intervals after the patient is discharged from the PACU. IV administration of narcotics to young patients needs to be done in small incremental doses by experienced personnel.

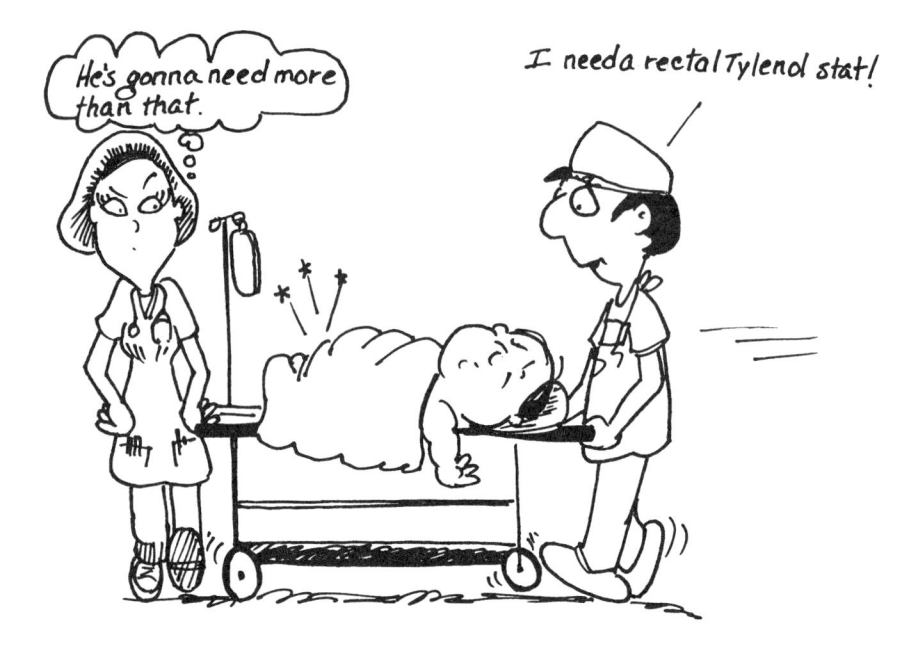

Many experienced clinicians prefer the use of morphine in 0.05 mg/kg increments every 10 to 15 minutes until pain is controlled (Table 2). Morphine has been a kinder, gentler drug in that it comes on slower and lasts longer than fentanyl. Therefore, respiratory depression (if it occurs) occurs gradually and with ample warning signs (e.g., sedation) before the onset of apnea. As adjunctive agents, ketorolac, 0.5 to 1.0 mg/kg IV (not for use in patients at high risk for postoperative bleeding), or a single dose of rectal acetaminophen, 30 mg/kg, are useful although better administered before arrival in the PACU because of their longer time to onset.

Experience with children is necessary to enable care providers to differentiate the behavioral responses of young children that are due to pain from those that are the result of anxiety, anger, and fear. Comforting measures such as being cuddled, parental presence, a favorite blanket, or a pacifier can be invaluable tools to enhance IV agents and to provide a smooth PACU stay.

Finally, pain unresponsive to analgesic agents should alert the clinician to perioperative complications such as ischemic pain from a limb cast that is too tight, lower abdominal pain from a distended bladder, chest pain with a pneumothorax, or shoulder pain from unsuspected rupture of a hollow viscus.

Continuous Intravenous Infusion

In children who have moderate to severe pain and who are unable to take oral medica-

TABLE 2. Opioid analgesics

Drug	Dosage	Form
Fentanyl[a]	1 µg/kg	IV
Morphine[a]	0.05–0.1 mg/kg	IV
Meperidine[a]	1 mg/kg	IV
Codeine	1.5 mg/kg q4h	PO:15-mg, 30-mg, 60-mg tablets; syrup 15 mg/ml
Oxycodone	0.15 mg/kg	PO: 5-mg tablets, syrup 5 mg/ml

[a]Titrate to effect, watching for respiratory depression; avoid intramuscular injection if at all possible!

tions, opioids may be administered by continuous IV infusion. After a therapeutic blood level (as manifested by clinical effect) is achieved, an infusion rate can be chosen to maintain that level. It is still necessary to closely observe patients on continuous infusions because, if excessive drug accumulates, respiratory depression will ensue. Many hours may elapse before this occurs, because the administered dose per hour in a continuous infusion is small and the rate of increase in the blood opioid level is slow. In patients without ventilatory support who are less than 1 year of age, respiratory monitoring and frequent nursing assessment are necessary safety measures. These patients, especially those younger than 1 month, may have immature ventilatory responses to hypoxia and hypercarbia and, if overdosage occurs, may be at a greater risk for respiratory depression than older children.

Choice of Opioid for Intravenous Infusion. Morphine is the opioid most frequently used for postoperative analgesia. It has been extensively studied in most age groups of children, although few data exist for premature infants. In full-term infants less than 1 month of age, morphine clearance is about one third that in older children and one half that in adults. The elimination half-life is correspondingly prolonged, about three times that in adults (2). Serum levels of 10 to 25 ng/ml are analgesic (3). This level is usually achieved with an infusion rate of 5 to 15 µg/kg per hour after a loading dose of 25 to 75 µg/kg.

Patient-Controlled Analgesia

"Pain is real when you get other people to believe in it. If no one believes in it but you, your pain is madness or hysteria."
—Naomi Wolf

Patient-controlled analgesia (PCA) is a preferred method of providing pain relief after the anesthesia block wears off or if the child, parents, surgeon, and anesthesiologist decide that regional anesthesia or nurse-administered IV medication is not the technique of choice. Our experience has been that continuous IV infusions or PCA works much better than as-needed IM injections. To receive PCA, patients usually should to be about 6 years old, although some "record setting" young children (e.g., 4-

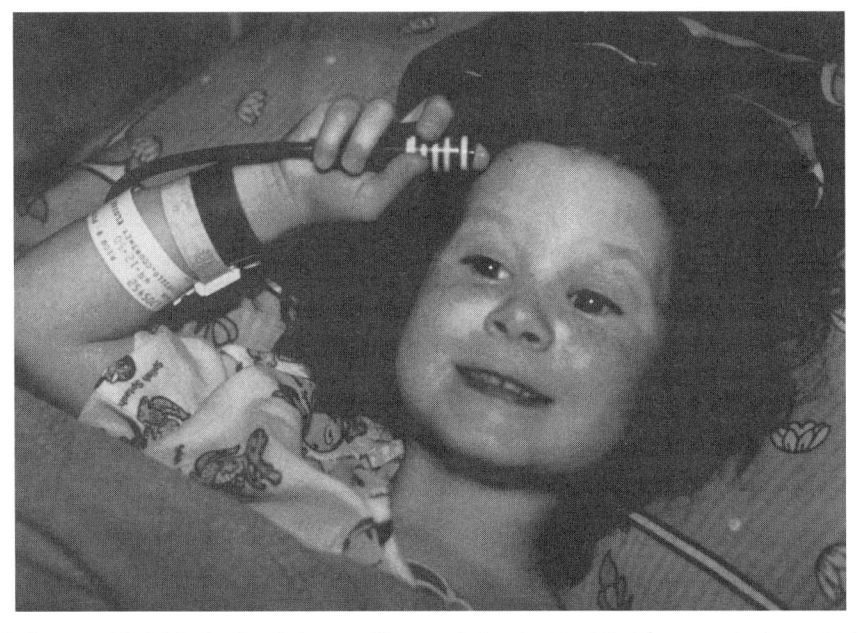

FIG. 3. A 4-year-old child who is *status post* lower abdominal incision for a urologic procedure. She was very happy to be able to give her own pain medications via the PCA button.

year-olds) have been successfully treated with PCA (Fig. 3).

In adults, pain scores with PCA are similar to regularly scheduled IM injections every 4 hours while awake. The same should be true for children. (Besides, how many of you would prefer IM injections every 4 hours? That's what we thought!) If we don't use PCA because we determine that the child is not suitable (or the parents are not suitable—a bigger problem), then another mode of delivery is IV PRN (as needed) infusions—morphine 0.1 mg/kg over 20 minutes or even continuous opioid infusions (see continuous intravenous infusion). Again, many of us use morphine throughout the hospital as the standard opioid; therefore, the entire hospital staff is familiar with the drug.

A sample set of orders for PCA is shown in Table 3. This order form is basically a simple modification of the same format used for adults. Suitability for PCA of children may be assessed by the child's understanding of a Visual Analogue Scale—a 10-cm line with 0 (no pain) at one end and 10 (worst pain) at the other end of the scale or the facial scale (see Fig. 1). In addition, the child may be asked to rank three pains—a mosquito bite, falling up the stairs, and falling off a bicycle going fast down a hill. Scores are expected to be low, medium, and high. If the child ranks all three test questions at one end of the scale, he or she is unsuitable for PCA because of a lack of understanding that there are grades of pain. We also caution the parents very strongly—if they push the button for the child, the safety mechanism is bypassed and the child could receive an overdose of medication. Therefore, in some respects, assessment of the parents for suitability is more important than assessment of the child. Most children do very well with the pain button after a few hours.

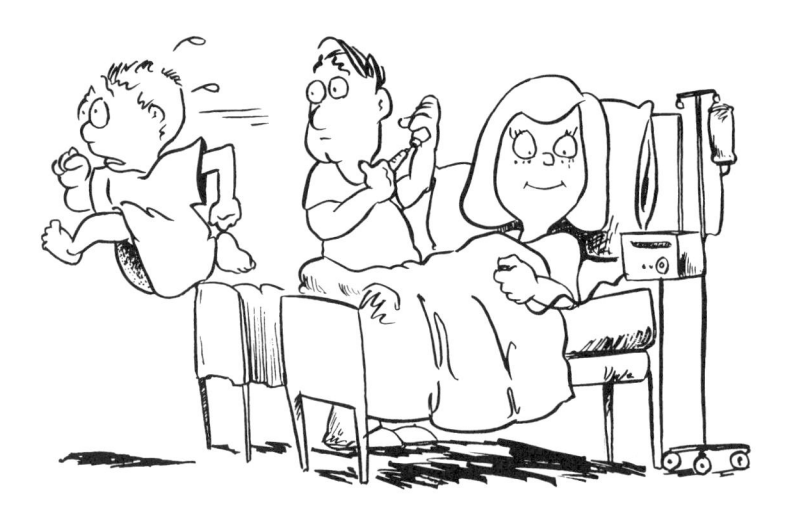

All nurses should be trained in PCA use, setup, and assessment. In fact, a pain assess-

TABLE 3. *Patient-controlled analgesia orders[a]*

1. Discontinue previous pain medications. All pain medications to be written by the Anesthesia Pain Service.
2. Morphine, 1 mg/ml, in PCA syringe.
3. Morphine, 0.02 mg/kg per dose.
4. Lockout time 15 minutes.
5. Keep pain scores!

PCA, patient-controlled analgesia.
[a]Patient receives bolus morphine titrated to analgesia in postanesthesia care unit (PACU) before receiving pain treatment button. Patient reassessed by Anesthesia Pain Service 2 hours after leaving PACU, and dosage is adjusted according to pain score.

TABLE 4. *Nonopioid analgesics*

Drug	Dose	Forms available
Acetaminophen	10–15 mg/kg PO q6h Maximum 2600 mg/d 45 mg single dose	Tablets: 80 mg Syrup: 32 mg/ml Suppositories: 120, 325, 650 mg
Ibuprofen	10–20 mg/kg PO q6h	Tablets: 300, 400 mg Syrup: 100 mg/5 ml
Ketorolac	0.5 mg/kg IV to load* 0.5 mg/kg q8h** intramuscularly or q6h intravenously	Parenteral form used intramuscularly or intravenously

* Maximum dose=30 mg   **Limit use to 48 hours

ment score is required on the vital signs sheet, next to the respiratory rate—that is how important we feel it is.

Nonsteroidal Anti-inflammatory Drugs

Pharmacologic management of mild to moderate postoperative pain may begin, unless there is a contraindication, with a nonopioid analgesic, such as acetaminophen or an NSAID. Moderately severe to severe pain is usually treated with an opioid as a first-line drug, but acetaminophen and NSAIDs constitute an excellent part of a balanced pain management program. Even though they are not sufficient themselves to control pain, acetaminophen or NSAIDs can significantly decrease the amount of opioid necessary for complete pain control. This decreased need for opioids means decreased opioid side effects. Of course, all NSAIDs must be used with care or avoided completely in patients with thrombocytopenia, coagulopathies, or where postsurgical bleeding might be critical. However, acetaminophen does not alter platelet function, and there is some evidence that ketorolac has less effect on platelet function than does aspirin. In addition, ketorolac is the only parenteral NSAID approved by the Food and Drug Administration (FDA) (Table 4).

A special word about ketorolac: Like many other drugs, ketorolac is not FDA-approved for use in children. And, we have already mentioned that children do not like shots. However, there is *experience* with this drug used orally and intravenously in children. If you are going to choose ketorolac in children, we recommend administering it intramuscularly only in anesthetized patients. Use the IV route if the child is awake.

One possible analgesic regimen is rectal acetaminophen, administered just after induction of anesthesia but before the surgical incision. This allows the analgesic properties of the nonopioid analgesic to begin the beneficial effect as the surgery begins. There are no rectal NSAIDs available in the United States at this time; however, premedication with an oral NSAID might be useful.[a]

In general, PRN use of medications is not a good way to treat pain, and NSAIDs are no exception. As a matter of fact, patients treated with a PRN schedule have analgesic blood levels of drugs for only 30% of the dosing interval; they are suffering most of the time. In a study done in England, rectal diclofenac was compared with caudal bupivacaine in a group of children scheduled for lower abdominal surgery (4). It was found that pain at 1 hour postoperatively was present 40% of the time in patients given diclofenac and 0% in patients given bupivacaine. However, there was no difference in pain at 2 and 4 hours postoperatively. These differences may be accounted for by the slow rectal absorption of diclofenac. It was not surprising, therefore, to find that IV ketorolac administered intraoperatively (0.9 mg/kg) was as effective as IV morphine (0.1 mg/kg) administered to chil-

---

[a]Ed. Note (JMB): We mix midazolam and ibuprofen as a premedication for selected patients (e.g, prior to dental restorations).

dren to provide postoperative pain relief (5). Furthermore, there was less nausea and vomiting in the ketorolac patients.

Subsequent studies have confirmed that ketorolac is as effective as both meperidine (Jolene Bean, unpublished data) and morphine (6) in providing postoperative pain relief in children. In the most recent study, IV ketorolac (1 mg/kg loading dose and 0.5 mg/kg every 6 hours) was safe and cost-effective when given as part of a fractionated unit dosing system (7).

These and other studies have led to the rational use of NSAIDs in the treatment of postoperative pain in children. Ketorolac (0.5 mg/kg, up to 30 mg) may be administered IV to children 45 minutes before the estimated completion of surgery. Ketorolac is given every 6 hours IV in the same dose for 48 hours if needed. Once the child has begun to take oral fluids, ketorolac is discontinued and ibuprofen given 10 mg/kg every 6 hours (around the clock, not PRN). Although ketorolac may have a narcotic-sparing effect, it is not effective for severe pain. Therefore, patients may have a standing order for morphine 0.1 mg/kg every 3 hours PRN for severe pain. Narcotic requirements are substantially reduced by the concomitant use of the NSAIDs.

Because NSAIDs work at the periphery, there are no central or ventilatory suppressant effects. Reports of gastrointestinal, renal, and coagulation side effects are extremely rare.

Gastrointestinal Side Effects

The inhibition of prostaglandins has a desirable effect on pain relief, but an undesirable effect on the gastric mucosa (mucosal protection is diminished). However, symptoms of heartburn and gastritis have been reported to be much less severe in children than in adults. With the acute use of NSAIDs (1 to 3 days) gastrointestinal complaints in children are rare. No episodes of gastritis were documented in 3420 doses given to 383 pediatric patients (7).

Renal Side Effects

The kidney is dependent on prostaglandins only in the presence of renal insufficiency. Therefore, it is not surprising to find that most reports of renal effects associated with NSAIDs have been in patients who have associated risk factors (e.g., hypovolemia and renal tumor) or who become dehydrated (8). In well-hydrated noncritically ill patients, renal complications are unlikely with the acute use of NSAIDs.

Bleeding and NSAIDs

The inhibition of platelet thromboxane and platelet aggregation may lead to prolonged bleeding time with the use of NSAIDs. Only aspirin, however, produces an irreversible inhibition of platelet aggregation. With the other NSAIDs, platelet aggregation inhibition resolves in 24 hours after discontinuation of the drug. In a study by Jolene Bean at the Scott and White Clinic, ketorolac, 0.75 mg/kg, given to children for pain increased bleeding times, but resulted in no evidence of clinical bleeding (unpublished data). Likewise, there were no episodes of clinically significant bleeding in the previously mentioned large series (6). Therefore, NSAIDs may be used in routine surgical patients with little fear of causing significant coagulopathy or bleeding. NSAIDs are best avoided in patients at risk for significant perioperative bleeding (e.g., tonsillectomy) and those with preexisting coagulation defects.

REGIONAL ANESTHESIA TECHNIQUES

Caudal Block

Anatomic Differences between Child and Adult

There are anatomic differences between the infant and the adult that are important to consider in performing a caudal block. In the infant, the spinal cord ends at about L3, whereas in the adult, the spinal cord ends at about T12 (Fig. 4). More important, the dural sac of the infant may extend distally to S3, whereas the dural sac of the adult usually ends higher at about S1. Therefore, inadver-

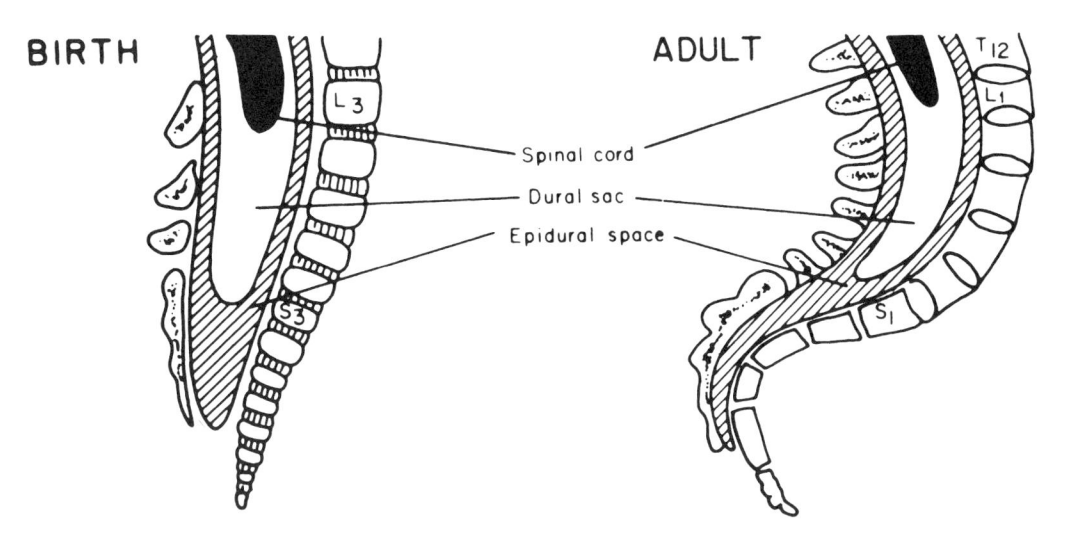

FIG. 4. Anatomic differences between infant and adult important in performing a caudal block.

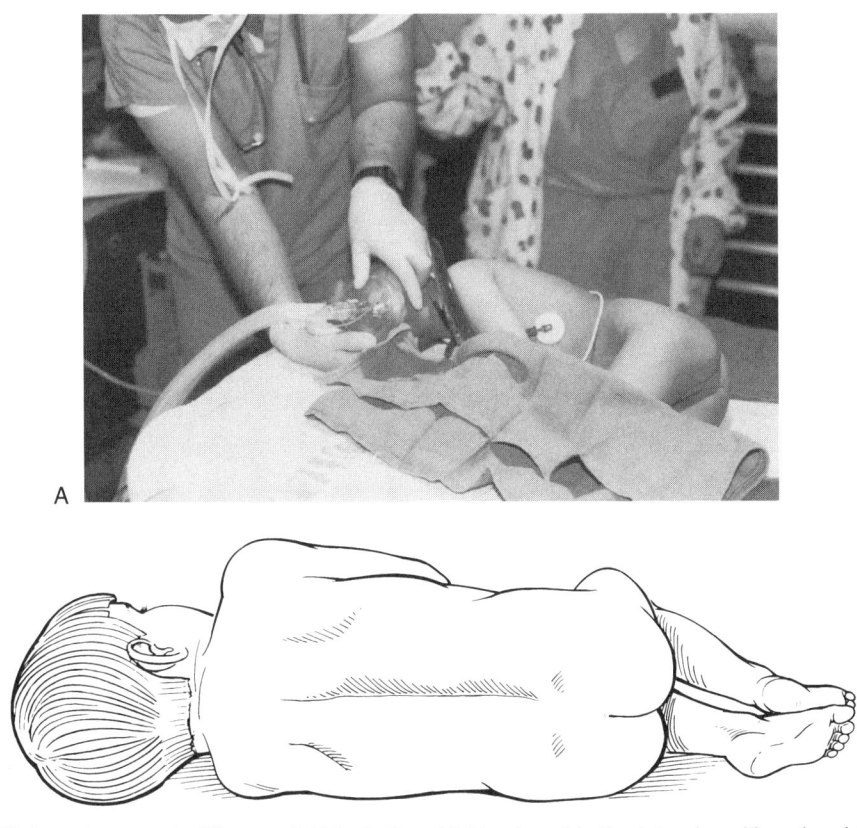

FIG. 5. Before placement of the caudal block, the child is placed in the lateral position: the child's right side down for left-handed clinicians **(A)** and the child's left side down for right-handed clinicians **(B)**.

tent subdural or wet tap is unfortunately easier in the younger patient.

Equipment

For a one-shot caudal block, a 23-gauge butterfly needle connected by extension tubing to a syringe of appropriate size may be used. For many experienced clinicians, this equipment and an alcohol swab is all the paraphernalia that is needed for a one-shot caudal block in infants and children. Alternatively, one may use either a blunt-tipped "B" bevel and a T-piece extension or simply a blunt-tipped needle connected to a syringe.

Technique for the One- or Two-Shot Caudal Block

After the child is placed in lateral position (Fig. 5), the sacral hiatus is identified (Fig. 6). The sacral hiatus, which is situated at the lower end of the sacrum, is extremely easy to identify in infants and young children. The large bony processes on each side are called

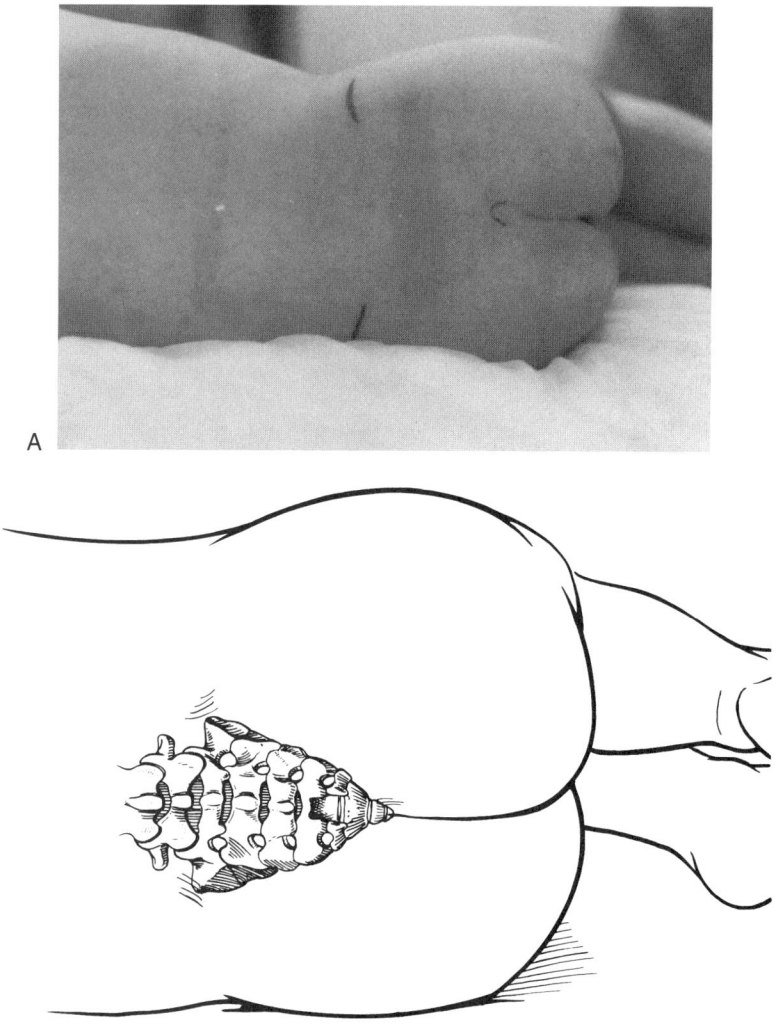

FIG. 6. (A) The sacral hiatus (the lower marking in **A**) is at the bottom of an equilateral triangle formed by the two posterior iliac crests and the sacral hiatus. **(B)** The large bony processes on each side of the sacral hiatus are called *cornua*. The coccyx is just caudal to the sacral hiatus.

the cornua. The coccyx lies immediately caudal to the sacral hiatus. The hiatus is covered by the sacrococcygeal membrane. In infants and prepubertal children, these landmarks are easily palpable or even visible through the skin because of the absence of the large sacral pad of fat which usually develops at puberty. The cornua and the sacrococcygeal membrane that lies between the two cornua feels much like two knuckles on a clenched fist with the sacrococcygeal ligament in the space between the two knuckles. Asepsis is maintained either by wearing gloves or by palpating the skin through a sterile alcohol swab (Fig. 7).

The caudal space is entered using a short (1-inch) 23-gauge needle, which has been attached to a syringe containing the appropriate volume of local anesthetic solution (Fig. 8). The needle is placed exactly in the midline and inserted at ~45-degree angle to the coronal plane perpendicular to all other planes (Fig. 9A). When using the "butterfly" needle technique, the needle is held as one would hold a pencil. As the needle is advanced, the bevel should be facing anteriorly to minimize the chance of piercing the anterior sacral wall (the most common reason for inadvertent intravascular or intraosseous injection). A distinct "pop" is felt as the sacro-

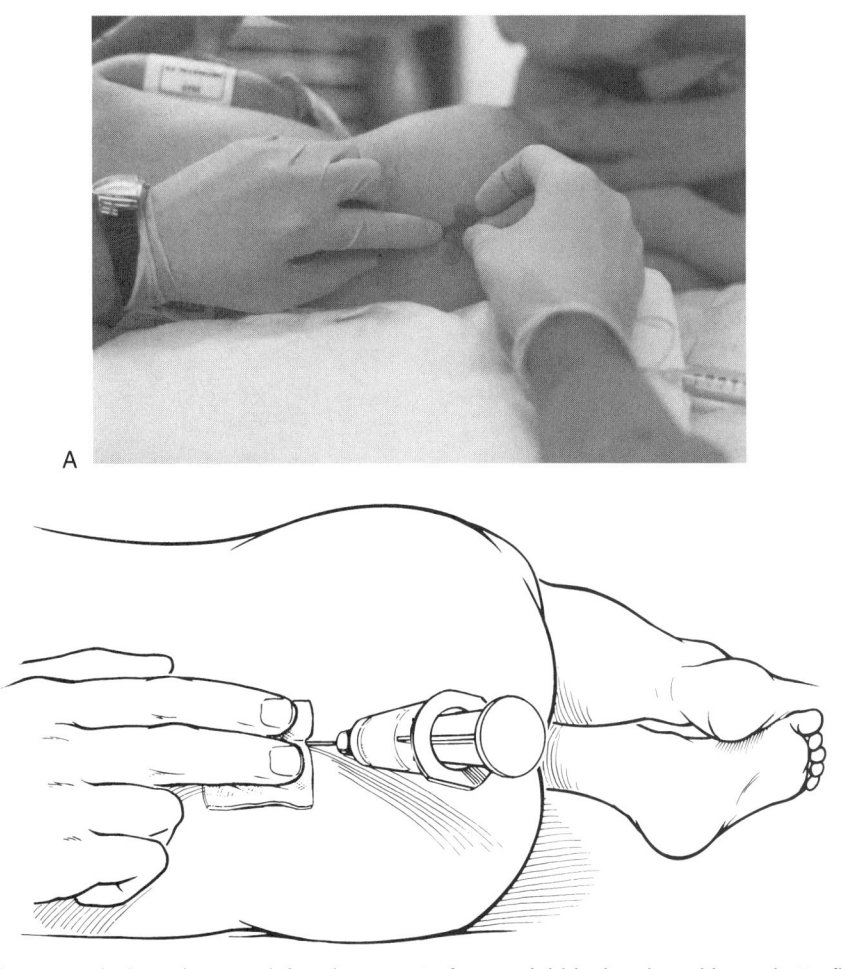

FIG. 7. Proper technique (see text) for placement of a caudal block using either a butterfly needle **(A)** or a short-bevel needle and syringe **(B)**.

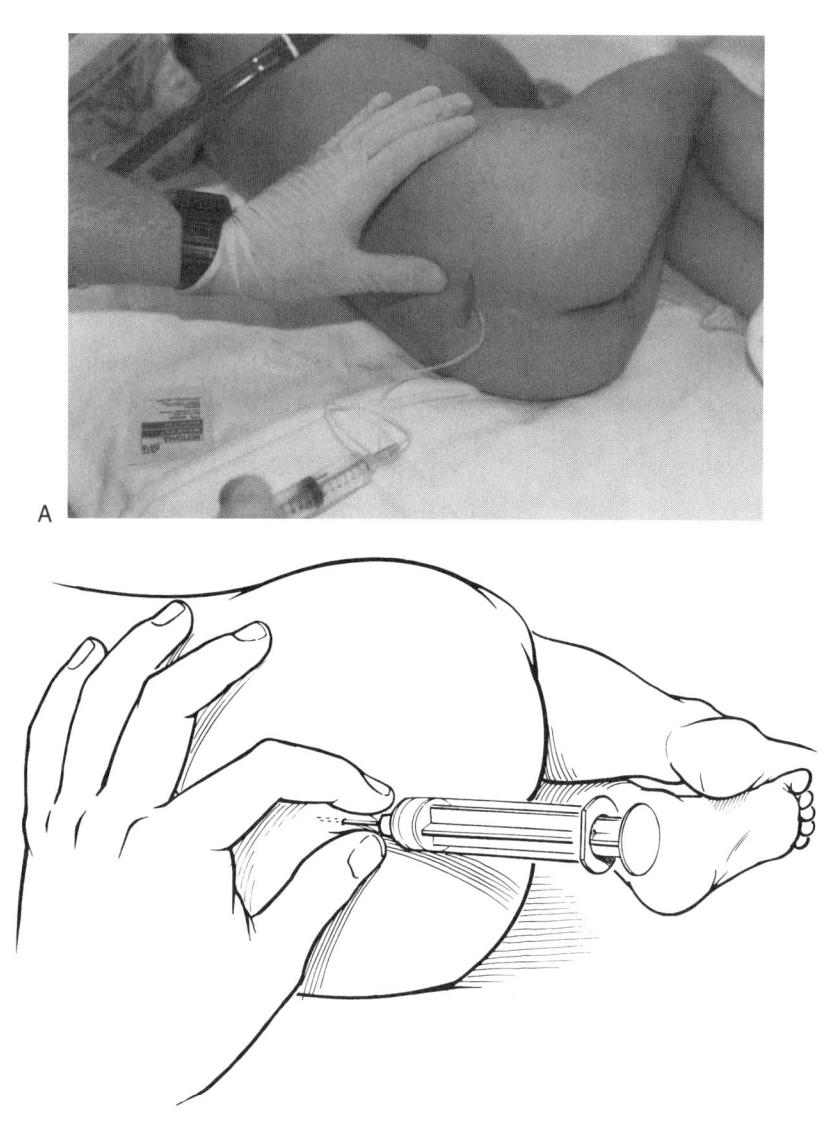

FIG. 8. (A) During injection of local anesthesia in a caudal block, skin overlying the needle is palpated to rule out subcutaneous injection. **(B)** Using a needle and syringe for a caudal block, the apparatus is stabilized as shown.

coccygeal membrane is pierced. In children and older infants, the angle of the needle may be lowered to ~15 degrees and advanced an additional 1 to 2 mm to ensure that all the bevel surface is in the caudal space (Fig. 9B). In small infants, advancement of the needle after the "pop" may be unnecessary and will increase the chances of dural puncture. After repeatedly demonstrating the absence of blood or cerebrospinal fluid after attempted aspiration (as well as disconnecting the syringe and extension tubing to allow flow of blood by gravity), the appropriate amount of local anesthetic is injected and the child is placed in the supine position. An easy way to remember the procedure is by the three words "knuckle, pencil, pop." These three words indicate the three major components of the technique; that is, the anatomy feels like a *knuckle,* hold the needle like a *pencil,* and you will feel a very pronounced *pop.*

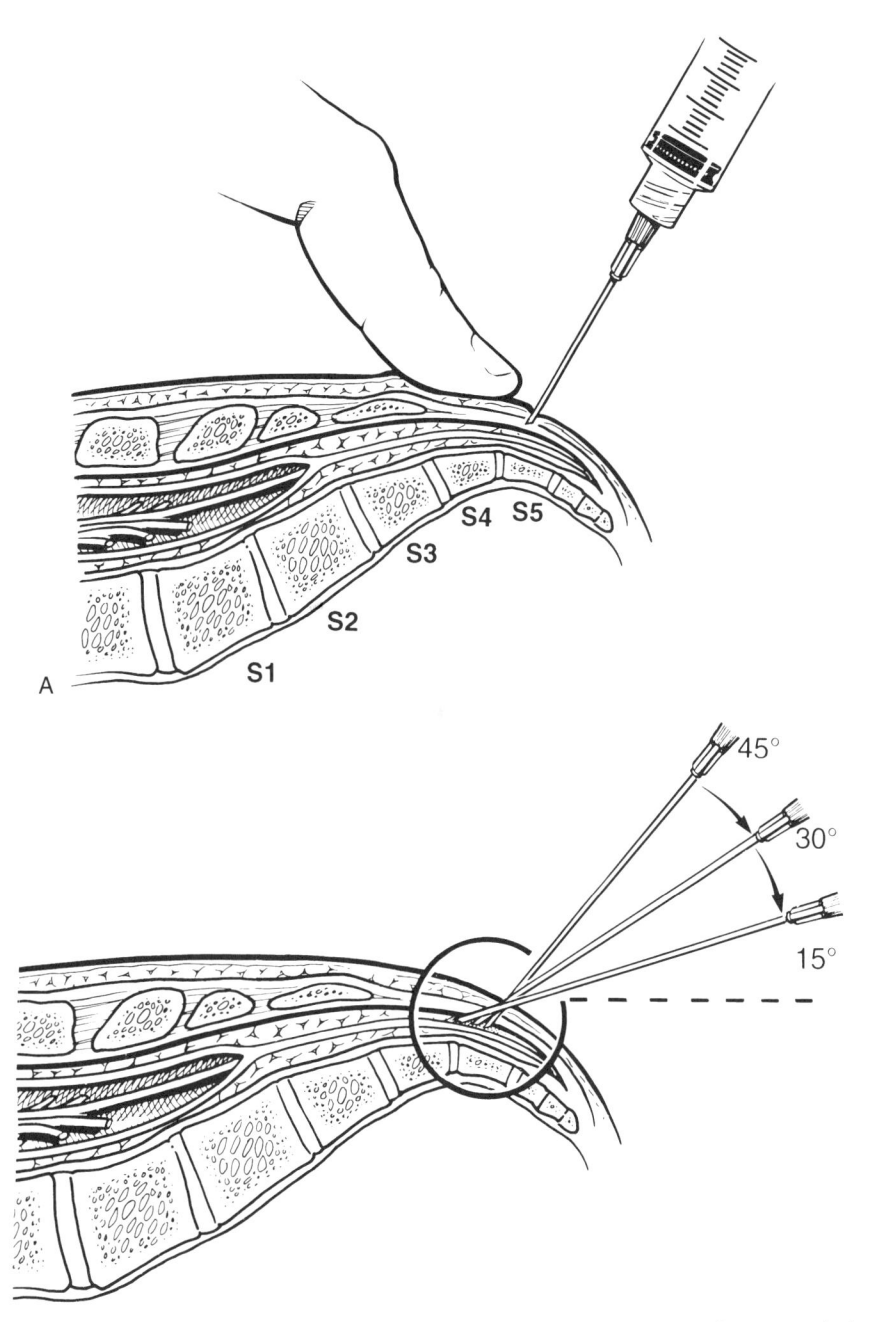

FIG. 9. In the caudal block, the needle is inserted at a ~45-degree angle to the coronal plane perpendicular to all other planes **(A)**. After the definite "pop" is felt, the angle is dropped to ~15° and the needle advanced a few millimeters, with care not to advance it too far (i.e., into the dural sac) **(B)**.

TABLE 5. *Maximum recommended dosages of local anesthetics in children*

Local anesthetic	Maximum dosage (mg/kg)
Lidocaine[a]	7.0
Bupivacaine[b]	3.0
Tetracaine	1.5
Procaine	10.0
Mepivacaine	7.0
Ropivacaine	3.0

[a]Lidocaine is short-acting—approximately 90 minutes. [b]Bupivacaine is long-acting—approximately 180–600 minutes.

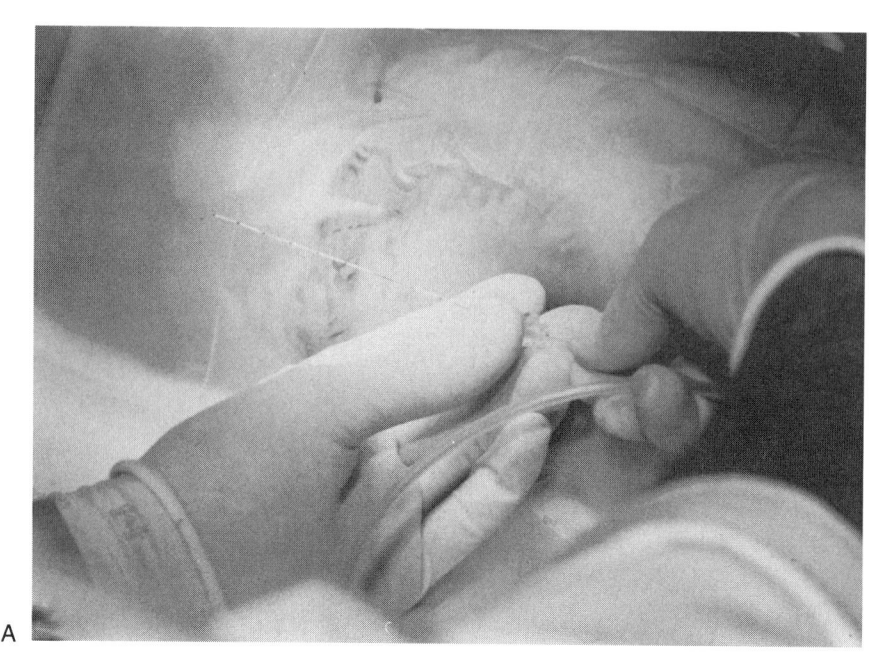

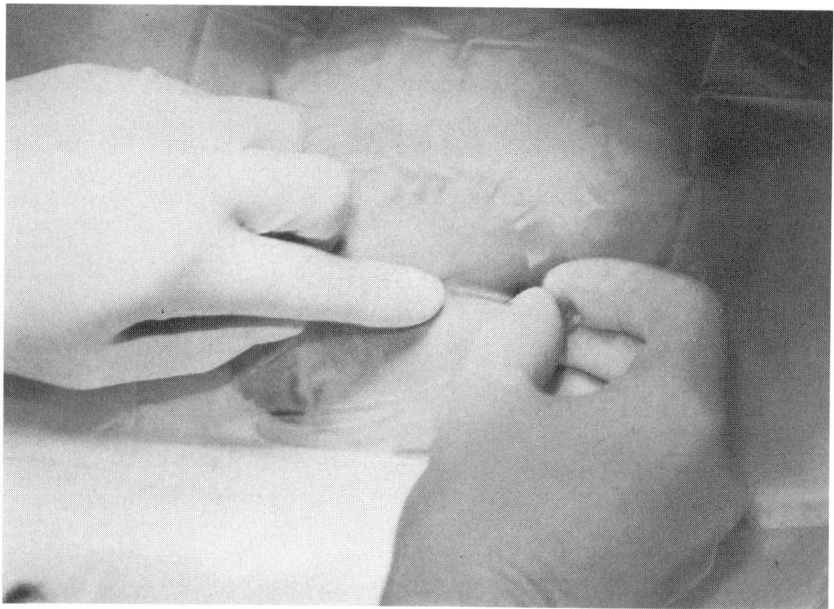

FIG. 10. (A) For placement of a caudal catheter for continuous infusion, the estimated length is first "eyeballed" against the child's back, noting at what length the distal tip will need to be. **(B)** The sacral hiatus is palpated, and a needle is inserted into the caudal space.

The variables that determine the quality, duration, and extent of a caudal block are volume, total dose, and concentration of the drug. As for volume: 0.5 ml/kg will result in an adequate sacral block, 1.0 ml/kg will produce a block of the lower thoracic nerves, and 1.25 ml/kg will reach the midthoracic region. The total dosage should always be checked to ensure that it is within the acceptable safe dose limit of the drug (Table 5).

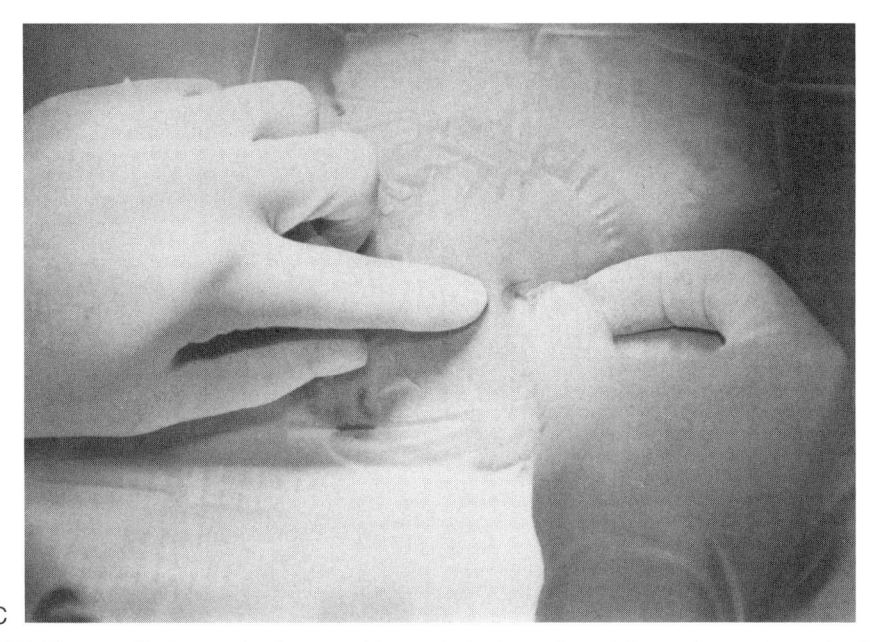

(C) The needle is now in place and is ready for insertion of the catheter shown in A.

Either bupivacaine (0.125% to 0.25%) or ropivacaine (0.2%) may be used. A 0.125% bupivacaine solution will produce the same quality and duration of postoperative analgesia as a 0.25% concentration (8). Moreover, the more dilute solution results in less motor blockade. The addition of epinephrine may increase the duration of bupivacaine or ropivacaine (9) and is of benefit as a test dose. Whereas epinephrine as a test dose will not reliably produce tachycardia in children unless preceded by atropine (10), intravenous epinephrine will produce T-wave elevation on the ECG if injected inadvertently **(see Signs and Symptoms of Local Anesthetic Toxicity).**

The duration of postoperative analgesia following a caudal block can be substantially prolonged by using preservative-free morphine. The duration of pain relief provided by caudal analgesia is substantially longer with caudal morphine (range 10 to 36 hours) than with bupivacaine (range 4 to 8 hours) (11). However, there may be a risk of respiratory depression after epidural morphine. Children are observed in the hospital for 24 hours after receiving a caudal block with morphine. Krane and associates (12) reported good pain relief in a study comparing caudal morphine, caudal bupivacaine, and IV morphine for postoperative pain relief after genital, urinary, or lower extremity orthopaedic surgery. Krane (13) recommends a morphine dose of 50 µg/kg to provide adequate pain relief and reported respiratory depression requiring naloxone only in patients receiving larger doses. We frequently use morphine, 50 µg/kg, with or without bupivacaine, for postoperative analgesia in patients. We continue to avoid the use of caudal narcotics in our ambulatory patients.

Continuous Postoperative Caudal Analgesia

In selective cases in which pain is expected to be continuous for 24 hours or to be more severe, a caudal catheter is placed for the continuous infusion of local anesthetics. In this technique, the skin is prepped and sterilely draped, and the catheter insertion length is estimated by "eyeballing" it against the child's back so that the catheter tip will be at the desired dermatomal level—usually at the level of the surgical incision (Fig. 10A). The sacral hiatus is palpated, and a 17-gauge Crawford needle is inserted into the caudal space in the same fashion as the butterfly technique described previously (see Fig. 10B). Through this Crawford needle (see Fig. 10C), we insert a 20-gauge Theracath spring-wired epidural catheter (Arrow, EC-05000, Reading, PA). The catheter is then advanced to the desired dermatomal level and secured into place.

After negative aspiration, 0.5 ml/kg of local anesthetic is injected (usually preoperatively), and a constant infusion of local anesthetic and fentanyl is infused. We use a

TABLE 6. *Pediatric epidural order sheet*

Date: _____ Time: _____
Insertion site: _____

1. No systemic opioids (narcotics) unless approved by pain service. Urology patients may receive oxybutynin (Ditropan) as needed.

2. Epidural solution check one.
   ___ 1. Bupivacaine 0.1%
   ___ 2. Fentanyl 2 mcg/ml with bupivacaine 0.1%
   ___ 3. Other (specify) _____

3. Epidural infusion rate: _____ cc/hr
   (Usual rates are 0.1-0.5 cc/kg/hr)

4. If the patient has no bladder catheter, may straight-cath p.r.n. for urinary retention greater than _____ hours.

5. Patient assessments:
   a. HR, BP, objective pain and sedation scores (see scoring system below) q 2h. Record objective pain and sedation scores on "FLOW SHEET - PROGRESS RECORD"
   b. RR q 1h for the first 24 hours, then q 2h (unless unusual concern)
   c. Discontinue infusion and page pain service Dr. _____ bpr # _____) if:
      I. Somnolence (Excessive sleepiness)
      II. RR < 12 (age > 8 Years); RR < 14 (ages < 8)
      III. BP systolic < 80 (ages < 12 months)
          BP systolic < 90 (ages > 12 months)
      IV. No movement in toes or ankles
   d. Page pain service STAT, apply oxygen, stimulate, and turn off infusion if:
      i. Cyanosis
      ii. Severe unresponsiveness
      iii. RR < 8 or apnea
      iv. BP systolic < 65
   e. Continuous pulse oximetry monitoring   Page Pain Service if < _____.

6. For pruritus. (choose one)

   ___ Diphenhydramine (Benadryl)
       0.5 mg/kg x _____ kg = _____ mg iv
       over 20 minutes q 6 h p.r.n.,
       hold for somnolence
   ___ Naloxone (Narcan)
       0.002 mg/kg x _____ kg = _____ mg iv
       over 20 minutes q 2 h p.r.n
       (for use with epidural opioids only)

7. For nausea: (choose one)

   a. _____ Diphenhydramine (Benadryl)
              0.5 mg/kg x _____ kg = _____ mg iv
              over 20 minutes q 6 h p.r.n.,
              hold for somnolence *along with*
              Perphenazine (Trilafon)
              0.015-0.025 mg/kg x _____ kg = _____ mg iv
              over 20 min q 6h, hold for somnolence
   b. _____ Naloxone (Narcan) 0.002 mg/kg x _____ mg iv
              over 20 minutes q 2h p.r.n.
              (for use with epidural opioids only)
   c. _____ Prochlorperazine (Compazine)
              _____ mg po   pr   im   (circle one)
              1 q 6h p.r.n.

8. Turn patient from side to side q 4h or prn and pad heels appropriately

9. Inspect epidural site for redness, infection, bleeding, and/or contamination and catheter for kinking and/or dislodgment q 4h

Physician's Signature:
   Ordered by _____ MD
   Anesthesiology Resident
   BPR # _____
   Approved By _____ MD
   Anesthesiology Attending
   BPR # _____

Patient gets 0-2 points for each of five categories (max. 10)

OBJECTIVE PAIN - DISCOMFORT SCALE*			
POINTS	0	1	2
BP	10% Pre-op	10-20% Pre-op	20-30 Pre-op
Crying	No crying	Crying, but responds to tender loving care (TLC)	Crying, does not respond to TLC
Movement	none	restless	thrashing
Agitation	patient asleep or calm	mild	hysterical
Verbal eval. or body lang.	patient asleep or no pain	mild pain (cannot localize)	moderate pain verbally or by pointing

Sedation score: 1 = wide awake
                 2 = drowsy
                 3 = dozing
                 4 = awakens when roused
                 5 = asleep

combination of fentanyl (2 µg/ml) and bupivacaine (0.1%). The initial epidural infusion rate is 0.1 to 0.5 ml/kg/hour titrated to patient response. We then use a customized pediatric epidural order sheet (Table 6). This order sheet requires frequent and periodic patient assessments of respiratory rate, heart rate, and blood pressure as well as objective pain and sedation scores. Infusion is discontinued if somnolence occurs or if respiratory rate falls below a prescribed limit.

Pruritus frequently occurs and can be treated with naloxone, 2 µg/kg IV over 20 minutes. It is often necessary to repeat this dose of naloxone (up to three times). If pruritus persists, benadryl, 0.5 mg/kg, is given. This inevitably cures the itching. For nausea, either diphenhydramine, naloxone, or prochlorperazine may be prescribed. Some experienced clinicians suggest that caudal catheters be limited to a time period of 2 days. After that period, the incidence of complication, particularly infection, increases.

Ilioinguinal and Iliohypogastric Nerve Block

This simple block produces effective postoperative pain relief for patients receiving hernia repair, hydrocelectomy, and orchiopexy. The ilioinguinal nerve runs between the transverse and internal oblique muscles. The iliohypogastric nerve runs superficial to the inguinal muscles close to the anterior superior iliac spine.

Both nerves can be blocked easily by infiltration of the abdominal wall in the area medial to the anterior superior iliac spine (Fig. 11). A 25 gauge needle is used to puncture the skin 1 cm medial to the anterior superior iliac spine just above the inguinal ligament. Three fan-shaped injections are made as the needle is withdrawn plus a subcutaneous wheal. One may use either 0.5% bupivacaine and a dose of up to 2 mg/kg with 1:200,000 epinephrine (14) or a more dilute 0.25% bupivacaine solution in a dose of 2 mg/kg (15).

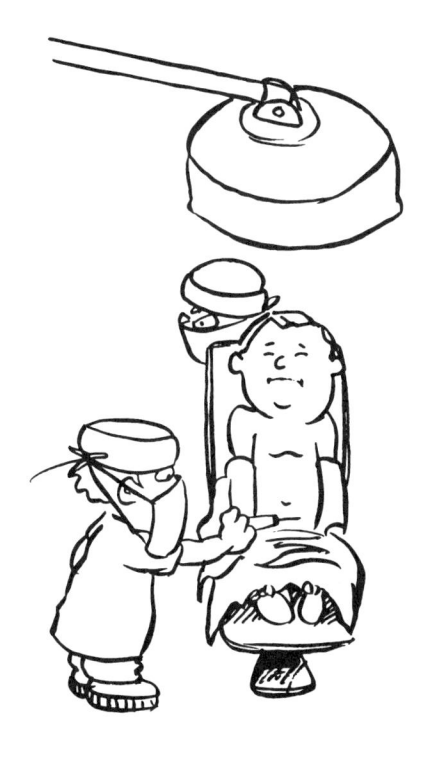

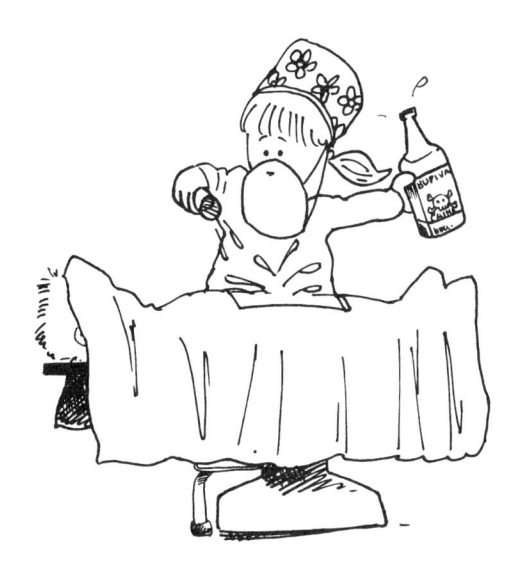

The Splash Block

A variation of the ilioinguinal-iliohyhpogastric block is bupivacaine instillation or the "splash block." It is administered at the

246   CHAPTER 10: PERIOPERATIVE PAIN MANAGEMENT

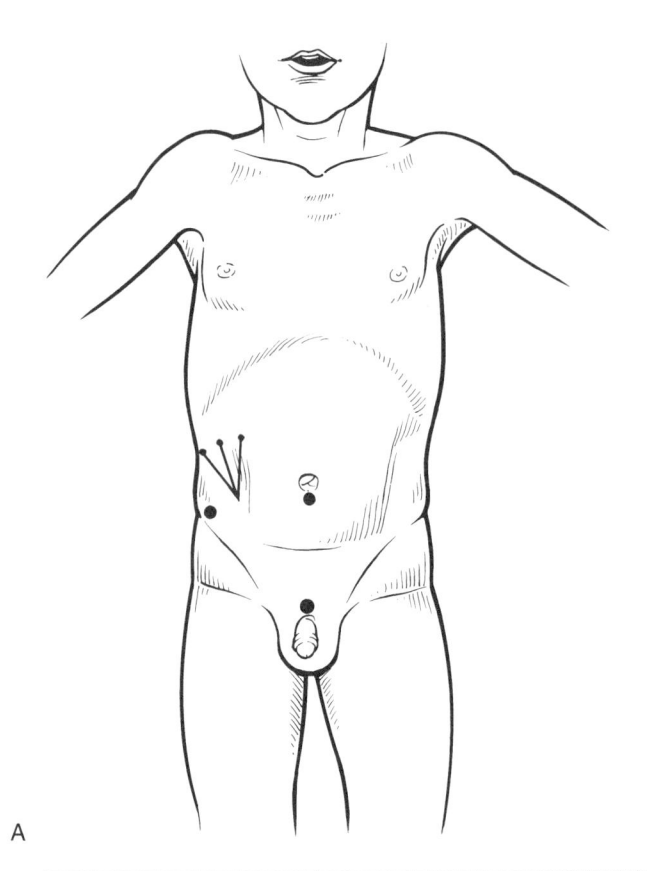

FIG. 11. (A) Location of the injection site for an ilioinguinal iliohypogastric nerve block. **(B)** An 18-month-old infant getting his nerve block.

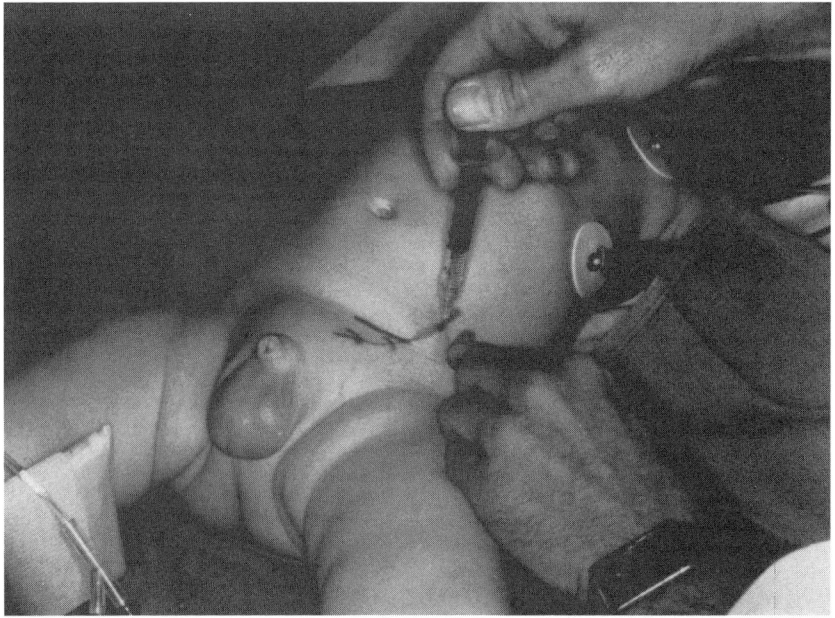

end of the surgical dissection, for example, just before starting closure of a hernia repair. The surgeon is asked to instill 5 to 10 ml of 0.25% bupivacaine into the wound, wait 1 minute, and then start the closure. The local anesthetic will be absorbed by the muscle layers as well as the exposed nerves, and the pain relief is every bit as good as that achieved with more formal blocks. Easy for all concerned! It is important to be certain that the surgeon waits for precisely 1 minute before aspirating or blotting out the local anesthetic. It should be regarded as a wound irrigation, but must stay in place long enough to be absorbed.

Postcircumcision Pain Relief with Local Anesthetics

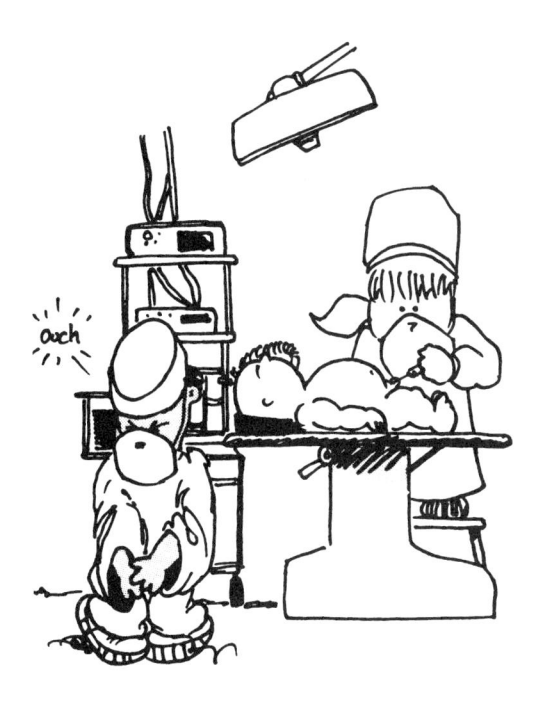

Subcutaneous Ring Block

Pain relief for circumcision may be achieved with topical local anesthetic, dorsal penile nerve block, or a subcutaneous ring block. The latter block was described by Broadman and associates (16) and consists of subcutaneous infiltration of the base of the penis with 0.25% bupivacaine.

Dorsal Penile Nerve Block

The dorsal penile nerve block involves two injections of 1 to 2 ml local anesthetic at the 10:30 and 1:30 positions instilled deep to Buck's fascia to block each of the paired nerves (17) (Fig. 12). To avoid nicking the penile artery and subsequent hematoma formation, a short 25-gauge needle is inserted through the skin and gently advanced to the hub of the needle or until the symphisis pubis bone is gently touched. One should avoid jamming the needle against the bone because this may cause a barb to be formed on the needle. This barb will then act as a hook and may tear the soft tissues, especially vascular tissue or the artery. This block provides good analgesia in most cases. In a recent study, dorsal nerve block and caudal block were found to be equally efficacious in blocking pain after circumcision (18). Children who received a nerve block, however, voided and stood unaided earlier and had a lower incidence of vomiting than those who received a caudal block.

Topical Lidocaine

Topical lidocaine has also been successfully used to produce penile analgesia during circumcision of children. In two recent studies, lidocaine spray, ointment, or jelly was found to be effective in reducing pain and bypassed the need for postoperative analgesics (19,20). Lidocaine jelly also proved effective after hospital treatment for such pain.

Upper Extremity Blocks

Interscalene Block of the Brachial Plexus

Anatomy. Blockade of the nerve roots and trunks is preferable when proximal block of the shoulder is desired. The interscalene block

248   CHAPTER 10: PERIOPERATIVE PAIN MANAGEMENT

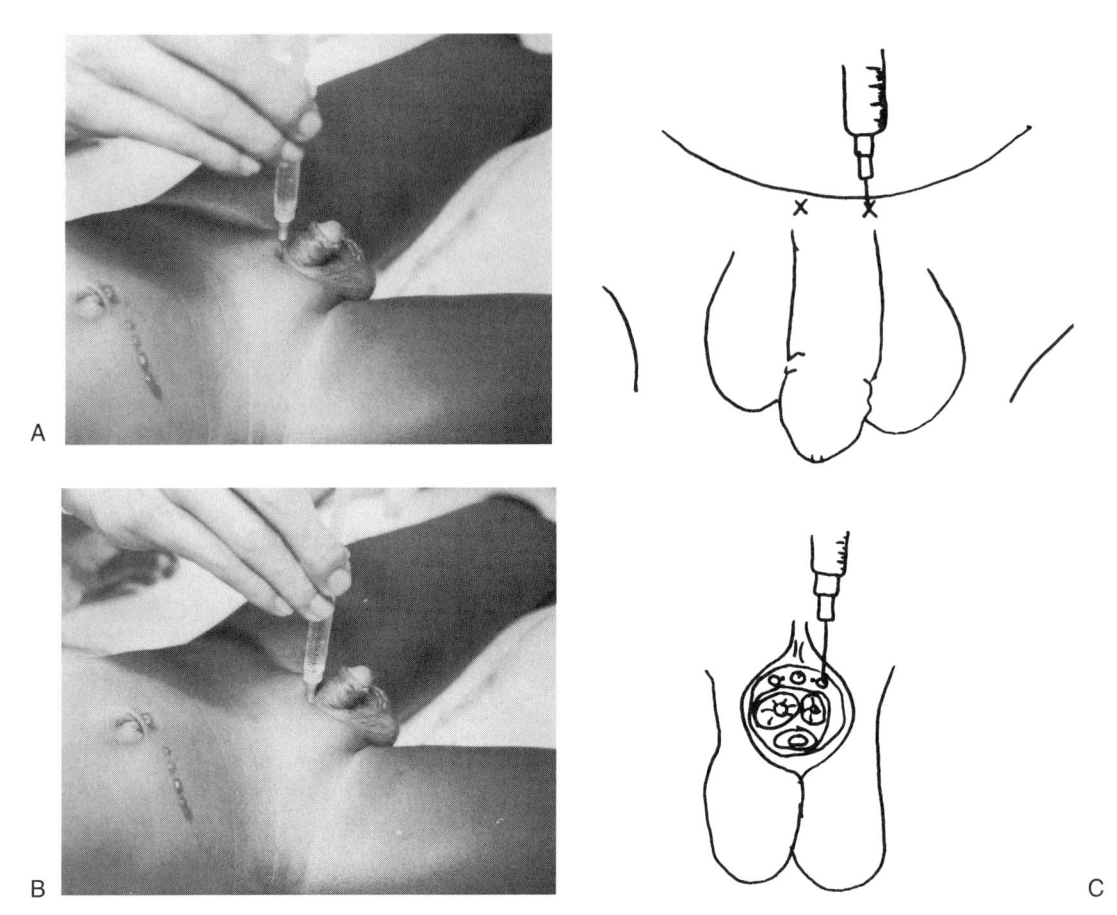

FIG. 12. Dorsal penile nerve block: **(A)** With the base of the penis as a clock face, the needle is inserted at 10:30 and 1:30 (shown here) and advanced in a plane perpendicular to the skin. **(B)** The short 25-gauge needle is gently advanced until the hub is reached or until the needle tip gently touches the pubic bone. **(C)** Local anesthetic is injected around the dorsal penile nerves as the needle is withdrawn.

was developed by Winnie as an alternative to the supraclavicular approach because of the lower risk of pneumothorax (21,22).

The roots and trunks are ensheathed in the fascia of the anterior and middle scalene muscles in the region known as the interscalene space. This triangular-shaped space extends from the emergence of the roots from their grooved transverse processes to the point at which its trunks pass behind the clavicle (21). This groove lies on the superior surface of the transverse process of the cervical vertebrae. The groove separates the transverse processes into anterior and posterior tubercles, which are origins for the anterior and middle scalenes. Vital adjacent structures including the external jugular, the phrenic and vagus nerve branches, and the carotid artery and stellate ganglion are susceptible to injury or dysfunction.

Technique. The patient lies supine with head rotated to the side opposite the side to be treated. Paresthesias are preferred in adults; however, adequate blockade can be obtained by guidance with a nerve stimulator. The head is lifted to palpate the posterolateral border of the sternocleidomastoid. The interscalene groove is palpated by rolling the fingers back over the border of the sternocleidomastoid and onto the belly of the anterior scalene to the groove. A line extended from the cricoid laterally to intersect the interscalene groove should be opposite the transverse process of C6. The external jugular vein often overlies this point of intersection. A 23-gauge 3-inch regional block needle is inserted at a 45-degree angle slightly caudad and backward (22). While using the nerve stimulator, the clinician advances the needle until motor activity in the arm is obtained. If bony contact is made at a deep location, then it is likely that the vertebral body has been contacted and the needle should be withdrawn and redirected posteriorly. Digital pressure above the level of injection should encourage downward spread.

Limitations. Relatively large volumes of local anesthetic are required. The lower trunk and thus the ulnar nerve may be missed. Potentially serious side effects can occur. It is a difficult block to perform in small children, who generally have poorly defined cervical anatomy.

Supraclavicular Approach to the Brachial Plexus

The Kuhlenkampf method in which the first rib is used as a landmark is less satisfactory than Fortin's method in which the brachial plexus is brought toward the surface by placing a roll under the child's shoulders. The shoulders are pushed back on the table, the subclavian artery is palpated, and the needle is inserted lateral to the artery. A nerve stimulator is used to elicit electrical stimulation of the nerves. Usually, mechanical stimulation of the nerve (paresthesia) is not tolerated in the awake child. The supraclavicular approach attempts to block the brachial plexus at the level of the divisions. The ulnar, antebrachial, and medial antebrachial nerves may not be well anesthetized.

Complications. Complications encountered in the supraclavicular approach to the brachial plexus in decreasing order of frequency are stellate ganglion block and Horner's syndrome > laryngeal nerve block (superior laryngeal bilaterally and the recurrent laryngeal on the right side) > phrenic nerve block > pneumothorax (23,24). Systemic toxicity and total spinal, a high epidural, and allergic reactions can occur but are very rare.

Applications. Open- or closed-shoulder reductions, most arm or forearm procedures, and acute exacerbations of chronic or recurrent disease can be managed with the supraclavicular approach. Indwelling catheters can be used in the acute perioperative period but are not usually stable; thus, long-term use is difficult.

Parascalene Block of the Brachial Plexus

Dalens and colleagues (25), in 1987, described a new approach to the brachial plexus in children. The aims of the approach are to penetrate the sheath where the three trunks are formed and to provide a vector of insertion that is distant to vital structures such as the great vessels, the subarachnoid, the stellate ganglion, vagus and phrenic nerves, and the apical pleura.

Anatomy. The landmarks are (a) the midpoint of the clavicle, (b) the posterior border of the sternocleidomastoid, and (c) Chassaignac's tubercle (C6). A line is drawn from the midpoint of the clavicle to Chassaignac's tubercle. The site of puncture is the junction of the lower and the upper two thirds of this vertical line. The point of insertion should lie at least 1.5 cm above the upper limits of the subclavian artery pulsations. An insulated-block needle is connected to a nerve stimulator, and stimulation of the limb is elicited.

Technique. The patient is positioned with a roll under the shoulders to move the brachial plexus to a more anterior position. The head of the child is rotated away from the side to be blocked. The needle is inserted at right angles to the skin and advanced until there is motor activity (twitches) of the hand. If no twitches can be elicited on the first attempt, the needle is withdrawn and redirected laterally until a response is obtained. The brachial plexus is usually located 0.7 to 3 cm from the skin's surface (24).

Limitations. The limitations of the parascalene approach are similar to those previously mentioned for the interscalene approach; however, the lower branches are blocked more than 50% of the time. With the interscalene approach, the lower branches are blocked about 33% of the time (24).

Complications. There are few complications with this approach, given the route and level of approach. Most major structures are avoided, which adds to the safety of this approach.

Indications. The technique can be applied in situations in which the interscalene approach is appropriate. The frequency of utilization is limited in infants; however, in older children, this block can be beneficial, especially in shoulder dislocations. Horner's syndrome may still occur and persist for several hours. This must be taken into consideration in the event that head trauma or change of mental status has occurred as part of the initial presentation. Patients requiring neurologic examination are not candidates for interscalene or parascalene blockade.

Axillary Approach to the Brachial Plexus

The axillary approach has gained more favor than other techniques of brachial plexus blockade in children. It is safe and easy to perform.

Anatomy. The axillary artery can be palpated at the junction of the pectoralis major and the coracobrachialis muscles when the arm is abducted and externally rotated 90 degrees. The trunks of the brachial plexus pass behind the clavicle. They unite and form the three cords that surround the second part of the axillary artery. Next, the cords divide into the three terminal branches close to the third part of the artery. The ulnar nerve lies medially, the radial nerve lies posteriorly, and the median nerve lies lateral to the axillary artery.

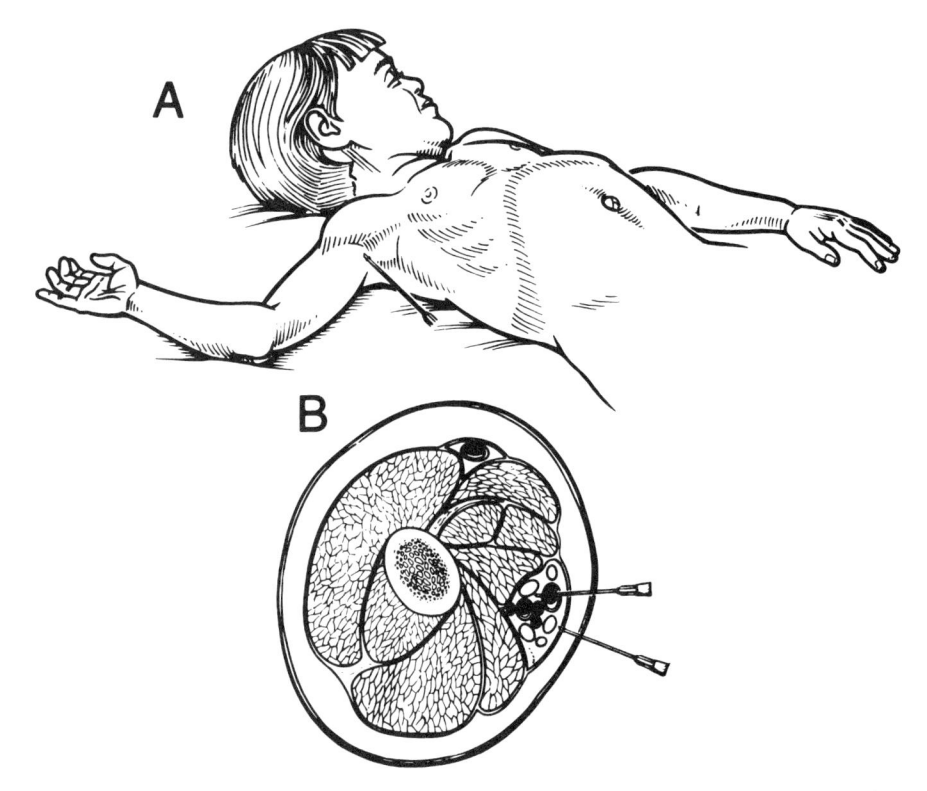

FIG. 13. **(A)** Position of the child for brachial plexus block. **(B)** Anatomic landmarks and needle position for the transarterial approach.

The terminal branches may vary slightly in position with regard to the axillary artery.

Axillary blockade of the brachial plexus has been reported to have a failure rate as high as 30%. It was proposed that the nerves and vessels are separated by discrete fascial septa and required several injection sites for adequate blockade (26). In 1987, however, Partridge and associates (26) examined 18 cadavers and found that although septa did exist, the spread of injected dye was immediate.

Technique. Several techniques are routinely used by practitioners and include the transarterial approach (Fig. 13), the two-injection procedure, and several perivascular approaches (Fig. 14). In general, all the approaches use needle insertion just below the pectoralis, where it is crossed by the coracobrachialis. All of the techniques also use distal occlusion of the axillary artery and sheath in an effort to force the spread of local anesthetic cephalad to involve the cords and possibly the trunks.

The perivascular technique is described. A tourniquet is placed just below the axilla. A 22- or 23-gauge blunt-tip block needle is inserted at right angles to the skin toward both the upper edge of the axillary artery and the humerus. Muscle twitches are sought and, although they increase the success rate of adequate blockade, nerve stimulation is not mandatory. A pop or click is usually appreciated as the needle enters the axillary sheath. Such detection of tissue transduction does not guarantee proper needle location within the neurovascular sheath. Penetration of the sheath is easily recognized by the transmission of arterial pulsations. A single injection is performed at the upper edge of the axillary artery.

Complications. Arterial puncture, whether accidental or deliberate, is undesirable and

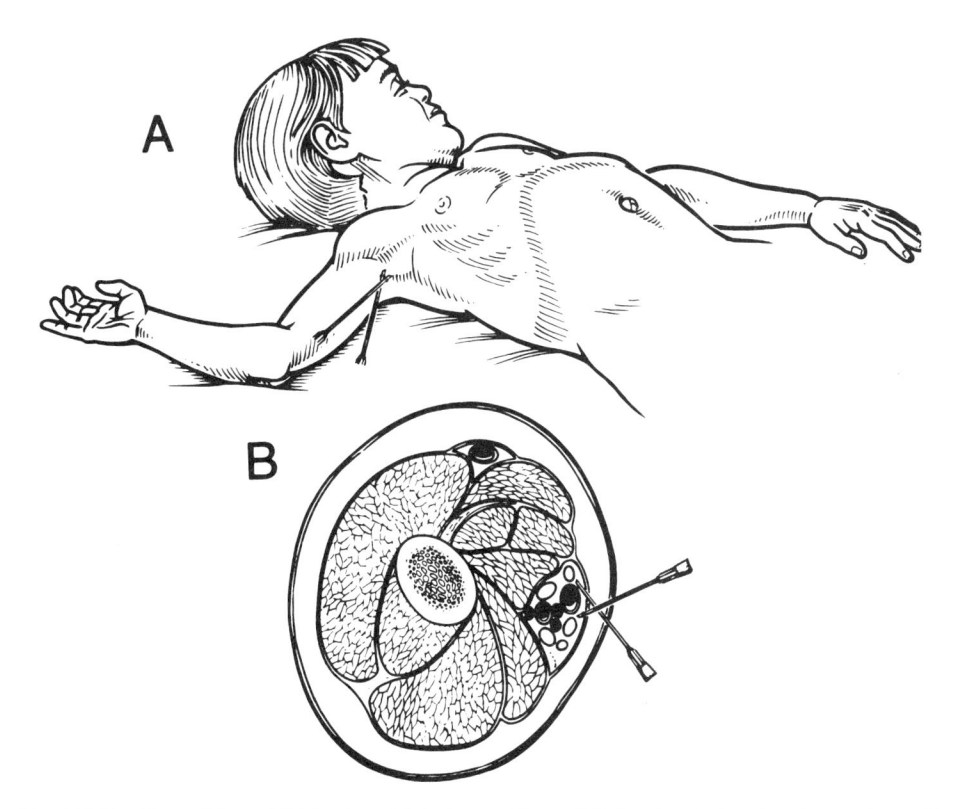

FIG. 14. (A) Position of the child for brachial plexus block. **(B)** Anatomic landmarks and needle position for the perivascular approach.

may result in transient vascular insufficiency. Intravascular injection of local anesthetic can cause systemic toxicity. The technique should be avoided in patients with preexisting vascular compromise or risk of developing such compromise.

Limitations. The axillary approach to the brachial plexus may not reliably block the musculocutaneous, intercostobrachial, or medial cutaneous nerves. Positioning requires the patient to abduct and externally rotate the arm, which may be painful or impossible in an awake child and often requires general anesthesia, especially in smaller children.

Applications. Procedures of the upper extremity that do not require anesthesia of the shoulder are appropriate. Continuous infusions via indwelling catheters have been used for traumatic hand injuries in the intraoperative and postoperative periods (27).

Continuous Brachial Plexus Nerve Block Using the Axillary Approach

Continuous brachial plexus nerve block via the axillary approach is easily inserted, has low morbidity, and is suitable for orthopedic or plastic surgical repairs of the hand or forearm (17). The axillary approach to the brachial plexus is accomplished in the supine child by abducting the child's arm to 90 degrees. A tourniquet applied near the site of the injection promotes proximal spread of local anesthetic and enhances the chances of successful block of the musculocutaneous nerve. The axillary artery is easily

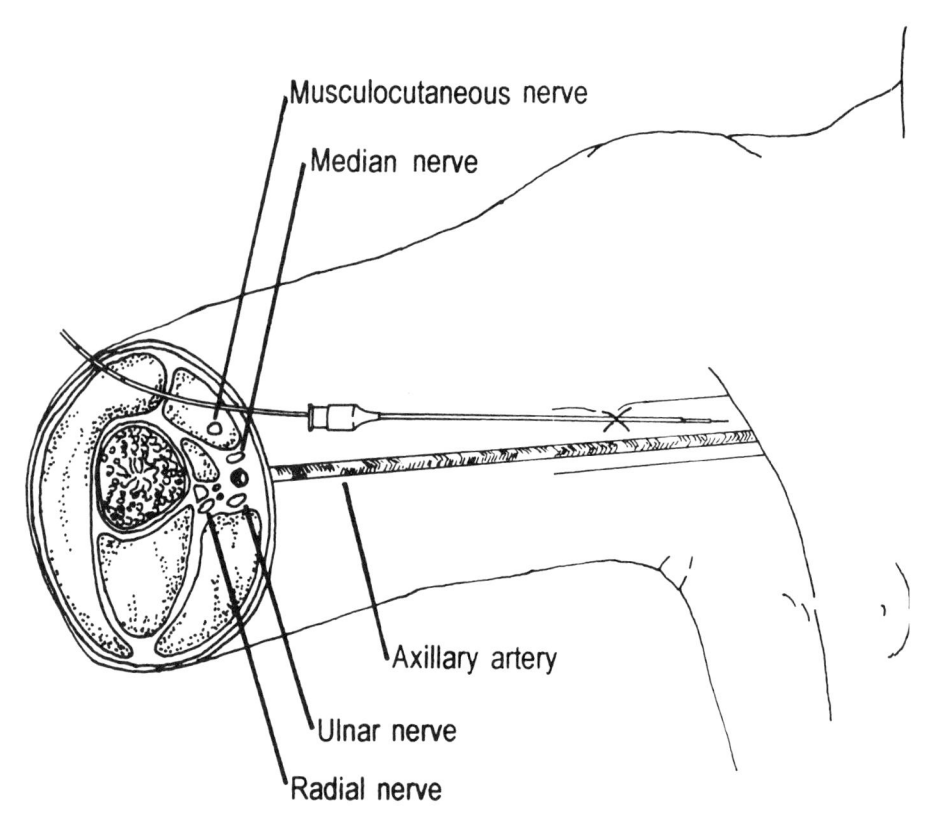

FIG. 15. Anatomic relation of nerves and arteries in the axilla important in the insertion of needle and catheter into the axillary sheath. The lines above and below the axillary artery represent lines drawn on skin (see text) and the approximate confines of the axillary sheath. (Reprinted with permission, from Badgwell JM: Anesthesia and Analgesia for Minor Injuries to Children. In *International Anesthesiology Clinics.* Winter 1994/Vol. 32:1, p. 142)..

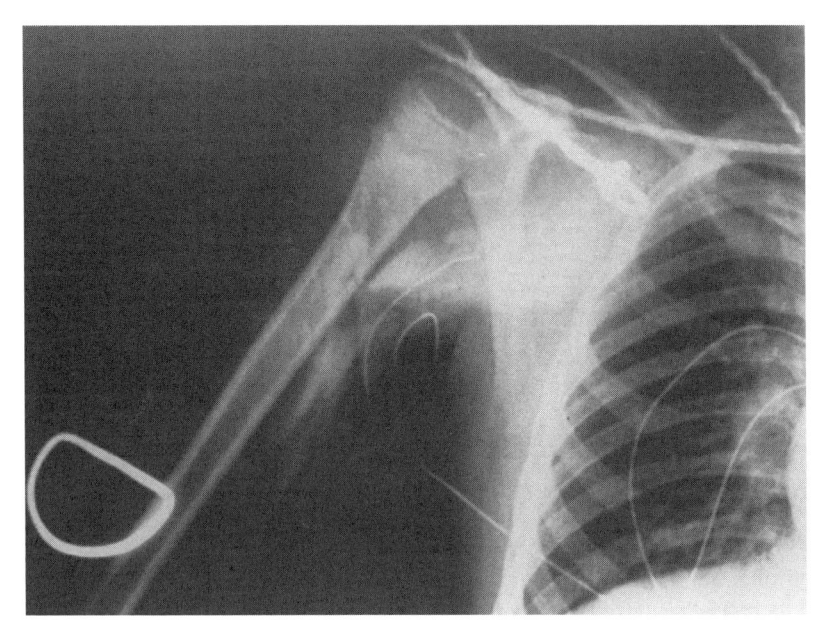

FIG. 16. X-ray film showing radiopaque dye injected through the catheter into the axillary sheath of a 9-year-old boy. Injection of radiopaque dye through a Crawford needle had been performed earlier in the technique (see text). (Reprinted with permission, from Badgwell JM: Anesthesia and Analgesia for Minor Injuries to Children. In *International Anesthesiology Clinics*. Winter 1994/Vol. 32:1, p. 143).

palpated in children at the junction of the pectoralis major and the coracobrachialis muscle when the arm is abducted and externally rotated. The artery and the plexus lie more superficially in children than in adults. The axillary artery is palpated and marked with a pen at the site of injection with an "X" and on either side of the artery with lines. The area is then sterilized, prepped, and draped. A nick is made in the skin with a 18-gauge needle to allow for ease of insertion of a blunt needle and to allow for a better feel of the pop as the blunt needle goes through the axillary sheath. An appropriate-sized blunt needle is then inserted at a 45-degree angle into the skin nick and advanced forward until a distinct pop is felt as the needle pierces the axillary sheath (Fig. 15).

Aspiration is performed to confirm that the needle has not entered a blood vessel. At this point, the angle of the needle is dropped to 15 degrees and then advanced slightly. Five milliliters of iohexol (Omnipaque) dye is then injected, and fluoroscopy of the axillary sheath is performed (Fig. 16). An outline of the axillary sheath confirms correct needle placement. Then a nerve stimulator is attached to the needle and stimulated with 0.5 mA current. This low-voltage current elicits motor movement of the hand only if the needle is inadvertently within the body of a nerve. Therefore, no motor movement of the hand is further evidence of correct needle placement.

If a single injection is to be performed, the medication is injected after needle placement. When using 1% mepivacaine, we inject 0.7 ml/kg. When using 0.25% bupivacaine, we inject a slightly smaller volume (0.5 ml/kg). The placement of a catheter for continuous infusion of local anesthetic provides excellent pain relief postoperatively and sympathetic blockade that may improve circulation after microvascular procedures. For a continuous axillary catheter, we insert a 20-gauge Theracath spring-wire epidural catheter (Arrow, EC-05000, Reading, PA) through a 17-gauge Crawford needle using the insertion technique previously described (see Fig. 1). After the catheter is inserted, we again aspirate, inject with 5 ml of iohexol, and stimulate the metal stylet of the catheter. Because the stylet is insulated by the catheter, 0.5-mA current stimulation of the stylet will elicit motor movement of the hand if the catheter is properly placed. The initial dose of bupivacaine is 0.5 ml/kg, followed by an infusion of 0.125% bupivacaine at 0.15 ml/kg/hour.

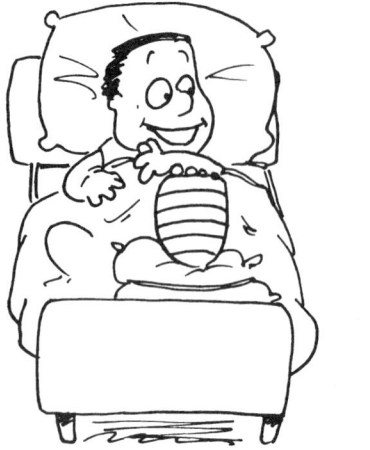

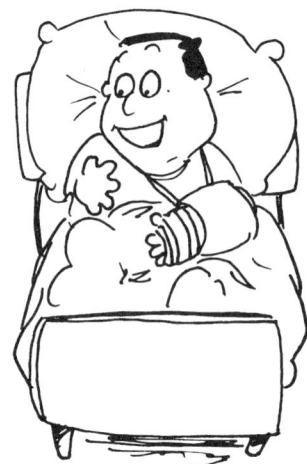

Lower Extremity Blocks

Psoas Compartment Block

Anatomy. The roots of the lumbar plexus emerge from their foramina into a fascial plane between the quadratus lumborum posteriorly and the psoas muscle anteriorly. The lumbar plexus is formed inside the psoas muscle from the anterior rami of the four upper lumbar nerves. The branches of the plexus emerge from the lateral and medial borders of the psoas. The lumbosacral trunk has contributions from the fourth and fifth lumbar nerves. This trunk passes down the pelvis and joins the anterior rami of the first, second, third, and fourth sacral nerves as they emerge from their anterior sacral foramina. Thus, a posterior approach through the quadratus lumborum will result in anesthetic being placed close to the lumbosacral plexus.

Technique. The technique was developed by Chayen and associates (28) and reported in 1976. The technique is as follows: the posterior superior iliac spine and the spinous process of the fourth lumbar vertebra are located by draw-

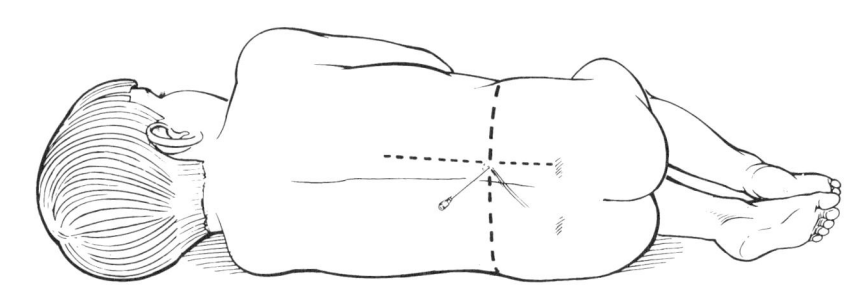

FIG. 17. Before psoas compartment block, the posterior superior iliac spine (PSIS) and the spinous process of the fourth lumbar vertebra are located by drawing a line connecting the iliac crests. The site of puncture lies at the midpoint between the PSIS and the spinous process of the fourth lumbar vertebra.

ing a line connecting the iliac crests (Fig. 17). The site of puncture lies at the midpoint between the PSIS and the spinous process of the fourth lumbar vertebra. A loss-of-resistance technique can be used; however, a nerve stimulator is recommended. Motor stimulation of the foot should be sought. Penetration of the intrathecal space is possible. Careful aspiration before injection is mandatory, and fractionation of the injection is important. This approach avoids the multiple punctures required for more peripheral blockade of the nerves supplying the lower extremity. The sciatic nerve may require separate blockade.

Limitations. The psoas compartment block approach may result in epidural blockade and thus has the potential of being a major conduction block. Therefore, this procedure should be reserved for inpatient surgery.

Complications. Intravascular injections and systemic toxicity have occurred. Total spinal blocks from inadvertent intrathecal injection are rare, but possible.

Applications. The psoas compartment block can be used in patients for hip procedures whose epidural space may be difficult to enter, and it can be considered as an alternative to midline epidural analgesia. A catheter can be placed to provide continuous infusion analgesia. There is a 90% success rate with this technique when a nerve stimulator is used.

Lateral Femoral Cutaneous Nerve Block

The use of the lateral femoral cutaneous nerve block had not been described in pediatrics until 1986 when McNicol (29) found the block to be 96% successful in children for postoperative pain relief.

Anatomy. The lateral femoral cutaneous nerve is purely sensory. It arises from the lumbar plexus from segments L2 and L3 and innervates the skin of the outer aspect of the thigh (Fig. 18). The nerve enters the thigh deep to the inguinal ligament and continues deep to the fascia lata.

Technique. A line is drawn from the anterior superior iliac spine to the spine of the pubic bone. The puncture site lies where the line is transacted at the junction of the lateral and medial thirds. Local anesthetic is deposited inferomedially to the anterior supe-

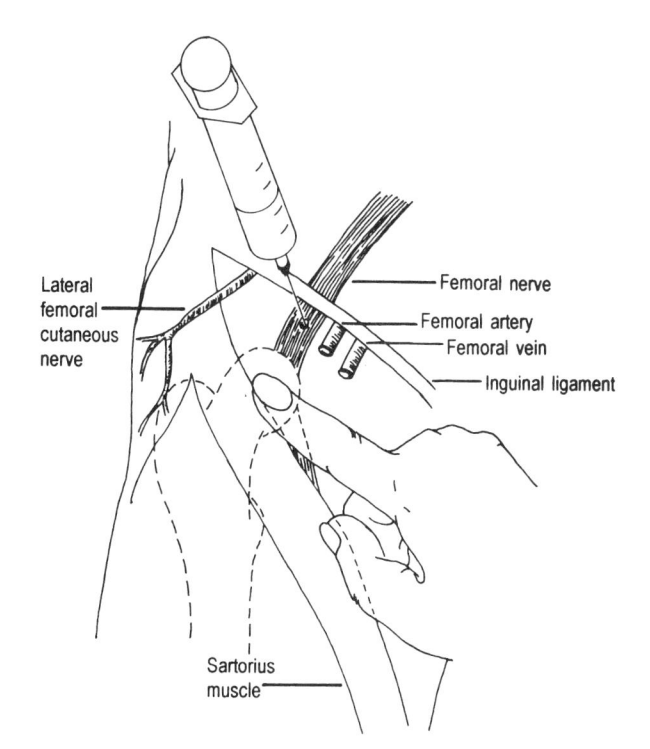

FIG. 18. Anatomic relations of the femoral area important in performing either a femoral nerve block, 3-in-1 inguinal paravascular nerve block, lateral femoral cutaneous nerve block, or fascia iliaca compartment block (see text). (Reprinted with permission, from Badgwell JM: Anesthesia and Analgesia for Minor Injuries to Children. In *International Anesthesiology Clinics.* Winter 1994/Vol. 32:1, p. 144).

rior iliac spine and inferiorly to the inguinal ligament. The local anesthetic is deposited in a fan-like fashion. The needle should pass deep to the fascia lata, and injection is performed as the needle moves parallel with the skin.

Complications. Inadvertent 3-in-1 blockade has occurred with the lateral femoral cutaneous nerve block (30). In general, it is a very safe and easy block to perform.

Limitations. The lateral femoral cutaneous nerve block often requires the use of other nerve blocks to provide adequate relief.

Applications. Split-thickness skin graft sites or other procedures limited to the distribution of the area supplied by the nerve are favored.

Femoral Nerve Block

Anatomy. The femoral nerve arises from segments L2-L4 and is a mixed motor and sensory nerve that supplies sensation to the front and part of the inside of the thigh. It is the most important nerve supplying sensation to the periosteum of the femoral shaft, and its motor component supplies the extensor muscles of the knee. The femoral nerve divides deep to the inguinal ligament and lies lateral to the femoral artery.

Technique. The anesthesiologist may find it more comfortable to stand on the opposite side of the side to be blocked. The femoral artery pulsation is identified near the middle of the inguinal ligament (Fig. 19). A 23-gauge regional block needle with an attached syringe is inserted perpendicular to the skin 0.5 to 1.0 cm lateral to the femoral artery. The local anesthetic may be deposited in a focal region just lateral to the femoral artery, or the anesthetic is injected in a fan-shaped direction while the needle is moved in and out a few millimeters at a time. Aspiration should be performed before each injection.

Complications. Femoral artery hematoma formation and residual femoral nerve dysfunction are possible complications from fan-like injections. Some anesthesiologists prefer a single injection just lateral to the femoral artery and below the inguinal ligament.

Limitations. The femoral nerve block cannot usually be used alone for upper thigh procedures. It is often combined with the lateral femoral cutaneous and obturator nerve blocks for adequate analgesia.

Applications. Continuous infusion catheters can be placed and provide good postoperative relief (31). Examinations of femur fractures can

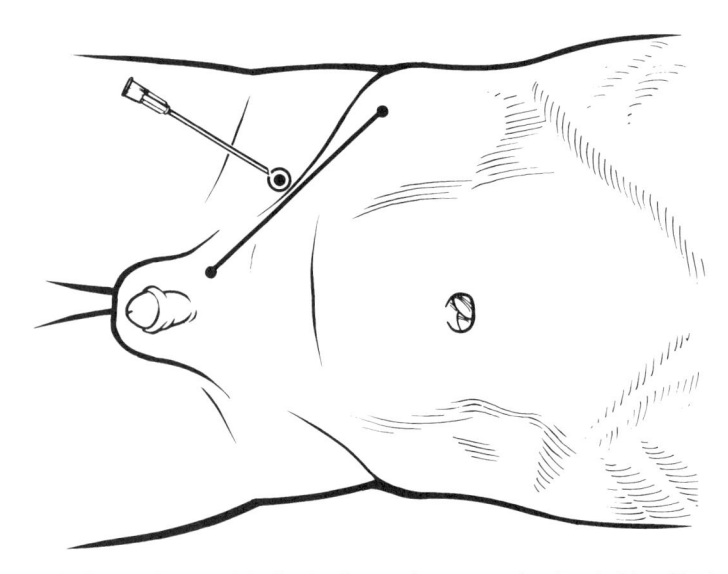

FIG. 19. Important in femoral nerve block, the femoral artery pulsation is identified near the middle of the inguinal ligament.

be performed with this block, especially when heavy sedation is contraindicated. The block has been used to treat bone pain in sickle cell crisis. Severe quadriceps spasms can be successfully managed with continuous infusions.

Fascia Iliaca Compartment Block

In 1989, Dalens and colleagues (32) developed a compartment block that has been proposed as a superior blocking technique to the 3-in-1 block, as described by Winnie (33). Dalens' cadaveric studies supported the hypothesis that if sufficient amounts of a solution were injected posterior to the fascia iliaca, there would be spread of solution along the inner surface with resultant anesthesia of the femoral, lateral femoral cutaneous, genitofemoral and obturator nerves.

Anatomy. The fascia iliaca is a complex fascial sheath. Medially, it attaches to the vertebral column and upper sacrum. Rostrally, it blends with the fascia covering the quadratus lumborum, and laterally and caudally, it attaches to the inner iliac crest. At the level of the femoral triangle, the fascia iliaca becomes narrow and is covered by the fascia lata and forms the roof of the lacuna musculorum and the lacuna vasorum. The femoral, lateral femoral cutaneous, and obturator nerves run a significant distance close to the inner aspect of the fascia iliaca (32). The genitofemoral and ilioinguinal nerves also pass posterior to the fascia iliaca and can be blocked with a single injection.

Technique. To perform the fascia iliaca block, a blunt 22- or 23-gauge regional needle with a syringe attached is needed. A line is drawn from the anterior superior iliac spine to the pubic tubercle. This line is divided into thirds and marks the location of the inguinal ligament. The puncture site is 0.5 to 1 cm below at the junction of the lateral and middle thirds. A loss-of-resistance technique is used. A loss of resistance will be appreciated twice (33). The first is the fascia lata, and the second is the fascia iliaca. The technique is reported to have a 90% success rate, even in the hands of the novice. The likelihood of blockade of the lower extremity nerves with this technique is as follows: femoral nerve blockade 99%, lateral femoral cutaneous nerve 90%, obturator nerve 75%, and the upper branches of the lumbar plexus 50% (34).

Complications. The fascia iliaca compartment block is an easy and reliable block, which does not place any vital structures at risk. Unless rapidly acting agents are used, profound anesthesia may not occur until 30 minutes or more after the completion of the block.

Limitations. The sciatic nerve is not blocked with this technique; therefore, this compartment block is not appropriate as a sole anesthetic when blockade of the sciatic nerve is needed (e.g., in the knee joint).

Applications. Femoral osteotomies, femoral rodding procedures, split-thickness skin grafts, and related procedures are amenable. Surgical anesthesia of the iliac crests and hip may be variable, since these areas are predominantly supplied by the lumbar plexus (L1-L3).

Sciatic Nerve Block

The sciatic nerve is the largest nerve in the body. It is derived from the sacral plexus and is composed of two nerves—the tibial and the common peroneal nerves that are enclosed in a common sheath. The sciatic nerve emerges from the pelvis through the sciatic foramen and reaches the back of the thigh between the greater trochanter and ischial tuberosity.

There are three approaches to the sciatic nerve. The posterior approach is the classic approach still used to date. Other approaches include the lateral approach and the anterior approach (35).

Anatomy. The fascial components of the buttocks and thigh are multicompartmentalized. The aponeuroses of the fascia lata, fascia cribrosa, fascia iliaca, and gluteal fascia are definitive (unlike the compartments of the axillary sheath) and prevent the spread of local anesthetic between adjacent compartments. The thigh is further divided into a single anterior and two posterior compartments. The sciatic nerve lies in the medial posterior compartment deep in the subgluteal space.

Approaches

1. Anterior. The sciatic nerve is approached anteriorly while the child lies supine. A line is drawn from the anterior superior iliac spine to the pubic tubercle. This line is divided into thirds. Next, a line is drawn perpendicular to the junction of the inner and middle thirds. The needle angle is parallel with the inguinal ligament and projects from the end of the perpendicular line down to the greater trochanter. A nerve stimulator is used to assess movement of the foot and leg.
2. Lateral. This approach penetrates the subgluteal space and approaches the nerve close to the ischial tuberosity. The needle is inserted horizontally toward the posterior aspect of the femur at the level of the greater trochanteric prominence. The insertion site is approximately 3 cm dorsal to the greater trochanter. The needle is inserted until bony contact is made; then the needle is walked dorsally toward the ischial tuberosity. A nerve stimulator is used, and movement of the foot is sought.
3. Posterior. The posterior approach is the classic technique used for sciatic nerve block. Several variations exist. Traditionally, the patient lies in the lateral decubitus position with the side to be blocked positioned up. The thigh is flexed to 90 degrees, and the following landmarks are defined. A line is drawn connecting the posterior superior iliac spine and the greater trochanter, and the midpoint of the line is located. The sciatic nerve should be found in a line drawn perpendicular to the midpoint approximately 2 to 5 cm distal to the point of intersection. Again, a nerve stimulator is used, and motor activity of the foot should be detected. In children, a line is drawn from the greater trochanter to the distal end of the coccyx. The sciatic nerve lies at the midpoint of this line.

A loss of resistance technique can be used with any of the approaches described above for blockade of the sciatic nerve. Reliable blockade is best obtained with the guidance of a nerve stimulator.

Intravenous Regional Blocks

The technique of IV regional block was first described by August Bier in 1908 and has been applied to pediatric anesthesia since 1967, when Gingrich described the use of the Bier block for upper extremity procedures in children (36). This technique has found increasing popularity for the setting of upper extremity fractures in emergency wards and obviates the delays associated with the use of general anesthesia. A lack of cooperation in young children and the pain of manipulation during exsanguination limits the application of this technique in the very young; however, descriptions of use in children as young as 3 years of age can be found (36).

The Bier block was originally described without exsanguination of the extremity. Today, the common practice is to elevate and apply an Esmarch bandage to the limb before the inflation of the tourniquets (37). Double tourniquets are preferred, but a single-cuffed tourniquet can be used. Many agents have been administered; however, lidocaine is the drug of choice because of its relatively low systemic toxicity. Lidocaine is the only agent advocated for operative use.

Technique. A butterfly needle or IV catheter is placed distally in the affected extremity, and the limb is elevated to aid venous drainage. Next, an Esmarch bandage may be applied in a circumferential fashion from the distal to proximal aspect of the extremity. A double-cuffed tourniquet system is then applied, and the proximal cuff is inflated to 200 to 240 mm Hg and the Esmarch is removed. The local anesthetic is infused. After about 5 to 7 minutes, the distal cuff is inflated (now the upgoing cuff region is anesthetized), and the proximal cuff is deflated.

Complications. Dizziness, nausea, vomiting, hypertension, bradycardia, and arrhythmias have occurred. The incidence of sequevacalae is higher with agents such as bupivicaine.

Applications. Emergency department procedures for the forearm and elbow fractures are very appropriate. There may be characteristics of a plexus block when higher concentrations of local anesthetic are used. Consequently, the block may last for a prolonged period of time after deflation of the cuff. In general, however, the anesthetic effects are short-lived after deflation of the tourniquet. The brevity of the block makes it amenable to outpatient procedures. Low-dose or "mini-dose" lidocaine at 1.0 to 1.5 mg/kg has provided good to excellent anesthesia (38,39).

SUMMARY

Regional anesthetic techniques for children have been widely advocated for postoperative and procedural pain management. A large number of clinical series have reported excellent efficacy and safety. Several trials have found either improved analgesia or reduced side effects in patients treated with regional analgesia compared with control groups of patients receiving systemic opioids.

Most of the peripheral blocks that are used in adults can be applied in the pediatric population. Anatomic and physiologic differences must be taken into account. Peripheral nerve blocks can be performed safely and effectively in children of all ages. The cognitive development of the child must be considered when determining the conditions under which the block will be performed (i.e., sedation or general anesthesia). Except in older children, light sedation can increase perceptual distortion and may lead to combativeness. Deep sedation or light general anesthesia is often required. The end-result is a child who has been spared the emotional trauma and stress of the surgical environment with the benefit of often profound perioperative analgesia.

COMPLICATIONS OF EPIDURAL AND SPINAL ANESTHESIA

Although complications of regional anesthetic techniques in infants and children are rare, they do occur. The severity of complications may vary from relatively minor (e.g., infection) to very serious (e.g., cardiovascular collapse). Here, we will examine the gamut of complications associated with regional procedures in children and discuss the toxicity of local anesthetics and neuraxial opioids including predisposing factors, diagnosis, and therapy.

Incidence

The incidence of serious complications secondary to regional techniques and local anesthetics is very low, and no deaths have been reported. This is true even for very small infants. Murrell and coworkers (40) reported no complications in a series of term newborns and former preterm infants undergoing primarily abdominal procedures by combined epidural and light general anesthesia. A report of 2 years' experience from the Alberta Children's Hospital reveals that the majority of complications associated with the use of regional anesthesia techniques were minor and easily remedied (41). The few serious complications (e.g., seizures, cardiovascular collapse) were related to children with toxic plasma concentrations of bupivacaine (2.1 to 5.5 µg/ml). A survey from 12 well-established pediatric pain services worldwide will report results from 44,348 total regional anesthetic procedures in children (Sang and Berde, unpublished data, 1995). Of these procedures, only 24 were complicated by respiratory depression, 11 by convulsions, and 34 by noncritical events (infection, nerve root lesion, heel sores, and retained catheter). Seventy-three percent of the patients who experienced convulsions received continuous epidural bupivacaine doses of more than 0.5 mg/kg/hour. Only one serious cardiovascular complication (cardiac arrest) was reported.

Very rarely, serious cardiovascular complications may occur from other causes. For example, venous air embolism during caudal and epidural catheter placement in children have been reported (42,43). Most complications, however, are associated with excessive dosing of local anesthetics or opioids (44–47). Therefore, complications can be made extremely rare by limitation of bupivacaine dosing to no more than 0.4 to 0.5 mg/kg/hour and by limiting neuraxial opioids to recommended doses **(see Complications Related to Neuraxial Opioids)**.

Local Anesthetic Toxicity

Signs and Symptoms of Local Anesthetic Toxicity

The signs and symptoms of local anesthetic toxicity increase as plasma concentrations of local anesthetics increase (Fig. 20). As plasma and central nervous system tissue concentrations increase, symptoms of lightheadedness and dizziness occur and may progress to visual and auditory disturbances (e.g., diplopia and tinnitus). As plasma levels of local anesthetic continue to rise, excitation occurs and grand mal seizures may result. The end point of central nervous system depression is respiratory depression leading to respiratory arrest.

In anesthetized patients, the first signs of toxicity are frequently cardiovascular. In infants, the first objective sign of inadvertent intravascular injection of bupivacaine plus epinephrine is T-wave change on the electrocardiogram (ECG) (48) (Fig. 21). When 2-week-old piglets are given IV local anesthetic with or without epinephrine, or epinephrine alone, T-wave elevation occurs after epinephrine-containing solutions but not after bupivacaine or lidocaine alone (49) (Fig. 22). Therefore, adding epinephrine (1:200,000) to local anesthetic solution and continuous monitoring of the ECG provides an early warning marker (T-wave elevation) that may be used as a signal to discontinue the administration of local anesthetic. T-wave elevation is a more reliable marker of toxicity than heart rate increase, which requires prior atropine administration (50).

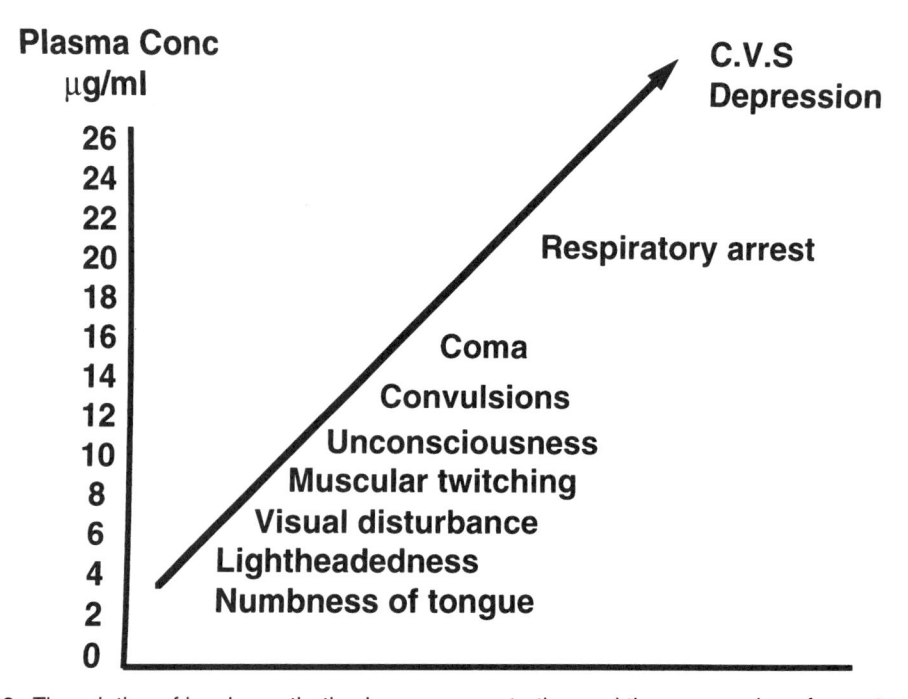

FIG. 20. The relation of local anesthetic plasma concentration and the progression of symptomatology in an awake patient. In anesthetized children, the earliest signs of local anesthetic toxicity are cardiovascular.

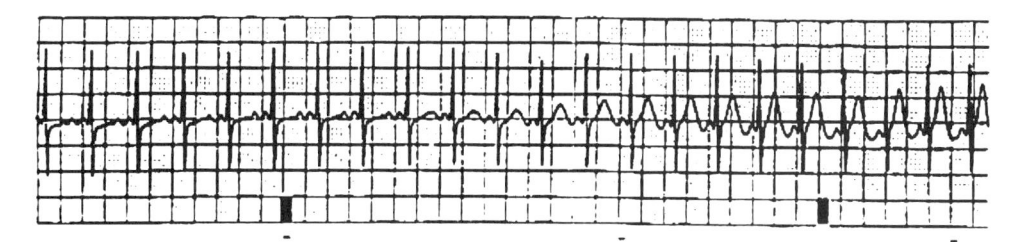

FIG. 21. The electrocardiogram from an 8-month-old infant during combined light general anesthesia and regional analgesia. A few seconds after the caudal administration of 1 ml 0.125% bupivacaine with epinephrine (1:200,000), T-wave elevation was observed and the injection discontinued. Aspiration revealed blood in the administration tubing. The T-wave elevation quickly returned to baseline, and caudal analgesia was continued after repositioning the needle.

Whereas the potential range for central nervous system toxicity of bupivacaine in adults is 3 to 5 µg/ml (51), the toxic threshold for children has not been demonstrated. Plasma bupivacaine concentrations after absorption from caudal bolus injections of 2.5 mg/kg of 0.15% bupivacaine result in blood levels ranging from 0.55 to 1.93 µg/ml (52) and caudal injection of 1.25 mg/kg bupivacaine followed by infusion of 0.2 mg/kg/hour result in plasma concentrations well below adult toxic levels (0.3 to 0.8 µg/ml) (53). By contrast, high plasma concentrations and cardiovascular toxicity may result from inadvertent intravascular injection of

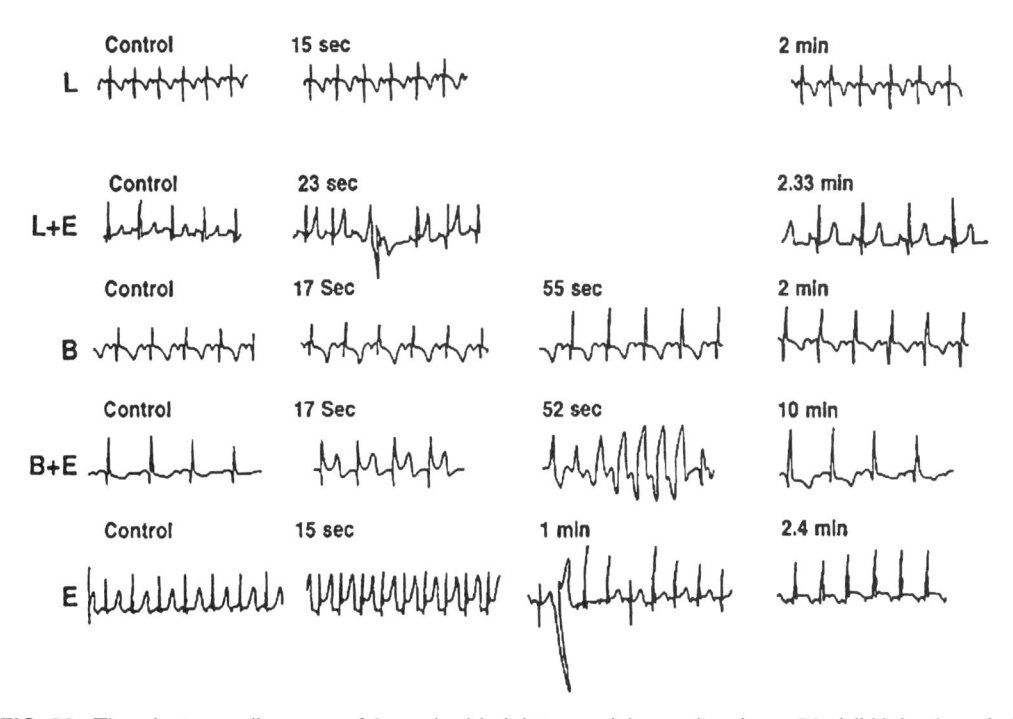

FIG. 22. The electrocardiograms of 2-week-old piglets receiving a slow (over 30 s) IV injection of either lidocaine (5 mg/kg) *(L)*, lidocaine with epinephrine (1:200,000) *(L + E)*, bupivacaine (2.5 mg/kg) *(B)*, bupivacaine with epinephrine *(B + E)*, or epinephrine alone *(E)*. The addition of epinephrine caused T-wave changes and ectopic beats that resolved. T-wave changes did not occur after local anesthetics alone.

these doses. Because local anesthetics redistribute throughout the body quickly, most toxic reactions are self-limited as plasma levels rapidly decrease. Therefore, serious complications may be prevented if injection of local anesthetic solution is discontinued when T-wave elevation appears on ECG.

Ropivacaine, a new local anesthetic agent has much less cardiac toxicity than bupivacaine. Therefore, fewer cardiac complications may occur during regional techniques as use of this drug grows. We know that inadequate airway management and subsequent hypoxia/hypercarbia may predispose pediatric patients to life-threatening cardiovascular complications after inadvertent intravascular injection of lidocaine and epinephrine (54). We also know that infants during light general anesthesia by face mask have an increased incidence of hypercarbia and dysrhythmias compared with the incidence of these complications in children with tracheal tubes (55). Finally, infants experience a higher incidence of adverse respiratory events than children (56) or adults. Therefore, infants are at increased risk of local anesthetic toxicity, particularly those infants managed with face mask anesthesia. These data emphasize the importance of maintaining a patent airway during regional anesthesia procedures in infants and children.

A complete list of factors known to be integral in enhancing and producing local anesthetic agent toxicity include age (57), volatile anesthetic agents (57), hypoxia (58), hypercarbia (59), rapid rate of infusion (59), or a combination of these factors (59).

Treatment of Toxicity

After intravascular injection of local anesthetic, cardiovascular toxicity is biphasic, consisting of an early pressor response, followed by a late response in which arterial blood pressure is decreased as a result of peripheral vasodilation and direct myocardial depression. Likewise, there is an early ECG response (e.g., T-wave changes), which may progress to more overt signs of myocardial irritability (e.g., ectopic beats). In a similar biphasic response, heart rate may initially increase and then decrease, eventually leading to asystole and cardiac arrest. Whereas treatment of early phase toxicity is usually simple (e.g., by allowing the drug to redistribute), toxicity that progresses to the late phase is often refractory to treatment and frequently fatal.

Convulsions may be controlled with lorazepam or midazolam (0.05 mg/kg incrementally until seizures stop), sodium thiopental (2 to 3 mg/kg), or propofol (2 mg/kg) (60). Succinylcholine may be administered if needed for control of the airway, although seizures may persist unless anticonvulsant medication is given. If the toxic response includes vasodilation and hypotension, treatment includes fluid loading with lactated Ringer's solution and the administration of phenylephrine (0.1 µg/kg/min). If life-threatening ventricular dysrhythmias occur as a result of bupivacaine, IV phenytoin (5 mg/kg) may be effective in restoring sinus rhythm (61). If cardiovascular collapse ensues, it is recommended by the American Heart Association to administer epinephrine (62). Recently, however, the advisability of epinephrine to treat bupivacaine-induced cardiovascular collapse has been questioned (63).

Based on current literature and a study in dogs, Feldman and colleagues (64) concluded that the use of epinephrine to treat cardiovascular collapse after local anesthetic should be reexamined. The potential problems with using epinephrine in this situation are (a) epinephrine may be ineffective (64) or (b) the dysrhythmogenic effect of epinephrine may be detrimental in efforts to restore sinus rhythm and cardiac output (63).

Are there vasopressor drugs, other than epinephrine, that may be more beneficial in the treatment of local anesthetic–induced hypotension and cardiovascular collapse? Heavner and associates (65) investigated the success of resuscitative attempts with different cardioactive drugs (amrinone, dopamine, norepinephrine, epinephrine, and isoproterenol) after bupivacaine-induced asystole in rats. The most important conclusion from this study was that when all factors were considered, norepinephrine may be the drug of choice for treating bupivacaine-induced asystole. By the measures used, norepinephrine, epinephrine, and isoproterenol were equieffective. What tipped the scale in favor of norepinephrine, however, was the absence of ventricular dysrhythmias after norepinephrine. Although extrapolation of this information to clinical situations in children must be done cautiously, the favorable outcomes with norepinephrine suggest that further investigation should be considered. In the latter study, the dose of norepinephrine used was 20% of the epinephrine dose (65).

Complications Related to Neuraxial Opioids

Respiratory depression can be a serious complication when opioids are combined with local anesthetic solutions. Although clinical respiratory depression usually occurs within the first 6 hours after the administration of epidural or intrathecal morphine, respiratory depression may occur up to 18 hours after morphine administration (65). The incidence of respiratory depression appears to be correlated with opioid dose, age, and supplemental systemic opioids. In a study of 138 children receiving 70 µg/kg caudal morphine, 11 developed respiratory depression (66). Ten of these 11 cases occurred in infants ≤ 1 year of age, and all 10 received supplemental parenteral opioids. In Sang's multi-institutional survey, 12 of 13 incidences of respiratory depression were associated with single-shot epidural morphine doses of greater than 50 µg/kg and 7 of 13 children received supplemental IV opioids or sedatives. Therefore, for epidural morphine, we recommend limiting bolus doses to no more than 50 µg/kg and infusions to no more than 5 µg/kg/hour and the avoidance of systemic opioids. If additional analgesia is required, acetaminophen or ketorolac should be considered.

Respiratory depression may also occur with intrathecal morphine. In the multicenter study, four cases of respiratory depression occurred and all four had received supplemental systemic opioids.

When neuraxial opioids are administered to children, monitoring with pulse oximetry or apnea monitors and continuous nursing assessment is recommended. The hallmark of impending respiratory depression is increasing sedation and decreasing depth of respirations. Airway resuscitative equipment and naloxone should be immediately available and naloxone administered for respiratory depression (1 to 2 µg/kg with repeated doses as necessary).

Lawhorn and Brown (66) compared epidural morphine (80 µg/kg) with epidural morphine plus butorphanol (40 µg/kg) in 20 children and found equal analgesia with significantly less pruritus, nausea, and oxygen-hemoglobin desaturation (SpO_2 < 90%) in the butorphanol group. In a study of 46 pediatric orthopedic patients, Lee and Rubin (67) found that 2 µg/kg clonidine significantly prolonged the analgesia compared with bupivacaine (0.25%) alone, and it was not associated with respiratory depression.

Pruritus, urinary retention, nausea, and vomiting occur frequently after neuraxial opioids. Pruritus is treated with naloxone (1.0 µg/kg, repeated as necessary) with or without diphenhydramine (0.5 mg/kg). Nausea and vomiting are treated with naloxone, metoclopramide (0.15 mg/kg), or ondansetron (0.1 mg/kg).

Complications Related to Technical Factors

Epidural catheters may cause nerve injury by nerve or dural penetration. Because most regional procedures in children are performed with the child asleep, the elicitation for paresthesia is not possible. Therefore, anesthetized children may be at increased risk for nerve injury during general anesthesia. Fortunately, the incidence of nerve injury is low and can be minimized by a microvoltage nerve stimulator to identify needle-tip location (e.g., during axillary plexus block) (68).

It is noteworthy that a review of the pediatric literature reveals no reports of residual neurologic sequelae from indwelling epidural catheters. By contrast, a devastating residual neurologic sequela—cauda equina syndrome—has been reported after continuous lidocaine spinal anesthesia with microcatheters in adults (69). Although experience with continuous spinal anesthesia using microcatheters in the pediatric population is limited, Payne and Moore (70) used bupivacaine 0.5% and subarachnoid microcatheters in 10 children <5 years of age for major abdominal surgery and achieved excellent surgical conditions, cardiovascular stability, and absence of motor or sensory deficits. Despite these favorable results, however, it was predicted that microcatheter infusions might place children at an increased risk for infection and durocutaneous fistula formation (70).

The infection rate associated with epidural procedures in children is extremely low. For epidural catheters, the infection rate was 0.04% in the multicenter study and 0.5% in the Canadian study (41). There have been no serious infections reported from single-caudal epidural injections including a review of 3500 children in which the "no-touch technique" (alcohol swab only) was used (71). The risk of infection, however, is potentially increased during continuous epidural injections. What should be done when a child with an indwelling catheter develops a fever? We recommend the evaluation of each case individually and leaving the catheter in place if a clear source for the fever (other than the catheter) is found or removing the catheter if a patient is septic or if the source of infection is unclear.

Leakage around the catheter frequently causes premature discontinuation of epidural infusions. In Wood's review of 190 infusions, the most common cause of leakage was drainage of local anesthetic solution around the entry site of the catheter (41). Leakage of cerebrospinal fluid around the catheter has not been reported.

Urinary retention after a single caudal injection of bupivacaine may be treated with parental reassurance as children almost always void within 24 hours. The time to first micturition after a single-shot caudal injection is about 5.5 hours and is unrelated to drug concentration at clinical doses (72). The addition of neuraxial opioids to local anesthetics, however, may make urinary retention more problematic (73).

Spinal Subarachnoid Anesthesia

Previously reported experience with spinal anesthesia is primarily in former preterm infants (74). Hypoxemia may complicate this procedure because of airway obstruction caused by undue flexion if care is not taken to extend the infant's neck. Most authors recommend a 22-g 1½-inch styletted spinal needle inserted in a midline position at either L4-5 or L5-S1 interspace. A low approach is necessary because the spinal cord of the neonate may extend as far as L3. A dosage of 1.5 to 2.0 mg hyperbaric tetracaine is the minimum effective dose for spinal anesthesia in infants, regardless of weight. Therefore, 0.5 to 0.6 mg/kg of 1% tetracaine mixed with 1 ml of $D_{10}W$ should provide adequate analgesia for inguinal surgery in most small ex-premature infants. If the spinal fails to provide adequate anesthesia, infiltration of the incision with additional local anesthetic provides a safe alternative. Supplementation with ketamine or anesthetics may put the child at risk for postoperative apnea (75).

Miscellaneous Complications

When children are receiving epidural infusions, care must be taken to prevent decubitus ulcers, heel sores, and compression nerve palsies. These precautions are especially true for children with orthopedic procedures, who may be limited in their ability to reposition themselves. These children may be protected by adequate padding of bed rails and nursing instructions for frequent patient turning.

As a final mention of complications, we should remember that the child with combined regional and very light general anesthesia is at risk for intraoperative awareness (76). Therefore, all conversation in the operating room should be pleasant and positive.

REFERENCES

1. McGrath PJ, Johnson G, Goodman JT, et al: CHEOPS: a behavioral scale for rating post-operative pain in children. In: Fields HL, Dubner R, Cervero F (eds). *Advances in pain research and therapy,* vol 9. New York: Raven Press 1985:395–402.

2. Lynn AM, Slattery JT: Morphine pharmacokinetics in early infancy. *Anesthesiology* 1987;66:136–139.
3. Lynn AM, Opheim KE, Tyler DC: Morphine infusion after pediatric cardiac surgery. *Crit Care Med* 1984;12:863–866.
4. Moores MA, Wandless JG, Fell D: Paediatric postoperative analgesia: A comparison of rectal diclofenac with caudal bupivacaine after inguinal herniotomy. *Anaesthesia* 1990;45:156–158.
5. Watcha MF, Jones MB, Lagueruela RG, et al: Comparison of ketorolac and morphine as adjuvants during pediatric surgery. *Anesthesiology* 1992;76:368–372.
6. Maunuksela EL, Kokki H, Bullingham RE: Clinical Trials and Therapeutics: comparison of intravenous ketorolac with morphine for postoperative pain in children. *Clin Pharmacol Ther* 1992;52:436–443.
7. Houck CS, Wilder RT, McDermott, Berde CB: Intravenous ketorolac in children following surgery: safety and cost savings with a unit dose system. *Anesthesiology* 1993;79:A1137.
8. Wolf AR, Valley RD, Fear DW, et al: Bupivacaine for caudal analgesia in infants and children: the optimal effective concentration. *Anesthesiology* 1988;69:102–106.
9. Warner MA, Kunkel SE, Offord KO, et al: The effects of age, epinephrine, and operative site on duration of caudal analgesia in pediatric patients. *Anesth Analg* 1987;66:995–998.
10. Desparmet J, Mateo J, Ecoffey C, Mazoit X: Efficacy of an epidural test dose in children anesthetized with halothane. *Anesthesiology* 1990;72:249–251.
11. Jensen BH: Caudal block for post-operative pain relief in children after genital operations. A comparison between bupivacaine and morphine. *Acta Anaesth Scand* 1981;25:373–375.
12. Krane EJ, Jacobson LE, Lynn AM, et al: Caudal morphine for postoperative analgesia in children: a comparison with caudal bupivacaine and intravenous morphine. *Anesth Analg* 1987;66:647–653.
13. Krane EJ: Delayed respiratory depression in a child after caudal epidural morphine. *Anesth Analg* 1988;67:79–82.
14. Shandling B, Steward DJ: Regional analgesia for postoperative pain in pediatric outpatient surgery. *J Pediatr Surg* 1980;15:477–480.
15. Hannallah RS, Broadman LM, Belman AB, et al: Comparison of caudal and ilioinguinal/iliohypogastric nerve blocks for control of post-orchiopexy pain in pediatric ambulatory surgery. *Anesthesiology* 1987;66:832–834.
16. Broadman LM, Hannallah RS, Belman AB, et al: Postcircumcision analgesia: a prospective evaluation of subcutaneous ring block of the penis. *Anesthesiology* 1987;67:399–402.
17. Soliman MG, Tremblay NA: Nerve block of the penis for postoperative pain relief in children *Anesth Analg* 1978;57:495–498.
18. Vater M, Wandless J: Caudal or dorsal nerve block? A comparison of two local anesthetic techniques for postoperative analgesia following day case circumcision. *Acta Anaesthesiol Scand* 1985;29:175–179.
19. Tree-Trakarn T, Pirayavaraporn S: Postoperative pain relief for circumcision in children: comparison among morphine, nerve block and topical analgesia. *Anesthesiology* 1985;62:519–522.
20. Tree-Trakarn T, Pirayavaraporn S, Lertakyamanee J: Topical analgesia for relief of post-circumcision pain. *Anesthesiology* 1987;67:395–399.

21. Winnie AP, Colins VJ: The subclavian perivascular technique of brachial plexus anesthesia. *Anesthesiology* 1964;25:353–363.
22. Winnie AP: Interscalene brachial plexus block. *Anesth Analg* 1970;49:455–466.
23. Al-Khafaji JM, Ellias MA: Incidence of Horner syndrome with interscalene brachial plexus block and its importance in the management of head injury. *Anesthesiology* 1986;64:127.
24. Dalens BJ: Section 1: Upper limb blocks. In: Dalens BJ (ed). *Pediatric regional anesthesia*. Boca Raton: CRC Press. 1990:205–281.
25. Dalens B, Vanneuville G, Tanguy A: A new parascalene approach to the brachial plexus in children: comparison with the supraclavicular approach. *Anesth Analg* 1987;66:1264–1271.
26. Partridge BL, Katz J, Bernirschke J: Functional anatomy of the brachial plexus sheath: implications for anesthesia. *Anesthesiology* 1987;66:743–747.
27. Rosenblatt R, Pepitone-Rockwell F, McKillop MJ: Continuous axillary analgesia for traumatic hand injury. *Anesthesiology* 1979;51:565–566.
28. Chayen D, Nathan K Chayen M: The psoas compartment block. *Anesthesiology* 1976;45:95–99.
29. McNicol LR: Lower limb blocks for children. Lateral cutaneous and femoral nerve blocks for postoperative pain relief in paediatric practice. *Anaesthesia*. 1986;41:27–31.
30. Sharrock NE: Inadvertent "3-in-1 block" following injection of the lateral cutaneous nerve of the thigh. *Anesth Analg* 1980;59:887–888.
31. Rosenblatt RM: Continuous femoral anesthesia for lower extremity surgery. *Anesth Analg* 1980;59:631–632.
32. Dalens B, Vanneuville G, Tanguy A: Comparison of the fascia iliaca compartment block with the 3-in-1 block in children. *Anesth Analg* 1989;69:705–713.
33. Winnie AP, Ramamurthy S, Durrani Z: The inguinal paravascular technic of lumbar plexus anesthesia: the "3-in-1 block." *Anesth Analg* 1973;52:989–996.
34. Dalens BJ: Blocks of nerves of the lower lumbar plexus supplying the lower extremities. In: Dalens BJ (ed). *Pediatric regional anesthesia*. Boca Raton: CRC Press, 1990:283–311.
35. Dalens B, Tanguy A, Vanneuville G: Sciatic nerve blocks in children: comparison of the posterior, anterior, and lateral approaches in 180 pediatric patients. *Anesth Analg* 1990;70:131–137.
36. Fitzgerald B: Intravenous regional anaesthesia in children. *Br J Anaesth* 1976;48:485–486.
37. Rosenberg PR, Heavner JE: Multiple and complementary mechanisms produce analgesia during intravenous regional anesthesia. *Anesthesiology* 1985;62:840–841.
38. Juliano PJ, Mazur JM, Cummings RJ, McCloskey WP: Low dose lidocaine intravenous regional anesthesia forearm fractures in children. *J Fed Orthop* 1992;12:633–635.
39. Bolte RG, Stevens PM, Scott SM, Schunk JE: Mini-dose Bier block intravenous regional anesthesia in the emergency department treatment of pediatric upper-extremity injuries. *J Fed Orthop* 1994;14:534–537.
40. Murrell D, Gibson PR, Cohen RC: Continuous epidural analgesia in newborn infants undergoing major surgery. *J Pediatr Surg* 1993;28:548–652.
41. Wood CE, Goresky GV, Klassen KA, et al: Complications of continuous epidural infusions for postoperative analgesia in children. *Can J Anaesth* 1994;41:7:613–620.

42. Guinand JP, Borbeen M: Probable venous air embolism during caudal anesthesia in a child. *Anesth Analg* 1993; 76:1134–1135.
43. Schwartz N, Eisenkraft JP: Probable venous air embolism during epidural placement in an infant. *Anesth Analg* 1993;76:1136–1138.
44. Matsumiya N, Dohi S, Takahashi H, et al: Cardiovascular collapse in an infant after caudal anesthesia with a lidocaine-epinephrine solution. *Anesth Analg* 1986;65:1074–1076.
45. Agarwal R, Gutlove DP, Lockhart CH: Seizures occurring in pediatric patients receiving continuous infusion of bupivacaine. *Anesth Analg* 1992;75:284–286.
46. McCloskey JJ, Haun SE, Deshpande JK: Bupivacaine toxicity secondary to continuous caudal epidural infusion in children. *Anesth Analg* 1992;75:287–290.
47. Ved SA, Pinosky M, Nicodemus H: Ventricular tachycardia and brief cardiovascular collapse in two infants after caudal anesthesia using a bupivacaine-epinephrine solution. *Anesthesiology* 1993;79:1121–1123.
48. Freid EB, Bailey AG, Valley RD: Electrocardiographic and hemodynamic changes associated with unintentional intravascular injection of bupivacaine with epinephrine in infants. *Anesthesiology* 1993;79:394–398.
49. Darrow EJ, Badgwell JM, Heavner JE, Reese S: Bupivacaine and epinephrine act synergistically to produce ventricular arrhythmias in young pigs. *Anesthesiology* 1994;81:A1357.
50. Desparmet J, Mateo J, Ecoffey C, Mazoit X: Efficacy of an epidural test dose in children anesthetized with halothane. *Anesthesiology* 1990;72:249–251.
51. Mather LE, Long GJ, Thomas J: The intravenous toxicity and clearance of bupivacaine in man. *Clin Pharmacol Ther* 1971;12:935–943.
52. Mazoit JX, Denson DD, Samii K: Pharmocokinetics of bupivacaine following caudal anesthesia in infants. *Anesthesiology* 1988;68:387–391.
53. Desparmet J, Meistelman C, Barre J, Saint-Maurice C: Continuous epidural infusion of bupivacaine for postoperative pain relief in children. *Anesthesiology* 1987;67:108–110.
54. Rice LJ, Broadman LM: Caudal anesthesia and cardiovascular collapse in an infant. *Anesth Analg* 1987;66:694.
55. Rolf N, Coté CJ: Persistent cardiac arrhythmias in pediatric patients: effects of age, expired carbon dioxide values, depth of anesthesia, and airway management. *Anesth Analg* 1991;73:720–724.
56. Cohen M, Cameron C, Duncan P: Pediatric anesthesia morbidity and mortality in the perioperative period. *Anesth Analg* 1990;70:160–167.
57. Badgwell JM, Heavner JE, Kytta J: Bupivacaine toxicity in young pigs is age dependent and is affected by volatile anesthetics. *Anesthesiology* 1990;73:297–303.
58. Heavner JE, Dryden CF Jr, Sanghani V, et al: Severe hypoxia enhances central nervous system and cardiovascular toxicity of bupivacaine in lightly anesthetized pigs. *Anesthesiology* 1992;77:142–147.
59. Heavner JE, Badgwell JM, Dryden CF Jr, Flinders C: Bupivacaine toxicity in lightly anesthetized pigs with respiratory imbalances plus or minus halothane. *Reg Anesth* 1995;20:1:20–26.
60. Heavner JE, Arthur J, Zou J, et al: Comparison of propofol with thiopentone for treatment of bupivaciane-induced seizures in rats. *Br J Anaesth* 1993;71:715–719.
61. Maxwell LG, Martin LD, Yaster M: Bupivacaine-induced cardiac toxicity in neonates: successful treatment with intravenous phenytoin. *Anesthesiology* 1994;80:682–686.
62. American Heart Association: *Textbook of advanced cardiac life support.* Dallas American Heart Association, 1987.
63. Heavner JE, Mather LE, Pitkanen M, Shi B: Should epinephrine be used to treat local anesthetic-induced cardiotoxicity? *Anesthesiology* 1994;80:1179–1180.
64. Feldman HS, Arthur GR, Pitkanen M, et al: Treatment of acute systemic toxicity after the rapid intravenous injection of ropivacaine and bupivacaine in the conscious dog. *Anesth Analg* 1991;73:373–384.
65. Heavner JE, Pitkanen MT, Shi B, Rosenberg PH: Resuscitation from bupivacaine-induced asystole in rats: comparison of different cardioactive drugs. *Anesth Analg* 1995;80:1134–1139.
66. Lawhorn CD, Brown RE Jr.: Epidural morphine with butorphanol in pediatric patients. *J Clin Anesthesiol* 1994;6:91–94.
67. Lee JJ, Rubin AP: Comparison of a bupivacaine-clonidine mixture with plain bupivacaine for caudal analgesia in children. *Br J Anaesth* 1994;72:258–262.
68. Schaub L, Badgwell JM, Mian T: Continuous brachial plexus blockade in a child. *Pain Sympt Manag* 1991;6:164.
69. Rigler ML, Drasner K, Krejcie TC, et al: Cauda equina syndrome after continuous spinal anesthesia. *Anesth Analg* 1991;72:275–281.
70. Payne KA, Moore SW: Subarachnoid microcatheter anesthesia in small children. *Reg Anesth* 1994;4:237–242.
71. Broadman LM: Pediatric regional anesthesia. *Clin Anesth Updates* 1992;3:2:1–14.
72. Wolf AR, Valley RD, Fear DW, et al: Bupivacaine for caudal analgesia in infants and children: the optimal effective concentration. *Anesthesiology* 1988;69:102–106.
73. Lejus C, Roussiere G, Testa S, et al: Postoperative extradural analgesia in children: comparison of morphine with fentanyl. *Br J Anaesth* 1994;72:156–159.
74. Abajian JC, Mellish RW, Browne AF, et al: Spinal anesthesia for surgery in the high-risk infant. *Anesth Analg* 1984;63:359–362.
75. Welborn LG, Rice LJ, Hannallah RS, et al: Postoperative apnea in former preterm infants: prospective comparison of spinal and general anesthesia. *Anesthesiology* 1990;72:838–842.
76. Standen PJ, Hain WR, Hosker KJ: Retention of auditory information presented during anaesthesia: a study of children who received light general anaesthesia. *Anaesthesia* 1987;42:604–608.

11

Anesthesia for Procedures in and around the Airway

Lynne Ferrari

"I have just returned from Boston. It is the only thing to do if you find yourself up there."
—Fred Allen

The anesthetic management of the child who is having surgical procedures in the airway is particularly challenging. The restricted spaces of the pediatric airway require an understanding of airway dynamics, anatomy, and physiology as well as the use of specialized equipment. Perhaps more than any other surgery, procedures in the airway require communication and cooperation between surgeon and anesthesiologist.

ANESTHESIA FOR TONSILLECTOMY AND ADENOIDECTOMY

If you are caring for children, you are doing lots of tonsillectomies. Tonsillectomies are one of the most frequently performed procedures in the United States today (1). Tonsils are removed for treatment of chronic or recurrent tonsillitis, peritonsillar abscess, and obstructive tonsillar hyperplasia (2). Tonsils are frequently removed in children with valvular heart problems, since recurrent bacteremia secondary to infected tonsils increases the risk of endocarditis. Children requiring tonsillectomies often have more serious concomitant conditions such as chronic airway obstruction resulting in obstructive sleep apnea, CO_2 retention, cor pulmonale, failure to thrive, swallowing disorders, and speech abnormalities (3).

Large amounts of adenoidal tissue (which may or may not accompany large tonsils) present their own set of problems. Nasopharyngeal obstruction due to adenoidal hyperplasia may result in failure to thrive, speech disorders, obligate mouth breathing, and orofacial deformity including dental abnormalities. Although removal of the adenoids is usually accompanied by tonsillectomy, chronic or recurrent purulent adenitis and recurrent otitis media with effusion secondary to adenoidal hyperplasia are often treated by adenoidectomy alone.

Preoperative Considerations

Parents should be questioned for the presence of a recent upper respiratory infection, tonsillitis, current use of antibiotics, antihistamines, or other medicines, especially over-the-counter medications, which might contain aspirin or aspirin-like compounds. The physical examination should begin with observation of the patient, especially noting the presence of audible respiration, mouth breathing, nasal quality of the speech, and chest retractions. Children scheduled for tonsillectomy and adenoidectomy are often mouth breathers and have long faces, retrognathic mandibles, and high arched palates—the result of chronic nasopharyngeal obstruction (4). Extension of inflammation into the lower respiratory tract may produce edema and bronchospasm. Therefore, wheezing, rales, or stridor heard on chest auscultation may indicate airway obstruction from either bronchospasm or hypertrophied tonsils and adenoids.

The importance of laboratory examination is constantly being reevaluated. Documentation of preoperative hematocrit and coagulation parameters, however, is still valid. Many nonprescription cold medications and antihistamines contain aspirin, which may affect platelet function. Chest radiographs and electrocardiograms are not required unless specific history of abnormalities in these areas is elicited, such as recent pneumonia, bronchitis, upper respiratory infection, or history consistent with obstructive sleep apnea or cor pulmonale.

Obstructive Sleep Apnea

"He was a tubby little chap who looked as if he had been poured into his clothes and had forgotten to say when!"

—P.G. Wodehouse

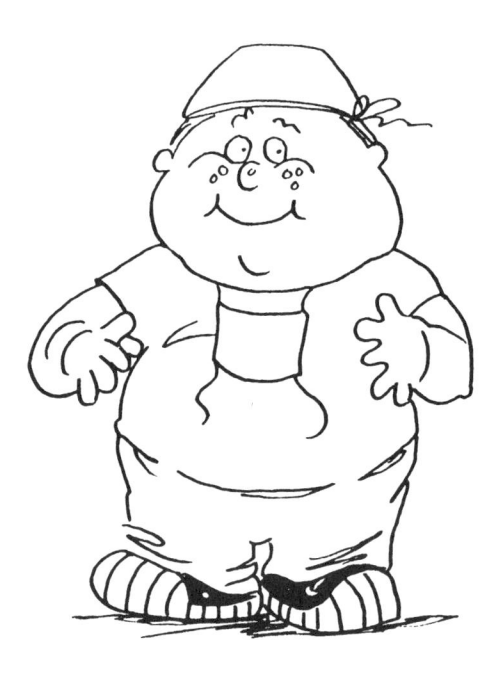

Apnea in the pediatric population usually brings to mind premature and ex-premature infants. Older infants and children, however, may develop apneic episodes during sleep as a result of tonsillar hypertrophy, commonly known as obstructive sleep apnea (OSA) (5). Some children with OSA have normal size tonsils. Children with OSA may have a range of symptoms from relatively benign mouth breathing and snoring at night to a full-blown Pickwickian syndrome. The following are common signs of OSA:

- Obesity
- Cor pulmonale
- Daytime somnolence
- Night-time snoring and apnea
- Enuresis
- Behavioral problems

Children with OSA usually experience (a) difficulty breathing while awake (despite only mild-to-moderate tonsillar enlargement) and (b) complete but transient airway obstruction during sleep. Children with OSA do not sleep well at night and may be grumpier than the average child during the day, a tip-off that the child has more serious complications (e.g., cor pulmonale).

The diagnosis of sleep apnea syndrome will probably have been made by the otolaryngologist or the child's pediatrician. The diagnosis of sleep apnea syndrome is confirmed by the presence of one or more of the following findings during graphic recordings of respiration during a period of natural sleep: Apnea determined by complete cessation of airflow on auscultation, oxygen desaturation (measured by pulse oximetry) to less than 90%, obstructive apnea determined by the absence of respiration for a minimum of 10 seconds accompanied by paradoxic movement of the rib cage and abdomen, and nasopharyngoscopic or cinefluoroscopic documented upper airway obstruction (6). For the anesthesiologist, it is merely a matter of asking the right questions. However, there are some tip-offs such as the following when the diagnosis is suspected but not confirmed.

- Labored respiration, especially during sleep (when pharyngeal muscles are relaxed)
- Obesity (a compounding factor in two thirds of patients with obstructive sleep apnea)
- Behavioral disturbances (from lack of sleep at night)
- Snoring (probably the best predictor of OSA)

Cor Pulmonale

"It ain't over till it's over."

—Yogi Berra

Pulmonary hypertension and cor pulmonale are the most critical complications associated with OSA (7,8). *Surgery does not immediately solve problems associated with cor pulmonale.* The child's physiology gradually returns to normal in the postoperative period (9). A review of the physiology of OSA will help to explain why this is true.[a]

Physiology of Upper Airway Obstruction

Chronic Alveolar Hypoventilation. The physiology of upper airway obstruction leading to cor pulmonale is well known (10–12). Upper airway obstruction with decreased minute volume ventilation, whether intermittent or continuous, leads to pulmonary ventilation-perfusion abnormalities and chronic alveolar hypoventilation. Hypercapnia and hypoxia ensue, which cause respiratory acidemia resulting in pulmonary artery vasoconstriction. This, in turn, leads to increased right ventricular work and cardiac hypertrophy. Continued pulmonary artery hypertension causes right ventricular dilation, followed by eventual failure and cor pulmonale.

Pulmonary Vasoconstriction. Pulmonary vasoconstriction in response to respiratory acidemia occurs by means of two mechanisms: (a) acute vasoconstriction, which occurs within minutes, and (b) long-term structural remodeling of the pulmonary vascular bed with hypertrophy of the muscle of the medium and small pulmonary arteries.

The acute vasoconstriction phase is reversible, but many features of the long-term muscular hypertrophy are not. Thus, even with relief of upper airway obstruction, some cases of pulmonary artery hypertension may not be completely reversible (12). Increased PCO_2 levels may persist after relief of upper airway obstruction (13). This increase suggests either fatigue or training of the respiratory control center to increased PCO_2 levels, which may represent a form of tachyphylaxis to chronic hypercapnia. The chronically hyposensitized respiratory center can require time (up to 4 days or longer) to regain normal responsiveness to CO_2 after relief of upper airway obstruction (14).

Resetting the Respiratory Control Center. It is well established that patients with chronic hypercapnia have a respiratory center that is stimulated primarily by hypoxia. Administration of oxygen with removal of the hypoxic drive in these patients abolishes the stimulus to ventilation. This can result in respiratory arrest (10,11,15,16). Children with severe cor pulmonale and CO_2 retention secondary to tonsil and adenoid hypertrophy fall into this category. Relief of upper airway obstruction does not immediately change the chronically sensitized respiratory center, and administration of oxygen to these patients can result in respiratory arrest.

Management Recommendations. The preceding information has led to the formulation of management recommendations based on the abnormal physiology of these patients (Fig. 1). Patients with severe OSA and resultant cor pulmonale are evaluated preoperatively with an arterial blood gas. Patients with normal PCO_2 (~35 to 45 mm Hg) are defined as mild cor pulmonale, and those with increased PCO_2 (>50 mm Hg) are defined as severe cor pulmonale. All patients are admitted preoperatively for an anesthesia consultation and treated for their cor pulmonale appropriately. After tonsillectomy/adenoidectomy, patients with elevated PCO_2 levels may be left intubated and ventilated mechanically in the intensive care unit (ICU) until the PCO_2 level has normalized.[b] These patients are then carefully extubated and observed. Alternately, pa-

---

[a]Ed. Note (JMB): It is interesting that children with OSA are not necessarily obese, one third of them being normal or small for age (5).

[b]Ed. Note (JMB): These recommendations are based on published otolaryngology literature (17). In terms of keeping patients with high PCO_2 intubated postoperatively, these recommendations may be a bit aggressive (or, conservative, depending on your point of view) than many of us actually practice. The point, however, is well taken. Kids with OSA and severe cor pulmonale need special attention.

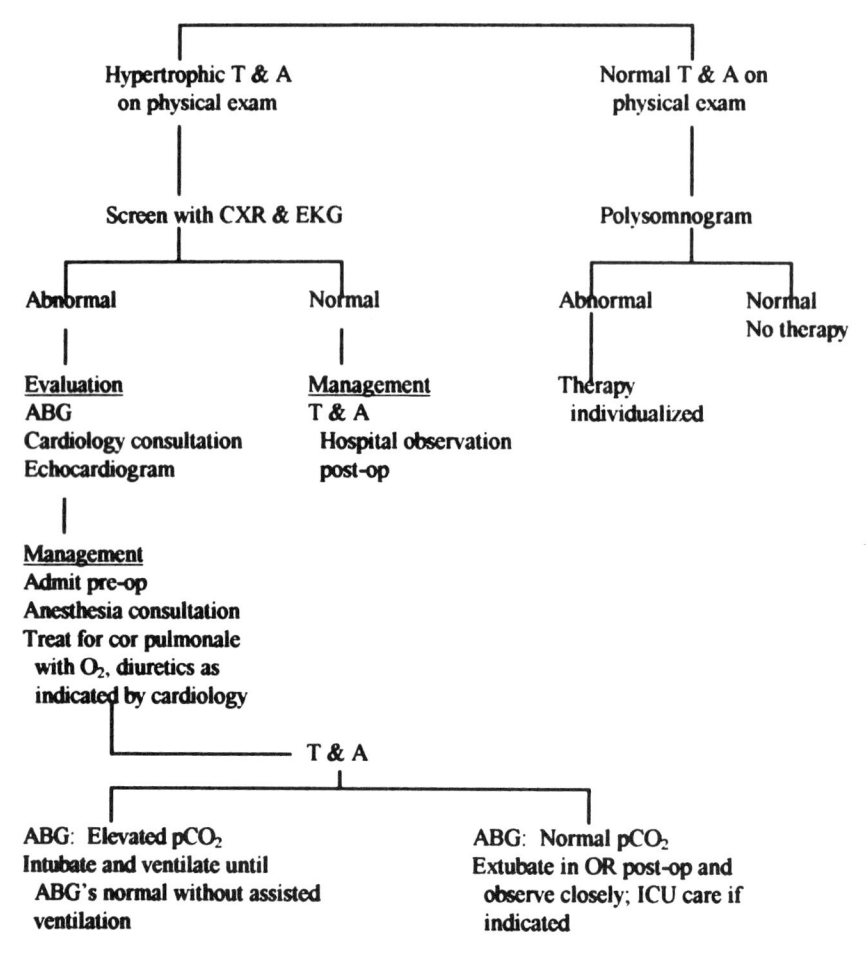

```
                    Hypertrophic T & A                       Normal T & A on
                    on physical exam                         physical exam
                           |                                        |
                    Screen with CXR & EKG                    Polysomnogram
                    ┌──────┴──────┐                          ┌──────┴──────┐
                Abnormal        Normal                   Abnormal         Normal
                    |              |                         |         No therapy
                Evaluation     Management                 Therapy
                ABG            T & A                      individualized
                Cardiology consultation   Hospital observation
                Echocardiogram            post-op
                    |
                Management
                Admit pre-op
                Anesthesia consultation
                Treat for cor pulmonale
                with O₂, diuretics as
                indicated by cardiology
                    └──────────────── T & A
                                ┌──────┴──────┐
                    ABG: Elevated pCO₂           ABG: Normal pCO₂
                    Intubate and ventilate until Extubate in OR post-op and
                    ABG's normal without assisted observe closely; ICU care if
                    ventilation                  indicated
```

FIG. 1. Recommendations from the otolaryngology literature for the management of the patient with a history of obstructive sleep apnea. (The editors feel that postoperative airway management with continued intubation in the patient with elevated PCO₂ is an *option* that should be considered, but is not mandatory in all such cases.) (Reprinted with permission, from International Journal of Pediatric Otorhinolaryngology, Vol. 16, Brown OE, Manning SC, Ridenour B / Cor pulmonale secondary to tonsillar and adenoidal hypertrophy: management considerations, p. 138, 1988, with kind permission from Elsevier Science Ireland Ltd, Bay 15 K, Shannon Industrial Estate, Co. Clare, Ireland.)

tients (particularly those with normal PCO₂ levels) may be extubated in the operating room postoperatively and closely observed. If there is any respiratory distress, they are reintubated and managed as patients with severe cor pulmonale.

Neurocognitive Defects in OSA

Children with OSA also may have neurocognitive defects and seizure disorders, the result of a variable degree of asphyxial brain injury during apneic episodes. Therefore, it is very important to document the child's neurocognitive skills and seizure status before surgery so that a decrement in the child's neurologic status is not attributed to a lack of anesthetic skill.

ANESTHETIC MANAGEMENT

The following are anesthetic goals for tonsillectomy and adenoidectomy:

- Induce unconsciousness in an atraumatic manner.

- Provide a quiet surgical field.
- Secure intravenous (IV) access to provide fluids and medications.
- Produce rapid emergence from anesthesia.
- Awaken the patient with reflexes intact.
- Protect the airway after surgery.

Premedication may be given at the discretion of the anesthesiologist. *Children with OSA, very large tonsils, or intermittent obstructive symptoms may occasionally receive sedative premedication, but they should be closely observed after administration of the premedication.* An oral benzodiazepine with or without antisialagogue is effective premedication for frightened children. Sedative premedication with midazolam often enhances a smooth transition to unconsciousness, preventing crying and struggling, which may be especially hazardous in an already compromised airway. Parental presence in selected cases may also help to provide a smooth induction of anesthesia **(see Chapter 2)**.

Induction of Anesthesia for Tonsillectomy

Anesthesia may be induced by means of a volatile agent, oxygen, and nitrous oxide by mask or by use of an IV agent. How does one decide what each child should get? Most of the time the decision is made for you. If you're lucky, the child will already have a line in place at the beginning of induction. Then, an IV induction including preoxygenation can be easily done. Preoxygenation is done so that if obstruction occurs, there is more time to comfortably manage the airway.

On the other hand, there are certain 3- to 5-year-old children who are scheduled for tonsillectomy who are not cooperative, who won't let you start an IV line, and for whom an inhalation induction can be the only method of induction. These children can be a real challenge. The administration of oral midazolam may be effective in calming the child and smoothing out the induction. Even when all goes well, children with large tonsillar and adenoidal tissues develop upper airway obstruction very soon after induction. Usually, this problem can be managed by the placement of an oral airway, but insertion of airway insertion presents a twofold problem: (a) getting the patient deep enough to tolerate the oral airway and (b) managing airway obstruction if it occurs **(see also Chapter 2)**.

In the best circumstances, inductions for tonsillectomy in children may be difficult and should be done in the operating room with the surgeon standing by ready to help if an emergency airway is deemed necessary. Placing a small amount of local anesthetic on the tongue after induction may anesthetize the tongue and oral pharynx so that the child will tolerate an oral airway at lighter levels of anesthesia.

The inhalation induction of anesthesia begins with relatively high-flow nitrous oxide and oxygen, then a slow increase of halothane or sevoflurane, and decreasing the nitrous oxide. As a general rule, when 3% inspired halothane is achieved, nitrous oxide is turned off. IV insertion is accomplished as soon as the patient will tolerate venipuncture.

After the successful placement of an IV, there are two options open to the anesthesiologist. One is to continue the inhalation induction and eventually intubate under deep volatile anesthetic agent. Alternatively, IV anesthetic agents and muscle relaxants can be used to facilitate intubation. To augment either inhalation or IV techniques, lidocaine can be applied topically to the larynx and vocal cords, that is, with 5 mg/kg lidocaine using either (a) 4% lidocaine by a 3-ml syringe and no. 22 needle (bent at a 45-degree angle) or a 22-gauge plastic IV catheter injected around the tonsillar bed or (b) a 10% lidocaine atomizer (1 puff = 10 mg; therefore a 10-kg child may receive 5 puffs).

Despite endotracheal intubation, blood in the pharynx may enter the trachea during the surgical procedure. Aspiration of blood and saliva may be minimized by doing the following:

- Packing the supraglottic area with petroleum gauze
- Inserting a cuffed endotracheal tube

- Inserting an endotracheal tube that does not allow a peritracheal leak.[c]

Blood and secretions present in the oral pharynx may be suctioned at the conclusion of surgery while the child is deeply anesthetized. Likewise, gastric decompression with an oral gastric tube may be performed at the end of surgery while the patient is deeply anesthetized to relieve gastric distention and remove any blood that may have entered the stomach during surgery. Blood in the stomach is a rare finding at the conclusion of tonsillectomy, unless there is a bleeding tonsil **(see Deep Extubation)**. By contrast, removal of gas may help to prevent postoperative nausea and vomiting.

Extubation

Intact airway reflexes are of utmost importance in preventing aspiration, laryngospasm, and airway obstruction. Which extubation technique—awake or deep—is most appropriate for children after tonsillectomy? (Also, see **Chapter 6** for further discussion of awake versus deep extubation.)

Deep Extubation. If important caveats are considered, children's tracheas following tonsillectomy may be extubated while the children are deeply anesthetized. "Deep extubation" is a colloquial expression describing tracheal extubation while a patient is deeply anesthetized but spontaneously breathing. If performed correctly, this method of tracheal extubation decreases the likelihood that tracheal stimulation by the endotracheal tube will cause coughing or bucking. Extubating the trachea under a deep plane of anesthesia allows the child to wake up gradually and smoothly. Obviously, this technique for extubation does not completely eliminate the risk of coughing, aspiration, and laryngospasm.

The most important key to successful deep extubation is the training of those involved in the patient's postoperative care. For example, the postanesthesia care unit nurses are required to be proficient in airway management of children, especially those who have been extubated during a deep plane of anesthesia. Nurses must be trained to not suction the oropharynx (unless absolutely necessary) and to not stimulate the patient, but rather to allow the patient to awake spontaneously and peacefully. Nurses should be instructed that children may still develop airway complications, but by allowing children to awaken peacefully without stimulation or suction, children should awake without these complications.

In general, it is advisable not to do a deep extubation after tonsillectomy in children who have OSA. Although the tonsils have been removed, the CO_2 response curve has not been reset. Therefore, these children will not respond to hypercarbia and may only respond to hypoxemia, if at all. Therefore, children with OSA who are to be extubated should be extubated when fully awake. Furthermore, posthypoxic-postobstructive pulmonary edema may occur as a result of unintentional premature extubation followed by laryngospasm and pulmonary edema. Efforts to prevent this problem include allowing the child to awaken peacefully.

Peacefully Awake Extubation. This peaceful awakening is an awake extubation technique preceded by topical application of local anesthetics to the tonsillar bed **(see Induction of Anesthesia for Tonsillectomy)**. Furthermore, a dose of IV lidocaine (1.5 mg/kg) is administered at the end of the tonsillectomy to further attenuate adverse airway responses. As a part of this peaceful awakening technique, the anesthesiologist is advised not to perform suction of the oropharynx but rather to lay the child on the side of the gurney in the time-honored tonsil position (lateral position with the head slightly down). At that point, one merely waits it out. During the waiting-out period, the anesthesiologist should be ever present to manage airway complications, if

---

[c]Ed. Note (JMB): It is well known that most pediatric anesthesiologists have traditionally insisted on a peritracheal gas leak. Others feel that a leak is not necessarily dangerous. It appears that this would be one instance in which a leak may place the patient at a disadvantage.

they occur. Postanesthesia care unit nurses are given the same set of instructions regarding suction and stimulation precautions as for deep extubation.

It should be noted also that children with cleft palate are very amenable to a peaceful awakening extubation. Children with cleft palate, like those with OSA, are better off if they did not go through the trial of a deep extubation. During the cleft palate procedure, many of the tissues are edematous and swollen, and therefore many of the same airway problems are present as they are with post-tonsillectomy patients.

Tonsillectomy and Adenoidectomy: Outpatient or Inpatient?

Although outpatient (same-day discharge) tonsillectomy and adenoidectomy may be safely and appropriately performed, the ultimate decision as to an inpatient or outpatient setting is a medical one and must be left to the attending anesthesiologist and responsible surgeon. Table 1 lists some of the conditions that may warrant overnight observation in an appropriate hospital setting after tonsillectomy and adenoidectomy (18).

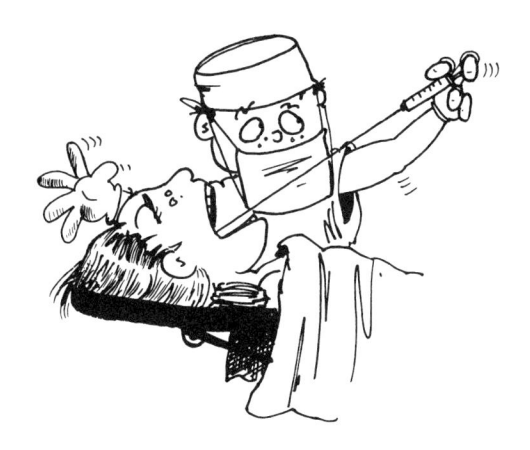

Complications

Pain

Pain is usually minimal after adenoidectomy but may be severe after tonsillectomy. Postoperative pain is decreased by instillation of local anesthesia intraoperatively. Infiltration of the peritonsillar space with local anesthetic and epinephrine not only provides postoperative analgesia, but also it has been shown to be effective in reducing intraoperative blood loss (19–21). Furthermore, infiltration with local anesthesia has been shown to produce a pre-

TABLE 1. *Tonsillectomy and adenoidectomy inpatient guidelines*

Recommendations of the American Academy of Otolaryngology—Head and Neck Surgery Pediatric Otolaryngology Committee

Condition 1.	Age 3 years or less
Condition 2.	Abnormal coagulation values with or without an identified bleeding disorder in the patient or family
Condition 3.	Evidence of obstructive sleep disorder or apnea due to tonsil or adenoidal hypertrophy
Condition 4.	Systemic disorders that put the patient at increased preoperative cardiopulmonary, metabolic, or general medical risk
Condition 5.	Child with craniofacial or other airway abnormalities including, but not limited to, syndromic disorders such as Treacher Collins syndrome, Crouzon's syndrome, Goldenhar's syndrome, Pierre Robin anomalad, C.H.A.R.G.E. association, achondroplasia, and most prominently, Down's syndrome, as well as isolated airway abnormalities such as choanal atresia and laryngotracheal stenosis
Condition 6.	When the procedure is being done for acute peritonsillar abscess
Condition 7.	When extended travel time, weather conditions, and home social conditions are not consistent with close observation, cooperativeness, and ability to return to the hospital quickly at the discretion of the attending physician

(Reproduced with permission, from Brown OE, Cunningham MJ: Tonsillectomy and Adenoidectomy In Patient Guidelines: Recommendations of the AAO-HNS Pediatric Otolaryngology Comitee. American Academy of Otolaryngology—Head and Neck Surgery Bulletin. September 1996, p. 13.)

emptive analgesia that may provide pain-free recovery for up to 1 week (22).

Postoperative pain management is still an uncertain problem in these children who have had tonsillectomy, especially those with OSA. Many feel that narcotics may depress the patient's ability to ventilate; therefore, the classic story is to avoid narcotics so that patients can breathe better. However, that leaves these children in considerable discomfort, which nonsteroidal anti-inflammatory drugs (NSAIDs) will not manage. Therefore, in the postoperative period, as the child awakens, doses of morphine in 0.05 mg/kg increments may be titrated. NSAIDs are avoided because of their potential to cause increased bleeding. Patients with a history of OSA should be admitted to the hospital rather than have their pain undertreated. If there is a question of sleep apnea, they are kept in an ambulatory surgery unit for approximately 4 hours after surgery until the level of consciousness, and so on, allows a joint decision by anesthesiologists and otolaryngologists as to whether or not the child can be discharged.

The Bleeding Tonsil

"Perhaps catastrophe is the natural human environment, and even though we spend a good deal of energy trying to get away from it, we are programmed for survival amid catastrophe."
—Germaine Greer

The most serious complication of tonsillectomy is postoperative hemorrhage which occurs in 0.1% to 8.1% of patients[d] (23). Approximately 75% of postoperative tonsillar hemorrhage occurs within 6 hours of surgery. The remaining 25% occurs within the first 24 hours of surgery, although occasionally bleeding may be noted on the sixth postoperative day (when the scab breaks free) (24,25). Sixty-seven percent of postoperative bleeding originates in the tonsillar fossa, 27% in the nasopharynx, and 7% in both. Initial attempts to control bleeding may be made using pharyngeal packs and electrocautery. If this fails, patients must return to the operating room for exploration and surgical hemostasis.

Preoperative Evaluation. During post-tonsillectomy hemorrhage, large volumes of blood may be swallowed. Since the amount of blood swallowed is often unknown and can be considerable, blood pressure must be checked with the patient in both the upright and supine positions to assess for orthostatic changes as an indication of decreased intravascular volume.

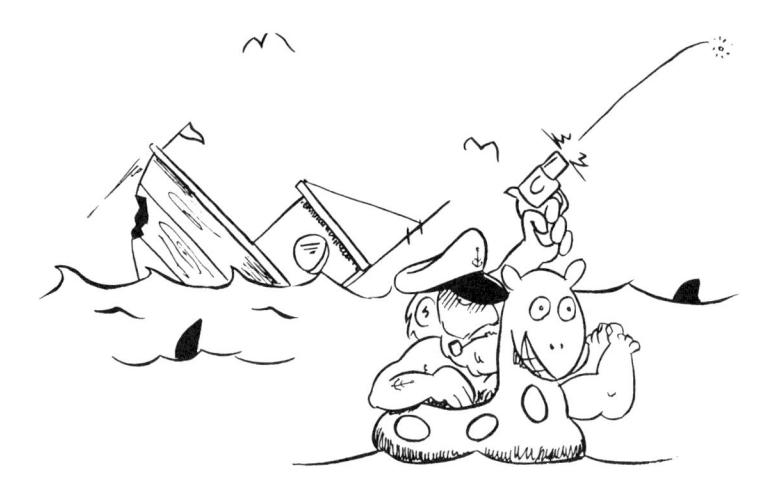

The presence of orthostatic hypotension indicates that blood volume is decreased by 20% to 30%, and supine hypotension indicates blood volume may be decreased by 30% or more. A quick check of the patient's hema-

---

[d]Ed. Note (JMB): I'm glad I don't practice in this latter group.

tocrit only tells us a lot about the ratio of red blood cells to everything else, but very little about intravascular volume. Intravascular volume should be restored with crystalloid, albumin, fresh frozen plasma, or red blood cell therapy until the heart rate has returned to normal and blood pressure is within an acceptable range. The decision to surgically correct post-tonsillectomy bleeding is based on clinical findings. Therefore, the added trauma of a preoperative hematocrit is unnecessary. It is better measured after the child has been anesthetized.

Induction of Anesthesia. A variety of laryngoscope blades and endotracheal tubes as well as suction apparatuses should be prepared in duplicate, since blood in the airway may impair visualization of the vocal cords and cause plugging of the endotracheal tube.

There are a couple of don'ts that are important to remember in dealing with these patients:

- Don't suction the stomach preoperatively. This may dislodge a clot and increase bleeding.
- Don't overlook preexisting conditions (e.g., asthma).

Induction of anesthesia begins with a consideration of full stomach (remember all the blood that was swallowed). Therefore, a rapid-sequence induction accompanied by cricoid pressure and a styletted endotracheal tube are essential. Intravenous access is mandatory in these patients and must be achieved regardless of the circumstances. Intravenous access may be obtained with a small 24-gauge catheter and then a larger vein may be sought intraoperatively. A cut-down of a superficial vein should be performed, if necessary, and even femoral or intraosseous infusion considered. Induction agents appropriate for these children include the following:

- *For the patient who has adequate blood volume and normal blood pressure:* sodium thiopental or propofol used with succinylcholine and rapid-sequence induction, or a nondepolarizing muscle relaxant with ventilation provided during cricoid pressure for a modified rapid-sequence induction.
- *For the patient who has borderline volume status:* ketamine (2 mg/kg) and succinylcholine administered intravenously in a rapid sequence.

It is appropriate to use either a cuffed (26) or uncuffed endotracheal tube in a child with a bleeding tonsil provided an appropriate leak is maintained.[e] Cuff or no cuff, the stomach may be suctioned to remove blood from intraoperative bleeding or bleeding that occurred preoperatively. These patients are probably best extubated awake, but experienced anesthesiologists may choose to perform "deep" extubations after adequate suction of gastric contents.

If bleeding continues postoperatively, one should look for a bleeding diathesis—either von Willebrand's disease or a similar condition. Antifibrinolytic adjuncts, such as DDAVP (desmopressin acetate), have been shown to be helpful, especially in patients who have von Willebrand's disease and persistent bleeding after tonsillectomy. Children who have had a bleeding tonsil repaired should be observed overnight so that further complications may be managed appropriately.

Postoperative Nausea and Vomiting

Nausea and vomiting after tonsillectomy can occur in up to 60% of patients. This is due to the combined effect of irritant blood in the stomach, interference of the gag reflex by edema, and stimulation of receptors af-

---

[e]Ed. Note (JMB): This is one of those areas in which pediatric anesthesiologists like to wax poetically (and controversially). To leak or not to leak, that is the question. I suppose the best advice is to place a tube that goes in easily without trauma and that allows positive-pressure ventilation at appropriate inflating pressures (20 to 30 cm H_2O). If the tube allows an excessive leak (e.g., at pressures lower than desired inflating pressures), it should be replaced with a larger tube. On the other hand, if the tube goes in easily without undue force, but no leak is present, leave it in.

fecting the chemoreceptor trigger zone. Postoperative administration of meperidine increases the probability of emesis, and other analgesic agents should be substituted for it. Antiemetic agents such as droperidol, 0.05 to 0.075 mg/kg, metoclopramide, 0.15 mg/kg, and ondansetron, 0.1 mg/kg, have been effective in controlling postoperative emesis in pediatric patients. Dehydration from poor oral intake as a result of nausea, vomiting, or pain should be offset by vigorous IV hydration during surgery to restore intravascular volume. If children cannot take oral fluids because of vomiting or if vomiting is so severe that it requires frequent administration of antiemetics, admission to the hospital may be indicated.

Special Considerations

Peritonsillar Abscess (Quinsy Tonsil)

Peritonsillar abscess, or quinsy tonsil, is a condition that may require immediate surgical intervention to relieve airway obstruction. An acutely infected tonsil may undergo abscess formation, producing fever, pain, and a large, tense mass in the lateral pharynx, which interferes with swallowing and breathing. Trismus is often an associated finding and is due to inflammation causing limited movement of the muscles of the jaw, face, and neck as well as local nerve compression by the mass itself. Initial treatment consists of needle decompression of the abscess followed by IV antibiotic therapy. If this is ineffective, surgical drainage with or without tonsillectomy and continued antibiotic administration is warranted. Despite the presence of trismus, a rapid-sequence IV induction and intubation may be accomplished since the trismus will resolve after anesthesia. Although the airway may seem severely compromised, the peritonsillar abscess is fixed laterally and usually does not interfere with ventilation of the patient by mask after induction of general anesthesia. Visualization of the vocal cords is not routinely impaired, since the pathology is supraglottic and well above the laryngeal inlet. Laryngoscopy and intubation should be gentle because the tonsillar area is tense and friable; if the abscess is ruptured, spillage of purulent material into the trachea can occur.

Retropharyngeal Abscess

Retropharyngeal abscess requires slightly different anesthetic management than does peritonsillar abscess. Whereas peritonsillar abscess may be drained under local anesthesia, a retropharyngeal abscess requires general anesthesia for surgical drainage. Furthermore, the lesion may compromise the airway and produce large amounts of exudate, especially if ruptured prematurely. In these patients, nasotracheal intubation is contraindicated. The trachea may be intubated under careful direct laryngoscopy.

Special Considerations for Children With Atlantoaxial Instability

Children with Down's syndrome often present for tonsillectomy. In fact, many may have OSA. In one study, 41 of 53 children with Down's syndrome had an abnormal polysomnogram (sleep study) (27). These children are a particular risk because of the well-known association of Down's syndrome and atlantoaxial instability. The laxity of the ligaments of the cervical spine as well as the immaturity of odontoid process in children make them especially prone to C1-C2 subluxation. Up to 31% of patients with Down's syndrome and achondroplasia may have atlantoaxial instability. Surgical intervention in children with atlantoaxial instability places these children at increased risk because of the potential for neurologic injury during neck manipulation (especially extension), which is required for tracheal intubation and positioning during tonsillectomy **(see also pages 400–401).**

Neurologic injury is also of concern in children with short stature syndrome including achondroplastic dwarfs in whom C1-C2 subluxation and stenosis of the spinal canal may be present (28). In this group of children, somatosensory evoked potential monitoring of the upper extremity may be used to evaluate the integrity of sensory conduction (28). In this manner, the neck of the anesthetized child with atlantoaxial instability can be monitored in an effort to minimize jeopardy to the integrity of the cervical spine and associated structures.

OTHER EAR, NOSE, AND THROAT SURGERIES

The anatomy of the ear and its associated structures in children are predisposed to many pathologic conditions that require surgical intervention. General anesthesia for the ear has its own set of unique considerations.

Myringotomy and Placement of Ventilation Tubes

Chronic serous otitis in children can lead to hearing loss, and drainage of accumulated fluid in the middle ear is simple and effective therapy. Myringotomy creates an opening in the tympanic membrane through which fluid can drain. The insertion of a small plastic tube through this incision serves as a stent for the ostium and allows for continued drainage of the middle ear. Myringotomy and tube insertion constitute a relatively short procedure, and anesthesia may be accomplished with a potent inhalation agent—oxygen and nitrous oxide administered by mask. Premedication is not recommended because most sedative drugs used for premedication far outlast the duration of the surgical procedure. The presence of a parent in the operating room during anesthetic induction is often more effective than premedication. Nevertheless, it is acceptable to administer an oral analgesic in the preoperative period in anticipation of postoperative discomfort. Oral acetaminophen with or without codeine administered preoperatively will be absorbed and have its peak effect in the postoperative period when analgesic requirement is greatest (29).

Patients with chronic otitis frequently have accompanying recurrent upper respiratory infections, and eradication of middle ear fluid resolves the concomitant upper respiratory infection. No significant differences in perioperative morbidity exist in children presenting for minor surgery with uncomplicated upper respiratory infection who are having general anesthesia administered by face mask (30). Since endotracheal intubation is avoided, the criteria for cancellation of surgery and anesthesia are unique. If endotracheal anesthesia cannot be avoided, the risk increases significantly. Endotracheal intubation performed in a child with an acute upper respiratory infection increases the risk for perioperative complications such as coughing, laryngospasm, bronchospasm, breath-holding, stridor, and oxygen saturation below 95%; atelectasis increased up to sevenfold (31). It is recommended that children with upper respiratory infection symptoms have oxygen saturation measured by pulse oximetry before induction of general anesthesia and have supplemental oxygen administered postoperatively (32).

Middle Ear and Mastoid Surgery

Tympanoplasty and mastoidectomy are two of the most common otologic procedures performed in children and involve surgical identification and preservation of the facial nerve. This requires isolation of the nerve by the surgeon and verification of its function by means of electrical stimulation. This is both safest and easiest if muscle relaxation is avoided and a volatile agent is the primary anesthetic. If a narcotic-relaxant technique is chosen, however, at least 30% of muscle response, as determined by a twitch monitor, should be preserved. The anesthesiologist must be vigilant in ensuring that damage to nerves, muscles, and bony structures does not occur.

Bleeding must be kept to a minimum during surgery of the small structures of the middle ear. Relative hypotension, keeping the mean arterial pressure 25% below baseline, is effective. When inhaled nitrous oxide is used, it diffuses along a concentration gradient in to air-filled middle ear spaces more rapidly then nitrogen moves out owing to differences in blood solubility (33). During procedures in which the eardrum is replaced or a perforation is patched, nitrous oxide should be discontinued or, if not possible, limited to maximum of 50% before the application of the tympanic membrane graft to avoid pressure-related displacement. After nitrous oxide is discontinued, it is quickly reabsorbed, creating a void in the middle ear with resulting negative pressure. This negative pressure may result in serous otitis, disarticulation of the ossicles in the middle ear, especially the stapes, and hearing impairment, which may last up to 6 weeks postoperatively.

The use of nitrous oxide may cause a high incidence of postoperative nausea and vomiting. This is a direct result of negative middle ear pressure during recovery. The vestibular system is stimulated by traction placed on the round window by the negative pressure that is created. Although all patients have the potential for nausea and vomiting postoperatively, children <8 years of age seem to be most affected. If the use of nitrous oxide cannot be avoided, vigorous use of antiemetics is warranted.

JUVENILE LARYNGEAL PAPILLOMATOSIS

Preoperative Considerations

The most common pediatric laryngeal tumor is papilloma, caused by the human papilloma virus. It is rarely malignant and often regresses spontaneously after puberty. The effects of local invasion, however, warrant prompt treatment. The most common early symptom is hoarseness, and the diagnosis is made by direct laryngoscopy. If left untreated, papillomatosis may result in more severe symptoms of aphonia and respiratory distress. As with all chronic obstructive processes, these conditions may eventually lead to right ventricular hypertrophy, pulmonary hypertension, and cor pulmonale (34). Tracheostomy may be elected to secure the airway in a severely compromised child, but this is a measure of last resort and may cause seeding of papilloma virus to the lower larynx and trachea.

The only effective treatment of papillomatosis is surgical removal of lesions. Lesions may be removed by sharp excision or laser vaporization (35). Despite successful removal of lesions, laryngeal papillomatosis is characterized by numerous relapses and recurrences of papilloma requiring repeated resection. To avoid repeated surgeries, recombinant interferon alfa or ribavirin may be administered (36,37). Because ribavirin can cause anemia, children who have had this therapy should have a preoperative hemoglobin measurement.

Laryngeal scarring, edema, fibrosis, and web formation may occur in children who have had prior laser treatment for papillomatosis (38). Therefore, it is helpful to evaluate airway dynamics and function (if possible) before induction of anesthesia. Prior anesthetic records may be helpful as well, but they might not accurately predict the current respiratory status.

Induction of Anesthesia

Preoperative sedation should be administered carefully (if at all) and the child continuously monitored, since even minimum diminution of pharyngeal tone and respiratory drive may worsen airway obstruction. Induction of anesthesia is begun after appropriate monitors have been placed (a pulse oximeter and precordial stethoscope may be all that the child will allow). An IV catheter is inserted and secured.[f]

Anesthesia is induced on an operating room table elevated to about a 75-degree an-

---

[f]Ed. Note (JMB): Many of us would insist on an IV before inducing anesthesia in patients with juvenile laryngeal papillomatosis. Many others may insert an IV line after the inhalation induction of anesthesia.

gle to facilitate diaphragmatic excursions and to minimize gravitational effects on the compromised larynx. Inhalation induction by mask is accompanied by assisted ventilation and the application of 3 to 5 cm H_2O of continued positive airway pressure. Gentle assisted positive-pressure ventilation is beneficial in both phases of respiration because it augments tidal volume with each inhalation and acts as a stent to open the laryngeal inlet on exhalation. The early insertion of the appropriate-sized oral airway accompanied by gentle jaw thrust provides optimal airway position to facilitate inhalation induction and to rapidly achieve a depth of anesthesia sufficient to permit assisted ventilation. Potential for disaster occurs when the child with a partially obstructed airway enters the excitation stage of anesthesia and mask ventilation becomes impossible. If this occurs, the head and mask are repositioned in an attempt to restore airway patency. If repositioning fails to restore patency, it may be necessary to intubate the trachea with a styletted endotracheal tube or a rigid bronchoscope. Transtracheal catheter ventilation is extremely hazardous in children (Fig. 2). Exhaled volume may have no pathway for egress, and barotrauma may ensue. Furthermore, transtracheal ventilation may cause dissemination of the virus to the lower airway.

When the appropriate depth of anesthesia has been obtained, IV access (if not already present) can be easily accomplished. The administration of an antisialagogue is appropriate when the IV is started because even small amounts of secretions can obstruct the surgeon's view of the larynx. Spontaneous or assisted ventilation should be maintained until control of the airway is secured and the ability to deliver positive-pressure controlled ventilation has been demonstrated.

Airway Management and Ventilation Techniques

Airway management and ventilation techniques are considered suitable for laser surgery, provided that patients remain immobile and the laser beam can be directed at a target that is entirely still and in full view. To meet these criteria, two categories of airway management exist for laser surgery: with and without an endotracheal tube.

With an Endotracheal Tube

The choice of endotracheal tube used during laser surgery can affect the safety of the technique. All standard polyvinyl chloride endotracheal tubes are flammable and can ignite and vaporize when in contact with the laser beam. Red rubber endotracheal tubes do not vaporize but instead deflect the laser beam when wrapped with reflective metallic tape. The unwrapped cuff below the vocal cords is not protected from laser injury. Cuffed endotracheal tubes should be inflated with sterile saline to which methylene blue has been added so that if a laser spark strikes the cuff and burns a hole, it will be readily detected by the blue dye and extinguished by the saline (39). Nonreflective flexible metal endotracheal tubes are specifically manufactured for use during laser surgery. However, the outer diameter of each size of the metal laser tube is considerably greater than its polyvinyl chloride counterpart, making it too large for ventilation of infants and small children.

Without an Endotracheal Tube

Apneic Technique. This technique is preferred by some surgeons because the advantage is the absence of an endotracheal tube, which may obscure the surgical field. In this technique, the child is anesthetized and rendered immobile by using a muscle relaxant or deep inhalation of a volatile agent. The trachea is not intubated, and the airway is given over to the surgeon, who uses the laser for very brief periods. In between laser applications, the patient is ventilated by mask. Because apnea is a component of this technique, it is prudent for the patient to be ventilated with 100% oxygen. Although this technique has been widely used with safety, there is a greater potential for debris and resected material to enter the trachea.

Oxyscope. In this technique, a Lindholm or Benjamin suspension laryngoscope fitted with an oxygen insufflation port (the oxyscope) is inserted into the larynx. The volatile anesthetic gas is mixed with oxygen and administered through the side port. Anesthesia may be maintained without muscle relaxant in the spontaneously breathing patient. In the absence of muscle relaxant, however, vocal cord movement may prevent adequate surgical conditions. To avoid vocal cord motion, a muscle relaxant may be given and the lungs ventilated with supraglottic jet ventilation. The advantage of using a muscle relaxant is a quiet surgical field. Jet ventilation or spontaneous ventilation through an oxyscope may not provide adequate oxygenation for pulmonary disease in patients with poor pulmonary compliance or small airway disease (40). Therefore, an alternative technique is needed in these patients. Further disadvantages of ventilation through an oxyscope are related to the lack of a tracheal tube (e.g., absence of complete control of the airway, no protection from laryngospasm, no protection from debris entering the airway, and inadequate scavenging).

It should be noted that although supraglottic jet ventilation is a safe and effective technique, the use of transtracheal ventilation (e.g., jet ventilation through a copper or plastic catheter inserted past the vocal cords) is hazardous in children. This is because the egress of gas is restricted and the child is placed at high risk for barotrauma (Fig. 2).

Anesthetic Maintenance

If a technique of suspension laryngoscopy and jet ventilation has been chosen, a short-acting muscle relaxant (e.g., mivacurium) may provide optimal conditions. Since ventilation may be intermittent, the mainstay of the anesthetic should be an IV rather than volatile agent. Propofol infusion may decrease the requirement for inhaled volatile agent, and the vocal cords may be sprayed with 4% lidocaine to decrease reactivity. Oxygen may be delivered alone or mixed with air or helium. If the child has been paralyzed, the trachea should be intubated at the conclusion of the surgical procedure. Then, the child should be allowed to emerge from anesthesia and to be extubated when fully awake. If a technique of spontaneous ventilation has been chosen, the child need not be intubated and should be allowed to emerge from anesthesia with careful mask ventilation.

Laser Considerations

The laser (*l*ight *a*mplification by *s*timulated *e*mission of *r*adiation) provides precision in targeting airway lesions, causes minimal bleeding and edema, and preserves integrity of surrounding structures to promote rapid healing. The CO_2 laser is the most widely used in medical practice and has particular application in the treatment of laryngeal or vocal cord papillomas, laryngeal webs, resection of redundant subglottic tissue, and coagulation of hemangiomas. Energy emitted by a CO_2 laser is absorbed by water or the water contained in blood and tissues. Human tissue is about 80% water, and laser energy absorbed by tissue water rapidly increases the temperature, denaturing protein and causing vaporization of the target tissue. The thermal energy of the laser beam cauterizes capillaries as it vaporizes tissues; therefore, bleeding is minimal and little edema occurs postoperatively.

Safety Precautions

Misdirected laser beams may cause injury to a patient or to unprotected operating room personnel. Because the eyes are especially vulnerable to laser injury, all operating room personnel should wear laser-specific eye goggles with side protectors to prevent injury, and the eyes of patients undergoing laser treatment must be protected by taping the eyes shut, followed by the application of wet gauze pads to the eyelids, which are then covered by a metal shield.

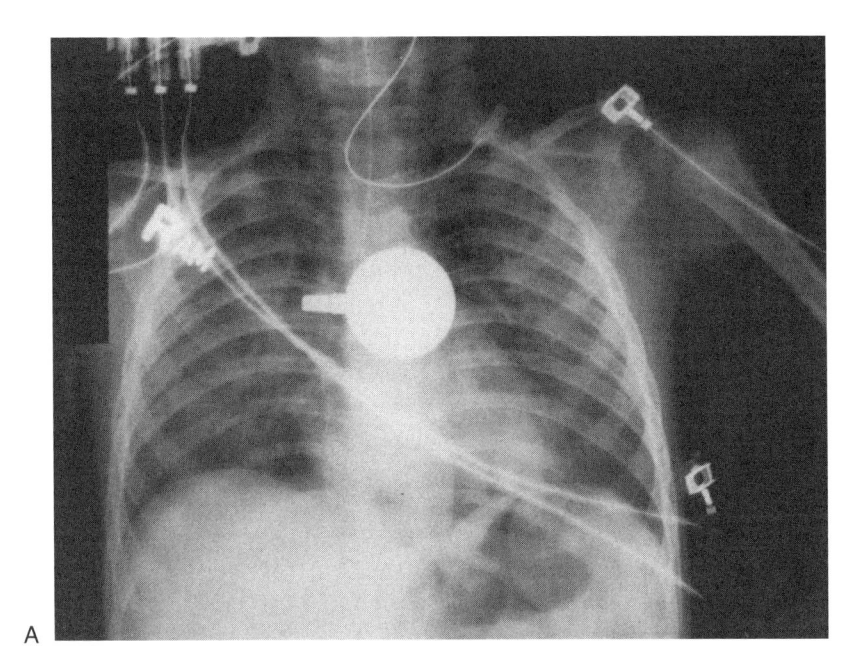

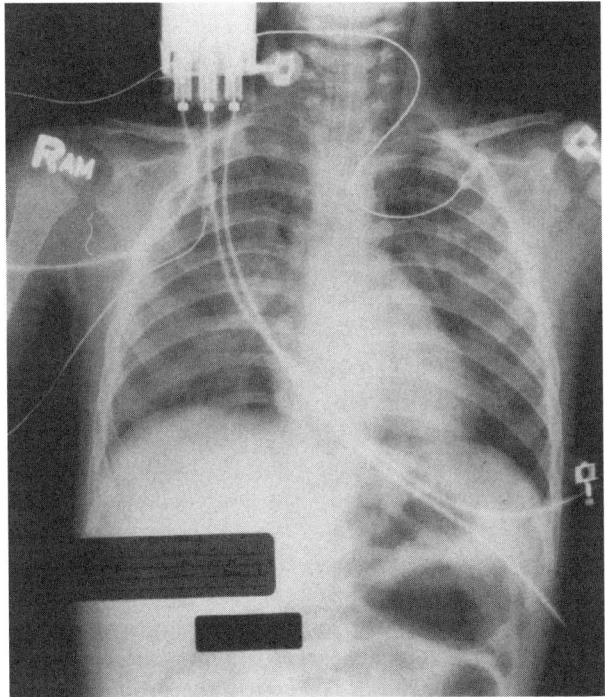

FIG. 2. (A) An inspiratory chest radiograph in a 10-month-old infant with a pneumomediastinum after only two jets of transtracheal jet ventilation. Barotrauma resulted from the inability of gas to escape. We now recommend only supraglottic placement of the ventilating catheter when jet ventilation is used. **(B)** An expiratory film in the same infant.

Laser radiation increases the temperature of absorbent material; therefore, flammable objects such as surgical drapes must be kept away from the path of the laser beam. Wet towels should be applied to exposed skin of the face and neck when laser is being used in the airway to avoid cutaneous burns from deflected beams. Laser smoke plumes may cause damage to the lungs, and interstitial pneumonia has been reported with long-term exposure. In addition, it has been postulated that during laser application cancer cells and virus particles (41) including HIV are vaporized and the resultant smoke plume, if inhaled, may be a vehicle for spread. Therefore, extreme care should be taken to suction smoke at the surgical site.

Suction of smoke can be easily accomplished by taping or holding a suction tubing at the proximal end of the suspension laryngoscope or bronchoscope. In addition, the use of specially designed small-bore filter masks for filtering of laser smoke is recommended.

Airway Emergencies

Upper airway emergencies may be life-threatening, and rapid respiratory failure can occur in patients suffering from croup, epiglottitis, or foreign body aspiration. Few clinical situations are more challenging to the anesthesiologist, since the anatomy of the pediatric airway renders it more susceptible to obstructive complications when compromised. In the presence of airway edema, greater proportional changes in the cross-sectional area of the infant airway compared with that of the adult result in increased airway resistance and work of breathing. The relatively large tongue of the infant worsens airway obstruction, and the detrimental impact of critical narrowing is compounded by the elasticity of the child's airway. Children with laryngeal obstruction may demonstrate collapse of the extrathoracic trachea distal to the site of obstruction during inspiration because of the compliant nature of the trachea in children.

Epiglottitis

Acute epiglottitis is one of the most feared infectious diseases in children and is the result of *Haemophilus influenzae* type B (42). It can progress with extreme rapidity from sore throat to obstruction to respiratory failure and death if proper diagnosis and intervention is not rapid. Although epiglottitis has been reported in very young children and adults, children are most susceptible between 2 and 7 years of age. Before the child's second birthday, vaccination against *H influenzae* type B polysaccharide is now recommended with the expectation of conferring immunity before the greatest period of vulnerability.

Characteristic signs and symptoms of acute epiglottitis include sudden onset of fever, dysphagia, drooling, thick muffled voice, and preference for the sitting position with the head extended and thrust forward. Supraglottitis may be a more appropriate designation, since it is the tissues of the supraglottic structures from the vallecula to the arytenoids, which are involved in the infectious process. The airway pressure differential on inspiration resulting from negative pressure inside and atmospheric pressure outside the extrathoracic airway and causing slight narrowing is exaggerated in the patient with airway obstruction. This dynamic collapse of the airway may become life-threatening in the crying, agitated child, and every attempt should be made to keep the child calm. Blood drawing, IV insertion, and excessive manipulation of the patient as well as sedation should be avoided before securing the airway to prevent the possibility of total obstruction. Retractions, labored breathing, and cyanosis may be observed in cases in which respiratory obstruction is present. However, in the early stages the child may be pale and toxic without respiratory distress. Direct observation of the epiglottis should not be attempted in the unanesthetized child and should be restricted to the operating room.

If the clinical situation allows, oxygen should be administered by mask and lateral radiographs of the soft tissues in the neck obtained. Thickening of the arytenoepiglottic folds as well as swelling of the epiglottis may be noted. Radiographic examination should be carried out only if skilled personnel and adequate equipment accompany the patient at all times. The child with severe airway compromise should proceed from the emergency room directly to the operating suite accompanied by the anesthesiologist and surgeon. Parental presence in this situation may calm an anxious and frightened child (43).

In most cases of epiglottitis, an artificial airway is established by means of endotracheal intubation (44). In some centers where personnel experienced in the management of the compromised pediatric airway are not available, tracheostomy is a less favored but acceptable alternative.

In the operating room, the child is kept in the sitting position while monitors are placed. A pulse oximeter and precordial stethoscope are essential. If it is felt to be helpful, one parent may accompany the child and remain in the operating room during the induction of general anesthesia. The operating room must be prepared with equipment and personnel for laryngoscopy, rigid bronchoscopy, and tracheostomy. Anesthetic induction is accomplished by inhalation of 100% oxygen and increasing concentrations of volatile anesthetic agent, which has traditionally been halothane; however, the advent of sevoflurane may change this practice. After loss of consciousness occurs, IV access should be secured and the child lowered into the supine position. Laryngoscopy followed by oral endotracheal intubation is then accomplished without the use of muscle relaxants. The endotracheal tube chosen should be at least one size (0.5 mm) smaller than would normally be chosen; a stylet is often useful.

After the surgeon has examined the larynx, noting the appearance of the epiglottis, arytenoepiglottic folds, and surrounding tissues, the endotracheal tube may be changed to a nasotracheal tube and secured. Tissue and blood cultures are taken, and antibiotic therapy is initiated. The child is then transferred to the intensive care unit for continued observation and radiographic confirmation of endotracheal tube placement. Sedation is appropriate at this time. Extubation is usually attempted 48 to 72 hours later in the operating room, when a significant leak around the nasotracheal tube is present and visual inspection of the larynx by flexible fiberoptic bronchoscopy confirms reduction in swelling of the epiglottis and surrounding tissues.

Laryngotracheobronchitis

Laryngotracheobronchitis (LTB), or croup, is usually encountered in children < 3 years of age. However, it can occur as early as 6 months and as late as 6 years of age. The cause is usually viral and the onset more insidious than that seen in epiglottitis. The child presents with low-grade fever, inspiratory stridor, and a barking cough.

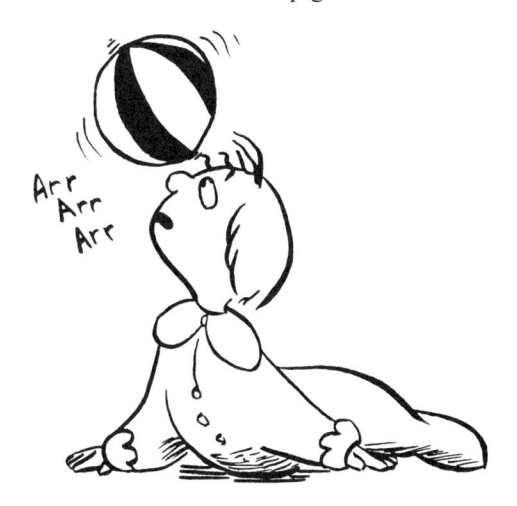

Radiologic examination confirms the diagnosis, and subglottic narrowing of the airway column secondary to circumferential soft tissue edema produces the characteristic "steeple" sign. Treatment includes cool, humidified mist, and, in the 6% of patients who require admission to the hospital, oxygen therapy is usually administered via tent. More severe cases of laryngotracheobronchitis are accompanied by tachypnea, tachycardia, and cyanosis, and racemic epinephrine administered by nebulizer is beneficial. The use of corticosteroids has been surrounded by a great deal of controversy, but current opinion is that a short course of corticosteroids may be beneficial. In rare circumstances, thick secretions are present in the airway, and the child requires intubation to allow pulmonary toilet and suctioning to be carried out. Management in the intensive care unit and extubation are carried out in the same fashion as for epiglottitis (43,44).

CONGENITAL STRIDOR

Preoperative Considerations

Stridor is the result of breathing during turbulent airflow secondary to an obstructed airway. It may occur either during inspiration, which is due to obstruction of the upper airway, or during exhalation, which is due to obstruction of the lower airway (Fig. 3). Obstructive lesions of the midtrachea cause biphasic stridor. The age of onset may aid in determining the cause since vocal cord paralysis is often present at birth, whereas laryngotracheomalacia develops early in infancy and cysts or masses of the vocal cords usually develop later in childhood. Symptomatic improvement may occur in specific positions, and this information should be sought in the history both to elucidate the cause and to be used during anesthetic induction to decrease the effects of obstruction on the airway. Physical examination should note the general condition of the child and the degree of airway compromise. Laboratory examination may include a chest radiograph, hemoglobin, or barium swallow to identify lesions that may be impinging on the trachea. Computed tomography (CT), magnetic resonance imaging (MRI), and pulmonary function testing (including flow-volume loops) are helpful if available but are not routinely obtained in the pediatric population.

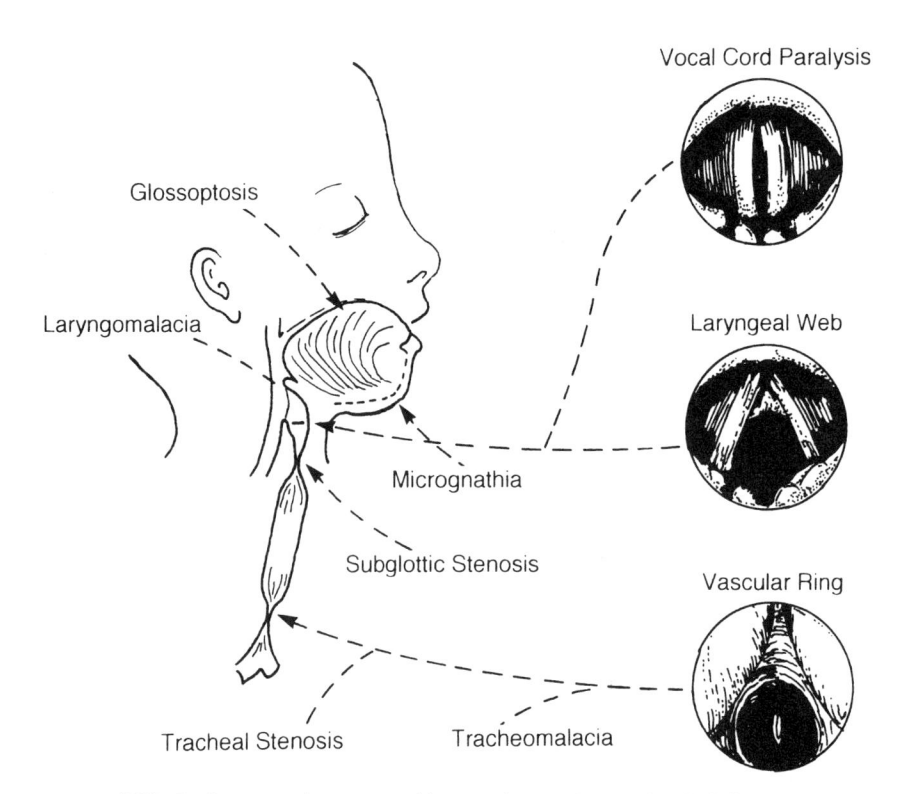

FIG. 3. Causes of upper and lower airway obstruction in infants.

Anesthetic Management

Anesthetic induction is best accomplished by inhalation of volatile agents by mask after which the examination of the airway begins. Small infants may be brought into the operating room unpremedicated. However, if premedication is necessary in the older child, caution should be used since respiratory depression and worsening of airway obstruction may occur. After placement of appropriate monitors, pulse oximeter probe, blood pressure cuff, electrocardiograph electrodes and precordial stethoscope, inhalation induction by mask is accomplished with 100% oxygen and increasing concentrations of a nonirritating volatile agent (halothane or sevoflurane). Patients should be placed in a position that facilitates ventilation—often the sitting position. After sufficient depth of anesthesia has been obtained, IV access should be secured. An antisialagogue is often administered to decrease secretions that may interfere with visualization of the airway.

FOREIGN BODY ASPIRATION

The following are the major concerns in the anesthetic management of a foreign body in the airway:

- Control of the airway
- Solution of the problem
- Full stomach
- Potential difficult airway

The child with a foreign body in the airway will present either electively or emergently. The child presenting electively will have had no food or drink and, if infected, will be treated with antibiotics and possibly bronchodilators. The patient who presents as an emergency generally must be considered as having a full stomach and may well need the institution of antibiotics, bronchodilators, and other aids. However, the basic principles of airway management are essentially the same. There have been many discussions and disagreements among anesthesiologists about whether or not it is possible to decrease the possibility of aspiration in emergency surgery by waiting a specific length of time after the emergency event. The consensus today is that there is nothing to be gained by waiting, since one still must assume that the stomach is full but that there may be a progression of the process (pneumonia) so that there may be more risks in waiting. Histamine-2 (H_2) blockers have never shown to be of value in this situation. Furthermore, it is probably unnecessary to worry too much about aspiration. It has been shown that 43% to 57% of children will not empty their stomachs even after 12 hours after a meal. In a study by Tiret and colleagues (45), a very low incidence of aspiration across the board was observed in children. Therefore, the risk of aspiration should not be the controlling factor. For these reasons, all foreign bodies should be managed emergently since there is nothing to be gained from waiting.

Preoperative Evaluation

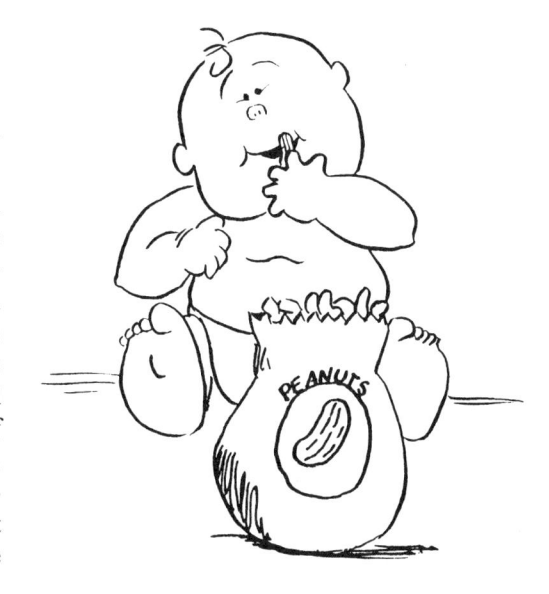

The drawing of the baby eating peanuts should send shivers up your spine and make you see red. Aspiration of a foreign body is a major cause of morbidity and mortality in children and peanuts are the worst offenders (46,47). Any history of coughing, cyanosis, refractory wheezing, or choking while eating (e.g., on peanuts, popcorn, jelly beans, and hot dogs) should suggest the possibility of foreign body aspiration. Physical findings include decreased breath sounds, tachypnea, stridor, wheezing, and fever. Foreign body aspiration is most common in toddlers 1 to 4 years old. The clinical presentation emcompasses a wide spectrum of clinical scenarios, from the child who has had an elective bronchoscopy to rule out a foreign body to the child in severe respiratory distress due to upper airway obstruction, reactive bronchospasm, or hyperinflation of the lung.

Most (95%) foreign bodies lodge in the right mainstem bronchus. Persistent cough or wheezing that does not get better with medical treatment may be the only presenting signs. Some foreign bodies are identifiable on radiologic examination; however, 90% are radiolucent and air trapping, infiltrate, and atelectasis are all that are noted. If the foreign body completely obstructs a bronchus or creates a ball valve phenomenon, distal hyperinflation from gas trapping may occur; a hyperinflated lung during expiratory phase may be seen on chest x-ray. The more distal the object in the airway, the more atelectatic changes are noted.

A foreign body lodges in the trachea (about 5% of airway foreign bodies) if it is too large to pass the carina. The signs of a tracheal foreign body range from a cough and abnormal voice to complete airway obstruction in the case of laryngeal foreign bodies. Any sharp object or any object causing acute upper airway obstruction with cyanosis and an inability to maintain ventilation requires emergency removal (46). Peanuts should be removed promptly, since peanut oil can cause an inflammatory response and subsequent pneumonitis (47). Also, peanuts tend to fragment and crumble over time, making removal extremely difficult.

Anesthetic Management

Preoperative Preparation

Unless the foreign body is life-threatening and needs immediate removal, several minutes can be taken to discuss the problem with the child and the parents. Sedative premedications may be used cautiously if the child can be closely monitored in close proximity to airway management equipment and to the operating room where the foreign body removal will take place.

If the patient has an IV line in place before the induction of anesthesia, matters are simpler. Atropine or glycopyrrolate may be given to reduce secretions and assist in bronchodilation of the patient. Antibiotics may be given if the patient is febrile or septic. If the child has asthma, high-dose corticosteroids and bronchodilators may be necessary.

Available Approaches

The approach to the anesthetic management of children with a foreign body depends on the level, degree, and duration of obstruction. A child who aspirates a foreign body while eating (almost always the case) further challenges the anesthesiologist by the presence of a full stomach. As previously discussed, waiting for the stomach to empty is impractical and unnecessary in the acute situation; however, it is acceptable in the stable situation.

The anesthetic technique for the retrieval of a foreign body of the airway depend on several factors:

- The preferences and skill of the surgeon
- The preferences and skill of the anesthesiologist
- Unrecognized factors

Some surgeons are extremely fast and talented, and all they need for the removal of a foreign body or for a diagnostic endoscopy is 1 or 2 minutes of paralysis. This can be accomplished with IV anesthesia, propofol, and succinylcholine or mivacurium in which there is rapid onset and rapid offset of the anesthetic and relaxant. For most patients, however, a longer and more complicated anesthetic is required.

Induction Techniques

If the child has recently eaten, full stomach precautions must be taken and anesthesia should be induced intravenously (topical EMLA cream may be applied to the skin before IV insertion in small children) by rapid sequence and gentle cricoid pressure maintained during intubation. If the child has not recently eaten, anesthesia may be induced by inhalation of 100% oxygen in halothane by mask. Inhalation induction can be prolonged secondary to obstruction of the airway and *nitrous oxide should be avoided* to reduce air trapping distal to the obstruction.[g] After induction, the anesthesiologist either (a) intubates the trachea with an endotracheal tube and gives over the airway to the surgeon, who will replace the endotracheal tube with a rigid bronchoscope or (b) gives over the airway for direct insertion of the bronchoscope.

MAINTENANCE OF ANESTHESIA

The remainder of the anesthetic technique falls into three categories: (a) patient spontaneously breathing, (b) patient anesthetized and paralyzed with controlled ventilation, and (c) a contingency plan.

The approach to a foreign body of the airway involves the consummate team approach with anesthesiologist and surgeon working out a technique for the endoscopy, which includes the surgical and anesthetic needs during endoscopy. The overriding issue to consider is the control of ventilation and oxygenation.

---

[g]Ed. Note (JMB): The use of nitrous oxide is controversial. What follows is the Fritz Berry technique for the induction of anesthesia in these patients. Note the use of nitrous oxide. The technique of induction of anesthesia for the child with a foreign body is one that the anesthesiologist does best and one that allows the gentle separation of parent and child. Many of these children already have an IV line in place; therefore, an IV induction can be accomplished. If the child has no IV line in place, the most frequently used alternative is an inhalation induction with high-flow nitrous oxide and halothane. Nitrous oxide and oxygen are delivered at 7 L and 3 L/min, respectively, and then nitrous oxide is discontinued and the concentration of halothane increased as tolerated. If an IV line has not been started, then a line should be started as soon as possible after the induction of anesthesia. An option in the extremely uncooperative child is the administration of intramuscular ketamine, 3 mg/kg, followed by either an IV or an inhalation technique.

Maintenance of Ventilation

One of the major controversies in the anesthetic management of foreign body aspiration is whether to control ventilation or to allow spontaneous respiration during bronchoscopy. Some endoscopists prefer a spontaneously ventilating patient to prevent dislodgement of the foreign body as it is being retrieved from the airway. Others prefer a paralyzed patient and motionless airway. Regardless of the technique used, the clinical problem to overcome is that these children have very irritable airways. Therefore, in both of these ventilation techniques, the use of topical lidocaine (3 to 4 mg/kg divided between the laryngeal structures and the tracheal mucosa) is helpful to suppress airway reflexes and prevent coughing and bronchospasm.

Spontaneous Ventilation

One of the advantages of the maintenance of spontaneous ventilation is that there is less barotrauma to the airway, so that there is a decreased chance of dislodgement of the foreign body with control of ventilation. The technique is to continue the inhalation induction, increasing the concentration of halothane up to 4% to 5% inspired while decreasing the nitrous oxide. The eye signs are of great aid in addition to the muscle relaxation of the masseter muscle and the abdominal muscles. When the patient is deeply anesthetized, laryngoscopy is performed and 4 to 5 mg/kg of 4% or 10% lidocaine sprayed on the epiglottis, vocal cords, and larynx. If the patient coughs, if the heart rate increases, or if the child moves during the laryngoscopy, it is evident that the anesthetic depth is not sufficient and more time needs to be taken to deepen the anesthetic. During this time period, ventilation is gently assisted to increase the depth of anesthesia.

One of the problems with allowing the patient to breathe entirely spontaneously is that the patient will autoregulate the depth of anesthesia. *Autoregulation* means that the patient will decrease tidal ventilation, thereby decreasing alveolar ventilation and slowing the induction of an adequate depth of anesthesia. However, with gentle assisted ventilation and some positive end-expiratory pressure (PEEP), the depth of anesthesia may be increased. At this point, the surgeon may introduce a rigid ventilating bronchoscope that has a side arm attachment for oxygen and anesthetic. High concentrations of inspired halothane and 95% oxygen are required because anesthetic and oxygen are diluted with room air by a Venturi effect.

Spontaneous ventilation should be preserved until the location and nature of the foreign body have been determined. Monitoring of adequate ventilation through a bronchoscope requires careful attention. Hypoxia and hypercarbia due to inadequate ventilation are caused by an excessively large leak around the bronchoscope or, more frequently, by inability to provide adequate gas exchange through a narrow-lumen bronchoscope fitted with an internal telescope. These conditions are remedied by frequent removal of the telescope and withdrawal of the bronchoscope to the midtrachea allowing effective ventilation. Bronchospasm may occur during examination of the respiratory tract and should be treated with increasing depths of anesthesia, nebulized albuterol, or IV bronchodilators. Although rare, pneumothorax should be suspected if acute deterioration during the procedure occurs.

Patients are carefully monitored using pulse oximetry and capnography. The importance of end-tidal CO_2 measurement is to determine the placement of the bronchoscope in the trachea as well as to monitor the frequency and depth of ventilation. The absolute number is of little value, since the primary monitor of adequacy of ventilation in this case is oxygen saturation.

When do you worry about decreasing oxygen saturation? This is often a difficult clinical question because many children who have aspirated a foreign body also have pneumonia, intrapulmonic shunting secondary to infection, or lower airway obstruction, making it difficult to achieve high oxygen-hemoglobin saturations. The baseline saturation in these children may be in the range of 95% to 96% and during periods of bronchoscopy may drop even lower (85% to 90%). If oxygen saturation as an arbitrary number can be maintained steadily in the high 80s and low 90s, this is acceptable. However, if a saturation has been at 95% and steadily drops to 85% and then to 80%, intervention is required. One may need to remove the telescope, ventilate through the bronchoscope, and administer gentle PEEP along with the 100% oxygen and halothane. If the bronchoscope is in the bronchus, it may have to be withdrawn into the trachea to allow reoxygenation and reanesthetizing the patient.

These patients often have little oxygen delivery system reserves; their oxygen saturation drops rapidly and their $PaCO_2$ rises rapidly as well. Clinical vigilance is essential. Attention is placed on symmetric chest excursion, breath sounds, and oxygen saturation. As in all airway cases, communication between the endoscopist and the anesthesiologist is very important. Both parties must cooperate in the care of the airway. If the endoscopist is taking too long to grasp the object with the bronchoscope in a distal airway and ventilation is inadequate, the endoscopist needs to retreat momentarily to the midtrachea so the patient can be ventilated. The combination of light anesthesia, hypoxia, and hypercarbia may produce a situation ripe for ventricular ectopy, particularly premature ventricular contractions (PVCs).

If PVCs occur during the procedure, carry out the following:

- Ensure oxygenation.
- Improve ventilation.
- Change to isoflurane.
- Administer IV lidocaine, 1.5 mg/kg[h]

If PVCs occur, it is probably wise to change the anesthetic agent from halothane to isoflurane. The value of halothane is its greater solubility and slower equilibrium. For example, when using halothane, if there is interruption of ventilation, the depth of anesthetic will not change as rapidly as with isoflurane. The added value of halothane, however, must go by the wayside if serious PVCs occur. Sevoflurane and desflurane are very insoluble and not great choices for airway surgery because of the rapid changes of depth that occur with changes in ventilation.

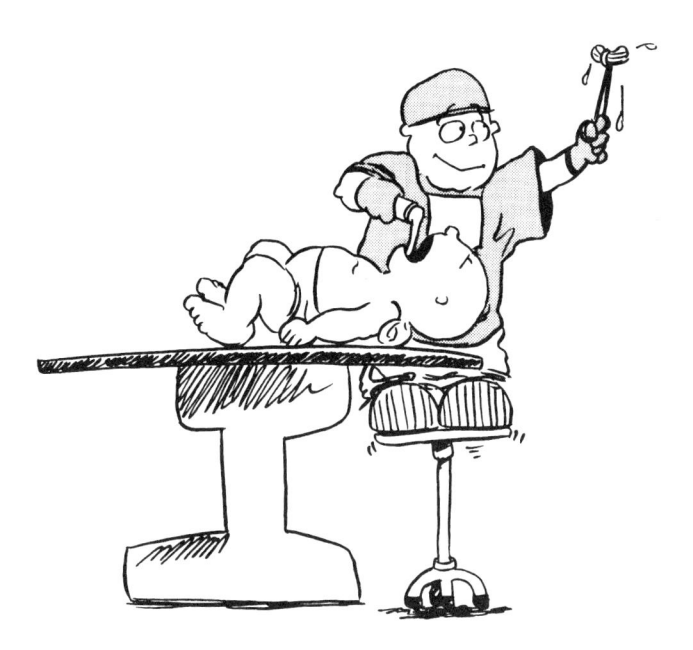

The Moment of Truth. The moment of truth comes when the surgeon secures the foreign body with forceps. At this point, attempts are made to extract the foreign body from the airway. At times the foreign body can be brought within the bronchoscope and removed. At other times it will not fit completely in the bronchoscope, and so the bronchoscope with forceps and the foreign body are then removed together. The issue is what is the best way to get the foreign body through the vocal cords, which may respond to the stimulation. If the patient is becoming light, as evidenced by an increasing heart rate and respiratory rate and an increase in muscle tone, a form of "midcourse correction" is to be followed. At this point, the anesthetic is to be deepened or the patient is paralyzed because if the child coughs or bucks, the foreign body may become fragmented with a resulting obstruction of bronchi and disaster. Therefore, the anesthesiologist is ready to give a dose of succinylcholine 1 mg/kg, lidocaine 1½ mg/kg, ketamine 1 mg/kg, or propofol 1 mg/kg. If there is any question, muscle paralysis is usually the best answer at this point.

When the foreign body is within the grasp of the forceps, the upper airway and glottis need to be quiet and relaxed. The spontaneously ventilating patient may need to be deepened or the manually controlled patient will need to be apneic. Supplemental IV lidocaine (1 mg/kg) is helpful to attenuate the airway reflexes. When the foreign body is retrieved, the forceps and the bronchoscope may need to come out as a unit. It is very important for the airway to be adequately anesthetized so the foreign body is not dislodged from the forceps by a cough or a closing glottis.

At times, particularly if the foreign body is vegetable matter, such as a peanut, there may be considerable swelling and edema around the site of the foreign body. Topical epinephrine diluted 1 to 10,000 or 1 to 100,000 will greatly reduce the swelling and edema and will facilitate the removal of the foreign body. The epinephrine needs to be given as a dilute

---

[h]Ed. Note (JMB): Lidocaine is administered when all treatable underlying causes (e.g., hypoxia, hypercarbia, and others) have been ruled out or treated.

solution. Vaponephrine, diluted 1 to 5, is useful for this purpose. After removal of the foreign body, the endoscopist should look again to make sure that all the material has been removed. If the child has a history of a full stomach, then after the endoscopist has completed the observation, the child should be intubated, the stomach decompressed, and the airway extubated while the child is awake. β-agonist bronchodilators such as albuterol or terbutaline may help with postoperative wheezing. Upper airway edema and secondary stridor from airway manipulation may be treated by racemic epinephrine inhalation or by prophylactic corticosteroid therapy (dexamethasone 0.5 mg to 1 mg/kg).

Opinions vary about the use of decadron to reduce inflammation associated with endoscopy. However, high-dose corticosteroids have been shown to be effective in other situations that are similar; therefore, most clinicians would administer a dose of 0.5 to 1 mg/kg of decadron as soon as the IV line is started. If the child develops postintubation, postinstrumentation croup, the addition of decadron may help to minimize this. In addition, racemic epinephrine should be considered to reduce upper airway edema.

Controlled Ventilation and Muscle Relaxation

Surgeons and anesthesiologists at some institutions prefer that patients lie completely motionless during removal of a tracheobronchial foreign body. Therefore, a technique that involves muscle relaxation and control ventilation is often indicated and, in my opinion, is usually appropriate. In this technique, anesthesia is induced either with IV or inhalation agents, and an IV line is started. The patient is given a short-acting muscle relaxant, either atracurium (0.3 to 0.5 mg/kg) or mivacurium (0.3 to 0.6 mg/kg) intravenously. A light level of general anesthesia using an inhalational agent plus topical anesthetization of the airway usually provides adequate analgesia, amnesia, and anesthesia. The advantage of this technique is that the so-called moment of truth is avoided because the surgeons have a completely motionless field.

Another advantage of this technique is that less total anesthetic is given, resulting in a more rapid recovery. The downside risk of this technique is that the foreign body (a) may be pushed further into the tracheobronchial tree, making removal more difficult, or (b) may be pushed into a ball-valve position, creating a hyperinflated lung.[i]

The Contingency Plan

As always, the anesthesiologist must have a contingency plan. Even though one's preferred technique may be spontaneous ventilation, if the child becomes desaturated and remains so, the contingency plan should include control of ventilation with or without muscle relaxation.

After the Foreign Body Is Out

After the foreign body is extracted, the usual technique is to reintubate the patient and let him or her awaken on the endotracheal tube and then extubate when the patient is in control of his airway reflexes. Examination of the entire tracheobronchial tree is carried out to detect any additional objects or fragments. Often vigorous irrigation and suctioning distal to the obstruction are required to remove accumulated secretions and prevent the possibility of postobstructive pneumonia. Corticosteroids are administered if inflammation of the airway mucosa is observed. Close observation of the patient postoperatively is required so that intervention may be early in the event of respiratory

---

[i]Ed. Note (JMB): It has been the editor's experience that this technique using control ventilation has provided satisfactory anesthesia without complication for many patients. To me, the issue of blowing the peanut further down the tube is overrated. Doubtless, the child has screamed and cried, taking in large inspired tidal volumes of air at maximum velocity. It is hard to imagine that controlled positive-pressure ventilation will move the peanut more than that. Furthermore, most patients with tracheobronchial foreign bodies present for removal days or weeks after aspiration. Therefore, the peanut is most likely fixed in place by the time we see the patient.

compromise secondary to airway edema or infection that may ensue.

ANTERIOR MEDIASTINAL MASSES

The most common anterior mediastinal masses in children are teratomas, masses of thymic origin, lymphomas (40% are Hodgkin's or non-Hodgkin's lymphoma), and angiomatous tumors (48,49). Children with anterior mediastinal masses may be scheduled to receive an anesthetic for tumor biopsy before chemotherapy or radiation therapy or surgical resection.

Children with anterior mediastinal masses may develop severe cardiopulmonary compromise, including cardiac arrest and death, upon induction of anesthesia (50–56). Cardiac arrest is frequently due to airway obstruction associated with loss of airway patency or compression of critical structures such as the pulmonary artery by an anterior mediastinal mass. In some patients, a change from the sitting to the supine position results in loss of airway. To make matters worse, the application of positive airway pressure may not always overcome extrinsic airway compression and loss of airway. Usually, the obstruction may be resolved with endotracheal intubation, although insertion of the tube down to the carina or, if a mass is distal to the carina, selective mainstem intubation may be required. Rigid bronchoscopy, however, is occasionally needed to relieve the obstruction. Severe airway obstruction may require selective intubation of each mainstem bronchus: the left side through a tracheostomy and the right side through a cuffed oral endotracheal tube positioned just below the tracheostomy stoma. Emergency sternotomy may be required to achieve adequate ventilation and venous return.

Preoperative Evaluation

Particularly ominous are signs and symptoms of marked airway obstruction, especially in the child who refuses to lie down. Anteroposterior and lateral chest radiographs, CT scans of the chest, and cardiac echocardiogram are helpful in assessing airway and cardiac compression. The CT scan is particularly helpful for planning airway management strategy. Flow-volume loops would be helpful but are often unattainable in children. Fortunately, information gained in the flow-volume loop is usually obvious from history and physical examination. For example, positional stridor or delayed exhalation is usually clinically apparent.

Anesthetic Management

An algorithm for management of the child with an anterior mediastinal mass is presented in Figure 4 (57). In children with enlarged cervical nodes, biopsy is best performed under local anesthesia. Unfortunately, when cervical nodes are absent, a mediastinal biopsy is required. In the symptomatic patient, 24 hours of corticosteroids and mediastinal radiation therapy is begun before biopsy (43). Most patients improve with this therapy and biopsy is then performed.

Careful preparation is necessary for a general anesthetic for biopsy or tumor resection. Most important, a strategy is devised for positioning the endotracheal tube. Sedative premedication is avoided. Anesthesia is induced with the patient in the semi-Fowler position; oxygen and halothane are used with the patient breathing spontaneously. Intubation is performed without the aid of muscle relaxants and the tube positioned as determined during the preoperative evaluation.

As with any other difficult airway, the key to successful management of these difficult patients is careful planning and preparation, with a backup plan readily available for each step. If the airway becomes obstructed, positive pressure is applied. If positive pressure does not relieve the obstruction, the child is placed in the lateral or prone position. If obstruction is still not relieved, a rigid bronchoscope (set up before induction) is passed beyond the obstruction, at which point ventilation and oxygenation should improve. If obstruction still persists, two alternatives remain: median sternotomy or femorofemoral bypass. Equipment for sternotomy or bypass must have been made available at the time of induction.

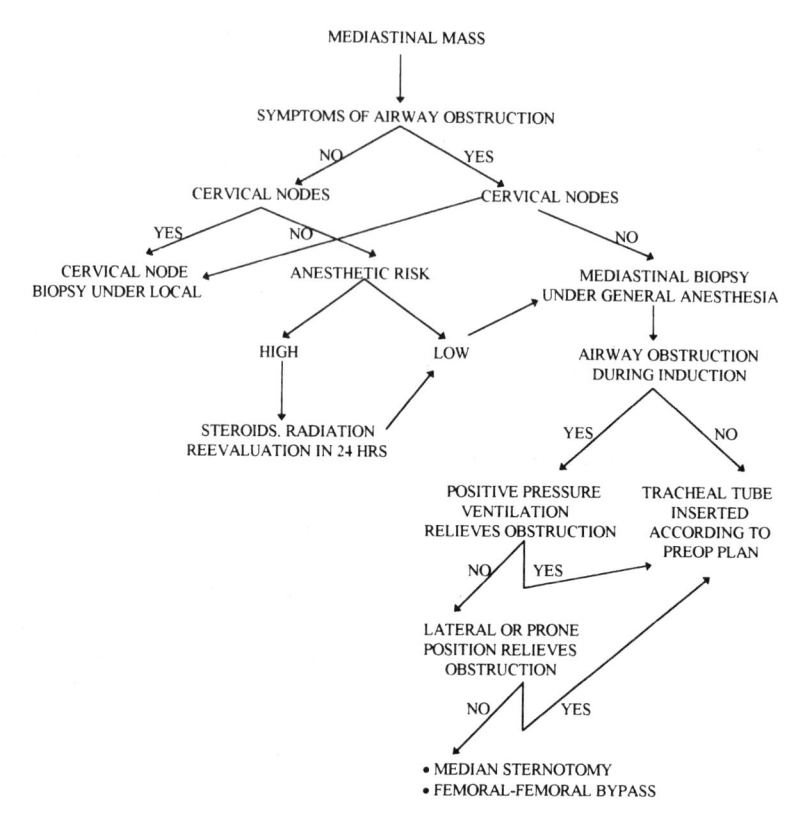

FIG. 4. An algorithm of the management of anterior mediastinal mass.

REFERENCES

1. Brodsky L: Modern assessment of tonsils and adenoids. *Pediatr Clin North Am* 1989;36:1551–1569.
2. Berkowitz RG, Zalzal GH: Tonsillectomy in children under 3 years of age. *Arch Otolaryngol Head Neck Surg* 1990;116:685–686.
3. Lieberman A, Tal A, Brama I, Sofer S: Obstructive sleep apnea in young infants. *Int J Pediatr Otorhinolaryngol* 1988;16:39–44.
4. Smith RM, Gonzalez C: The relationship between nasal obstruction and craniofacial growth. *Pediatr Clin North Am* 1989;36:1423–1434.
5. Guilleminault C: Obstructive sleep apnea: the clinical syndrome and historical perspective. *Med Clin North Am* 1985;69:1187–1203.
6. Chaban R, Cole P, Hoffstein V: Site of upper airway obstruction in patients with idiopathic obstructive sleep apnea. *Laryngoscope* 1988;98:641–647.
7. Noonan JA: Reversible cor pulmonale due to hypertrophied tonsils and adenoids: studies in two cases. *Circulation* 1965;32:(Suppl II):164.
8. Cayler GG, Johnson EE, Lewis BE, et al: Heart failure due to enlarged tonsils and adenoids: the cardiorespiratory syndrome of increased airway resistance. *Am J Dis Child* 1969;118:708–717.
9. Bland JW Jr, Edwards FK: Pulmonary hypertension and congestive heart failure in children with chronic upper airway obstruction. New concepts and etiologic factors. *Am J Cardiol* 1969;223:830–837.
10. Luke MJ, Mehrizi A, Folger GM Jr, Rowe RD: Chronic nasopharyngeal obstruction as a cause of cardiomegaly, cor pulmonale, and pulmonary edema. *Pediatrics* 1966;37:762–768.
11. Mullens PD, Nagaraj HS, McMurray GT: Upper airway obstruction resulting in cor pulmonale. *J Ky Med Assoc* 1965;76:223–226.
12. Perkin RM, Anas NG: Pulmonary hypertension in pediatric patients. *J Pediatr* 1984;105:511–522.
13. Bland JW Jr, Edwards FK: Pulmonary hypertension and congestive heart failure in children with chronic upper airway obstruction: new concepts of etiologic factors. *Am J Cardiol* 1969;23:830–837.
14. Massumi RA, Sarin RK, Pooya M, et al: Tonsillar hypertrophy, airway obstruction, alveolar hyperventilation and cor pulmonale in twin brothers. *Dis Chest* 1969;55:110–114.
15. Fujioka M, Young LW, Girdany BR: Radiographic evaluation of adenoidal size in children: adenoid-nasopharyngeal ratio. *Am J Radiol* 1979;133:401–407.
16. Noonan JA: Reversible cor pulmonale due to hypertrophied tonsils and adenoids: studies in two cases. *Circulation* 1965;2(Suppl):164.
17. Brown OE, Manning SC, Ridenour B: Cor pulmonale secondary to tonsillar and adenoidal hypertrophy: management considerations. *Int J Pediatr Otorhinolaryngol* 1988;16:131–139.

18. Cunningham MJ: Tonsillectomy and Adenoidectomy Inpatient Guidelines: Recommendations of the AAO-HNS Pediatric Otolaryngology Committee. American Academy of Otolaryngology—Head and Neck Surgery Bulletin. American Academy of Otolaryngology—Head and Neck Surgery 15(9):13–15, Sept 1996.
19. Woolf CJ, Chong MS: Preemptive analgesia: treating postoperative pain by preventing the establishment of central sensitization. *Anesth Analg* 1993;77:362–379.
20. Linden BE, Gross CW, Long TE, Lazar RH: Morbidity in pediatric tonsillectomy. *Laryngoscope* 1990;100: 120–124.
21. Fairbanks DN: Uvulopalatopharyngoplasty complications and avoidance strategies. *Otolaryngol Head Neck Surg* 1990;102:239–245.
22. Jebeles JA, Reilly JS, Gutierrez JF, et al: The effect of pre-incisional infiltration of tonsils with bupivacaine on the pain following tonsillectomy under general anesthesia. *Pain* 1991;47:305–308.
23. Denlon JV: Anesthesia and eye, ear, nose, and throat surgery. In: Miller RD (ed). *Anesthesia,* 4th ed. New York: Churchill Livingstone, 1994:2185–2196.
24. Carithers JS, Gebhart DE, Williams JA: Postoperative risks of pediatric tonsilloadenoidectomy. *Laryngoscope* 1987;97:422–429.
25. Conclasure JB, Grahm SS: Complications of outpatient tonsillectomy and adenoidectomy. A review of 3340 cases. *Ear Nose Throat J* 1990;69:155–160.
26. Yemen TA: Clinical Experience with cuffed-endotracheal tubes in children. Presented at the Society of Pediatric Anesthesia/American Academy of Pediatrics Section on Anesthesiology Annual Meeting in Tampa Bay, Florida, February 1996.
27. Marcus CL, Keens TG, Bautista DB, et al: Obstructive sleep apnea in children with Down syndrome. *Pediatrics* 1991;88:132–139.
28. Cunningham MJ, Ferrari LR, Kearse LA, McPeck K: Intraoperative somatosensory evoked potential monitoring in achondroplasia. *Paediatr Anaesth* 1994;4:129–132.
29. Tobias JD, Lowe S, Hersey S, et al: Analgesia after bilateral myringotomy and placement of pressure equalization tubes in children: acetaminophen versus acetaminophen with codeine. *Anesth Analg* 1995;81:496–500.
30. Tait AR, Knight PR: The effects of general anesthesia on upper respiratory tract infections in children. *Anesthesiology* 1987;67:930–935.
31. Cohen MM, Cameron CB: Should you cancel the operation when a child has an upper respiratory tract infection? *Anesth Analg* 1991;72:282–288.
32. DeSoto H, Patel RI, Soliman IE, Hanallah RS: Changes in oxygen saturation following general anesthesia in children with upper respiratory infection signs and symptoms undergoing otolaryngological procedures. *Anesthesiology* 1988;68:276–279.
33. Munson ES: Complications of nitrous oxide anesthesia for ear surgery. *Anesthesiol Clin North Am* 1993;11: 559–572.
34. Hawkins DB, Udall JN: Juvenile laryngeal papillomas with cardiomegaly and polycythemia. *Pediatrics* 1979; 63:156–157.
35. Rimell FL, Shapiro AM, Mitskavich MT, et al: Pediatric fiberoptic laser rigid bronchoscopy. *Otolaryngol Head Neck Surg* 1996;114:413–417.
36. McGlennen RC, Adams GL, Lewis CM, et al: Pilot trial of ribavirin for the treatment of laryngeal papillomatosis. *Head Neck* 1993;15:504–512.
37. Mattot M, Ninane J, Hamoir M, et al: Combined CO_2-laser and alfa recombinant interferon treatment in five children with juvenile laryngeal papillomatosis. *Acta Clin Belg* 1990;45:158–163.
38. Wetmore SJ, Key JM, Suen JY: Complications of laser surgery for laryngeal papillomatosis. *Laryngoscope* 1985;95:798–801.
39. Sosis MB, Dillon FX: Saline-filled cuffs help prevent laser-induced polyvinylchloride endotracheal tube fires. *Anesth Analg* 1991;72:187–189.
40. Weeks DB: Laboratory and clinical description of the use of jet-venturi ventilator during laser microsurgery of the glottis and subglottis. *Anesth Rev* 1985;12: 32–36.
41. Kashima HK, Kessis T, Mounts P, Shah K: Polymerase chain reaction identification of human papillomavirus DNA in CO_2 laser plume from recurrent respiratory papillomatosis. *Otolaryngol Head Neck Surg* 1991;104: 191–195.
42. Baxter JD, Pashley NR: Acute epiglottitis: 25 years of experience in management. The Montreal Children's Hospital. *J Otolaryngol* 1977;6:473–476.
43. Davis HW, Gartner JC, Galvis AG, et al: Acute upper airway obstruction: croup and epiglottitis. *Pediatr Clin North Am* 1981;28:859–880.
44. Battaglia JD, Lockhart CH: Management of acute epiglottitis by nasotracheal intubation. *Am J Dis Child* 1975;129:334–336.
45. Tiret L, Nivoche Y, Hatton F, et al: Complications related to anaesthesia in infants and children: a prospective survey of 40240 anaesthetics. *Br J Anaesth* 1988;61:263–269.
46. Kosloske AM: Bronchoscopic extraction of foreign bodies in children. *Am J Dis Child* 1982;136: 924–927.
47. Ward CF, Benumof JL: Anesthesia for airway foreign body extraction in children. *Anesth Rev* 1977;December:13.
48. Bower RJ, Kiesewetter WB: Mediastinal masses in infants and children. *Arch Surg* 1977;112:1003–1009.
49. Filler RM, Simpson JS, Ein SH: Mediastinal masses in infants and children. *Pediatr Clin North Am* 1979;26: 677–690.
50. Halpern S, Chatten J, Meadows AT, et al: Anterior mediastinal masses: anesthesia hazards and other problems. *J Pediatr* 1983;102:407–410.
51. Levin H, Bursztein S, Heifetz M: Cardiac arrest in a child with an anterior mediastinal mass. *Anesth Analg* 1985;64:1129–1130.
52. Bray RJ, Fernandes FJ: Mediastinal tumour causing airway obstruction in anaesthetised children. *Anaesthesia* 1982;37:571–575.
53. Amaha K, Okutsu Y, Nakamura Y: Major airway obstruction by mediastinal tumour. *Br J Anaesth* 1973;45: 1082–1084.
54. Todres ID, Reppert SM, Walker PF, Grillo HC: Management of critical airway obstruction in a child with a mediastinal tumor. *Anesthesiology* 1976;45: 100–102.
55. Keon TP: Death on induction of anesthesia for cervical node biopsy. *Anesthesiology* 1981;55:471–472.
56. Bittar D: Respiratory obstruction associated with induction of general anesthesia in a patient with mediastinal Hodgkin s disease. *Anesth Analg* 1975;54:399–403.
57. Ferrari LR, Bedford RF: General anesthesia prior to treatment of anterior mediastinal masses in pediatric cancer patients. *Anesthesiology* 1990;72:991–995.

12

Anesthesia for Infants and Children With Congenital Heart Disease

J. Michael Badgwell and Louis W. Elkins

"How else but through a broken heart may Lord Christ enter in?"
—Oscar Wilde

This chapter is intended to serve as a guide for the anesthesia in open and closed cardiac surgeries as well as for noncardiac surgeries and cardiologic procedures (e.g., cardiac catheterization) in children with congenital heart disease.[a]

It is arranged so that considerations are presented in the sequential order of perioperative events: preoperative assessment, preoperative operating room, equipment, and blood arrangements, premedication, perioperative management (e.g., induction of anesthesia, endotracheal intubation), cardiopulmonary bypass (CPB) management (going on and coming off), and postoperative care. Almost 90% of heart surgery in infants and children is performed because of the lesions listed in Table 1 (1). Therefore, after a general discussion of cardiac anesthesia, the focus will be on special management of anesthesia for these frequently occurring heart defects.

PREOPERATIVE ASSESSMENT

Children with congenital heart disease (CHD) may present with varying degrees of dyspnea, cyanosis, or failure to thrive. Infants or children with severe malformations may present with cardiac failure. Cardiac failure results from either the high pressures needed to compensate for obstruction (valve stenosis or coarctation) or high-volume flow through intracardiac (ventricular septal defect [VSD]) or extracardiac shunts (patent ductus arteriosus [PDA]). Dyspnea may result from cardiac failure or changes in pulmonary blood flow. To make matters worse, infants and children with CHD are very prone to repeated respiratory infections.

Conditions that cause increased blood flow to the lungs, if uncorrected, may eventually result in irreversible pulmonary hypertension. Pulmonary hypertension may be prevented by pulmonary artery banding or primary total repair during early life. Cyanotic conditions induce compensatory polycythemia, which may also lead to complications (see **Polycythemia**).

Evaluation of patients with CHD should include an independent physical examination, especially of the cardiovascular and respiratory systems, ear, nose, throat, teeth, and veins. It is essential to review the cardiology notes, echocardiogram, cardiac catheterization, and angiogram data. Although the pres-

---

[a] Ed. Note (JMB): This chapter is not intended to be an exhaustive review of everything known to man about pediatric cardiac anesthesia. It is intended to be a complete and concise description of how to do a well-managed pediatric cardiac anesthetic, with emphasis on practical issues in caring for the most common lesions. The advice proffered is done so with the understanding and agreement from you, the reader, that cardiac surgery in infants and children should be performed only where the most expert comprehensive medical and nursing care and all requisite facilities are available. This chapter is not intended to serve as a license in pediatric cardiac anesthesia for clinicians and hospitals that do not have support for this major undertaking.

Numerous abbreviations are used to describe conditions and related terms. For the reader's convenience, these abbreviations are presented separately in Table 2.

TABLE 1. Types of congenital heart defects

Type	Lesion	Incidence (%) in First Year of Life
Left-to-right shunt (acyanotic)	Ventricular septal defect	17
	Patent ductus arteriosus	7
	Endocardial cushion defect	5
	Atrial septal defect	3
	Truncus arteriosus[a]	2
Cyanotic	Transposition of the great vessels	11
	Tetralogy of Fallot	9
	Hypoplastic left heart syndrome	8
	Pulmonary atresia/stenosis	7
	Tricuspid atresia	3
	Total anomalous venous return[b]	3
Obstructive	Coarctation of the aorta	8
	Pulmonary stenosis	4
	Aortic stenosis	2

[a] Usually initially acyanotic but with the development of pulmonary vascular obstructive disease (PVOD), these patients become cyanotic.
[b] Although shunting may go both ways, this is usually a net R → L shunt and is usually a cyanotic lesion.

ence of an upper respiratory infection is often a debatable issue in noncardiac patients, it is much less debatable in the child with CHD (2). If a child with CHD has had a recent respiratory infection, elective surgery should be postponed for 2 to 6 weeks, if possible **(see The Child with a Runny Nose, Chapter 1)**.

A careful drug history is critical. Many patients with CHD take several medications regularly. Propranolol and other β-blockers should be discontinued the night before surgery. With rare exceptions, digitalis (3) and diuretics should be withheld on the day of surgery. If the patient requires oxygen therapy or maintenance of the sitting position during transit to the operating room, these should be specifically ordered.

Preoperative education is important in children with CHD. For example, children over 2 to 3 years of age should be taught about the oxygen tent, intravenous (IV) lines, chest drains, sedation, and controlled ventilation (when indicated).

PREMEDICATION

Children with CHD require adequate preoperative sedation to reduce excitement, anxiety, and crying (and thus reduce oxygen consumption). Therefore, preoperative sedation is ordered for all children >1 year or weighing >9 kg.

For children under 1 year of age weighing less than 9 kg, atropine may be administered by means of the following methods:

- Intramuscularly (IM), 30 minutes preoperatively
- IV, during induction (be cautious because the tachycardia that follows IV administration of atropine may be undesirable in patients with CHD)

Atropine may not be needed if pancuronium is given as the muscle relaxant.

Older children may receive one of the following regimens:

- Pentobarbital: 2 mg/kg IM, given 1.5 hours preoperatively; may be given rectally to children under 4 years and orally with a sip of water to older children
- Morphine: 0.1 to 0.2 mg/kg IM 1 hour preoperatively
- Midazolam: 0.5 to 0.75 mg/kg orally, or 0.1 mg/kg IV, 20 minutes preoperatively
- Atropine: (same as above)

These regimens of premedication do not usually cause significant decreases of oxygen-hemoglobin saturation levels preopera-

TABLE 2. *Glossary of abbreviations in congenital heart disease*

Heart conditions	
AS	aortic stenosis
ASD	atrial septal defect
CHB	complete heart block
HLHS	hypoplastic left heart syndrome
IHSS	idiopathic hypertrophic subaortic stenosis
LVH	left ventricular hypertrophy
PA	pulmonary atresia
PAPVR	partial anomalous pulmonary venous return
PDA	patent ductus arteriosus
PFO	patent foramen ovale
PS	pulmonic stenosis
RBBB	right bundle branch block
RVH	right ventricular hypertrophy
TA	tricuspid atresia
TAPVR	total anomalous pulmonary venous return
TGA	transposition of great arteries
TOF	tetralogy of Fallot
VSD	ventricular septal defect

Related terminology	
Ao	aorta
AV	atrioventricular
CO	cardiac output
CVP	central venous pressure
F_IO_2	inspired oxygen fraction
IPPV	intermittent positive-pressure ventilation
IVC	inferior vena cava
LA	left atrium
LV	left ventricle
PEEP	positive end-expiratory pressure
P_{AW}	peak airway pressures
PA	pulmonary artery
PV	pulmonary vein
PBF	pulmonary blood flow
PS	pulmonic stenosis
PVOD	pulmonary vascular obstructive disease
PVR	pulmonary vascular resistance
Q_P/Q_S	pulmonary to systemic blood flow ratio
Q_{sp}/Q_t	intrapulmonary shunt
RA	right atrium
RV	right ventricle
SaO_2	arterial oxygen hemoglobin saturation
$S_{PA}O_2$	pulmonary artery O_2 saturation
SV	stroke volume
SVC	superior vena cava
SVR	systemic vascular resistance
Δ_p/Δ_t	myocardial contractility
L → R	left to right shunt
R → L	right to left shunt

tively, even in the cyanotic patient (4). Nevertheless, careful observation of the patients with CHD after sedative premedication is prudent. A barbiturate may be ordered for the evening before surgery for children >8 years of age. For cyanotic children with a high hemoglobin (>16), maintenance IV fluids are ordered for the fasting interval.

SPECIAL PROBLEMS THAT MAY BE DISCOVERED AT PREOPERATIVE ASSESSMENT

Intracardiac Shunting

The clinician should be aware of intracardiac shunt that may be present. Right-to-left (R → L) shunts result in the following changes:

- Low arterial oxygen tension—only minimally improved by increasing the F_IO_2
- Delayed uptake of inhaled anesthetic agents
- Extreme danger of systemic emboli from venous air embolism
- Short arm-brain circulation time
- Danger of overdose with IV drugs
- Less efficient ventilation and gas exchange (large $PaCO_2 - P_{ET}CO_2$)

By contrast, left-to-right (L → R) shunts result in the following:

- Pulmonary vascular overperfusion, but good ventilatory efficiency and gas exchange initially
- Later pulmonary hypertension and congestive heart failure (eventually)

Outflow Obstructive Lesions

Lesions that restrict the outflow of blood from the heart (e.g., pulmonary or aortic stenosis) may result in the following conditions:

- Fixed cardiac output—and therefore the inability to compensate for changes in metabolic demand or peripheral vascular resistance
- Myocardial hypertrophy, with possible inadequacy of myocardial perfusion, especially to the subendocardium

- Congestive heart failure
- Sudden serious dysrhythmias

Other Special Problems Associated with CHD

Heart failure is common in infants with CHD and is worsened by drugs that depress the myocardium (e.g., halothane). Electrolyte disturbances may occur in infants and children with CHD. Serum potassium levels may be low, particularly in patients who have had prolonged diuretic therapy. Hypokalemia is especially bothersome in that it predisposes to cardiac dysrhythmias, particularly during hypothermia. In addition, due to metabolic demands that may outstrip supply, neonates with CHD frequently have low calcium and glucose levels.

Drug History

Drugs essential for therapy of infants and children with CHD may cause problems before, during, or after cardiac surgery. For digitalis, the therapeutic index is low—toxicity is an ever-present hazard, especially in young children. Because potassium levels may fall, hypothermia increases the risk of digitalis toxicity. Diuretics may deplete potassium, further increasing the risk of digitalis toxicity. Although β-adrenergic blocking agents may impair cardiac contractility, this is not usually a perianesthetic problem in these children.

Polycythemia

Polycythemia occurs as a compensatory response to hypoxia in some children with CHD (e.g., those with cyanosis). A high hematocrit level (>55) results in the following conditions:

- Increased viscosity of the blood and therefore increased cardiac work
- Increased tendency for thrombosis
- Increased risk of thrombosis if dehydration or venous stasis develops
- Possible coagulopathy—primarily thrombocytopenia
- Predisposition to cerebral abscess

Despite the dangers of polycythemia, these children are very dependent on a high hematocrit to ensure adequate oxygen transport. Hemodilution to normal hematocrit levels may be followed by severe cardiovascular collapse. In addition, lowering the hematocrit may also lead to increased R → L shunt. Hemodilution is indicated preoperatively only if there are signs of pathology from hyperviscosity (e.g., stroke). If done, hemodilution must be very carefully controlled and not taken to a hematocrit below 50%.

Patent Ductus Arteriosus

Some infants may be dependent on the patency of the ductus arteriosus as a route for shunting of blood until surgery can be performed (e.g., in transposition of great arteries with intact septum, interrupted aortic arch). In such infants, prostaglandins E_1 (PGE_1) are used to keep the ductus open (5). Infusion of PGE_1 (0.03 to 0.1 μg/kg/min) should be continued until the appropriate surgical procedure is completed.

Associated Malformations

Many children with CHD have additional defects (e.g., cleft palate, Down's syndrome, subglottic stenosis).

Sepsis

Sepsis is a major threat to the success of cardiac surgery. Great care must be taken to observe strict asepsis when inserting invasive monitoring or infusion lines.

Psychological Stress

Some children need repeated surgery, which imposes a severe psychological stress on them and their parents. In the final analysis, a very considerate, careful approach by the anesthesiologist is essential.

BLOOD SUPPLIES

During any type of cardiac surgery, blood must be immediately available. Even if the task of ordering blood is the responsibility of the surgical service, the anesthesiologist should ensure that adequate supplies of blood and blood products will be available by operation time. For pump cases, blood is administered as either fresh whole blood, modified whole blood, or packed red blood cells (PRBCs). Fresh whole blood is ideal but usually difficult to obtain and must be used within 24 hours after being drawn. Modified whole blood is fresh whole blood with the plasma components separated. When modified whole blood is requested, the matching unit (U) of plasma components (from the same donor) is sent with the blood. For most open heart surgery cases, modified whole blood or PRBCs is requested because fresh whole blood is more difficult to obtain. However, for major neonate repairs, such as arterial switch, fresh whole blood is requested. Examples of special requirements for cardiac patients are given in the following text.

For *nonpump cases* such as PDA ligation, coarctation of aorta, Blalock-Taussig shunt, order the following:

- 0 to 10 kg—1 U PRBCs
- 11 to 24 kg—2 U PRBCs
- >25 kg—3 U PRBCs

For atrial septal defect *(ASD) repair pump cases,* order the following:

- 3 U PRBCs

For *all other pump cases,* the following should be available:

- 0 to 10 kg—4 U PRBCs, fresh whole blood, or modified whole blood with matching platelets
- >10 kg—5 U PRBCs, fresh whole blood, or modified whole blood with matching platelets

For *cyanotic patients* with a hemoglobin >16 g/dl, plasma should be available.

For *all infants,* check that the blood to be supplied is <5 days old and tested for cytomegalovirus.

For *infants and children undergoing CPB,* ensure that PRBCs, fresh-frozen plasma, and platelets (1 U/5 kg) have been ordered.

For older children and those with high initial hematocrit, the cell saver may be used to conserve blood. In many of these children (e.g., those who have relatively minor surgery), blood transfusion may be avoided.

EQUIPMENT PREPARATION

All anesthesia and monitoring equipment are checked before bringing the patient into the operating room. Although most pediatric cardiac patients do not have coronary artery disease, ischemic injury may still occur, particularly after the insults of CPB and deep hypothermic circulatory arrest (6). In most cases, standard electrocardiography (ECG) with observation of the ST segment provides adequate information regarding the myocardial status. If available, calibrated ECGs and ST-segment trend analysis may provide even more sophisticated information. In addition, cardiac function may be evaluated and monitored in pediatric patients using pulmonary artery flotation catheters, transesophageal echocardiography, and transtracheal Doppler imaging.

Pulmonary Artery Flotation Catheters

In children as in adults, cardiac output may be determined using the thermodilution technique and a pulmonary artery flotation catheter **(see Chapter 3 for insertion techniques, complications, and so on)**. In patients with congenital cardiac lesions, however, pressure and cardiac output measurements may be inaccurate owing to high right-sided cardiac pressures or intracar-

ocardial function in children is the transesophageal echocardiography (TEE). This technology is now capable of producing M-mode, two-dimensional, and Doppler color-flow imaging, pulsed Doppler ultrasound, and continuous-wave steerable Doppler ultrasound. TEE equipment design is based on the concept of the flexible gastroscope with a transducer mounted at the tip. The direction of the ultrasound beam can be manipulated by the TEE controls, as with a gastroscope. Small probes now allow the use of this technology even in neonates and infants (8). The pediatric version is smaller, enabling its routine use in patients weighing as little as 2 kg. The biplane adult-sized probe, however, is suitable for use in children who weigh >8 kg. TEE has several important applications (9):

- Identification of regional wall motion abnormalities suggestive of myocardial ischemia
- Evaluation of left ventricular contractility and function
- Identification of residual intracardiac shunts after operative repair of CHD

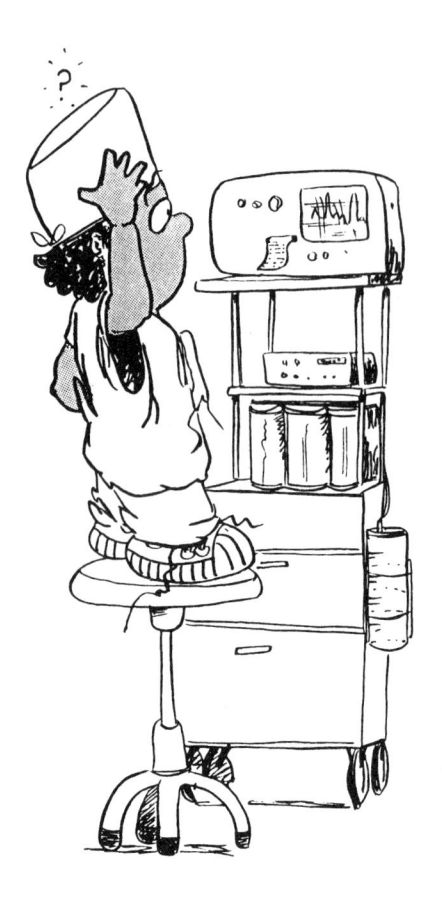

diac shunting. In these situations, cardiac output may be assessed in the light of other information such as arterial blood pressure and central venous pressure (CVP) measurements (including atrial catheters placed during surgery). Furthermore, information obtained from invasive monitors may be confirmed with clinical parameters (e.g., evaluation of peripheral pulses and perfusion, capillary refill,[b] urine output, and acid-base status).

- Detection of atrial thrombus or valvular vegetation
- Identification of intracardiac air before the discontinuation of CPB
- Residual flow obstruction
- Aortic dissection

Transesophageal Echocardiography

A recent technologic advance that has contributed much to the evaluation of my-

TEE imaging permits continuous assessment of ventricular function through the short-axis view. With alteration in the direction of the ultrasound beam, it can provide superior views of the mitral valve and mitral valve function compared with other approaches. Pediatric TEE facilitates intraoperative imaging of congenital cardiac malformations not visualized by standard transthoracic examinations and allows assessment of the adequacy of surgical intervention in newborns and small infants.

---

[b]Ed. Note (JMB): The reliability of this clinical tool (capillary refill) as a real-time monitor of cardiac function has been questioned (7). Recent studies have suggested that capillary refill as a clinical sign has a degree of specificity worse than a coin toss.

Contraindications and Disadvantages

Contraindications for TEE relate primarily to the size of the transducer probe relative to the size of the patient's esophagus. Such contraindications include unavailability of an appropriate-sized transducer probe, esophageal abnormalities such as strictures, fistulas, varices, and recent surgical procedures with suture lines that may be disrupted by passage of the TEE probe. One of the disadvantages of TEE in the pediatric population is associated with the use of the smaller TEE probe necessary for patients weighing <8 kg and the resultant decrease in image resolution. In addition, esophageal probes are less maneuverable in small patients and therefore less capable of imaging certain aspects of cardiac anatomy (10). Another limitation is that viewing the left pulmonary artery and left ventricular outflow tract from the esophagus may be difficult (11).

The issue of whether the anesthesiologist or the cardiologist should be responsible for reading TEE images remains controversial. Because the cardiologist may not be able to remain in the operating room at all times, it is useful for the anesthesiologist to understand cardiac imaging. Although a reasonable level of competence in use of the technique is not unreasonable for anesthesiologists, a cardiologist should be immediately available for times when anatomical diagnoses or surgical decisions must be based on echocardiographic findings.

Transtracheal Doppler Imaging

Another monitor of cardiovascular function in children is the transtracheal Doppler imaging. The transtracheal Doppler measures ascending aortic diameter and blood flow velocity and calculates cardiac output from these measurements (12). Proper probe positioning has been found to be essential to obtain good correlation with thermodilution values.

The ultrasound transducer probe located at the tip of an endotracheal tube is held against the anterior wall of the trachea by a special cuff. A small probe with a 3-mm transducer is available, which can be used for patients as small as 10 kg (13). Experience with the probe in the pediatric population, however, is limited.

The disadvantages of the transtracheal Doppler probe include its restriction to intubated patients and the fact that movement of the tube within the trachea combined with the high angle of incidence of the beam to the aortic blood flow introduces error in the assessment of cardiac output.

DRUG PREPARATION

There are as many ways to prepare drugs for a pediatric cardiac case as there are pediatric cardiac anesthesiologists. Table 3 is a list of basic drugs we have found useful in starting an open heart pediatric cardiac surgery.

Prepare vasopressors and inotropes in 60-ml syringes for use in continuous infusion pumps. If one uses the rule of three (i.e., amount of drug in mg per 50-ml syringe = 3 × the patient's weight in kg); 1 ml/hour will then

TABLE 3. *Drugs useful for starting pediatric open heart surgery*

Emergency drugs	Dilution
Sodium bicarbonate	7.5% solution: 20 ml
Atropine	Diluted to 0.1 mg/ml: 4 ml
Epinephrine	100 µg/ml and 10 µg/ml
Phenylephrine	100 µg/ml and 10 µg/ml
Ephedrine	2.5 mg/ml
Isoproterenol	20 µg/ml
Calcium chloride	100 mg/ml and 10 mg/ml
Other medications	**Dosage**
Atropine	10 µg/kg
Succinylcholine	2 mg/kg
Heparin	0.3 ml/kg (1:1000)
Ancef	25 mg/kg
Vecuronium or pancuronium	0.1 mg/kg
Amrinone or milrinone	10–15 µg/kg
Lidocaine	2 mg/kg
Fentanyl	Up to 100 µg/kg
Ketamine	1–3 mg/kg IV
	~8 mg/kg IM

IM, intramuscular; IV, intravenous.

equal 1 μg/kg/min. For example, in a 10-kg infant, infusions might include dopamine, 30 mg in 50 ml normal saline; sodium nitroprusside, 30 mg in 50 ml normal saline.

To avoid fluid overload in small infants, infusions may be concentrated to twice or triple strength.

Finally, the following medications are also made available: protamine, phentolamine mesylate, and dextrose 50%.

While preparing the room, it is a good time to check that preoperative medication has been given as ordered. Monitors including precordial stethoscope, blood pressure cuff, ECG, and pulse oximeter may then be arranged for later application. Temperature control may be especially poor in neonates with cyanotic CHD because they cannot respond to heat losses as well as normal infants can. Body temperature will fall rapidly if these infants are exposed to a cool environment. Therefore, a forced-air warming device is placed on the operating room table to be applied to children when they enter the operating room **(see Chapter 2)**.

ANESTHESIA FOR OPEN HEART SURGERY

Induction

If patients are adequately preoxygenated (i.e., completely denitrogenated) and if shunt flow hemodynamics are considered (Tables 4 to 11), different methods of induction of anesthesia do not markedly effect oxygen-hemoglobin saturation—even in cyanotic patients (14). Hence, if the technique is preceded by preoxygenation, the anesthesiologist may practice whatever technique he or she does best and seems most appropriate for a given patient. Therefore, before every induction, oxygen is administered by face mask. Often, the child is happier if the face mask is held slightly away from the face, using a high fresh gas flow. This technique, however, may not provide complete denitrogenation and may not be appropriate for cyanotic patients.

Anesthesia is induced with ketamine (3 to 5 mg/kg IM or 1 to 2 mg IV). Ketamine is relatively contraindicated in patients with suboptimal coronary perfusion (e.g., critical aortic stenosis or hypoplastic left heart) because ventricular fibrillation may develop. Intravenous induction may be useful in patients with R → L shunt, which slows inhalation induction. For most patients, IV thiopental given slowly (2 to 4 mg/kg) produces a smooth induction with minimal cardiovascular effects. Alternatively, particularly for the very unstable patient, fentanyl up to 30 μg/kg IV and diazepam up to 0.1 mg/kg IV may be administered for induction. Drugs given IV should be administered slowly in small doses. If a R → L shunt is present, IV agents act very rapidly, but if the circulation time is slow, the effect of these agents may be less rapid. If high-dose fentanyl is to be used, 50 to 100 μg/kg may be added to the IV drip chamber and infused over 15 to 30 minutes or given as intermittent boluses. In patients without IV access, anesthesia may be induced by mask inhalation of halothane or sevoflurane (after preoxygenation).

If hypotension occurs after induction of anesthesia, cardiotonic drugs may be needed to control cardiac shunt flow and to maintain oxygen-hemoglobin saturation (Table 12).

Endotracheal Intubation

For endotracheal intubation, the anesthesiologist may give succinylcholine (1 to 2 mg/kg IV) or an initial dose of nondepolarizing relaxant. After administration of muscle relaxant, the patient is ventilated until relaxation is adequate. Vecuronium (0.1 mg/kg) produces good conditions for intubation within 2 minutes. If fentanyl is to be used, pancuronium (0.1 mg/kg) may be given to offset the bradycardia-producing effect of fentanyl. Nondepolarizing agents may take longer for a full effect in patients with CHD (15). Therefore, a longer period of mask ventilation may be necessary before intubation is attempted, when using the nondepolarizing muscle relaxant agents. A cuffed endotracheal tube is used if size 6 mm or larger is required.

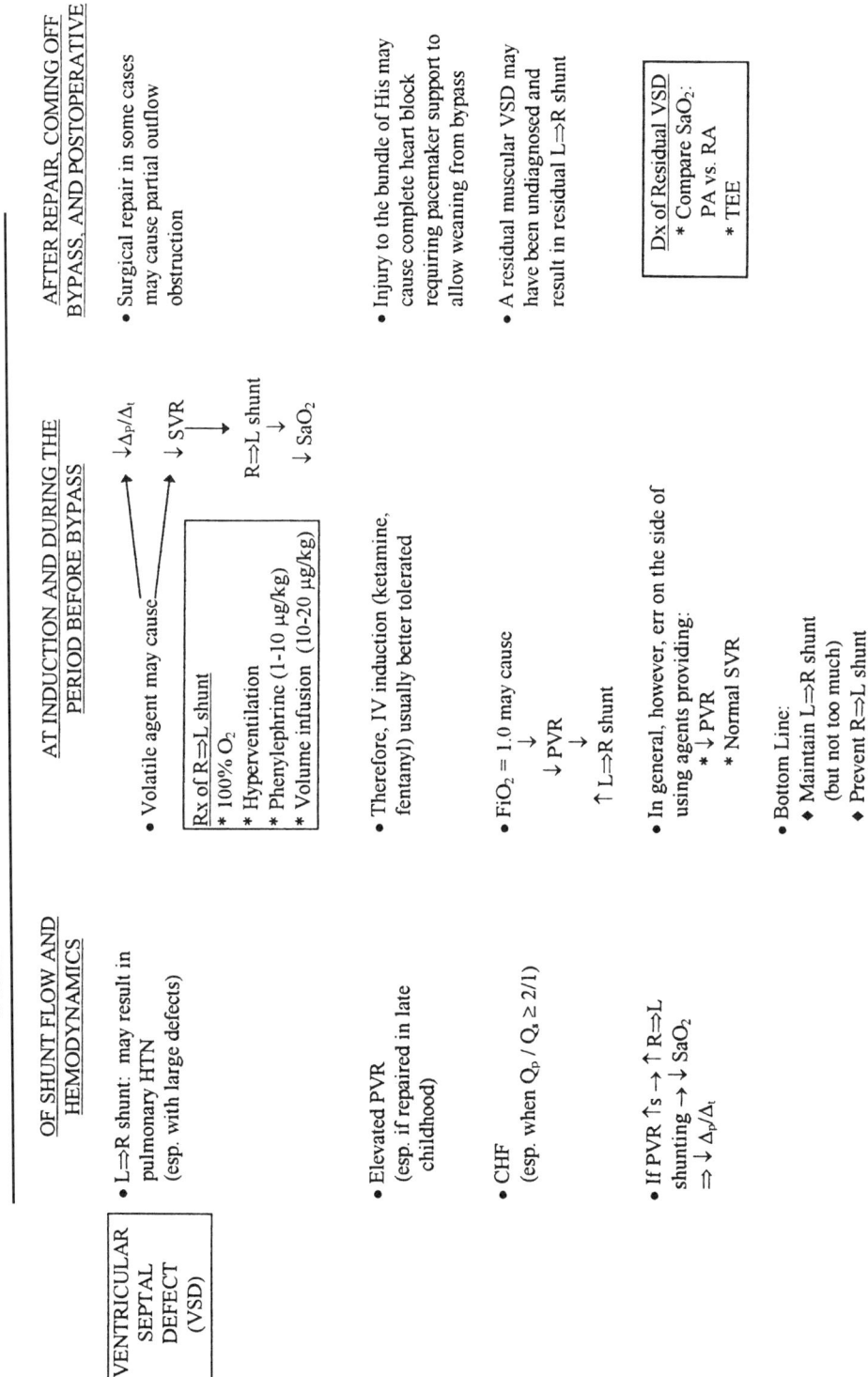

TABLE 4. Considerations for ventricular septal defect surgery

	OF SHUNT FLOW AND HEMODYNAMICS	AT INDUCTION AND DURING THE PERIOD BEFORE BYPASS	AFTER REPAIR, COMING OFF BYPASS, AND POSTOPERATIVE
VENTRICULAR SEPTAL DEFECT (VSD)	• L⇒R shunt: may result in pulmonary HTN (esp. with large defects) • Elevated PVR (esp. if repaired in late childhood) • CHF (esp. when $Q_p / Q_s \geq 2/1$) • If PVR ↑s → ↑R⇒L shunting → ↓ SaO_2 ⇒ ↓ Δ_p/Δ_t	• Volatile agent may cause ↓Δ_p/Δ_t / ↓ SVR → R⇒L shunt → ↓ SaO_2 Rx of R⇒L shunt * 100% O_2 * Hyperventilation * Phenylephrine (1-10 μg/kg) * Volume infusion (10-20 μg/kg) • Therefore, IV induction (ketamine, fentanyl) usually better tolerated • FiO_2 = 1.0 may cause → ↓ PVR → ↑ L⇒R shunt • In general, however, err on the side of using agents providing: * ↓ PVR * Normal SVR • Bottom Line: ♦ Maintain L⇒R shunt (but not too much) ♦ Prevent R⇒L shunt	• Surgical repair in some cases may cause partial outflow obstruction • Injury to the bundle of His may cause complete heart block requiring pacemaker support to allow weaning from bypass • A residual muscular VSD may have been undiagnosed and result in residual L⇒R shunt Dx of Residual VSD * Compare SaO_2: PA vs. RA * TEE

TABLE 5. Considerations for endocardial cushion effect

ENDOCARDIAL CUSHION DEFECT	OF SHUNT FLOW AND HEMODYNAMICS	AT INDUCTION AND DURING THE PERIOD BEFORE BYPASS	AFTER REPAIR, COMING OFF BYPASS, AND POSTOPERATIVE

• Consists of:
  ♦ ASD
  ♦ VSD
  ♦ Clefts in mitral and tricuspid leaflets
 	
• 30% are found in kids with Down's syndrome
 	
• Surgical repair:
  ♦ Division of common A-V valve
  ♦ Closure of ASD and VSD with single or double patch
  ♦ Mitral and (sometimes) tricuspid valves require repair of separated portions
	• Large L⇒R shunt
	  ♦ Magnitude controlled by PVR
	    (↓PVR → ↑L⇒R shunt)
	
	• High PBF
	  ↓
	  CHF + Pulmonary hypertension
	
	• Myocardial depressants, and ↓PVR + ↑L⇒R shunt are *poorly tolerated*
	
	• These patients have the same potential complications as ASD and VSD
	
	• Mitral valve may be severely regurgitant
	
	• Left anterior hemiblock may exist
	
	• Older children develop pulmonary vascular obstructive disease (PVOD)
		• Anesthetic considerations are similar for infants with large VSDs	One Or More Of The Following May Be Required Intra- Or Postoperatively:
			
			• Inotropic support for failing heart
			
			• Afterload reduction for mitral regurgitation
			
			• Measures to adjust PVR
			
			• Most frequent *postoperative* problems:
			  ♦ Residual VSD
			  ♦ Mitral insufficiency
			  ♦ Pulmonary hypertension
			
			• Measures to ↓PVR and prolonged IPPV are often necessary because pulmonary vascular beds are hyperreactive. (esp. those with PVOD)

TABLE 6. *Considerations for truncus arteriosus*

TRUNCUS ARTERIOSUS	OF SHUNT FLOW AND HEMODYNAMICS	AT INDUCTION AND DURING THE PERIOD BEFORE BYPASS	AFTER REPAIR, COMING OFF BYPASS, AND POSTOPERATIVE

• Consists of:
  ♦ Single great artery (SGA) gives rise to:
    ⇒ Coronary and pulmonary arteries (1 or 2) and systemic circulations
  ♦ Large VSD
 	
• Prognostic factors in survival:
  ♦ Reversibility of ↑ₐPVR: Hyperoxia → ↓PVR = good prognosis
  ♦ In children with "fixed" PVR:
    *Expect problems
    *Poor prognosis
 	
• Surgical repair:
  ♦ VSD is closed
  ♦ PA(s) is (are) detached
  ♦ Conduit placed between RV & PA(s)
  ♦ Truncal valvoplasty
 	
• Extracardiac anomalies frequent
  ♦ DiGeorge's syndrome
    ⇒ Calcium metabolism problems
    ⇒ Airway problems to small mouth, micrognathia
	• Complete mixing of systemic and pulmonary venous blood in SGA
	  ⇓
	  Mild ↓ SaO_2
	
	  ♦ PBF ≅ 1/PVR
	
	• PA orifice is seldom restrictive
	  Excessive PBF early in life as PVR ↓s ("pulmonary steal")
	  ↑SaO_2 ↓Q_s/Q_p
	    ↘ ↙
	  ↓ Systemic O_2 Transport
	    ↓
	  Lactic acidosis
	
	• These children may develop ⇒ PVOD
	
	• Truncal valve regurgitation
	  ↓
	  ↑RV and LV volume load
	  ↓
	  CHF
		• Anesthetic management:
		  ♦ *Control PBF*
		    *Keep low or normal
		  ♦ Support RV and LV
		
		• Induce with ketamine or fentanyl
		
		• Monitor calcium closely, replete PRN
		
		• PBF may ↑ with:
		  ♦ Anesthetic agents
		  ♦ Alkalosis
		  ♦ O_2 Administration
		
		• ↑PBF ⇒ ↓BP
		    ⇒ CHF
		
		• *Therefore*, take measures to ↑ PVR:
		  ♦ Mild acidosis
		  ♦ Titrate FIO_2 to SaO_2 = 85-90%
		  ♦ Avoid volatile anesthetic agents
		
		• Maintain normal or low SVR
		  ♦ To improve systemic perfusion
		  ♦ To decrease ⇑ PBF
			• Two most common problems
			  ♦ Persistent pulmonary hypertension
			  ♦ Poor Δ_p/Δ_t
			
			• Persistent PA Hypertension + RV failure ⇒ can be fatal; *Therefore*, after repair:
			  ♦ Provide normal Δ_p/Δ_t using inotropes
			  ♦ Lower the PVR
			    *Hyperventilation
			    *Oxygenation (FiO_2 = 1.0)
			    *Nitric Oxide
			
			• Residual VSD* (*Suspect residual VSD if patient not doing well)
			  Additional RV & LV loads
			    ↗ ↘
			  ↓BP ↓SaO_2
			
			• Truncal valve regurgitation
			  →
			  LV failure
			
			• Obstruction of the PA conduit
			  →
			  RV Hypertension

TABLE 7. Considerations for transposition of great vessels

TRANSPOSITION OF GREAT VESSELS (TGV)	OF SHUNT FLOW AND HEMODYNAMICS	AT INDUCTION AND DURING THE PERIOD BEFORE BYPASS	AFTER REPAIR, COMING OFF BYPASS, AND POSTOPERATIVE
• Basic defect ♦ RV→Aorta ♦ LV→PA ♦ Some have PS	• Mixing of pulmonary and systemic blood necessary through: ♦ VSD ↗ Naturally occurring ♦ ASD ↘ Created by balloon septostomy ♦ PDA - kept open with PGE₁ • Physiologic disturbance ♦ Inadequate mixing ♦ *Not* one of inadequate PBF • LA is usually volume overloaded	• LA⇒RA shunt improves SaO₂ • One of three surgeries available ♦ Atrial level (Mustard, Senning) Switches ♦ Great artery level (Jatene) ♦ Ventricular level (Rastelli)	• Postoperative problems differ by procedure • *Atrial Baffle* - creates these flows: ♦ Pulmonary venous blood →Tricuspid→RV→Ao ♦ Systemic venous return →Atrial septum→Mitral→LV→PA *RV works against high pressures *Postoperative problems ◊Baffle can obstruct venous return ⇒SVC syndrome (systemic venous hypertension) ⇒Pulmonary venous hypertension →Resp. failure →Poor ABG's →Pulmonary edema ↓ (Bloody fluid in ETT) →Low cardiac output

* Preoperative LV outflow obstruction, large PDA, or *restrictive* VSD*
    Poor LV ability
    ↓
    CHF
    (Huge support needed)

* Preoperative *nonrestrictive* VSD*
    Good LV ability
    (Minimal support needed)

• *Arterial switch* - arteries divided, reattached
♦ Coronary arteries reattached to NeoAo
± ⇒ myocardial ischemia or infarction

Prevention of MI in TGV
  * Inotropic support
  * ↑ Coronary perfusion pressure
  * Control HR
  * Rx with vasodilators

• Inotropic support needed depends on *ability of LV* to tolerate work

TABLE 8. Considerations for tetralogy of Fallot

	OF SHUNT FLOW AND HEMODYNAMICS	AT INDUCTION AND DURING THE PERIOD BEFORE BYPASS	AFTER REPAIR, COMING OFF BYPASS, AND POSTOPERATIVE
TETROLOGY OF FALLOT (TOF)	• Pathophysiology varies in severity	• *Normal systemic BP critical*	• Most patients have residual bi-ventricular dysfuntion * Need inotropic support

CONSISTS OF:
• VSD
• RV outflow obstruction
• Overriding aorta
• RVH
	• Some kids have "TET SPELLS" as response to stress
	
	"TET SPELL"
	↑RV obstruction and ↑PVR
	⇒
	↑R⇒L shunt
	⇒
	Severe cyanosis
	
	• PVR usually normal due to:
	  * PS
	  * R⇒L shunt
	
	• However, *vicious cycle may occur*:
	
	↓SaO$_2$, ↓pH
	↑R⇒L ← ↑PVR ← ↑catecholamines
	↑RVOT obstruction ← ↑Δ$_p$/Δ$_t$
	
	• If cyanotic, polycythemic:
	  * Preoperative hydration
		• Appropriate induction techniques
		  * Fentanyl, pancuronium
		  * Ketamine may be used if adequate ventilation is assured
		    [Ketamine + Hypoventilation
		    ⇒
		    ↑PVR[43]]
		
		• Rx of cyanotic ("TET") spells
		  * 100% O$_2$
		  * Hyperventilation
		  * Phenylephrine (1-10 μg/kg)
		  * Volume infusion (10-20 ml/kg)
		  * Optional:
		    - Propranolol (5 μg/kg, ↑ dose PRN)
		    - Esmolol infusion (100-200 μg/kg/min, no loading dose)
			• Some patients may have
			  * RBBB
			  * Residual pulmonic obstruction, and shunting
			    ⇒
			    ↓RV function
			
			• S$_{PaO_2}$ > 80% with FiO$_2$ of ~ 0.5 = L⇒R shunt and Q$_p$/Q$_s$ > 1
			⇒
			May lead to complications following bypass

TABLE 9. *Considerations for hypoplastic left heart syndrome*

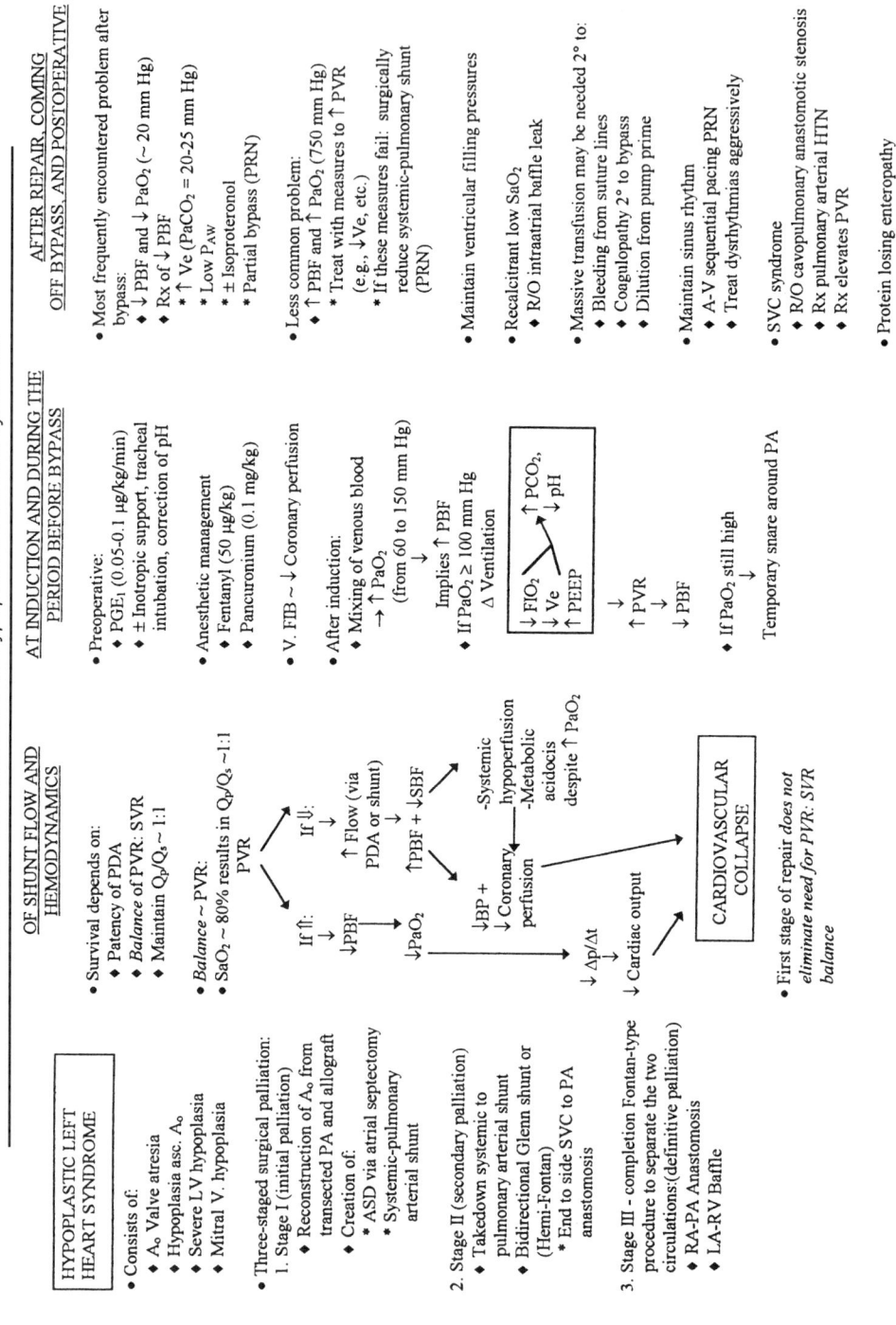

HYPOPLASTIC LEFT HEART SYNDROME	OF SHUNT FLOW AND HEMODYNAMICS	AT INDUCTION AND DURING THE PERIOD BEFORE BYPASS	AFTER REPAIR, COMING OFF BYPASS, AND POSTOPERATIVE
• Consists of: ◆ A₀ Valve atresia ◆ Hypoplasia asc. A₀ ◆ Severe LV hypoplasia ◆ Mitral V. hypoplasia • Three-staged surgical palliation: 1. Stage I (initial palliation) ◆ Reconstruction of A₀ from transected PA and allograft ◆ Creation of: * ASD via atrial septectomy * Systemic-pulmonary arterial shunt 2. Stage II (secondary palliation) ◆ Takedown systemic to pulmonary arterial shunt ◆ Bidirectional Glenn shunt or (Hemi-Fontan) * End to side SVC to PA anastomosis 3. Stage III – completion Fontan-type procedure to separate the two circulations (definitive palliation) ◆ RA-PA Anastomosis ◆ LA-RV Baffle	• Survival depends on: ◆ Patency of PDA ◆ *Balance* of PVR: SVR ◆ Maintain $Q_p/Q_s \sim 1:1$ • *Balance* ~ PVR: ◆ $SaO_2 \sim 80\%$ results in $Q_p/Q_s \sim 1:1$ PVR If ⇑: ↓PBF ↓PaO_2 ↓BP + ↓ Coronary perfusion ↓Δp/Δt ↓ Cardiac output If ⇓: ↑Flow (via PDA or shunt) ↑PBF + ↓SBF -Systemic hypoperfusion -Metabolic acidosis despite ↑PaO_2 **CARDIOVASCULAR COLLAPSE** • First stage of repair *does not eliminate* need for PVR: SVR balance	• Preoperative: ◆ PGE_1 (0.05-0.1 μg/kg/min) ◆ ± Inotropic support, tracheal intubation, correction of pH • Anesthetic management ◆ Fentanyl (50 μg/kg) ◆ Pancuronium (0.1 mg/kg) • V. FIB ~ ↓ Coronary perfusion • After induction: ◆ Mixing of venous blood → ↑PaO_2 (from 60 to 150 mm Hg) → Implies ↑PBF ◆ If $PaO_2 \geq 100$ mm Hg Δ Ventilation ↓FIO_2 ↑PCO_2, ↓Ve ↓pH ↑PEEP → ↑PVR → ↓PBF ◆ If PaO_2 still high Temporary snare around PA	• Most frequently encountered problem after bypass: ◆ ↓PBF and ↓PaO_2 (~20 mm Hg) ◆ Rx of ↓PBF * ↑Ve ($PaCO_2$ = 20-25 mm Hg) * Low P_{Aw} * ± Isoproterenol * Partial bypass (PRN) • Less common problem: ◆ ↑PBF and ↑PaO_2 (750 mm Hg) * Treat with measures to ↑PVR (e.g., ↓Ve, etc.) * If these measures fail: surgically reduce systemic-pulmonary shunt (PRN) • Maintain ventricular filling pressures • Recalcitrant low SaO_2 ◆ R/O intraatrial baffle leak • Massive transfusion may be needed 2° to: ◆ Bleeding from suture lines ◆ Coagulopathy 2° to bypass ◆ Dilution from pump prime • Maintain sinus rhythm ◆ A-V sequential pacing PRN ◆ Treat dysrhythmias aggressively • SVC syndrome ◆ R/O cavopulmonary anastomotic stenosis ◆ Rx pulmonary arterial HTN ◆ Rx elevates PVR • Protein losing enteropathy ◆ Pleural effusions ◆ Ascites

TABLE 10. *Considerations for pulmonic stenosis/atresia*

PULMONIC STENOSIS / ATRESIA	OF SHUNT FLOW AND HEMODYNAMICS	AT INDUCTION AND DURING THE PERIOD BEFORE BYPASS	AFTER REPAIR, COMING OFF BYPASS, AND POSTOPERATIVE

• Encompasses a *spectrum* of lesions:
 ♦ Asymptomatic mild PS:
   * RV dilates slowly
   * Cardiac failure appears late
 ♦ Severe PS
   * Systolic gradient RV to PA:
   ⇒ ↑ RV pressure ⇒ RV hypertrophy ⇒ RV failure
 	
 • Surgical procedures:
 ♦ P. valvotomy if:
   * RV well developed
   * PA is present
 ♦ Systemic - pulmonic shunt if:
   * RV not developed
 	
 • PBF ~ PDA
 	
 • ASD or patent foramen ovale is virtually always present in PA
	• Severity of symptoms ~ degree of ↓ PBF and ↓ CO
	
	 • Peak pressure on RV cath data shows *severity of stenosis*:
	 ♦ Mild: ≤ 50 (mm Hg)
	 ♦ Moderate: RV = LV
	 ♦ Severe: RV > LV
	
	 • *Primary hemodynamic goal is to maintain PBF*
	 ♦ Therefore, *prevent*:
	   * ↑ PVR
	   * ↓ SVR
	   * ↓ PDA flow → ↓ PaO$_2$
	   * PGE$_1$ infused to maintain PDA
	
	 • ↑ Heart Rate:
	 ♦ ↓ Diastolic filling time → ↓ CO
	 ♦ ↑ outflow obstruction and ↓ RV filling
	
	 • Underdeveloped RV requires high filling pressures
	 ♦ If RV dilated → Tricuspid valve regurgitation
		• Maintain stable HR
		 ♦ Prevent tachycardia
		 ♦ Prevent bradycardia
		   * Neonate cannot ↑ stroke volume to compensate for ↑ HR
		
		 • Maintain adequate filling volume to maintain RV filling pressures
		
		 • Maintain myocardial contractility
		
		 • After induction, phenylephrine (0.5-1.0 µg/kg/min or .01-0.05 mg/kg/dose) may be needed to maintain SVR
			• Goal of surgical therapy is to improve oxygenation and ↓ RV afterload
			
			 • In immediate postoperative period, there may be:
			 ♦ R⇒L shunting
			   ⇓
			   ↓ PaO$_2$
			
			 • With infant's growth and ↑ RV compliance → PaO$_2$ ↑s
			
			 • If ↓ PaO$_2$ persists:
			 ♦ ± PGE$_1$ infusion

TABLE 11. *Considerations for congenital left ventricular outflow obstruction*

	OF SHUNT FLOW AND HEMODYNAMICS	AT INDUCTION AND DURING THE PERIOD BEFORE BYPASS	AFTER REPAIR, COMING OFF BYPASS, AND POSTOPERATIVE
CONGENITAL LEFT VENTRICULAR OUTFLOW OBSTRUCTION (e.g., CRITICAL AORTIC STENOSIS)	• LV outflow tract obstruction: $\Rightarrow$ LV failure $\Rightarrow$ Poor systemic perfusion $\Rightarrow \downarrow$ BP $\Rightarrow$ Pulmonary congestion	• These patients *do not tolerate*: ♦ Myocardial depressants ♦ Rapid heart rates	• Residual stenosis $\Rightarrow \downarrow$ Myocardial performance
Types of A_o Stenosis: • Valvular ~70% • Subvalvular ~20% • Supravalvular ~10%			
Consists of: • Thickened and rigid A_o valves • Variable fusion of valvular commissures • ± Endocardial fibroelastosis of left ventricle • ± Abnormalities of mitral valve	• $\downarrow$ Coronary perfusion + $\uparrow$ LV pressure $\Downarrow$ *Borderline coronary perfusion*	• Ventricular fibrillation may occur with surgical manipulation of heart • Defibrillator should be available • Mitral regurgitation may continue	• Aortic regurgitation may occur • If obstruction adequately relieved: ♦ Myocardial function improved by: * $\downarrow$ Afterload (cautiously) * Inotropic agents (Especially, if A_o regurgitation occurs) * Maintain adequate preload
Treatment choices: • Valvotomy under direct vision • Balloon angioplasty	• Systemic blood flow may be partly supported by R $\Rightarrow$ L flow through PDA ♦ Infusion of PGE_1 may help maintain systemic flow		

TABLE 12. *Doses and effects of cardiotonic drugs*

Agent	Doses (IV)	Peripheral vascular effect	Cardiac effect	Conduction system effect
Noncatecholamines				
Digoxin (total digitalizing dose)	20 µg/kg premature 30 µg/kg neonate (0–1 mo) 40 µg/kg infant (<2 y) 30 µg/kg child (2–5 y) 20 µg/kg child (>5 y)	Increases peripheral vascular resistance 1–2+; acts directly on vascular smooth muscle	Inotropic effect 3–4+; acts directly	Slows sinus node; decreases AV conduction
Calcium chloride	10–20 mg/kg/dose (slowly)	Variable; probably depends on serum ionized Ca^{2+} level	Inotropic effect 3+; depends on ionized Ca^{2+}	Slows sinus node; decreases AV conduction
Calcium gluconate	30–60 mg/kg/dose (slowly)			
Nitroprusside	0.3–5 µg/kg/min	Donates nitric oxide group to relax smooth muscle and dilate pulmonary and systemic vessels	Indirectly increases cardiac output by decreasing afterload	Reflex tachycardia
Amrinone	1–3 mg/kg loading dose; 5–20 µg/kg/min maintenance	Systemic and pulmonary vasodilator; platelet and toxic effects not well established in neonates	Increases cardiac output in neonates and infants	Minimal tachycardia

		Peripheral vascular effect		Cardiac effect			
Agent	Doses (IV)	Alpha	Beta2	Delta	Beta1	Beta2	Comment
Catecholamines							
Phenylephrine	0.1–0.5 µg/kg/min	4+	0	0	0	0	Increases systemic resistance, no inotropy; may cause renal ischemia; useful for treatment of TOF spells
Isoproterenol	0.05–0.5 µg/kg/min	0	4+	0	4+	4+	Strong inotropic and chronotropic agent; peripheral vasodilator; reduces preload; pulmonary vasodilator; limited by tachycardia and oxygen consumption
Norepinephrine	0.1–0.5 µg/kg/min	4+	0	0	2+	0	Increases systemic resistance; moderately inotropic; may cause renal ischemia
Epinephrine	0.03–0.1 µg/kg/min 0.2–0.5 µg/kg/min	2+ 4+	1–2+ 0	0 0	2–3+ 4+	2+ 3+	Beta2 effect with lower doses; best for blood pressure in anaphylaxis and drug toxicity
Dopamine	2–4 µg/kg/min 4–8 µg/kg/min >10 µg/kg/min	0 0 2–4+	0 2+ 0	2+ 2+ 0	0 1–2+ 1–2+	0 1+ 2+	Splanchnic and renal vasodilator; may be used with isoproterenol; increasing doses produce increasing alpha effect
Dobutamine	2–10 µg/kg/min	1+	2+	0	3–4+	1–2+	Less chronotropism and arrhythmias at lower doses; effects vary with dose similar to dopamine; chronotropic advantage compared with dopamine may not be apparent in neonates

Reprinted with permission, from reference 23

Equipment Placed on the Patient after Intubation

After induction, the following are placed in position:

- Esophageal stethoscope
- Noninvasive blood pressure cuff
- Rectal (or bladder) and esophageal (or tympanic membrane) temperature probes
- A large-bore IV infusion line **(see Chapter 3)**
- An arterial line, usually in the right radial artery, and a double-lumen CVP line, usually via the external or internal jugular vein (the second lumen can be used for vasoactive drug infusion)
- Urinary catheter for measurement of urine output perioperatively and postoperatively
- Nasogastric tube
- +/−Electroencephalogram electrodes connected to a cerebral function monitor

Line Placement

For pump cases, two large-bore peripheral IVs are inserted: one large IV in the saphenous vein (for blood components) and one in a vein on the dorsum of the hand (Fig. 1). In the large blood IV line, two stopcocks are placed near the anesthesia team so that blood products may be pumped in and measured using 50-ml syringes.

Next, a central venous line is inserted, most commonly in the right internal jugular vein **(see Chapter 3)**. Preferably, a double-lumen catheter is used. The distal lumen of the catheter is connected to the CVP monitoring line, and bolus medications are injected in this line at the distal stopcock. The proximal lumen of the catheter is used for continuous medication infusions. A carrier infusion is connected to this line as well as a manifold system IV adaptor to accommodate multiple-infusion lines.

After all the lines are established, the patient should be positioned on the table with the assistance of the circulating nurse. All lines are brought up to the head of the table, and an ether screen frame is placed. A blue towel is placed at the head of the table. All IV and arterial lines are labeled and placed on top of the towel. All other lines (e.g., breathing circuit, monitoring cables) are kept below the towel.

Controlled Ventilation

Ventilation is controlled with a volume-cycled ventilator. Normocarbia is maintained and confirmed by end-tidal and serial arterial blood gas analysis. It is important to avoid respiratory alkalosis (16), because it results in the following:

- Reduces cardiac output
- Causes vasoconstriction and increases systemic resistance
- Shifts the hemoglobin-oxygen (Hb-O2) dissociation curve to the left
- Decreases myocardial blood flow
- Decreases serum potassium level
- Favors development of dysrhythmias
- Decreases cerebral blood flow

$PaCO_2$ should be in the physiologic range (35 to 40 mm Hg). Note that end-tidal CO_2 is a satisfactory means to monitor $PaCO_2$ in acyanotic patients but may underestimate the $PaCO_2$ in children with cyanotic CHD (17). One should be aware of the possible effects of intermittent positive-pressure ventilation on shunts. High intrathoracic pressures are avoided, but the lung volume is maintained as necessary by the use of positive end-expiratory pressure (PEEP). Pulmonary vascular resistance is least at an optimal lung volume and increases at volumes above or below this optimal volume.

Maintenance of Anesthesia

Anesthetic Agents

Optimal myocardial function and cardiac output must be maintained during surgery. Therefore, agents that cause excessive my-

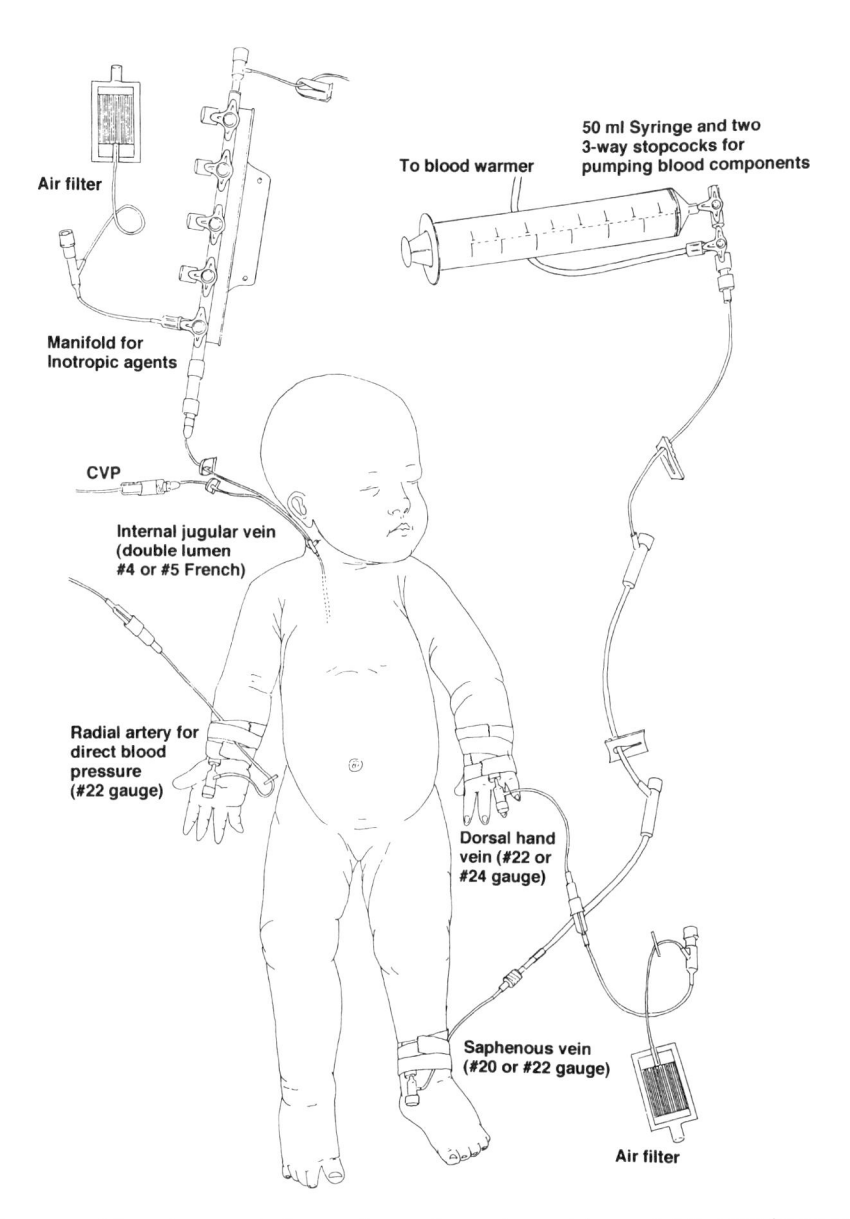

FIG. 1. Suggested line placement sites and vascular equipment for pediatric open heart surgery.

ocardial depression are generally avoided. Drugs that produce a controllable degree of myocardial depression (e.g., halothane) may be useful, however, when there is ventricular muscle obstructing blood flow (e.g., in tetralogy of Fallot).

Anesthesia may be maintained with a suitable mixture of nitrous oxide (N₂O) and O₂ to ensure an appropriate oxygen-hemoglobin saturation. Air plus O₂ is used in patients for whom N₂O may be contraindicated. It is rarely necessary to use more than 50% oxygen. If a large R → L shunt is present, increasing the F_IO_2 will have very little effect on the PaO_2. N₂O is avoided in the patient with pulmonary hypertension.

If myocardial function is good, isoflurane, 0.5% to 0.75%, or 0.5% halothane may be given, depending on the lesion. Volatile agents, if used, may be given in low concentrations and supplemented with generous doses of fentanyl (up to 100 mg/kg). Patients with cardiac failure who benefit from afterload reduction (e.g., VSD) may do well with isoflurane. Patients who may benefit from myocardial depression (e.g., tetralogy of Fallot) may do well with halothane.

Control of Intracardiac Shunting

Detrimental changes in cardiac shunts must be prevented. Patients who are dependent on systemic-to-pulmonary shunts (e.g., patients with tetralogy of Fallot) will desaturate if the systemic arterial pressure is allowed to fall. Therefore, drugs that have minimal effects on systemic vascular resistance are used in these patients (Tables 4 to 11).

Control of Cardiac Workload

Conditions that favor optimal myocardial perfusion must be maintained throughout surgery to avoid ischemic damage to the heart and subsequent impairment of cardiac function postoperatively. The duration of diastole and the diastolic pressure are important factors in maintaining perfusion of the myocardium, which is especially vulnerable if ventricular hypertrophy is present. The anesthesiologist is careful to avoid producing tachycardia, which shortens diastole and thus may impair myocardial perfusion. Blood and fluids are replaced in adequate volume to maintain the diastolic blood pressure.

During CPB, it is preferable to maintain a regular rhythm until aortic cross-clamping and cardioplegia administration. If ventricular fibrillation occurs, higher perfusion pressures are needed to ensure myocardial perfusion. The following steps are taken to minimize cardiac workload:

- Hypertension and tachycardia during anesthesia are prevented by ensuring adequate levels of analgesia and by use of vasodilators or β-adrenergic blockers when appropriate.
- Drugs that may produce hypertension (e.g., pancuronium) are given cautiously.
- Pulmonary hypertension must be controlled.

Some patients with large L → R shunts (e.g., VSD, truncus arteriosus, atrioventricular canal) are at risk for pulmonary hypertensive crises during and after surgery. It is important to prevent these crises because they are difficult to reverse. The following are standard measures that may be taken to prevent hypertensive crises:

- Minimal handling of the child
- Controlled hyperventilation ($PaCO_2$ = 25 to 30)
- Fentanyl infusion (e.g., 25 µg/kg loading dose plus 2 µg/kg/hour)
- Sodium nitroprusside infusion
- Phenoxybenzamine: 1 mg/kg loading dose followed by 1 mg/kg/day in divided doses
- PGE_1 infusion, 0.03 to 0.1 µg/kg/min (18)
- Avoidance of nitrous oxide

Use of Muscle Relaxants

Incremental doses of muscle relaxants are given as needed. The choice of muscle relaxant for use during maintenance of anesthesia should be influenced by the following:

- Vecuronium has very little effect on cardiovascular parameters and is probably the agent of choice for most infants and some children.
- If some decrease in afterload might be advantageous, D-tubocurarine is still a useful drug.
- Pancuronium, 0.1 mg/kg, may be used if high-dose fentanyl is used.

Maintenance of Fluid Balance

Fluid balance is adjusted to provide optimal cardiac filling pressures. Serial measurements of all relevant indices, including blood gas analyses, should be made throughout surgery to achieve these objectives. Maintenance fluids are given according to body weight to replace the calculated deficit during fasting (if any) and maintain urine output at >1 ml/kg/hour **(see Chapter 9)**. Additional fluid loading before CPB has not been shown to be advantageous.[c]

Many of these children are polycythemic preoperatively. If so, plasma is preferable to blood as a replacement fluid. A hematocrit of 35% to 40% by the end of surgery is usually desirable. A blood warmer is used for all infusions.

Blood loss from sponges, suction, drapes, and specimens are measured carefully and running totals maintained. It is seldom necessary to transfuse blood before CPB unless major blood loss occurs during dissection around the heart (e.g., during repeat operations). However, during venous cannulation in small infants, a significant volume of blood may be lost. One should always be prepared to replace this sudden blood loss.

In summation of fluid management, the goal of fluid management is to maintain the hematocrit at near-preoperative level and the intravascular volume high enough to maintain CVP. If the hematocrit is very high preoperatively, initial losses are replaced with plasma, but the clinician is cautioned against too much hemodilution before CPB.

MANAGEMENT OF CARDIOPULMONARY BYPASS

Prebypass Preparation

Prebypass systemic corticosteroids may help preserve myocardial tissue during ischemic arrest periods, but this is controversial. During dissection around the heart, blood pressure and ECG are watched closely. Dysrhythmias are common, although most are innocuous. If hypotension or dysrhythmias persist, the surgeon may be asked to desist (if possible) until the condition corrects itself.

Heparinization

Before surgery, the pump circuit is primed with heparin (250 U/100 ml of prime volume). Immediately before aortic cannulation, the surgeon will give heparin into the right atrium or ask for heparin to be given via the central line. A dose of 0.3 ml/kg of 1:1000 beef lung heparin (3 mg/kg or 300 U/kg) is administered from a fresh unopened vial. Dosage is verified with the perfusionist and staff. The drug is administered in the CVP line by connecting the syringe of heparin to the stopcock, aspirating until blood returns in the syringe, injecting the total dose, then flushing the CVP line many times. *It is absolutely critical that the correct dose of heparin is delivered into the central circulation before bypass.* If in doubt about the central line or if no central line is available, heparin should be given by the surgeon.

A repeat anticoagulant therapy (ACT), performed 3 minutes after heparin, should be three to four times the control ACT (usually 600 to 700 seconds). The surgeon should be restrained from further surgery until ACT is appropriate. When appropriate ACT is ensured, the surgeon is advised that the heart can be bypassed. Heparin has a larger volume of distribution and a more rapid plasma clearance in infants compared with adults (19). Therefore, larger doses may be required initially, and the level of heparinization should be checked frequently.

Insertion of Cardiac Venous Cannulas

Hypotension may occur when the cardiac venous cannulas are inserted. If this happens,

---

[c] Ed. Note (JMB): In other words, a preoperative fresh water drowning is not needed in these cases.

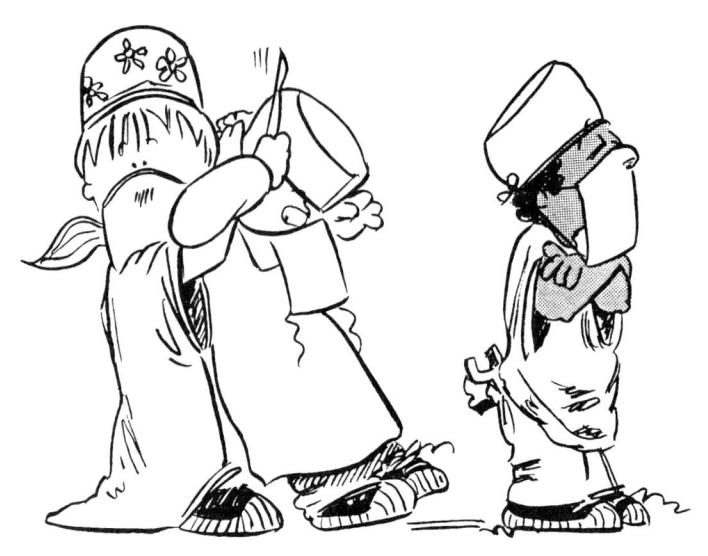

Waiting on the ACT to rise

volatile agents are discontinued and the inspired O₂ concentration increased until bypass has been instituted. Additional fluid infusion may also help to restore blood pressure. If the aorta is already cannulated, this fluid can be delivered from the pump. Close observation of the operative field is prudent at this time. Ventilation (lung expansion) is decreased to assist the surgeon with venous cannulation by providing for improved exposure of the surgical field.

Considerations During Cardiopulmonary Bypass

During CPB, the myocardium may be protected by a cardioplegic solution infused into the coronary circulation following aortic clamping (20). Controversy exists as to what is the most advantageous type of solution, but most solutions contain high levels of potassium with added dextrose and buffers. The addition of free-radical scavenger agents and calcium ion channel blockers has been suggested. Repeated doses of cardioplegia are normally used at 15- to 20-minute intervals. Remember that the heart has a great tendency to rewarm because of manipulation and heat from operating room lights. Therefore, during prolonged surgery, cold cardioplegic solutions should be repeated and a pericardial cooling bath used.

On initiation of CPB, ventilation is discontinued once the perfusionist reports that full flow is established. The lungs are ventilated a few times with air. All monitoring alarms should be placed on standby. Although they probably would not clot off anyway in a heparinized patient, all IVs should be turned to keep vein open (KVO) rates. Patent IV catheters are a must when coming off CPB. The urine output should be recorded and the urine volumeter emptied. The pump technicians take great pride in assuring their patients have good urine output during bypass. An additional dose of muscle relaxant should be given to patients undergoing circulatory arrest or other patients, if indicated.

Once the patient is on bypass, the pump flow should be increased to establish satisfactory perfusion. Indicators of adequate perfusion are the cerebral function monitor, urine output, and repeated acid-base studies. Note that in patients with cyanotic CHD, perfusion pressures may be low during early bypass. This is due to the increased vascular bed of the patient and the use of low-viscosity perfusate. High flows may be required initially, but the systemic pressure will increase progressively, especially as cooling progresses. The use of vasoconstrictors is not usually necessary. When the perfusion pressure is low, it is of vital importance that the superior vena cava (SVC) pressure should be at or near zero. Increase in SVC pressure may have an adverse effect on cerebral perfusion pressure.

During bypass, the lungs may be allowed to collapse. Although traditional approaches are to maintain continued oxygen flow through the lungs or even to inflate the lungs with continuous positive airway pressure (CPAP) of 5 to 10 cm H_2O, human and animal experience does not support any particular advantage for keeping the lungs inflated (21). In fact, one study showed that CPAP during bypass actually decreased subsequent arterial oxygenation (22).

Isoflurane (0.5%) is added to the oxygenator to continue anesthesia and improve perfusion, or additional doses of fentanyl are given. Remember that fentanyl is bound to the plastic of the CPB circuit, so blood levels fall precipitously on bypass. Cautiously add volatile agents to the oxygenator during hypothermic bypass as high blood levels may result. Volatile agents should be discontinued 15 minutes before the end of bypass. During bypass (partial and total), the ACT is repeated every 30 minutes and additional doses of heparin given as necessary to prolong the ACT to >600 seconds. Blood samples for acid-base, electrolyte, and hematocrit determinations are taken every 30 minutes and just before CPB is discontinued.

"Coming Off" Bypass

At approximately 10 minutes before coming off CPB, the blood warmer is primed with whole blood or modified whole blood. The Y-set is primed with the blood bag being held with the entrance ports pointing upward. The end of the transfusion line is connected to the distal stopcock of the double stopcock in the large-bore peripheral IV line. A 50-ml syringe is attached to the proximal stopcock. This setup will allow for rapid syringing of blood products. Blood is aspirated into the 50-ml syringe so that it is ready for immediate injection before coming off bypass. It is absolutely critical that all air be removed from the blood transfusion IV tubing.

The surgeon may insert pulmonary artery or left atrial monitoring lines (23). If so, these are connected over the drape to the appropriate pressure monitoring lines, air bubbles are removed, and the lines are zeroed. The surgeon may also insert pacing wires before cessation of bypass. If so, the wires are connected to a pacer over the drape, and ability of the pacemaker to capture is tested.

Before coming off bypass, additional dosages of fentanyl or pancuronium should be given as needed. During discontinuance of bypass, the following additional efforts may be performed to reduce the possibility of cerebral air embolism:

- The carotid arteries are compressed for 20 seconds. (Rarely done anymore).

- During the early post-bypass phase, N_2O is not given (N_2O might increase the danger if air emboli are present).

Inotropic and vasopressor infusions along with the carrier infusion are started approximately 5 to 10 minutes before coming off bypass (Table 12).

In many cases, sodium nitroprusside is infused at 1 to 2 µg/kg/min to reduce afterload before weaning from bypass. Administration of nitroprusside is very important for the patient with pulmonary hypertension (e.g., after repair of a VSD in a child with pulmonary hypertension) (24).

Atrial and pulmonary artery catheters placed intraoperatively give valuable information about preload and contractility and are helpful to guide fluid management and vasopressor administration. Furthermore, these catheters provide information helpful to control pulmonary versus systemic blood flow and to control intracardiac shunt direction (if a shunt still exists after surgery). For example, a patient who is stable after VSD repair and who has pulmonary hypertension (normal pulmonary artery pressure is one half to one third of systemic pressure) may benefit from afterload reduction.

Another example in which atrial pressure lines are helpful is when CPB is discontinued. At this time, blood is infused from the pump until the left atrial pressure is adequate (normal is 8 to 12 mm Hg, depending on the cardiac lesion). Preload may be carefully maintained at the desired pressure.

Improving Cardiac Output. After all but the most minor cardiac operations, a deterioration in cardiac function is to be expected. This deterioration progresses for the first few hours after surgery, probably associated with edema of the myocardium and other changes. The result is a decrease in compliance of the ventricles and a decrease in contractility. Therapy at this time must be directed to ensuring optimal filling pressure, producing optimal cardiac rate and rhythm, and reducing the afterload.

Optimal filling pressures are ensured through judicial administration of blood components and fluids. As the compliance of the ventricles is low in infancy and reduced in all patients after cardiac surgery, high filling pressure (8 to 12 mm Hg) will probably be required.

Optimal cardiac rate and rhythm are most effectively achieved by the use of inotropes (see following section) or sequential pacing when necessary. In children as in adults, sinus rhythm (i.e., atrial contraction) significantly augments cardiac output.

Afterload is reduced by the use of vasodilators. In patients with ventricular dysfunction, vasodilators increase cardiac output with little change in cardiac work or arterial blood pressure. When vasodilators are used, the preload must be maintained by infusion of appropriate fluids. Sodium nitroprusside is infused at rates starting at 1 to 2 µg/kg/min and increased up to 5 µg/kg/min as needed. Although rarely used today, phenoxybenzamine has been administered to produce a long-lasting adrenergic blockade. Some patients will not tolerate well left ventricular afterload reduction, for example, those with impaired right ventricular function (e.g., following tetralogy of Fallot repair).

Inotropic Agents. If a low cardiac output persists despite the latter measure, infusion of inotropic agents is necessary. To improve myocardial contractility, dopamine is infused at 5 to 10 µg/kg/min by infusion pump (25). In infants and children, dopamine has been shown to be effective in increasing cardiac output, but higher doses are required than in adults and the vasodilating effect is less than in adults. Hence, the concurrent infusion of a vasodilator is frequently indicated (26). The combined administration of dopamine and sodium nitroprusside may also be effective in reducing pulmonary vascular resistance in patients with pulmonary hypertension. Most often these agents are given as soon as the patient is weaned from bypass. Calcium is infused to maintain the serum calcium at a high normal level (1 to 1.2 mmol/dl). If serious low output persists despite the latter measure, an epinephrine infusion of 0.05 to 1 µg/kg/min may be needed.

Failure to Wean from Bypass

Failure to wean from bypass (e.g., hypotension and bradycardia despite inotropic support) may be attributable to one or more factors (including hypovolemia, cardiac conduction defects, and metabolic derangements). If volume status is restored (i.e., CVP = 10 to 15) and hypotension persists, pharmacologic manipulation of afterload and contractility may be indicated. If heart rate is slow or if sinus rhythm is absent, sequential pacing may be necessary. The dopamine infusion may be increased to 15 µg/kg/min if hypotension persists. Calcium infusion (~750 µg/kg/min) may improve performance in some patients, but calcium should not be given until the heart has resumed a good regular beat. Calcium is monitored closely to maintain the nonionized concentration at 1 to 1.2 mm/dl.

Management after Cardiopulmonary Bypass

Immediate Post-Bypass Period

In infants and small children, the endotracheal tube should be suctioned before coming off bypass. The surgeon is notified before tracheal suction so that bypass cannulas can be protected. Ventilation is reestablished with 100% oxygen. Monitoring alarms are reenabled. Usually, 10 mg/kg of calcium is administered during weaning. As the CPB is terminated, incremental bolus dosages (5 mg/kg) or infusions (~750 μg/kg/min) of calcium or epinephrine (1 to 5 μg/kg) may be needed to maintain blood pressure. The urine output during CPB is recorded and reported to the perfusionist.

Adequate preload is maintained by infusion of blood components. If available, left atrial pressure may be used to guide volume administration. The goal for left atrial pressure in most patients is approximately 12 mm Hg. Other indicators of volume status are the pulmonary artery diastolic pressure, CVP, systemic blood pressure, TEE data, and the visual appearance of fullness of the right atrium. Most patients require several 50-ml syringes of blood in the immediate postoperative period. To avoid citrate toxicity (hypotension that occurs when citrate in blood components binds calcium), administration of blood products may require additional incremental boluses or infusion of calcium.

Restoration of Coagulation

When the patient's condition is stable and the surgeon concurs, protamine is administered. The aortic cannula is generally left in place until 50% of the protamine dose is administered. Protamine is initially given on a 1:1 ratio with the total amount of heparin given or approximately 4 mg/kg. Because the perfusionist usually gives additional heparin in the pump prime as well as during bypass, the perfusionist should by asked for the total protamine dosage. The protamine is administered slowly over 10 to 15 minutes. At 20 minutes after CPB, blood samples are taken for coagulation studies, electrolytes, blood gases, and repeat ACT (27). Additional protamine (0.5 to 1.0 mg/kg) is given if indicated.

Treatment of Excessive Bleeding

In children with cyanotic CHD and in small babies in whom the pump-priming volume is large in relation to their blood volume, one may anticipate continued bleeding, owing to platelet and other factor deficiencies after a long pump run. All bleeding must be well controlled before the chest is closed. Not infrequently, however, excessive bleeding occurs, especially in infants with repeat cardiac surgery (28). Treatment of excessive bleeding is aimed at correcting hemostatic abnormalities identified by laboratory or on-site monitoring (e.g., thromboelastography [29]). If on-site monitoring is not available, while one is waiting for results from the laboratory, urgent treatment is directed toward correcting the most probable abnormality in that age group. In children <2 years of age, assuming proper surgical hemostasis and adequate heparin neutralization, fresh whole blood of less than 48 hours may be transfused (30,31). Fresh whole blood will restore coagulation factors toward normal, increase the number of functional platelets, and correct anemia simultaneously. If fresh whole blood is not available, treatment may be initiated empirically with platelets, followed by fresh frozen plasma if bleeding persists. Therapy is readjusted when laboratory results become available. In small neonates, in whom the dilution of coagulation factors and fibrinogen may be particularly severe, cryoprecipitates may be useful to avoid volume overload and further dilution of platelets (31).

Children >2 years of age are less susceptible to severe dilution coagulopathy, and there is no documented evidence that fresh whole blood is useful in this patient population (30). Accordingly, treatment of excessive bleeding in these children should be initiated with platelet concentrates, followed by fresh frozen plasma if bleeding remains uncontrolled.

If platelet count, prothrombin time (PT), and activated partial thromboplastin time (aPTT) are immediately available, transfusion of platelets may be considered when the platelet count is <100,000/µl, and cryoprecipitates (children <6 months) or fresh frozen plasma (children >6 months) may be transfused if bleeding is associated with a prolonged PT and aPTT (>1.5 normal values) (32). If bleeding is associated with both a decreased platelet count and a prolonged PT and aPTT, fresh whole blood may be transfused in children <2 years of age. For older children or when fresh whole blood is not available, initial therapy aims at correcting the platelet count. When fresh frozen plasma and PRBCs are transfused together, single-donor components should be administered, whenever possible, to decrease the risk of transmitting infectious diseases.

ε-Aminocaproic acid, 100 mg/kg, or tranexamic acid, 25 mg/kg, may be useful if there is evidence of significant fibrinolysis and bleeding remains uncontrolled. Finally, reoperation is considered when bleeding >5% of the estimated blood volume persists for more than 3 consecutive hours after operation or exceeds 10% of the estimated blood volume for any 1-hour period (33).

The treatment of excessive blood loss after pediatric cardiac operations is summarized as follows (28):

- Red blood cells are transfused to maintain the hemoglobin concentration at >10 mg/dl in children with acyanotic heart disease or with cyanotic heart disease when no residual shunt is expected after the operation. When correction of shunt is incomplete, a hemoglobin concentration of 12 mg/dl should be maintained.

  - If bleeding still exceeds 5% of estimated blood volume per hour during the second hour after CPB despite adequate neutralization and no suspicion of surgical bleeding, a platelet count, PT, and aPTT are obtained.

- If the platelet count is <100,000/mL and PT and aPTT are >1.5 times normal:
- In children <2 years of age, fresh whole blood is administered (if available) to achieve desired hemoglobin concentration.
- In children >2 years of age or if fresh whole blood is not available, transfuse in order:
  - Platelets: 1 U (<6 months) or 1 U/10 kg (>6 months)
  - Cryoprecipitate, 1 U (<6 months), or fresh frozen plasma 10 to 20 ml/kg (>6 months)
  - If the platelet count is less than 100,000/µL and PT and aPTT are <1.5 times normal, platelets are administered: 1 U (<6 months) or 1 U/10 kg (>6 months).
  - If the platelet count is >100,000/µl and PT and aPTT are >1.5 times normal, cryoprecipitate is administered, 1 U (<6 months), or fresh frozen plasma, 10 to 20 ml/kg (>6 months).
- When bleeding persists, the coagulation profile is reassessed. Consultation with a hematologist is encouraged at this point.
- Consider ε-aminocaproic acid, 100 mg/kg, or tranexamic acid, 25 mg/kg, if there is evidence of significant fibrinolysis and antifibrinolytics are not contraindicated.
- Reoperation should be contemplated when bleeding of >5% of estimated blood volume persists for more than 3 consecutive hours after the operation or exceeds 10% of the estimated blood volume for any 1-hour period.

Cardiac Tamponade

Cardiac tamponade is suggested by hypotension, increasing filling pressures (e.g., elevated CVP), and equalized filling pressures that occur rapidly after chest wall closure in a child who was previously stable. The treatment for cardiac tamponade is surgical reopening of the chest, usually to tie off a "surgical bleeder." Bleeding that is secondary to coagulopathy is rarely brisk enough to cause tamponade.

Management at the End of Surgery

At the end of surgery, after all but the simplest procedures (e.g., closure of ASD secundum), an endotracheal tube is left in for continuing positive-pressure ventilation or CPAP. Positive-pressure ventilation is usually continued for 12 to 48 hours. Therefore, muscle relaxants are not reversed usually.

A chest radiograph is obtained and examined carefully, looking for pneumothorax, hemothorax, atelectasis, and cardiac tamponade, and ensuring that the tip of the endotracheal tube is well above the carina. In addition, placement of all other indwelling lines is confirmed.

Transport to the Intensive Care Unit

Before transport, the patient's trachea is usually reintubated, since tubes almost always seem to fill with blood and secretions during cardiac surgery. During transportation to the intensive unit (ICU), a full bag of blood is attached to the IV line to ensure immediate availability in case of sudden hemorrhage. The patient is covered with warm blankets, given oxygen, and monitored with pulse oximetry. If the patient is still intubated, controlled ventilation is continued. Breath and heart sounds can be monitored by stethoscope, and ECG and arterial pressure are observed using transport monitors.

PROFOUND HYPOTHERMIA WITH CIRCULATORY ARREST

Profound hypothermia with circulatory arrest is used for some neonates and infants undergoing cardiac surgery (34). Hypothermia is usually achieved by means of bloodstream cooling on CPB. It is particularly advantageous for the following reasons: (a) the heart is still and exsanguinated, making more precise surgery possible, and (b) the cannulas can be removed from the operative field during repair, thus allowing for a clear surgical field.

It is disadvantageous in that the duration of CPB may be prolonged.

Anesthetic Management

Preoperative

Routine management is performed as above. One exception from the care described above for routine CPB is that the operating room may be kept cool (<20° C).

Perioperative

Induction and Intubation. Anesthesia may be induced and intubation performed as described above.

Maintenance. Anesthesia is maintained with appropriate concentrations of isoflurane, 0.5% to 0.75%, as tolerated, supplemented with large doses of fentanyl. Maintenance fluids are given to meet requirements and blood or plasma are given when indicated to replace losses. No dextrose-containing solutions are given because hyperglycemia may increase the danger of cerebral damage during total circulatory arrest (35). Large doses of fentanyl (>50 μg/kg) may limit the increase in blood glucose that occurs during hypothermic CPB (36). IV methylprednisolone (Solu-Medrol), 15 to 25 mg/kg, is given slowly, and heparin is administered as outlined **(see Heparinization)**. After CPB is begun, the difference between the esophageal temperature and the temperature of the pump's output should not exceed 10° C. Phentolamine, 0.2 mg/kg, may be administered to improve tissue perfusion, speed even cooling, and minimize acidosis on rewarming (37). Before CPB is discontinued, an incremental dose of relaxant is given. When the esophageal temperature is 16° C and the rectal temperature <20°

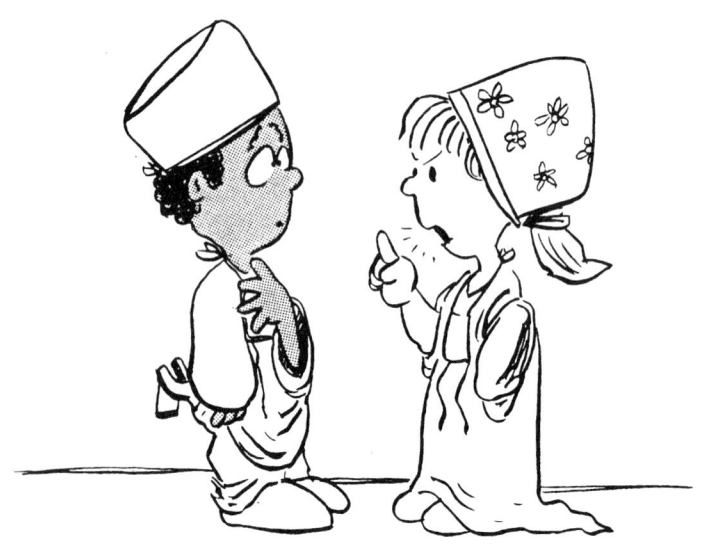

The Consultation

C, CPB is discontinued, blood is drained to the venous reservoir, and the venous cannulas are removed. Ice bags are packed around the head and the duration of circulatory arrest recorded. The lungs are kept inflated at 5 cm H_2O with an air-oxygen mixture.

When the repair is complete, the venous cannulas are replaced, and the patient is rewarmed until the esophageal temperature is 37° C. The temperature of the blood from the pump should never exceed 39° C, and the patient's temperature should not be raised above 37° C. The metabolic acidosis that is seen during rewarming should not be corrected (38). Excess administration of sodium bicarbonate may result in postoperative metabolic alkalosis (39). The rest of the procedure is as described for CPB management **(see Management of Cardiopulmonary Bypass)**.

Postoperative

A nasotracheal tube and controlled ventilation may be necessary for 24 to 48 hours. Routine postoperative cardiac care should be applied. Magnesium sulfate (1 meq/kg/24 hours) with potassium chloride (2 to 4 meq/kg/24 hours) is added to maintenance fluids given at a constant rate over each 24 hours.

Initial Management of Post-Bypass Patients in the Intensive Care Unit

The following is a brief outline of the intensive care necessary in the postoperative management of infants and children who have undergone cardiac surgery. For more detailed information regarding care of these patients in the ICU, the anesthesiologist may consult a standard text on postoperative cardiac care or perhaps consult with his or her pediatric intensivist.

Controlled Ventilation

Most patients benefit from a period of controlled ventilation (40) or PEEP or CPAP during the immediate postoperative period (41). Controlled ventilation is continued for patients who have the following:
- Hypoxemia despite a high F_IO_2
- Low cardiac output
- Pulmonary hypertension
- Diminished lung compliance

- Persistent dysrhythmias
- Hypothermia (<34° C)
- Continuing hemorrhage
- Inability to maintain adequate ventilation

Controlled ventilation permits the more liberal use of narcotic analgesics and hence a more comfortable early recovery phase. Furthermore, controlled ventilation assists in restoring the lung volume to normal and improves gas exchange (42). Levels of added oxygen and PEEP or CPAP can be reduced as the pulmonary status improves. Diuretic therapy may be indicated to reduce lung water. Special measures to control pulmonary vascular resistance may be required in patients with pulmonary hypertension.

The Tracheal Tube

During CPB, bloody secretions accumulate in the tracheal tube. Hence, a change of tracheal tubes (if not already done in the operating room) provides the child with a clean tube in the ICU. If controlled ventilation is to be prolonged, the orotracheal tube may be changed to a nasotracheal tube if the patient's condition is stable enough to tolerate it.[d] Alternatively, ventilation may be continued through an orotracheal tube if preferred by the nursing staff. After the tracheal tube situation is sorted out, adequate ventilation is confirmed by auscultating the chest. Appropriate inspired oxygen concentration is ordered, and ventilation and oxygenation are confirmed by blood gas determination.

Fluid and Electrolyte Therapy

Blood should be administered to maintain the hemoglobin level at near-normal levels (14 to 15 g/dl), especially when cardiac dysfunction is present. Acid-base status should be monitored and acidosis corrected by sodium bicarbonate infusions. Dextrose-containing electrolyte solutions should be infused at low maintenance rates:

- 5% dextrose plus 0.3 normal saline is given for older children.
- 10% dextrose plus 0.3 normal saline is given for infants (<1 month old) to provide dextrose at 4 to 6 mg/kg/min.
- Potassium chloride, 2 meq/kg/day, is added, provided that the urine output is >1 ml/kg/hour.
- Magnesium sulfate, 1 meq/kg/day, is added to the IV fluid regimen for infants after procedures under profound hypothermia.
- If urine output falls (<1 ml/kg/hour) in the presence of hypotension, fluid orders are reviewed to ensure an adequate intake. A fluid challenge may be administered, and, if there is no result, a diuretic is ordered (furosemide, 1 to 2 mg/kg IV).

Blood loss is checked by drainage tubes, and the nurses are instructed to replace this and further losses with appropriate components. If bleeding persists, coagulation studies are ordered. Based on the results of these studies, fresh frozen plasma or platelet concentrates are administered as indicated.

Pain Management

Before leaving the patient to the care of those in the ICU, the anesthesiologist assures that adequate analgesia and sedation have been considered. The following narcotic analgesic and sedative drugs may be ordered:

- Morphine may be given IV every 2 hours or, preferably, as a continuous infusion (10 to 30 µg/kg/min)
- Diazepam, 0.1 mg/kg IV every 2 hours as needed, or midazolam infusion
- Neurally applied opioids or local anesthetics **(see Chapter 10)**

---

[d]Ed. Note (JMB): It is preferable to change tubes at the end of the procedure, rather than pass a nasotracheal tube initially, which could cause nosebleed when the patient is heparinized.

MANAGEMENT OF ANESTHESIA FOR SPECIFIC LESIONS

Management of anesthesia for specific lesions revolves primarily around control and manipulation of shunt flow and hemodynamics during the preinduction, induction, and weaning from bypass periods. To make the guidelines for management convenient, outlines for management of each of the frequently occurring lesions are presented (Tables 4 through 11). Described are key considerations of shunt flow/hemodynamics and the critical periods before and immediately after bypass.

Ligation of Patent Ductus Arteriosus

Older Infants and Children

PDA as the sole lesion in older infants and children usually presents no problems, requiring only routine anesthetic management as for thoracotomy. Special requirements for careful monitoring, however, are required for (a) bradycardia during dissection near the vagus nerve and (b) change in pulse pressure after ligation (diastolic pressure may rise at this time).

Blood loss is usually minimal, seldom necessitating transfusion, but hemorrhage may be sudden and massive if a major vessel is torn. Therefore, a reliable large-bore IV infusion line (20-gauge cannula, if possible) should be established, and blood should be immediately available in the operating room.

Premature Infants and Neonates

Although PDA usually closes early in infancy, it may persist in some infants, particularly preterm infants weighing <1500 g and infants with respiratory distress syndrome (RDS), excessive fluid therapy, neonatal asphyxia, hypoxia, or acidosis. A PDA may result in a large L → R shunt, with pulmonary vascular engorgement and congestive heart failure. Clinical signs of PDA with congestive heart failure include tachypnea, hepatomegaly, and bounding pulses. Diagnosis of PDA is confirmed by the following:

- Auscultation of the typical murmur
- Radiographic evidence of increase vascularity
- Echocardiogram findings of a large left atrium: aorta ratio (>1.2:1)

PDA has been known to prevent weaning from ventilatory support of infants with RDS. Surgical exposure for a neonatal PDA is via a left thoracotomy (Fig. 2).

Preoperative Considerations

Medical Therapy. Administration of indomethacin, a prostaglandin inhibitor, 0.1 to 0.2 mg/kg orally, for several days may induce closure of PDA. Indomethacin may cause renal damage and suppress bone marrow and hence is contraindicated in patients with renal failure or coagulopathy. Very small infants (<1000 g) do not respond as well to indomethacin with closure of the PDA as do larger, less immature infants. Surgical treatment (ligation) is necessary if indomethacin therapy fails or is contraindicated.

Before surgery, arrangements are made to transfer the patient to the operating room in a transport incubator with a ventilator, if indicated. Sedative premedication is unnecessary in this age group.

Anesthetic Management

The operating room is heated, and all warming devices are positioned before transferring the patient to the operating table. The usual monitors are attached, and arterial catheter is usually not required. If the patient is intubated, the tracheal tube is firmly fixed and confirmed to be patent and well positioned.

Induction and Tracheal Intubation. If the infant is not intubated, atropine (0.02 mg/kg), fentanyl (50 µg/kg), and vecuronium (0.1 mg/kg) are given, and the infant ventilated with oxygen for 3 minutes followed by tracheal intubation. Anesthesia is maintained

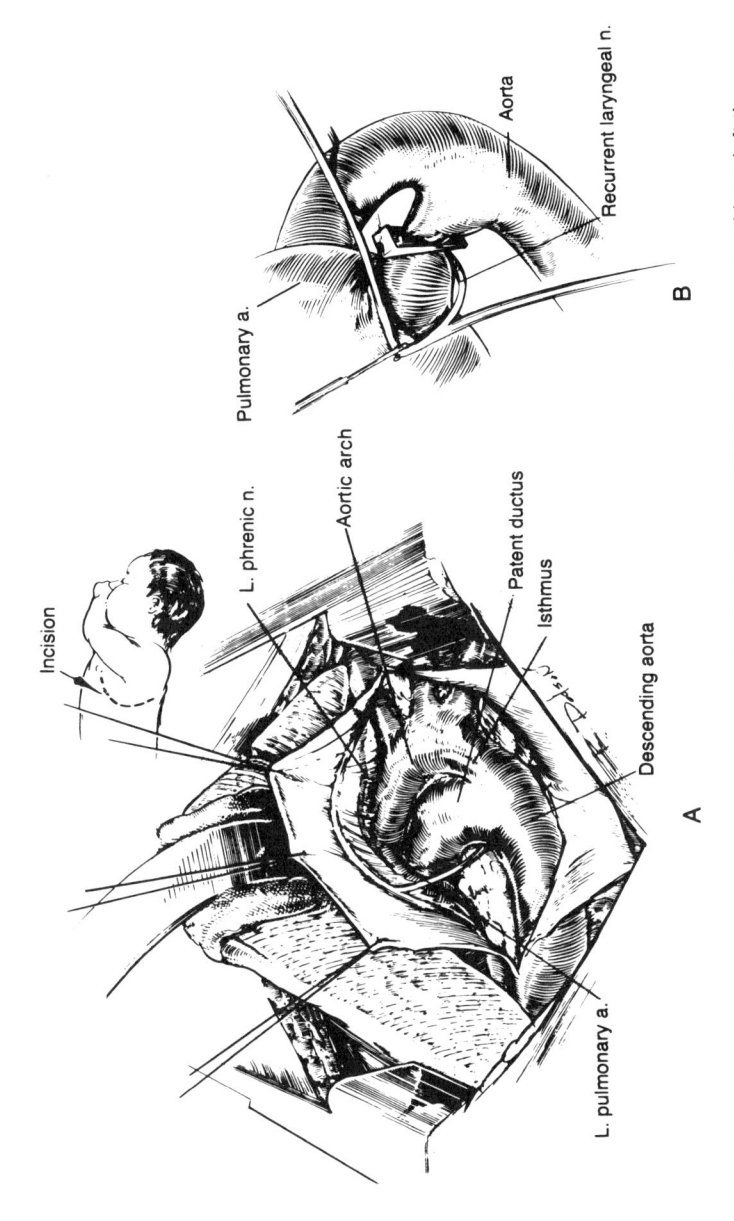

FIG. 2. (A) Surgeon's perspective of neonatal patent ductus (PDA) arteriosus exposed by a left thoracotomy with the pleura incised and mobilized. Note the relative sizes of the PDA and the aortic isthmus. **(B)** Surgical closure using a metal clip. (From Castañeda et al, ref. 23, with permission.)

with N₂O and O₂ with F₁O₂ appropriate to ensure O₂ saturation. Isoflurane (0.5% to 1.0%), fentanyl (10 to 12 μg/kg), or a combination of isoflurane and fentanyl is administered. Small doses of vecuronium (0.05 mg/kg) may be used to facilitate ventilation and to prevent movement. A reliable IV line should be ensured. Blood loss is usually minimal but can be catastrophic if a vessel is torn. Maintenance fluids are administered judiciously. Patients with PDA are often overhydrated preoperatively, but, just as often, these infants have been given diuretics and may be volume-depleted. Fortunately, they usually do not suffer significant third-space losses during surgery.

Postoperative Considerations

Continued ventilation is necessary for most infants with PDA with close attention to post-thoracotomy complications (e.g., atelectasis). Improvement in respiratory status after ligation of PDA depends on resolution of pulmonary vascular congestion and pulmonary disease (respiratory distress syndrome or bronchopulmonary dysplasia).

Rarely, the thoracic duct may be injured during PDA ligation, requiring drainage of the resulting chylothorax. Damage to the recurrent (left) laryngeal nerve is also a rare complication.

RESECTION OF AORTIC COARCTATION

Aortic coarctation is classified according to its site in relation to the ductus arteriosus (i.e., preductal or postductal). The preductal (infantile) type usually is accompanied by other anomalies (e.g., VSD or PDA) and may present as cardiac failure in an infant <6 months of age. The postductal (adult) type may be asymptomatic; it is usually diagnosed during investigation of hypertension in the upper limbs in preschoolers. By contrast, most infants with aortic coarctation have severe cardiac failure and are being treated with digoxin and diuretics and, possibly, assisted ventilation. Furthermore, associated anomalies are common in infants.

Anesthetic Management

Preoperative

Blood gases should be determined and abnormalities corrected, if possible. Supportive drugs (e.g., epinephrine, dopamine) are prepared in case they should be necessary during surgery. It is essential that normothermia be maintained before, during, and after surgery. Blood pressure cuffs are applied to the right arm and on a lower extremity. A reliable IV line is established at a site other than the left arm. Routine anesthetic management is followed. Anesthesia may be maintained with nitrous oxide, isoflurane, and fentanyl. An arterial line is placed into the right radial artery. Central venous access is often helpful, particularly if sodium nitroprusside is to be given to control blood pressure (see next section).

Intraoperative

Clamping the Aorta. Clamping the aorta could compromise the blood supply to the spinal cord. Therefore, optimal blood pressure should be maintained. While the aorta is clamped, severe proximal hypertension may occur and require treatment. During the period of aorta clamping, blood pressure is controlled, if necessary, by adjusting the inspired concentration of isoflurane. The systolic blood pressure in the arm should not be allowed to exceed 80 mm Hg in infants and 140 mm Hg in older children. Distal aortic pressure during clamping varies with the proximal pressure and should be maintained at a mean of 40 to 50 mm Hg to perfuse the spinal cord. In the very rare event that severe proximal hypertension cannot be controlled after aortic clamping or if the distal pressure is very low, a temporary shunt must be placed to bypass the site of anastomosis.

Unclamping the Aorta. One must be prepared to support the circulation when the clamps are removed. The surgeon will first remove the distal clamp and then slowly remove the proximal clamp. Blood pressure is monitored continuously. If hypotension develops, infusion of small amounts of fluid or cardiotonic drugs may be required. If this is unsuccessful, the surgeon is asked to partially reapply the proximal clamp briefly. The blood pressure may remain slightly lower for a while but is usually back above normal levels by the end of the operation. Sodium nitroprusside may be used to control this.

Although blood is made available for transfusions, surprisingly few infants and children require transfusion. Bleeding from collateral vessels is less profuse than in adults. In most cases, controlled ventilation is not required postoperatively, and the patient can be extubated at the end of the operation.

Postoperative

The postoperative course is usually stable. In the rare instance in which the patient is unstable, one may wish to transfer the infant to the ICU with a nasotracheal tube in place and control ventilation for a period of time. Most patients, however, do well. Nevertheless, these patients should be monitored continuously in the ICU, with special attention being paid to signs of blood loss, measuring chest drainage, and observing clinical hemodynamic indices. Hypertension usually persists for several days postoperatively and, if severe, may necessitate therapy with sodium nitroprusside or propranolol. Prevention of hypertension is essential to prevent arteritis and to help prevent postoperative bleeding. Rarely, the postoperative course is complicated by intestinal ileus due to mesenteric arteritis. In extreme cases, bowel resection may be required. Other rare, but serious, postoperative complications include paraplegia due to spinal cord ischemia during repair.

REPAIR OF VASCULAR RINGS AND TRACHEOMALACIA

Congenital anomalies of the great vessels may encircle or compress the trachea, bronchi, and esophagus (Fig. 3). Compression by these vascular rings may lead to stridor and difficulty with feeding during early infancy. The infant with a vascular ring often assumes a characteristic opisthotonic position. In addition, anomalous vessels may compress bronchi and cause gas trapping in individual lobes of the lung. Resultant emphysematous lobes may then compress adjacent lobes.

Infants and children with repaired tracheoesophageal fistulae may also have dyspnea during feeding. In these infants, an abnormally soft trachea is compressed against the aorta during swallowing. The onset of dyspnea during feeding in this condition usually occurs between 2 and 4 months of age. Aortopexy usually relieves symptoms, but in some patients insertion of an external stent to reinforce the trachea is necessary.

Special Anesthetic Problems

Infants and children with vascular rings and tracheomalacia may develop chronic respiratory infection with impaired pulmonary function and respiratory failure. In addition, vascular compression may result in emphysema of one or more lobes, compressing other lung tissue. If airway compression is at the level of the carina or main bronchi, a normally situated endotracheal tube will not relieve the obstruction. In these cases, endobronchial intubation may be required. Endotracheal intubation may be required preoperatively to relieve serious symptoms. Air trapping in a lobe due to vascular compression of the airway can often be alleviated by the application of PEEP. To the dismay of the well-intended anesthesiologist, the use of an esophageal stethoscope in infants with a vascular ring may cause acute airway obstruction.

Anesthetic Management

Optimal pulmonary status should be achieved by ordering intensive respiratory care. Bronchoscopy with endobronchial suction may be required. A method of induction and intubation that ensures a good airway

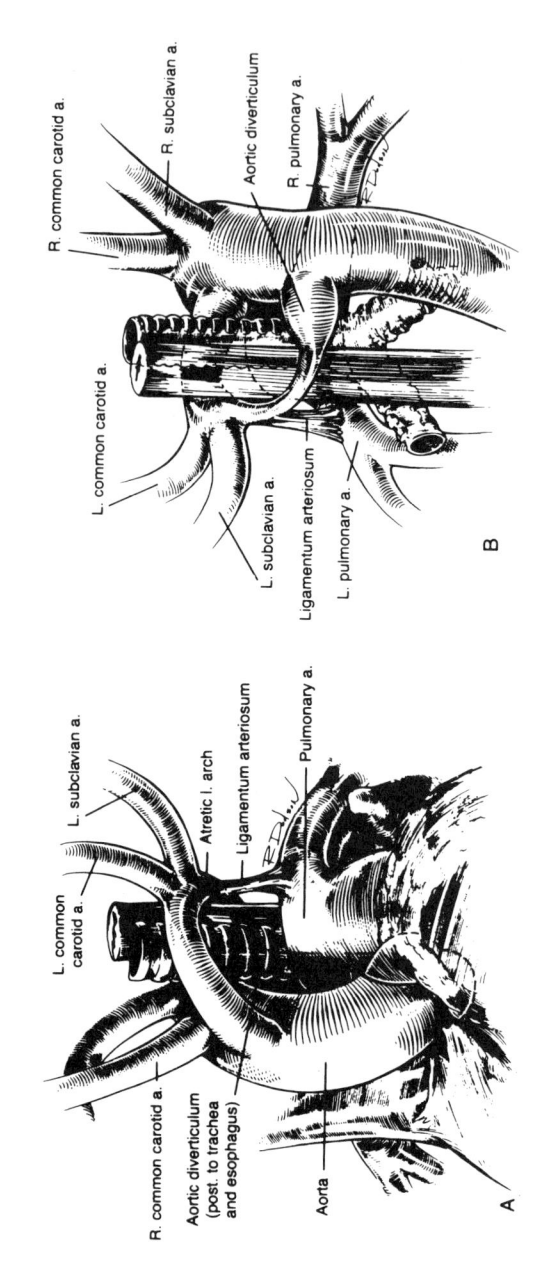

FIG. 3. The most common double aortic arch consists of a dominant right posterior aortic arch with a hypoplastic or atretic left anterior arch. The ligamentum arteriosum contributes to secondary tracheoesophageal compression and should be divided along with the left anterior arch. **(A)** Anterior view. **(B)** Posterior view. (From Castañeda et al, ref. 23, with permission.)

past the obstructing lesion is used. If the obstruction is low, one may choose to do one of the following:

- Pass into a main bronchus a long endotracheal tube with side holes for ventilating the other bronchus, *or*
- Ventilate the patient via a bronchoscope. The bronchoscope may be placed accurately under direct vision and adjusted perioperatively.

For aortopexy, a bronchoscope should be used to ensure that the compression is relieved. Compression of the trachea should always be assessed during spontaneous ventilation and coughing because if controlled ventilation is used, the trachea is held open and appears corrected in every case. If it is necessary to assess the airway during surgery, the larynx is sprayed with lidocaine before insertion of the bronchoscope. During the remainder of the operation, ventilation can be assisted or controlled. Muscle relaxants are not given. Because operations on the great vessels may be associated with serious bleeding, a reliable large-bore IV infusion route should be established.

Postoperative Anesthetic Management

A humidified croup tent is ordered for at least the first 24 postoperative hours. If residual obstruction persists, nasotracheal intubation is continued for 24 hours and the airway is reassessed. Partial obstruction may be improved by a small 1- to 2-inch-thick bolster placed below the shoulders. Racemic epinephrine or dexamethasone may be required for postinstrumentation croup.

SURGERY TO INCREASE PULMONARY BLOOD FLOW

Operations to increase pulmonary blood flow include the following:

- Blalock-Taussig procedure (subclavian artery anastomosed to pulmonary artery). A modified Blalock procedure using a synthetic graft between the vessels and preserving the continuity of the subclavian artery is most commonly performed.
- Glenn procedure (SVC anatomosed to pulmonary artery).
- Central shunt (main pulmonary artery to ascending aorta).
- Potts operation (left pulmonary artery anastomosed to descending aorta).[e]
- Waterston procedure (right pulmonary artery anatomosed to ascending aorta).[e]

The latter operations are performed for infants and children in whom right-sided cardiac lesions have decreased the pulmonary blood flow (e.g., tetralogy of Fallot, tricuspid atresia). Procedures are usually performed during infancy and may be followed by total correction of the defect at an older age.

Special Anesthetic Problems

Many patients with decreased pulmonary blood flow are severely hypoxemic and polycythemic. During surgery, one pulmonary artery is partly occluded so that the anastomosis can be completed; this causes a further temporary decrease in pulmonary blood flow. Patients with polycythemia may have a coagulation defect, although this is rarely a problem. In small infants, the narrow lumen of the new shunt is prone to thrombosis. This may be avoided by the use of a small dose of heparin and appropriate fluid therapy.

Preoperative Anesthetic Management

If possible, the patient should be in optimal respiratory condition with no active infection or recent history of upper respiratory tract infection. If the patient is taking digoxin, the morning dose is generally held (although some clinicians order the daily

---

[e]Ed. Note (JMB): These are mostly of historical importance now.

dose of digoxin to be given at 6:00 AM on the day of operation). If the patient is taking β-blocking agents, these should be continued up to the evening before surgery. Adequate sedation (including morphine for children >1 year or weighing >10 kg) is ordered. For patients with a hemoglobin of >16 g/dl during the preoperative fasting period, IV maintenance fluids are ordered. *An IV line is not placed in the arm on the side to be used for a subclavian shunt.*

Perioperative Anesthetic Management

Because most patients with decreased pulmonary blood flow have a R → L shunt, anesthesia is usually induced intravenously. For the Blalock-Taussig procedure, a blood pressure cuff is placed on the arm opposite the operative site. Anesthesia may be maintained with a volatile agent of at least 50% oxygen and fentanyl. Halothane may be used, since it tends to decrease the ventricular (right) contractility and hence obstruction to outflow. In patients with tetralogy of Fallot, if oxygen-hemoglobin desaturation occurs intraoperatively, it should be treated with propranolol, 0.5 mg/kg IV. If hypotension occurs with volatile agent administration, it may be necessary to substitute fentanyl.

Immediately before the pulmonary artery is clamped, 100% oxygen is given, the lungs are inflated well, and a further dose of relaxant is given. After the clamps are in place and if the patient's oxygenation appears stable, the surgeon may proceed with the anastomosis. If blood pressure falls or bradycardia occurs while the anastomosis is being performed, cardiotonic drugs (e.g., epinephrine, 1 to 5 µg/kg) may be necessary until the anastomosis and the clamps are removed. A modified Blalock anastomosis is usually performed with a synthetic graft. In small infants, it is usual to give a small dose of heparin (100 U/kg) to prevent thrombosis of the shunt. A bolus of fluid after the clamps are released may enhance flow through the shunt. In polycythemic patients, plasma or crystalloid may be given to replace blood loss and to decrease the hematocrit.

One should remain aware that once the shunt is established, the patient's pulmonary blood flow will be blood pressure–dependent. Thus, hypotension is to be avoided.

Postoperative Anesthetic Management

An audible new murmur indicates that the shunt is functioning. Extubation in the operating room is preferred. Intermittent positive-pressure ventilation is seldom necessary, and spontaneous ventilation with low intrathoracic pressure may improve flow through the new shunt. After shunt placement, left ventricular work is increased owing to increased left atrial and left ventricular end-diastolic pressure. Diastolic pressure is usually decreased by the low-pressure runoff provided by the shunt that could potentially compromise coronary blood flow and precipitate cardiac failure. Therefore, the child may require a larger digitalis dose than previously. If the anastomosis is small and considered likely to be blocked by thrombosis, heparin is ordered in suitable dosage for several days postoperatively.

SURGERY TO INCREASE INTRA-ATRIAL MIXING

The Blalock-Hanlon operation is a closed operation performed via a right thoracotomy, which creates a large ASD to allow intra-atrial mixing. It is usually performed in children with transposition of the great vessels and an intact ventricular septum. Patients with this condition often deteriorate soon after birth, as the ductus arteriosus (possibly the only route for mixing of pulmonary and systemic blood) starts to close. In modern practice, balloon septostomy has largely replaced the Blalock-Hanlon operation. A balloon septostomy is usually attempted initially but does not always create an adequate ASD. The patency of the ductus arteriosus can usually be maintained by a continuous infusion of PGE_1 until septostomy or the Blalock-Hanlon operation can be completed.

Special Anesthetic Problems

Infants who need increased intra-arterial mixing may have had recent attempts at balloon septostomy and therefore may not be in optimal condition. In addition, many of these infants are dependent on an infusion of PGE_1 that must be continued intraoperatively. During the actual creation of the defect, the cardiac output is reduced dramatically for a short period of time (about 30 seconds). Blood loss may be significant.

Preoperative Anesthetic Management

Acidosis and hypothermia, if present, should be corrected and the prostaglandin infusion continued. If bleeding occurred during attempted balloon septostomy, signs of hypovolemia may appear.

Perioperative Anesthetic Management

In general, these patients are managed as for the Blalock-Taussig operation except that the following is done before the atrial clamp is applied:

- Lungs are ventilated with 100% oxygen for 3 minutes.
- An incremental dose of muscle relaxant is given to ensure paralysis and to prevent ventilation during the time the atria are open.
- Sodium bicarbonate, 1 meq/kg, calcium gluconate, 10 meq/kg, and isoproterenol, 1 µg/kg, are infused just before clamping. This cocktail gives the myocardium a boost over the critical period.

As the clamp is applied to the atria to create the ASD, the lungs are allowed to collapse briefly. During closure of the atrium, the lungs are inflated with oxygen.

Postoperative Anesthetic Management

Usually, the patient's trachea can be extubated soon after the operation. Tracheal extubation is desirable to allow increased pulmonary blood flow. If intermittent positive-pressure ventilation is required, a low mean intrathoracic pressure is maintained. At the end of surgery, prostaglandin infusion may be discontinued. Oxygenation should be improved (PaO_2 = 40 mm Hg or higher). Intensive respiratory care, however, is required for several days.

SURGERY TO DECREASE PULMONARY BLOOD FLOW

Pulmonary artery banding is performed to decrease pulmonary vascular congestion in infants who have a large L → R shunt in an attempt to avoid pulmonary hypertension. Banding is usually performed as an emergency procedure in the newborn period.

Preoperative Anesthetic Management

Many patients with pulmonary vascular congestion are in severe congestive heart failure. Therefore, optimal control of cardiac failure is desirable. Measures to improve the infant's general status include intermittent positive-pressure ventilation for several hours before surgery.

Perioperative Anesthetic Management

Myocardial depressants (e.g., halothane) should be administered cautiously. A muscle relaxant (vecuronium) and narcotic analgesic (fentanyl) may be administered. The patient is monitored closely as the pulmonary artery band is applied. The systemic blood pressure should rise, but the saturation should not fall (i.e., no R → L shunt should occur). Oxygen-hemoglobin desaturation, if it occurs, indicates that the pulmonary artery band may be too tight. It is usual to also monitor the distal pulmonary artery pressure during banding. This pressure should fall to about 30% to 50% of systemic pressure.

Postoperative Anesthetic Management

Controlled ventilation may be required for several days. Although these patients often can be weaned and extubated within 24 hours.

CARDIOLOGIC PROCEDURES

Cardiac Catheterization

Cardiac catheterization is usually an elective procedure, and older children will benefit from preoperative teaching, a visit to the catheter laboratory, and familiarization with the process to be performed (44). Cardiac catheterization may be performed under general anesthesia (45) or with a combination of sedation plus local or regional analgesia. The following are important prerequisites for gathering reliable catheter data (45):

- Hemodynamic parameters should be maintained as constant and unchanged as possible.
- The inspired oxygen concentration should remain constant throughout the procedure: Room air is preferred if this is safe for the patient; otherwise, a constant optimum inspired oxygen concentration should be selected.
- The patient should be maintained in an optimal physiologic state (e.g., normothermic, well-hydrated, euglycemic).

Special Anesthetic Problems

These patients may be seriously ill and in cardiac failure. Their condition may further deteriorate during cardiac catheterization, especially if dysrhythmias occur. Furthermore, the contrast media used for angiograms may cause adverse effects (e.g., anaphylaxis).

Sedation

When the procedure is to be performed under sedation, the following technique has proved satisfactory:

- An IV route is established with local analgesia.
- Monitors are applied (ECG, pulse oximeter, blood pressure cuff and Doppler ultrasound, temperature probe).
- IV sedation is administered **(see Chapter 16)**.
- Small infants may be offered a brandy soother and often settle with this alone.
- Caudal analgesia may be useful for some children, especially if bilateral femoral catheterization is necessary or if large catheters are to be inserted (e.g., Gruentzig catheters).

General Anesthesia

If general anesthesia is preferred, the patient should be carefully monitored as previously described. A technique using endotracheal nitrous oxide and low concentrations of volatile agent in 40% oxygen with spontaneous ventilation is usually satisfactory.

Some forms of CHD are now being treated by therapeutic interventional cardiac catheterization (e.g., by balloon dilation of the stenotic valve or umbrella closure of the ASD or PDA). General anesthesia is usually preferred because the patient must be absolutely immobile and the need for urgent open operation if complications occur is a real possibility. A large-bore IV route suitable for rapid transfusion should be in place.

Cardioversion

Cardioversion is usually an emergency. The dysrhythmia may be severe, markedly reducing cardiac output and producing shock.

Preoperative Anesthetic Management

Oxygen (100%) is given by mask. One should ascertain whether the child has eaten recently and ensure that all equipment is prepared and checked. Precordial stethoscope, blood pressure cuff, and ECG are applied.

TABLE 13. Indications for endocarditis prophylaxis

Cardiac conditions

Endocarditis prophylaxis recommended
Prosthetic cardiac valves, including bioprosthetic and homograft valves
Previous bacterial endocarditis, even in the absence of heart disease
Most congenital cardiac malformations
Rheumatic and other acquired valvular dysfunction, even after valvular surgery
Hypertrophic cardiomyopathy
Mitral valve prolapse with valvular regurgitation

Endocarditis prophylaxis not recommended
Isolated secundum atrial septal defect
Surgical repair without residual 6 months after secundum atrial septal defect, ventricular septal defect, or patent ductus arteriosus
Physiologic, functional, or innocent heart murmurs
Previous Kawasaki disease without valvular dysfunction
Previous rheumatic fever without valvular dysfunction
Cardiac pacemakers and implanted defibrillators

Dental or surgical procedures

Endocarditis prophylaxis recommended
Dental procedures known to induce gingival or mucosal bleeding, including professional cleaning
Tonsillectomy or adenoidectomy
Surgical operations that involve intestinal or respiratory mucosa
Bronchoscopy with a rigid bronchoscope
Sclerotherapy for esophageal varices
Esophageal dilatation
Gallbladder surgery
Cystoscopy
Urethral dilatation
Urethral catheterization if urinary tract infection is present[a]
Urinary tract surgery if urinary tract infection is present[a]
Prostatic surgery
Incision and drainage of infected tissue[a]

Endocarditis prophylaxis not recommended[b]
Dental procedures not likely to induce gingival bleeding, such as simple adjustment of orthodontic appliances or fillings above the gum line
Injection of local intraoral anesthetic (except intraligamentary injections)
Shedding of primary teeth
Tympanostomy tube insertion
Endotracheal intubation
Bronchoscopy with a flexible bronchoscope, with or without biopsy
Cardiac catheterization
Endoscopy with or without gastrointestinal biopsy
Cesarean section

This table lists selected procedures but is not meant to be all-inclusive.

[a]In addition to the prophylactic regimen for genitourinary procedure, antibiotic therapy should be directed against the most likely bacterial pathogen.

[b]For patients who have prosthetic heart valves, a previous history of endocarditis, or surgically constructed systemic-pulmonary shunts or conduits, physicians may choose to administer prophylactic antibiotics even for low-risk procedures that involve the lower respiratory, genitourinary, or gastrointestinal tracts.

(Reprinted with permission from Dajani AS et al: Prevention of bacterial endocarditis: Recommendations by the Heart Association. JAMA 264:2919–2922, 1990.)

TABLE 14. Prevention of bacterial endocarditis[47]

Procedure	Drug	Dosage for children — Dosing regimen[a]
Dental and Upper Respiratory Procedures		*Standard Regimen*
	Amoxicillin	50 mg/kg PO 1 hr before procedure; then 25 mg/kg 6 hr after initial dose
		Amoxicillin / Penicillin—Allergic Patients
	Erythromycin or Clindamycin	Erythromycin ethylsuccinate, 20 mg/kg, or erythromycin stearate, 20 mg/kg, PO 2 hr before procedure; then half the dose 6 hr after initial dose; 10 mg/kg PO 1 hr before procedure and 5 mg/kg 6 hr after initial dose
	Drug	Dosing Regimen[b]
		Patients Unable to Take Oral Medications
	Ampicillin	IV or IM ampicillin, 50 mg/kg, 30 min before procedure; then IV or IM ampicillin, 25 mg/kg or PO administration of amoxicillin, 25 mg/kg 6 hr after initial dose
		Ampicillin/Amoxicillin/Penicillin—Allergic Patients Unable to Take Oral Medications
	Clindamycin	10 mg/kg IV 30 min before procedure and 5 mg/kg IV or PO 6 hr after initial dose
		Patients Considered High Risk and Not Candidates for Standard Regimen
	Ampicillin, gentamicin, and amoxicillin	IV or IM ampicillin, 50 mg/kg, plus gentamicin, 2.0 mg/kg (not to exceed 80 mg), 30 min before procedure; followed by amoxicillin, 25 mg/kg PO 6 hr after initial dose; alternatively, the parenteral regimen may be repeated 8 hr after initial dose
		Ampicillin/Amoxicillin/Penicillin—Allergic Patients Considered High Risk
	Vancomycin	20 mg/kg IV over 1 hr, starting 1 hr before procedure; no repeated dose necessary
	Drug	Dosage Regimen
Gastrointestinal and Genitourinary Procedures		*Standard Regimen*
	Ampicillin, gentamicin, and amoxicillin	IV or IM ampicillin, 50 mg/kg plus gentamicin, 2.0 mg/kg (not to exceed 80 mg), 30 min before procedure; followed by amoxicillin, 50 mg/kg PO 6 hr after initial dose; alternatively, the parenteral regimen may be repeated once 8 hr after initial dose
		Ampicillin/Amoxicillin/Penicillin—Allergic Patient Regimen
	Vancomycin and gentamicin	IV vancomycin, 20 mg/kg, over 1 hr plus IV or IM gentamicin, 2.0 mg/kg (not to exceed 80 mg), 1 hr before procedure; may be repeated once 8 hr after initial dose
		Alternate Low-Risk Patient Regimen
	Amoxicillin	50 mg/kg PO 1 hr before procedure; then 1.5 gm 6 hr after initial dose

Follow-up doses should be half the initial dose. Total pediatric dose should not exceed total adult dose.
[a] Includes those with prosthetic heart valves and other high-risk patients. Total pediatric dose of amoxicillin: < 15 kg, 750 mg; 15 to 30 kg, 1500 mg; and > 30 kg, 3000 mg (full adult dose).
[b] No initial dose is recommended in this table for amoxicillin (25 mg/kg is the follow-up dose). (Reprinted with permission from Dajani AS et al: Prevention of bacterial endocarditis: Recommendations by the Heart Association. JAMA 264:2919–2922, 1990.)

Perioperative Anesthetic Management

An IV line is secured and 100% oxygen is administered by face mask. Anesthesia is induced in the usual fashion with full-stomach precautions taken as necessary **(see Chapter 2)**. Methohexital (2 mg/kg) has proved to be an ideal induction agent in this situation because of its short duration of action. As soon as anesthesia has been induced and good oxygenation achieved, countershock can be applied. Methohexital (1 mg/kg) may be repeated, if necessary.

Postoperative Anesthetic Management

The period of recovery after cardioversion is short, but the patient should be monitored with pulse oximetry, blood pressure cuff, and ECG for several hours afterward.

ANESTHESIA FOR NONCARDIAC SURGERY IN THE CHILD WITH CHD

Infants and children with CHD frequently present (either before or after cardiac repair) for noncardiac surgery. Anesthetic management of these patients is not too much different from management of cardiac surgery, with the obvious exceptions (e.g., children for appendectomy usually do not require heparinization and CPB).

In general, the same principles that govern management at induction and maintenance (e.g., shunt flow manipulation and maintenance of desired hemodynamics) govern the anesthetic management of children with CHD for noncardiac surgery. Therefore, when managing a child with CHD, the guidelines expressed in Tables 4 through 11 may be followed to provide the patient with a hemodynamically stable anesthetic. Probably the most important aspect of management of these children is the prevention of bacterial endocarditis (see following text).

Bacterial Endocarditis Prophylaxis

Children with valvular disease, prosthetic valves, most forms of CHD, hypertrophic cardiomyopathy (idiopathic hypertrophic subaortic stenosis), and mitral valve prolapse, as well as postcorrection cardiac patients (Table 13), should receive antibiotics for bacterial endocarditis prophylaxis before surgery (47) (Table 14). Patients with repaired or corrected cardiovascular lesions continue to receive preoperative and postoperative antibiotic prophylaxis; only uncorrected secundum ASDs or surgical repair without residual beyond 6 months of secundum ASD, VSD, or PDA are generally excluded from prophylaxis. The children at highest risk for bacterial endocarditis are those with prosthetic valves, congenital aortic stenosis after valvotomy, and systemic-to-pulmonary anastomoses (Blalock-Taussig and others) (48). The current recommendations for prophylaxis in children are listed in Table 14. These should be implemented by the anesthesiologist if not ordered by the surgical team. Patients at highest risk should probably receive parenteral prophylaxis.

REFERENCES

1. Fyler DC: Report of the New England Regional Infant Cardiac Program. *Pediatrics* 1980;65(Suppl):376.
2. Steward DJ, Sloan IA: Recent upper respiratory infection and pulmonary artery clamping in the aetiology of postoperative respiratory complications. *Can Anaesth Soc J* 1969;16:57–60.
3. Soyka LF: Pediatric clinical pharmacology of digoxin. *Pediatr Clin North Am* 1981;28:203–216.
4. Stow PJ, Burrows FA, Lerman J, Roy WL: Arterial oxygen saturation following premedication in children with cyanotic congenital heart disease. *Can J Anaesth* 1988;35:63–66.
5. Silove ED: Pharmocological manipulation of the ductus arteriosus. *Arch Dis Child* 1986;61:827–829.
6. Bell C, Rimar S, Barash P: Intraoperative ST-segment changes consistent with myocardial ischemia in the neonate: a report of three cases. *Anesthesiology* 1989; 71:601–604.
7. Baraff LJ: Capillary refill: is it a useful clinical sign? *Pediatrics* 1993;92:723–724.
8. Ritter SB, Hillel Z, Narang J: Transesophageal real time doppler flow imaging in congenital heart disease: experience with a new pediatric transducer probe. *Dyn Cardiovasc Imag* 1989;9:92–96.

9. Lowe SV, Deshpande JK, Tobias JD: Perioperative monitoring. In: Kambam J (ed). *Cardiac anesthesia for infants and children.* St. Louis: CV Mosby, 1994.
10. Bolger A, Czer L, Freidman A: Intraoperative transesophageal color Doppler imaging: advantages and limitations. (Abstract). *J Am Coll Cardiol* 1988;11:217.
11. Greeley WJ, Ungerleider RM: Echocardiography during surgery for congenital heart disease. In: de Bruijn NP, Clements FM (eds). *Intraoperative use of echocardiography.* Philadelphia: JB Lippincott, 1991:129–156.
12. Abrams JH, Weber RE, Holmen KD: Continuous cardiac output determination using transtracheal Doppler: initial results in humans. *Anesthesiology* 1989;71: 11–15.
13. Notterman DA, Castello FV, Steinberg C, et al: A comparison of thermodilution and pulsed Doppler cardiac output measurement in critically ill children. *J Pediatr* 1989;115:554–560.
14. Laishley RS, Burrows FA, Lerman J, Roy WL: Effect of anesthetic induction regimens on oxygen saturation in cyanotic congenital heart disease. *Anesthesiology* 1986; 65:673–677.
15. Lucero VM, Lerman J, Burrows FA: Onset of neuromuscular blockade with pancuronium in children with congenital heart disease. *Anesth Analg* 1987;66: 788–790.
16. Murkin JM, Farrar JK, Tweed WA, McKenzie FN, Guiraudon G: Cerebral autoregulation and flow/metabolism coupling during cardiopulmonary bypass: the influence of $PaCO_2$. *Anesth Analg* 1987;66:825–832.
17. Burrows FA: Physiologic dead space, venous admixture, and the arterial to end-tidal carbon dioxide difference in infants and children undergoing cardiac surgery. *Anesthesiology* 1989;70:219–225.
18. Long WA, Rubin LJ: Prostacyclin and PGE_1 treatment of pulmonary hypertension. *Am Rev Respir Dis* 1987;136:773–776.
19. Cohen JA, Bethea HL, Rush WJ: Heparin kinetics during pediatric open heart operations. *Perfusion* 1986; 1:271–275.
20. Bull C, Cooper J, Stark J: Cardioplegic protection of the child's heart. *J Thorac Cardiovasc Surg* 1984;88: 287–293.
21. Stanley TH, Liu WS, Gentry S: Effects of ventilatory techniques during cardiopulmonary bypass on post-bypass and postoperative pulmonary compliance and shunt. *Anesthesiology* 1977;46:391–395.
22. Byrick RJ, Kolton M, Hart JT, Forbath PG: Hypoxemia following cardiopulmonary bypass. *Anesthesiology* 1980;53:172–174.
23. Hickey PR. Anesthesia for cardiovascular surgery. In: Castañeda AR, Jonas RA, Mayer JE, Hanley FL, eds. *Cardiac surgery of the neonate and infant.* Philadelphia: WB Saunders, 1994:74.
24. Faraci PA, Rheinlander HF, Cleveland RJ: Use of nitroprusside for control of pulmonary hypertension in repair of ventricular septal defect. *Ann Thorac Surg* 1980;29:70–73.
25. Lang P, Williams RG, Norwood WI, Castañeda AR: The hemodynamic effects of dopamine in infants after corrective cardiac surgery. *J Pediatr* 1980;96:630–634.
26. Stephenson LW, Edmunds LH Jr, Raphaely R, et al: Effects of nitroprusside and dopamine on pulmonary arterial vasculature in children after cardiac surgery. *Circulation* 1979;60:104–110.
27. Mattox KL, Guinn GA, Rubio PA, Beall AC Jr.: Use of the activated coagulation time in intraoperative heparin reversal for cardiopulmonary operations. *Ann Thorac Surg* 1975;19:634–638.
28. Guay J, George-Étienne R: Mediastinal bleeding after cardiopulmonary bypass in pediatric patients. *Ann Thorac Surg* 1996;62:1955–1960.
29. Martin P, Horkay F, Rajah SM, Walker DR: Monitoring of coagulation status using thromboelastography during paediatric open heart surgery. *Int J Clin Monit Comput* 1991;8:183–187.
30. Manno CS, Hedberg KW, Kim HC, et al: Comparison of the hemostatic effects of fresh whole blood, stored whole blood, and components after open heart surgery in children. *Blood* 1991;77:930–936.
31. Kern FH, Morana NJ, Sears JJ, Hickey PR: Coagulation defects in neonates during cardiopulmonary bypass. *Ann Thorac Surg* 1992;54:541–546.
32. Murray DJ, Olson J, Strauss R, Tinker JH: Coagulation changes during packed red cell replacement of major blood loss. *Anesthesiology* 1988;69:839–845.
33. Lake CL: Postoperative complications. In: Lake CL (ed). *Pediatric cardiac anesthesia,* 2nd ed. Norwalk, CT: Appleton & Lange, 1993:465–483.
34. Steward DJ, Sloan IA, Johnston AE: Anaesthetic management of infants undergoing profound hypothermia for surgical correction of congenital heart defects. *Can Anaesth Soc J* 1974;21:15–22.
35. Steward DJ, DaSilva CA, Flegel T: Elevated blood glucose levels may increase the danger of neurological deficit following profoundly hypothermic cardiac arrest. (Letter). *Anesthesiology* 1988;68:653.
36. Ellis DJ, Flegel TF, Steward DJ: Fentanyl reduces hyperglycemia in pediatric patients undergoing hypothermic cardiopulmonary bypass. *Anesthesiology* 1988;69A:740.
37. Bridges KG, Reichard GA Jr, MacVaugh H III, et al: Effect of phentolamine in controlling temperature and acidosis associated with cardiopulmonary bypass. *Crit Care Med* 1985;13:72–76.
38. Ellis RJ, Hoover E, Gay WA, Ebert PA: Metabolic alterations with profound hypothermia. *Arch Surg* 1974; 109:659–663.
39. Johnston AE, Radde IC, Steward DJ, Taylor J: Acidbase and electrolyte changes in infants undergoing profound hypothermia for surgical correction of congenital heart defects. *Can Anaesth Soc J* 1974;21:23–45.
40. Downes JJ, Nicodemus HF, Pierce WS, Waldhausen JA: Acute respiratory failure in infants following cardiovascular surgery. *J Thorac Cardiovasc Surg* 1970;59:21–37.
41. Gregory GA, Edmunds LH Jr, Kitterman JA, et al: Continuous positive airway pressure and pulmonary and circulatory function after cardiac surgery in infants less that three months of age. *Anesthesiology* 1975;43: 426–431.
42. Yates AP, Lindahl SGE, Hatch DJ: Pulmonary ventilation and gas exchange before and after correction of congenital cardiac malformations. *Br J Anaesth* 1987; 59:170–178.
43. Hickey PR, Hansen DD, Cramolini MD: Pulmonary and systemic hemodynamic responses to ketamine in infants with normal and elevated pulmonary vascular resistance. *Anesthesiology* 1985;62:287–293.
44. Naylor D, Coates TJ, Kan J: Reducing distress in pediatric cardiac catheterization. *Am J Dis Child* 1984;138: 726–729.

45. Manners JM, Codman VA: General anaesthesia for cardiac catheterisation in children: the effect of spontaneous or controlled ventilation on the evaluation of congenital abnormalities. *Anaesthesia* 1969;24:541–553.
46. Topkins MJ: Anesthetic management of cardiac catheterisation. *Int Anesthesiol Clin* 1980;18:59–69.
47. Committee on Rheumatic Fever, Endocarditis, and Kawasaki Disease of the Council on Cardiovascular Disease in the Young of the American Heart Association: prevention of bacterial endocarditis. Recommendations by the American Heart Association. *JAMA* 1990;264:2919–2922.
48. Kaplan EL, Rich A, Gersony W, Manning J: A collaborative study of infective endocarditis in the 1970's: emphasis on infections in patients who have undergone cardiovascular surgery. *Circulation* 1979;59:327–335.

13

Pediatric Neuroanesthesia: Beyond the Theory

Bruno Bissonnette

"The brain is not an organ to be relied upon. It is developing monstrously. It is swelling like a goitre."

—Alexander Blok
The Scythians, 1918

In pediatric neuroanesthesia, the selection of anesthetic technique has a profound effect on the attenuation of significant morbidity (1). As in adults with intracranial pathology, anatomic and physiologic factors may be manipulated for the benefit of the patient. In pediatrics, however, there is the added challenge of physiologic differences between developing children and their adult counterparts. The child is not simply a small adult. At birth, the central nervous system (CNS) development is incomplete and will not be mature until the end of the first year of life. Because of this delay in the maturation of the CNS, there are important pathophysiologic and psychological differences between adults and children. This chapter reviews the basic concepts necessary for understanding of the anesthetic problems related to children undergoing neurologic surgery and will then go beyond the basics to present concepts for guiding, in a very direct way, the clinical management of these patients.

NEUROPHYSIOLOGY

To understand how anesthetic actions affect the outcome of neuroanesthesia, it is helpful to review basic neurophysiology of the cerebral metabolism, cerebral blood flow, spinal fluid dynamics, spinal cord blood flow, and regulation.

Energetics of Cerebral Metabolism

The energy from glucose required to maintain and regulate the synaptic connections, voltage, and messenger systems is considerable (2). Glucose depletion rapidly leads to coma and eventually to brain death. Glucose storage capacity of the brain (glycogen stores) is sufficient to provide less than three minutes of normal rates of adenosine triphosphate consumption. Therefore, the brain is entirely dependent on blood circulation for the 120 g of glucose it requires each day. The cerebral metabolic rates for oxygen and glucose differ by age (Table 1).

TABLE 1. *Cerebral metabolic ($CMRO_2$) and blood flow (CBF) rates by age*

	Anesthetized infants (including newborns)	Children (6–36 mo)	(3–12 y)	Adults
$CMRO_2$ (ml/min/100 g)	2.3(4)		5.2	3.5
CMR glucose (mg/min/100 g)			6.8(3)	5.5
CBF (ml/min/100 g)	~40(6,7)[a]	90(5)	100(4)	50

[a]Estimated.

Cerebral Blood Flow, Cerebral Metabolic Rate, and Cerebral Blood Volume

Cerebral blood flow (CBF) is higher in children than adults (see Table 1). When cerebral metabolic rate (CMRO$_2$) rises (e.g., in the presence of fever or during seizure activity), CBF increases with a concomitant increase in cerebral blood volume (CBV), leading to a potential increase in intracranial pressure (ICP). Conversely, hypothermia and certain anesthetic agents that decrease CMRO$_2$ cause a reduction in CBF. During hypothermia, CMRO$_2$ and CBF decrease about 7% per degree centigrade (8). Children, like adults, have the capacity for cerebral autoregulation (e.g., maintenance of a constant oxygen delivery over a wide range of perfusion pressures). Adults maintain a constant CBF over a range of mean arterial pressures (MAP) between 60 and 150 mm Hg (Fig. 1). Although autoregulatory thresholds for infants and children are not well known, neonatal animal models suggest that the lower limit for autoregulation may be around 40 mm Hg of pressure with a suggested upper pressure limit of 90 mm Hg (9,10) (see Fig. 1). It is assumed that infants with MAP <60 mm Hg also autoregulate, since induced hypotension in these patients seems to be well tolerated (11,12). By contrast, neonates in severe distress may have altered autoregulation (13). The CBF changes passively with systemic blood pressure in these patients.

In children, as in adults, blood pressure alone is an insufficient measure of cerebral perfusion. Cerebral perfusion pressure (CPP) = MAP − central venous pressure (CVP) or MAP − ICP when ICP is > CVP. Anemia, hemodilution, or drugs which alter the rheologic properties of blood increase oxygen delivery by decreasing viscosity. Autoregulation is impaired or abolished by hypoxia (13), vasodilators (14), and variable concentrations of volatile anesthetics (15). However, as in adults, hyperventilation has been reported to restore autoregulation in the neonate (16). Intracranial pathology as the result of trauma, areas of inflammation surrounding tumor, and abscess or sites of focal ischemia also alter autoregulation (17). Autoregulation is easily impaired or lost in the newborn, and it may lead to the development of intraventricular hemorrhage, CNS damage, or death (18).

In infants and children, as in adults, the cerebrovascular reactivity to hypocarbia is a useful tool in reducing CBF, CBV, and ICP. The CBF varies linearly with PaCO$_2$ between 20 and 80 mm Hg (Fig. 2). A 1 mm Hg fall in PaCO$_2$ results in about 4% decrease in CBF. When arterial PCO$_2$ sampling is unavailable, end-tidal CO$_2$ may be used to guide ventilation management.

A study in anesthetized infants and children using transcranial Doppler ultrasonography has demonstrated that CBF velocity changes logarithmically with the end-tidal carbon dioxide pressure (P$_{ET}$CO$_2$) (19) (Fig. 3). The cere-

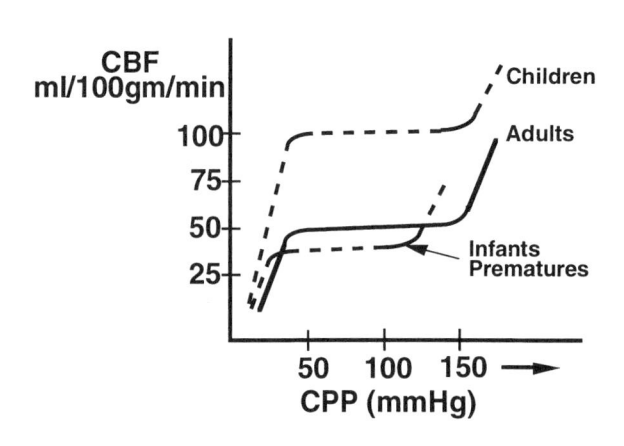

FIG. 1. The relation between the cerebral perfusion pressure (CPP) and the cerebral blood flow (CBF). The mean CBF is autoregulated between 50 and 150 mm Hg of CPP in adults. In children age 6 months to 12 years, CBF is autoregulated but at higher values than in adults, whereas premature and newborn infants have a CBF lower and the inferior and superior limits of cerebral autoregulation are different.

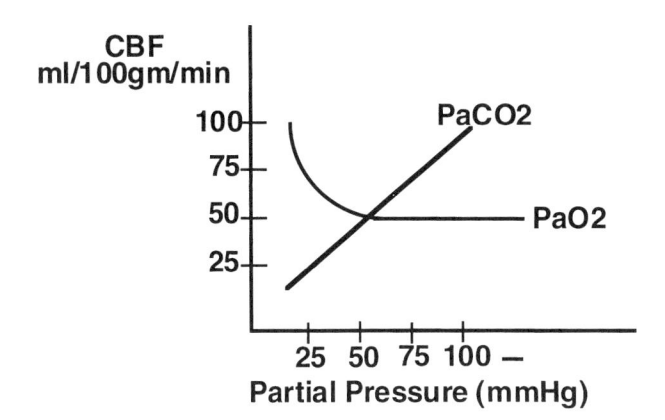

FIG. 2. The effect of CO_2 and O_2 on cerebral blood flow (CBF). In adults, the CBF varies linearly for any changes of $PaCO_2$ between 20 mm Hg and 80 mm Hg. However, the effect of a diminution in PaO_2 on CBF is not observed until it reaches 50 mm Hg where CBF increases exponentially.

brovascular response to hypoxia is not well studied in children. Adults show no change in CBF until PaO_2 falls below 50 mm Hg, at which time it begins to increase exponentially (Fig. 2).

Cerebrospinal Fluid

In both adults and pediatric patients, ICP is much more dependent on CBF and CBV than cerebrospinal fluid production. Reduction of cerebrospinal fluid production by one third has been shown to reduce ICP by only 1.1 mm Hg (20). It is therefore not surprising that drugs such as acetazolamide, which reduce cerebrospinal fluid production, have little effect on ICP except in patients whose intracranial compliance curve lies far to the right.

Spinal Cord Blood Flow

Spinal cord blood flow is controlled by the same factors as those for CBF (21,22). Spinal

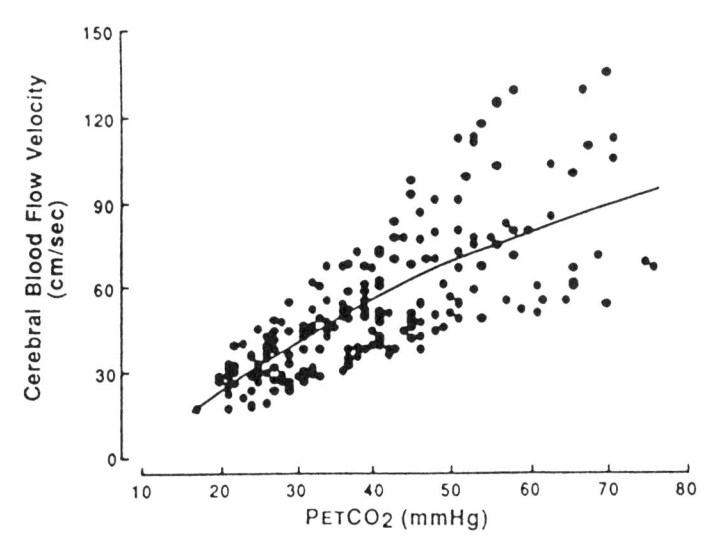

FIG. 3. Logarithmic relation between the end-tidal CO_2 and the cerebral blood flow velocity (CBFV) of the middle cerebral artery in children. This relation demonstrates that the ability to CO_2 to vasoconstrict and reduce CBFV is highly efficient in the low CO_2 range, whereas the effect of high CO_2 is more variable and not linear up to 80 mm Hg, as suggested in adults. (From Pilato et al, ref. 19, with permission.)

cord perfusion pressure (i.e., MAP–extrinsic pressure on the cord) describes the adequacy of spinal perfusion (23). Pressure exerted by local extrinsic mechanical compression such as tumor mass, hematoma, spinal venous congestion, and increased intraspinal fluid pressure influence the spinal cord perfusion pressure. The spinal cord blood flow autoregulates in the range of 45 to 180 mm Hg (21–25). The following conditions affect spinal cord blood flow:

- Blood pressure exceeding autoregulation limits (26)
- Severe hypoxia (27)
- Hypercapnia (25)
- Trauma that abolishes vascular reactivity (25)

PHARMACOLOGY OF IMPORTANCE IN PEDIATRIC NEUROANESTHESIA

Inhalational Anesthetic Agents

Nitrous Oxide

Nitrous oxide (N_2O) is not a total anesthetic in the absence of other inhalational agents (e.g., halothane or isoflurane) or intravenous anesthetics. When used alone in subanesthetic doses (e.g., 60% to 70%), N_2O causes cerebral excitement and metabolic stimulation accompanied by an increase in CBF (28). In infants and children anesthetized with 70% N_2O/30% O_2, fentanyl, and diazepam, CBF increases compared with the same anesthetic with an air/O_2 mixture (29). Increase in CBF is not associated with significant changes in MAP or heart rate or cerebrovascular resistance. Barbiturates, benzodiazepines, morphine, and hypocapnia *reduce the effect of* N_2O *to increase CBF* (30,31). By contrast, volatile anesthetic agents add to the increases in CBF (32). It seems prudent to avoid N_2O administration in the child with a "tight brain" (e.g., poor cerebral compliance). Furthermore, because of the ability of N_2O to increase $CMRO_2$, it would be unwise to continue administration in the presence of diminished cerebral perfusion.

Halothane

Halothane is a cerebral vasodilator that decreases cerebrovascular resistance and increases CBF in a dose-dependent fashion (33). Halothane remains an appropriate anesthetic agent when used with hyperventilation. The effect of halothane and hyperventilation on cerebral circulation, however, is limited even at 1.0 MAC (34,35). When normal CO_2 is maintained in children, CBF increases (measured as CBF velocity by transcranial Doppler imaging) between 0.5 MAC and 1.0 MAC but does not increase further at 1.5 MAC (35). When halothane concentration is decreased from 1.5 MAC to 0.2 MAC, CBF velocity remains higher at any given concentration achieved while increasing the MAC (36). This phenomenon is called *hysteresis of the cerebral vasculature* and may be important in patients with raised ICP (36). For example, there may be a persistent increase in CBV and ICP when backing off halothane concentration. Therefore, after one increases halothane concentration (e.g., to control an acute nociceptive response), one must remember that decreasing the halothane concentration after this transient situation will favor the maintenance of an increased CBF and CBV. In children, as in adults, halothane decreases cerebrovascular resistance, increases CBF, and increases ICP (37–41). Therefore, in patients known to have reduced intracerebral compliance, halothane should be avoided until the dura is open, particularly if ICP is not monitored.

Isoflurane

Isoflurane affects CBF less than halothane does at equivalent MAC doses (33) and provides a degree of "cerebral protection" (42). In addition, cerebral autoregulation is less affected by isoflurane than halothane (33), and isoflurane has minimal effects on the cerebrovascular reactivity to CO_2 (41). Between 0.5 MAC and 1.5 MAC isoflurane, CBF velocity does not change if CO_2 is kept normal (43). Furthermore, the hysteresis phenomenon does not occur with isoflurane as it does with halothane (44). In the presence of brain injury, however, isoflurane (45) and halothane (46) (as well as enflurane [47]) may increase ICP equally.

Sevoflurane

Sevoflurane has very fast recovery properties and is similar to isoflurane with respect to its effects on CBF, $CMRO_2$, and ICP (48). In animals, sevoflurane induces substantially smaller increases in ICP than isoflurane (49). Furthermore, sevoflurane may have a protective effect during incomplete ischemia (50). Therefore, sevoflurane has become a popular agent in neuroanesthesia.

Desflurane

In animals, desflurane increases CBF and decreases $CMRO_2$ (51). At 1.0 MAC, desflurane increases ICP significantly in neurosurgical patients with supratentorial mass lesions even in the presence of hypocapnia (52). As with sevoflurane, there are no available neuroanesthetic data for desflurane in children. One may predict, however, that the characteristics for both agents in adults will hold true for children as well.

Intravenous Anesthetics

Barbiturates

Barbiturates decrease CBF and $CMRO_2$ in a dose-dependent manner and are efficient in reducing ICP (53,54). A major problem with barbiturates in infants and small children is that they can significantly reduce myocardial contractility and systemic blood pressure. Therefore, barbiturates may reduce cerebral perfusion pressure (CPP). Barbiturates may be useful, however, in preventing an increase in ICP during laryngoscopy and tracheal intubation (55). Cerebral autoregulation and cerebrovascular reactivity to CO_2 is preserved with barbiturates, and cerebrospinal flow dynamics are not altered. With the exception of methohexital (which may activate seizure foci in patients with temporal lobe epilepsy [56]), barbiturates are effective in controlling epileptiform activity.

Etomidate

Etomidate has a direct vasoconstrictive effect on cerebral vasculature and reduces CBF (34%) and $CMRO_2$ (45%) without affecting myocardial function (57,58). After etomidate, cerebrovascular reactivity to CO_2 is maintained (57). Its suppression of the adrenocortical response to stress (59), however, and its ability to trigger myoclonic activities limit its use (60).

Droperidol

Because droperidol reduces CBF 40% without changing the $CMRO_2$ (61), it may be undesirable in patients with cerebrovascular disease or increased ICP. The combination of fentanyl and droperidol, however, has little effect on CBF.

Propofol

Propofol reduces CBF and $CMRO_2$ (62) and can reduce ICP, but concomitant reduction of MAP may diminish CPP (63).

Benzodiazepines

Benzodiazepines decrease CBF and $CMRO_2$ by approximately 25% and reduce ICP (64,65). Flumazenil, a benzodiazepine antagonist, reverses the beneficial effects of the benzodiazepines on CBF, $CMRO_2$, and ICP (64). Therefore, flumazenil should be used with caution in patients with high ICP or abnormal intracranial elastance.

Opioids

Opioid agents cause minor reduction or no effect on CBF, CMRO$_2$, and ICP (66). If the patient is experiencing pain, however, opioids can cause a modest reduction in these variables by an indirect effect on the sympathetic system. The use of fentanyl with N$_2$O in neuroanesthesia is associated with a decrease in CBF and CMRO$_2$. In neonatal animals, fentanyl does not affect cerebral circulation (67).

Ketamine

Ketamine has little effect on CMRO$_2$ however it is a potent cerebral vasodilator capable of increasing CBF by as much as 60% in the presence of normocapnia (68). It is not surprising that patients with increased ICP are likely to suffer clinical deterioration after administration of ketamine (69). Therefore, ketamine is contraindicated in children with decreased intracranial compliance.

Muscle Relaxants

In general, muscle relaxants have little effect on cerebral circulation (70). In adults, succinylcholine produces an initial decrease in ICP followed by an increase above baseline levels. Recent evidence, however, indicates that using succinylcholine to facilitate tracheal intubation in children does not cause any changes in CBF velocity and ICP (71). In addition, the increase in ICP and CBF associated with succinylcholine may be reduced by prior administration of general anesthesia or by administration of nondepolarizing muscle relaxants. Therefore, this drug is still appropriate for pediatric patients with increased ICP. These patients may benefit more from rapid control of the airway with hyperventilation than they will suffer from a slight increase in ICP caused by succinylcholine.

Pancuronium and atracurium in the presence of halothane have been shown to have no effect on CBV, ICP, or CMRO$_2$ (73). Large doses of d-tubocurarine, atracurium, or metocurine may show transient cerebrovascular dilatation owing to the histamine release and therefore could be responsible for a slight increase in ICP (74). In a study of patients with reduction in intracranial compliance, vecuronium caused a slight decrease in ICP, which was probably associated with a concomitant decrease in CVP (75).

PATHOPHYSIOLOGY OF INTRACRANIAL PRESSURE

The cranium is a closed space occupied by brain mass (70%), extracellular fluid (10%), blood (10%), and cerebrospinal fluid (10%). To maintain constant cranial volume, an increase in any one of these volumes must be offset by a reduction in the others. Brain mass is almost incompressible. Changes in cerebrospinal fluid volume is the primary buffer for increases in the other volumes. The ICP increases when intracranial volume can no longer be offset by decreased cerebrospinal fluid volume. An idealized pressure/volume relationship can be described to represent the intracranial compliance curve (Fig. 4). Normal ICP is between 8 to 18 mm Hg in adults and 2 to 4 mm Hg in children. Newborns normally have a positive ICP on the day of birth but may subsequently develop subatmospheric ICP in early life (76,77). Negative ICP is one of the factors that may promote intraventricular hemorrhage, especially in the under 2500 g premature infant.

Although the cranium is a rigid container, the pediatric patient with open fontanelles or suture lines may be able to compensate for a *slow and progressive* increase in intracranial volume by expansion of the skull. Suture lines, however, are difficult to separate and cannot compensate for *acute* increases in intracranial volume. In the older child, as in the adult, the skull is a rigid, nonexpandable container in which pressure depends on the total volume of brain substance, interstitial fluid, cerebrospinal fluid, and blood. A patient with normal ICP, yet at a noncompliant point on the curve, may experience a large and potentially dangerous increase in ICP owing to only a small change in volume. In infants and children, the ICP increases much faster than it does in adults. This rapid increase explains why a child can progress from neurologically well to moribund in a very short period of time (e.g., <30 minutes).

If the elevated ICP leads to a decrease in blood supply, cerebral ischemia may occur. To reduce the dire complications of elevated ICP, the anesthesiologist is often required to rapidly shift the patient's intracranial compliance curve to the right, change the slope of the patient's curve, or move the patient's compliance position to the left.

GENERAL ANESTHETIC CONSIDERATIONS

Preoperative Assessment

History and Physical Examination

The clinical presentation of the pediatric patient with intracranial hypertension varies according to age and duration of increase in ICP. Sudden massive increases in ICP, however, will cause coma in any age, even infants with open fontanelles and sutures. Neonates and infants with increased ICP often present with increased irritability, poor feeding, lethargy, bulging anterior fontanelle, dilated scalp veins, cranial enlargement or deformity, or lower extremity motor deficits. Clinical signs and symptoms, however, may be subtle. A history of headache on awakening is suggestive of reduced intracranial compliance caused by hypercapnia and vasodilatation during sleep. Increased ICP presenting in childhood is most frequently caused by tumor. As ICP reaches critical levels, vomiting, decreased level of consciousness, double vision due to oculomotor or gaze palsies ("sunset sign"), dysphonia, dysphagia, or gait disturbance associated with midbrain compression may develop. Assessment of cranial nerve function and the patient's ability to protect the airway must be evaluated. Injury to the third cranial nerve may result in ptosis. Injury to the sixth cranial nerve may produce a strabismus.

Auscultation of the patient's lungs may determine the presence of aspiration or pulmonary edema. Neurogenic pulmonary edema (78,79) (related to ischemia of the medulla and distortion of the brain stem [80,81]) is associated with a variety of intracranial pathologies including hemorrhage (82,83), head trauma (84), and seizure disorders (85). During the preoperative assessment of a neurologic pa-

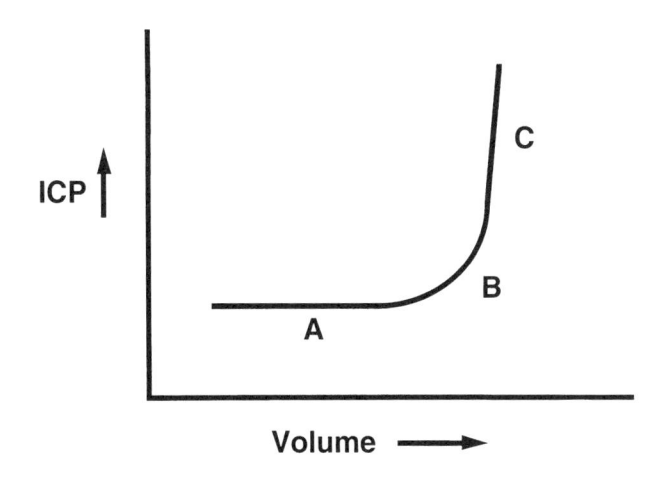

FIG. 4. A schematic drawing demonstrating the relation between the intracranial pressure and volume. Initially *(phase A)*, when the intracranial volume increases, the intracerebral pressure does not increase suggesting the presence of compensatory mechanisms. However, when the elastance of the system is limited *(phase B)*, a further increase in volume translates into a rise in pressure. Finally, when the compensatory mechanisms have been exhausted, a slight change in volume leads to an exponential increase in pressure *(phase C)*.

tient, one cannot exclude the possibility of spinal cord dysfunction. Disturbances of neurologic function arising from injury of the cervical spinal cord may affect the respiratory and cardiovascular centers.

Laboratory Tests

Laboratory tests may help diagnose the syndrome of inappropriate antidiuretic hormone (SIADH) as well as electrolyte abnormalities or volume contraction from protracted vomiting. Diabetes insipidus may result in hypernatremia. Disturbances in metabolism such as hypo- or hyperglycemia may also occur. The preoperative history and chart review may reveal the need for steroid supplementation in patients with a suppressed adrenal axis from prior steroid therapy aimed at reducing tumor edema. Neurosurgical patients may be receiving anticonvulsant medication. Recognition of seizure history as well as any potential drug interaction is important. Patients with a suprasellar tumor such as craniopharyngioma frequently have pituitary dysfunction and should therefore have a complete endocrine evaluation including thyroid and adrenal function studies.

Radiographic Imaging

The following four imaging modalities aid in the assessment of intracranial hypertension:

- Plain skull radiography
- Ultrasonography
- Computed tomography (CT) scan
- Magnetic resonance imaging (MRI)

Skull radiographs may show the "beaten copper sign" and splitting of the sagittal sutures caused by chronic increased ICP. In infants and young children, the cranial sutures should not exceed 2 mm and should not have bridges or closures (86). Ultrasonography of the brain is useful in premature infants and neonates because it is relatively inexpensive, it does not require sedation, and it can be performed at the bedside through the fontanelle. The real-time sector scanner can visualize virtually all parts of the brain (87).

In the past two decades, the development of CT scan and MRI has revolutionized the investigation of cerebral pathology. Therefore, it is important for neuroanesthesiologists to be familiar with these modalities of preoperative assessment and to insist on reviewing the films before proceeding with anesthesia. The preoperative evaluation of laboratory reports will help to identify neuroanesthetic considerations and will help to design the most appropriate anesthetic technique. Decisions regarding the use of mannitol or the identification of any highly vascularized tumors on the MRI are examples of how the analysis of these tests can help in the anesthetic preparation.

Premedication

The routine use of sedation in pediatric neurosurgical patients is best avoided. If sedation is used, one must assess ICP and monitor children continuously. Remember that a slight increase in CBV caused by even minimal respiratory depression could lead to a large disturbance in the state of consciousness of the child.

Exceptions to the "no sedation" rule include children with intracranial vascular lesions (with no increase in ICP) who may benefit from some degree of sedation to avoid precipitating a sympathetic surge and preoperative hemorrhage. Midazolam (0.5 mg/kg or chloral hydrate, 40 mg/kg, for small children) may be administered orally 1 hour before surgery. Once again, these premedications should be administered in the preoperative waiting area under constant "human" monitoring.

Patient Positioning

The anesthesiologist's preoperative visit should contribute helpful information regarding anticipated positioning needs. Furthermore, it is essential to communicate with the neurosurgeon before the procedure to coordinate the positioning requirements.

General rules for patient positioning in neuroanesthesia are the same as for other anesthetics (e.g., the eyes must be securely taped closed). If the patient is to be placed prone, the face, eyes, and other vulnerable areas should be padded with styrofoam sheeting to prevent the adverse effects of localized pressure. Because pulmonary ventilation may be compromised by incorrect positioning, chest excursion must be ensured (e.g., during prone position). The use of bolsters or a metal frame for the prone patient allows the diaphragm to move freely. The endotracheal tube should be taped securely in place, especially in prone patients whose secretions may loosen the tape.[a] Usually, a 10-degree head-up position is required to allow cerebral venous return and reduce venous congestion. Rotation of the head to one side may cause a reduction in cerebral venous return. If the head must be turned to facilitate surgical exposure, the trunk should also be turned to maintain the axial position and improve venous return. During any surgical procedure, it is important for the anesthesiologist to be able to inspect the endotracheal tube and circuit connection and have access for possible endotracheal suctioning and assessment. In addition, it is essential to be able to see a hand or foot during the surgery to assess the quality of peripheral perfusion, the adequacy of gas exchange, and temperature homeostasis and to correlate this information with the data gained by the electronic monitoring devices.

Monitoring

Basic monitoring for pediatric anesthesia is the same as for any case with the addition of a urinary catheter (if diuretics are to be given) and special neurologic monitoring. Very specialized neurologic monitoring has, over the past decade, increased in importance and is now contributing to improve the neurosurgical outcome (88). Recent technologic progress in monitoring now allows noninvasive monitoring of bioelectric signals, cerebral perfusion and flow velocity, brain tissue oximetry, and ICP. Monitoring for specific operations is discussed in later sections on specific Anesthetic Considerations.

General Principles of Induction of Anesthesia

Induction

An induction technique for a child with elevated ICP should be chosen to achieve rapid control of the airway and to allow hyperventilation. Systemic hypertension associated with laryngoscopy may be attenuated by the administration of intravenous lidocaine (1 mg/kg) at induction. If it is used in small infants, lidocaine should be given in the correct dose and slowly (over 60 seconds) to prevent cardiac dysrhythmias or cardiac arrest (89).

A rapid-sequence technique with intravenous thiopental (5 mg/kg), atropine (0.02 mg/kg), and succinylcholine (1.5 to 2 mg/kg) followed by manual hyperventilation (with rapid rate and low tidal volume) and tracheal intubation is appropriate for most cases. In cases of full stomach (e.g., recent feeding or delayed gastric emptying associated with increased ICP), cricoid pressure and manual ventilation can be performed without insufflation of the stomach (90,91). The use of low-pressure, fast-rate ventilation ("panting respiratory pattern") ensures control of $PaCO_2$ and eliminates the possibility of gastric distention. In neuroanesthesia, one need not shy away from the use of succinylcholine, despite the recent awareness of its potential adverse effects (e.g., hyperkalemic cardiac arrest in undiagnosed muscular dystrophy) (92). Succinylcholine has been used in thousands of Canadian infants and children over the years without a single death attributable to succinylcholine (93). Furthermore, the adminis-

---

[a] Ed. Note (JMB): We have found that nasotracheal tubes are a bit more secure than tubes inserted orally.

tration of thiopental before succinylcholine apparently reduces to zero the incidence of dire complications (94). It is important, however, to remember that hyperkalemia may occur after administration of succinylcholine in other clinical conditions:

- Closed head injury without motor deficits (95)
- Severe cerebral hypoxia (96)
- Subarachnoid hemorrhage (97)
- Cerebrovascular accident with loss of brain substance and paraplegia (98)

If in doubt, the administration of vecuronium, 0.4 mg/kg, has been shown to produce excellent intubating condition time similar to succinylcholine (99).

Anesthesia in patients without ready intravenous access may be induced via a small "butterfly" needle (25-gauge needle with wings), which can be inserted with minimal patient stress or hemodynamic fluctuation. Failing this, it may be less injurious in children with raised ICP to perform a skillful inhalation induction (with assisted ventilation to limit the increase in CO_2) than it is to subject them to a difficult intravenous placement or an awake intubation. In infants subjected to an awake tracheal intubation, the ICP increases owing to a reduction of the venous outflow from the cranium (71).

Maintenance

Anesthesia may be maintained with N_2O, isoflurane, and a suitable muscle relaxant. Intermittent positive-pressure ventilation is used to maintain mild hypocapnia (28 to 32 mm Hg). Administration of a single large dose of an opioid (e.g., fentanyl, 3 to 5 µg/kg) before scalp incision provides intraoperative analgesia with minimal risk of postoperative, neurologic, and respiratory depression. Deep levels of anesthesia are not needed after scalp reflection because the brain is unresponsive to incision or puncture. Furthermore, lighter anesthesia will allow monitoring of possible excessive brain tissue retraction that could lead to brain ischemia. Therefore, the clinician, assisted by monitoring equipment and his or her judgment, can guide the neurosurgeon to apply appropriate retraction pressure and thus to prevent tissue damage. In the final analysis, overly deep anesthesia is relatively contraindicated in children undergoing intracranial neurosurgical procedures.

Intracranial Pressure Control

Fluid Management

Fluid administration in the neurosurgical patient depends on the type of brain pathology. For example, a patient with increased ICP or increased brain mass or both requires a fluid administration regimen that must balance adequate intravascular volume against any effort to dehydrate the brain mass. By contrast, in a patient undergoing a ventricular shunt or repair of myelomeningocele, fluid management is mainly replacement of third-space losses. The goal of fluid management is to maintain an isovolemic, iso-osmolar, and relatively iso-oncotic intravascular volume and to maintain cerebral perfusion (100). The administration of lactated Ringer's solution (osmolarity: 273 mOsm/L) alone may lead to hemodilution, reduction of plasma osmolarity, and cerebral edema (101). If large volumes are to be infused, the use of sodium chloride (NaCl) 0.9% (osmolarity: 308 mOsm/L) is the fluid of choice to maintain intravascular iso-osmolality. The rapid administration of normal saline (10 ml/kg) has little effect on CBV and ICP and helps to maintain hemodynamic stability (102). Nevertheless, there is no single perfect protocol for fluid replacement in neurosurgical patients with increased ICP. Most anesthesiologists administer osmotic diuretic therapy at the beginning of anesthesia and measure the resulting diuresis **(see Diuretics to Reduce ICP).**

As diuresis and blood loss progress, volume is replaced with a mixture of crystalloid with colloid solutions. After an initial 20 ml/kg of crystalloid solution, the author recommends the use of a mixture of 3:1 normal saline with 5% albumin. Blood products are administered on the basis of hemodynamic instability associated with diminution of oxygen carrying capacity. Some neurologic procedures (e.g., resection of a vascular malformation) may require a large-bore intravenous access and the availability of blood products for massive volume replacement.

After a recent insult (primary lesion), the brain is vulnerable to a "secondary brain insult" (penumbral area) from hypotension, hypoxia, or ischemia. The penumbral area is a vulnerable territory in which cellular viability and function are time-dependent and will be preserved or restored only if CBF and collateral flow are maintained. Mechanical insult (e.g., retraction) (103) and ischemia (e.g., from hemodynamic instability) (104) threaten viability and function of the penumbral area.

Factors That Make Fluid Management Difficult

Efforts to dehydrate the brain are complicated by the requirement for maintaining adequate circulating blood volume **(see Diuretics to Reduce Intracranial Pressure)**. Furthermore, measurement of blood loss in most pediatric neurosurgical procedures is an inexact science. A substantial portion of the blood loss flows onto the drapes and thus is difficult to measure. To make matters worse, the addition of large amounts of irrigation solution makes it virtually impossible to assess blood loss accurately. A critical moment for blood loss in infants and small children is during scalp incision and reflection. Infiltration of the scalp with bupivacaine 0.125% (maximum dose = 3 mg/kg) with 1:200,000 epinephrine will help to reduce blood loss and the hemodynamic response to scalp incision and reflection (105). If the above maximum dosing is followed, bupivacaine blood concentrations will remain in the nontoxic range (106). Urine output in the presence of aggressive diuresis may be a misleading indicator of adequate volume replacement. In this situation, CVP monitoring will be more useful.

Pediatric patients, particularly neonates and infants, present the additional problem of glucose homeostasis. Dextrose-containing solutions are associated with a poorer neurologic outcome and are best avoided where possible, unless the presence of hypoglycemia has been confirmed (stressed neonates who have reduced glycogen stores) (107,108). Many infants from the intensive care unit may have high glucose loads in their parenteral nutrition. Abrupt cessation of these solutions may precipitate an insulin-induced hypoglycemia. In the final analysis, blood glucose levels should be sampled frequently in neurosurgical patients and normoglycemia maintained.

Diuretics to Reduce Intracranial Pressure

Mannitol

Mannitol (20% solution) remains the most popular diuretic used for reducing ICP and providing brain relaxation. Small doses (e.g., 0.25 to 0.5 g/kg) raise osmolality by 10 mOsm, enough to reduce cerebral edema and ICP (109). Larger doses produce a longer duration of action, but there is no scientific evidence that mannitol is capable of further reducing the ICP (109). Nevertheless, in the presence of cerebral ischemia, larger doses of mannitol (up to 2.0 g/kg) may be used, but this dose should be given with caution, especially in small infants and children. The onset of action with mannitol begins within 10 to 15 minutes and remains effective for at least 2 hours. Mannitol-induced vasodilatation affects intracranial and extracranial vessels and can transiently increase CBV and ICP while simultaneously reducing systemic blood pressure (110). In particular, children may experience transient hemodynamic instability (in the first 1 to 2 minutes) caused by the rapid administration of mannitol (111). Therefore, mannitol is given at a rate no greater than 0.5 g/kg over 20 to 30 minutes.

Subsequently, the period of hypotension is followed by an increase in cardiac index, blood volume, and pulmonary capillary wedge pressure, reaching peak values 15 minutes after infusion. Thus, mannitol should be administered with caution to children with congestive heart failure (a condition often associated with arteriovenous malformations) (112). After mannitol, changes in intravascular volume last for about 30 minutes when the central hemodynamic changes return to normal levels.

Loop Diuretics

Loop diuretics, furosemide and ethacrynic acid, may be useful in reducing brain edema by inducing a systemic diuresis, decreasing cerebrospinal fluid production, and resolving cerebral edema by improving cellular water transport (112). Furosemide reduces ICP without a transient increase in CBV or blood osmolality. However, it is not as effective as mannitol (113). The initial pediatric dose of furosemide should be 0.6 to 1.0 mg/kg if administered alone or 0.3 to 0.4 mg/kg if administered with mannitol. The administration of furosemide immediately before mannitol increases venous capacitance and reduces the transient increase in intravascular volume while providing effective dehydration. There is, however, a danger of electrolyte imbalance when producing profound dehydration (112). Furosemide should be given before mannitol to benefit from the increase in venous capacitance.

Corticosteroids

Corticosteroids are an important part of the therapeutic regimen in patients with increased ICP associated with brain tumors. Corticosteroids (dexamethasone, 0.1 mg/kg up to 10 mg administered during induction and every 6 hours for three doses) reduce edema around the tumor penumbral area, but may require hours or days to produce an effect.

Temperature Homeostasis

In some cases, the child's temperature is allowed, during surgery, to drift down to 33° to 34° C. Hypothermia reduces the $CMRO_2$ and may be useful in brain cell protection. It is *unnecessary to induce hypothermia in small children*. Neonates and infants are already prone to hypothermia because of their large surface area compared with body mass (114). In addition, core temperature falls immediately after induction of anesthesia owing to internal redistribution of body heat from the central compartment to the periphery. Finally, temperature decreases as heat is lost to the environment. At some point in the case, however, patients will need to be rewarmed and temperature homeostasis maintained. To achieve this goal, forced-air warming blankets and warming of intravenous fluids may be used. In addition, dry inspired gases may be warmed and moisturized with a heat exchanger (115,116). Temperature monitoring is essential, but the actual site for the probe is less important than its reliability (117). An esophageal or rectal probe placement is usually selected. The use of warmed fresh gases may contribute to falsely increase the esophageal temperature by about 0.35° C (118).

Venous Air Embolism

Venous air embolism may occur whenever the operative site is elevated above the heart, with the risk of air embolism increasing as the height difference increases. Air embolism occurs primarily in infants and children during procedures involving the skull (as in morcellation of the cranial vault, craniectomy for craniosynostosis and spinal cord procedures) (119,120). The incidence of air embolism during craniosynostosis repair in supine infants may be as high as 67%. Low blood pressure occurring without obvious reason may be explained by venous air embolism. The incidence of venous air embolism has been reduced considerably by the use of the prone position for posterior fossa surgery (121).

Venous air embolism most commonly occurs during the first hour of surgery, and detection depends entirely on the sensitivity of the monitors used (122). Less than 50% of cases of detected emboli produce systemic hypotension, but other systemic complications may occur. For example, an increase in right-sided pressure from air embolus may cause air to pass from the right side of the heart into the left via a septal defect causing paradoxical air embolus with the consequences of cerebral or myocardial infarction.

It is essential to take all measures to avoid air embolism. Meticulous avoidance of a negative pressure gradient and the routine use of intermittent positive-pressure ventilation are mandatory. On detection of air entrainment, the anesthesiologist must do the following:

- Advise the neurosurgeon to stop surgery.
- Flood the surgical field and compress the jugular veins to prevent further ingress of air.
- Ventilate with 100% oxygen.
- Attempt to withdraw air through the central venous catheter if present. Do not attempt to insert a catheter.
- Treat any hemodynamic complications.

Nitrous oxide must be discontinued. If hemodynamic instability persists, the patient should be turned and advanced cardiac resuscitation begun immediately. The application of cardiac compression is essential to break the air lock in the right ventricle out flow tract. Intravenous fluids, appropriate antiarrhythmic agents, and inotropic agents or vasopressors may be necessary and should be administered as needed. The benefit of a positive end-expiratory pressure (PEEP) of 10 cm H_2O to prevent an entry is controversial (124). When venous air is detected during craniotomy in children, it has been suggested that the success rate to aspiration of this air is between 38% and 60% (123).

Craniosynostosis

Sagittal synostosis accounts for about 50% of all craniosynostoses. Males predominate in most reported series. With fusion of the sagittal suture, the skull becomes scaphocephalic in appearance, resulting in an elongated anteroposterior dimension. Operative intervention is directed toward releasing the affected suture at an early age (<6 months) to prevent any damage associated with chronic ICP. The surgical repair might be a straightforward "strip craniectomy" with or without interposed Silastic sheeting wrapped around the cut bone edges or a cranial vault osteotomy for multiple suture synostosis (morcellation).

The following are special anesthetic considerations for infants with craniosynostosis: (a) increased ICP, (b) massive blood loss, and (c) venous air embolism.

Evidence of increased ICP will dictate the technique used for induction of anesthesia. A recent retrospective study of 74 infants with premature closure of a single suture line showed that 18% had a significant rise in ICP, whereas 38% had a slightly increased ICP measurement (125). Elevated ICP was seen more often when a midline suture was involved. This should be kept in mind during the preoperative assessment. The degree of blood loss is increased in patients with multiple-strip craniectomies and especially with older infants (>6 months), who have thicker bone tables. Blood loss either during or after surgery is often clinically significant. As a safe anesthetic conduct, cross-matched blood should always be available in the operating theater because blood replacement therapy is most often used. Communication with the surgical team is essential at all times. Special attention must be paid to the time when the neurosurgeon is removing the midline fused sagittal suture from the sagittal sinus because brisk venous bleeding and air embolism can occur. Most craniosynostosis surgery is performed when the infant is between 2 and 6 months of age, a period that coincides with normal physiologic anemia. For all patients, since bleeding can be early and brisk, it is mandatory for neuroanesthesiologists *not* to begin the surgical procedure until an adequate, large-bore, intravenous access for fluid and blood replacement has been obtained. Blood should be available at induction of anesthesia since transfusion will most often be required to maintain an acceptable hemoglobin level.

Simple suture craniectomy in the young child with normal ICP does not require arterial line placement. However, for those with elevated ICP or those undergoing extensive multiple suture procedures, the use of an indwelling arterial catheter is highly recommended. It is usual practice for the author to induce arterial hypotension (20% to 25% blood <preinduction MAP) during these procedures. Deliberate hypotension using halothane and controlled ventilation without PEEP has been demonstrated to be beneficial for children undergoing craniectomy for unilateral or bilateral craniosynostosis (126). In their study, estimated blood loss was decreased from 111 to 89 ml (mean) for all ages and from 133 to 72 ml (mean) for infants between 8 and 32 weeks of age compared with the normotensive control group.

Hydrocephalus

Hydrocephalus is characterized by an increased volume of cerebrospinal fluid within the ventricular system (Fig. 5). It is caused either by excessive production (choroid plexus papilloma), obstruction of cerebrospinal fluid pathway, or reduced reabsorption. The obstruction may lie within the ventricles themselves, within the subarachnoid space, or at sites of cerebrospinal fluid egress or absorption. In the newborn period and especially in premature infants, hydrocephalus is usually secondary to intraventricular hemorrhage. The most common neurosurgical operation for hydrocephalus today is the ventriculoperitoneal shunt (Fig. 6).

Ventriculoperitoneal shunts are prone to malfunction, and a ventriculoperitoneal shunt revision is a common operation in pediatric neurosurgery. In most patients (80%), a proximal end or ventricular catheter obstruction is found at the time of revision.

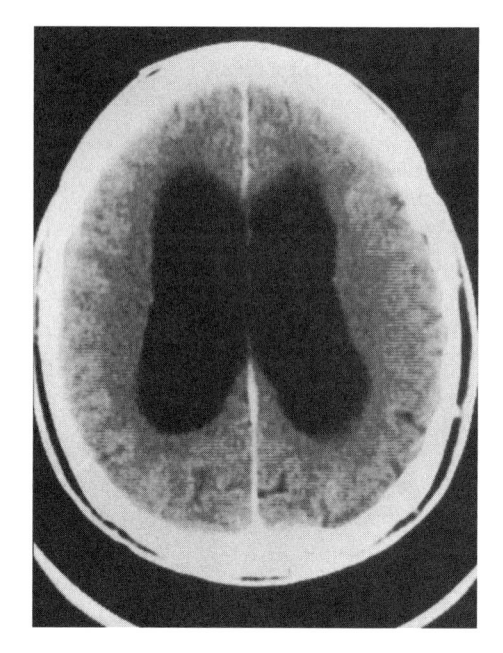

FIG. 5. Axial computed tomography scan of newborn baby with gross ventriculomegaly and hydrocephalus. The intracranial pressure is high, and periventricular edema is evident.

Preanesthetic assessment must include the following:

- Level of consciousness. Patients presenting for primary shunting, shunt revision, or shunt malfunction may exhibit severe elevations in ICP, which require aggressive treatment. Patients can evolve rapidly from an awake in neurologic status to stupor or coma within a short period of time **(see ICP Pathophysiology Section).**
- Full stomach. Evidence of vomiting or delayed gastric emptying are indications to induce anesthesia by a rapid-sequence technique.
- Coexisting pathology. Does the child have evidence of other significant organ system compromise (e.g., child with cerebral palsy who frequently aspirates)?
- Age-related pathophysiology. Is the patient likely to present problems with apnea, poor pulmonary compliance, or immature renal function?

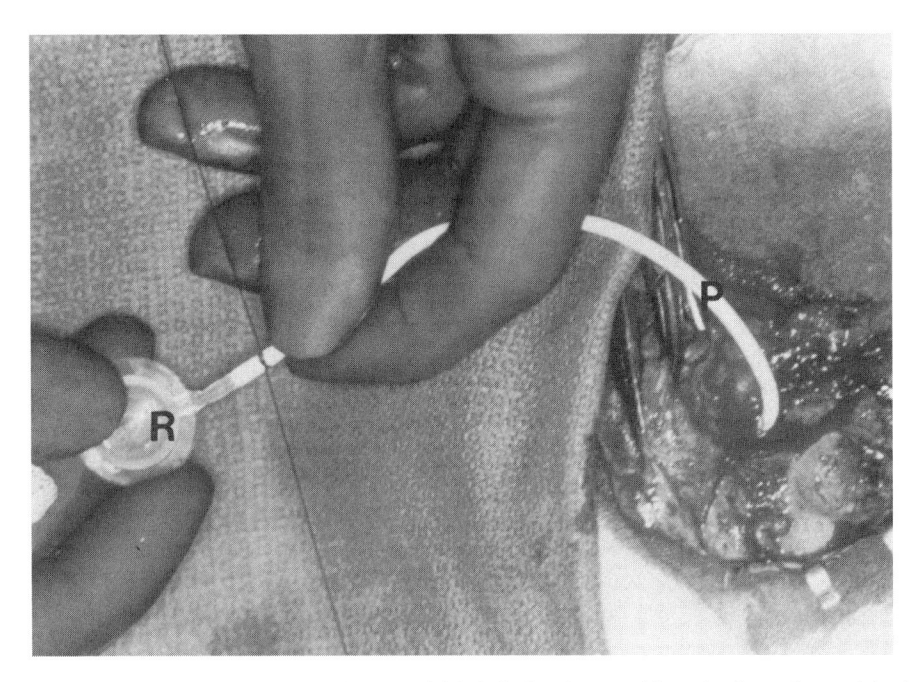

FIG. 6. Photograph of a ventricular catheter, which is being inserted into the lateral ventricle through a frontoparietal burr hole. A silk tie is placed around the connection between the valve system and the Silastic catheter before being inserted within a subcutaneous tunnel.

Induction and Intubation

Routine monitoring is most often used. However, arterial line placement is usually reserved for the patient with uncontrolled ICP and hemodynamic instability. Many patients with hydrocephalus have undergone many neurosurgical procedures. In the child without clinical evidence of elevated ICP, induction may proceed by face mask or intravenously; in children with increased ICP and delayed gastric emptying, a rapid-sequence induction is preferable.

Maintenance

Ventilation. After securing the airway, patients with increased ICP are hyperventilated to a PaCO$_2$ of between 28 and 30 mm Hg, whereas those with normal ICP are maintained at normocapnia. Spontaneous ventilation should be avoided to reduce the risk of pneumothorax during insertion of the subcutaneous guide.

Positioning. A supine position with the head turned or in a slightly lateral position is most often used. Careful attention to the patency of the cerebral venous return during positioning is essential to limit cerebral venous congestion. Therefore, neurologically compromised patients should be placed in a 30-degree head-up position with minimal neck rotation or flexion to improve venous drainage. Patients often have the shunt tubing placed posteriorly before coursing to the abdomen, and those patients are placed in a head-turned position to maintian the axial line. Patients should have an axillary roll in place and all extremities padded.

Anesthetic Agents. Anesthesia is usually maintained with a combination of N$_2$O in O$_2$ together with low concentrations of isoflurane or halothane. Narcotic supplementation can be used before skin incision in one unique dose. However, for infants and children stuporous at time of induction, the use of narcotic should be limited or avoided to reduce factors affecting the postoperative neurologic status and assessment. Although N_2O increases CBF in anesthetized pediatric patients (29), it has been suggested that this increase in CBF and $CMRO_2$ caused by N_2O is effectively blunted by hyperventilation and pretreatment with thiopental. Halogenated anesthetics may be used in low concentrations in patients with elevated ICP associated with hypocapnia.

Fluid Management. Fluid therapy is as per routine, since ventricular shunt procedures usually do not result in significant blood or third-space losses.

Body Temperature. Maintenance of body temperature is important during shunt procedures despite their relatively short duration. A large body surface area is exposed and prepared, particularly for ventriculoperitoneal shunting, and infants may cool rapidly.

Emergence

Anesthetic considerations for emergence are elimination of anesthetics, reversal of neuromuscular blockade, and delayed gastric emptying.

The trachea should be extubated once the patient is fully awake and has an appropriate gag reflex in order to protect the airway against emesis on emergence. Adequate reversal of neuromuscular blockade must be ensured if they were used. Although the use of gastric suctioning does not provide assurance against regurgitation, it may be appropriate to reduce gastric volume, which is often largely increased in patients with neurologic disorders. Unfortunately, patients undergoing shunt procedures are often neurologically impaired and have poor airway control under the best of circumstances. Therefore, they should be kept lying on the side opposite the site of the surgical incision and insertion of the ventriculoperitoneal shunt valve.

Postoperative Management

Supplemental oxygen should be given in the postoperative period. Neurosurgical patients in general and preterm infants <50 weeks' postgestational age in particular are liable to have abnormal respiratory patterns or apnea. Moderately hypothermic patients (33° to 34.5° C) should be actively rewarmed before tracheal extubation.

Analgesics should be used judiciously in neurologically impaired patients. Generous use of local anesthetic skin infiltration at the time of surgery can substantially reduce the requirement for postoperative analgesia. Patients without neurologic impairment before surgery can be given a routine postoperative pain regimen.

Intracranial Tumors

Neoplasms of the CNS account for a major proportion of all solid tumors in children <15 years of age (127). These neoplasms constitute the second most common neoplasm in children after leukemia. The classification of pediatric brain tumors is reported in Table 2. Primary brain tumors are responsible for 20% of all cancers in children and for 20% of childhood cancer deaths. In the United States in 1991, the annual incidence of brain tumors was 3.1 per 100,000 among children <15 years of age. Tumor incidence is slightly higher for males than females (1.2:1) (128,129). Almost two thirds of all childhood brain tumors arise in the posterior fossa with an unfortunate predisposition for midline structures. Although survival of children with brain tumors has improved, it remains very low for children <2 to 3 years of age at the time of diagnosis.

Brain tumors are expanding, space-occupying lesions, which lead eventually to an increased ICP accompanied by decreased CPP with the consequence of cerebral ischemia. Brain tumors are also frequently associated with hydrocephalus.

Anesthesiologists have an important role in the management of children with intracranial tumors. The following section describes an anesthetic approach for supratentorial and posterior fossa craniotomies.

TABLE 2. *Classification of pediatric brain tumors*

Central neuroepithelial tumors
   Astrocytoma—low and high grade
   Astroblastoma
   Choroid plexus papilloma and carcinoma
   Ependymoblastoma
   Ependymoma
   Ganglioglioma
   Medulloblastoma
      (primitive neuroectodermal tumor [PNET])
   Neuroblastoma
   Oligodendroglioma
   Subependymoma

Meningeal tumors
   Meningiomas
   Primary leptomeningeal melanoma
   Primary meningeal sarcoma

Maldevelopmental tumors
   Craniopharyngioma
   Dermoid tumor
   Epidermoid tumor
   Hamartoma
   Intracranial lipoma
   Rathke's cleft cyst

Germ cell tumors
   Choriocarcinoma
   Embryonal carcinoma
   Endodermal sinus tumor
   Germinoma
   Teratoma

Vascular tumors
   Arteriovenous malformation
   Capillary telangiectasia
   Cavernous malformation
   Venous angioma

Supratentorial Craniotomy

Supratentorial lesions account for about 40% to 45% of all pediatric brain neoplasms. Pediatric brain tumors often arise from midline structures including the hypothalamus, epithalamus and thalamus, and basal ganglia. These lesions are usually associated with obstructive hydrocephalus. The most common tumors in infants are hemispheric masses, such as astrocytomas (129). In infants, intracranial neoplasms have an incidence approximately twice that of the overall incidence in children (e.g., 37% compared with 16% to 24% (130). The relative incidence of hemispheric tumors is also higher after the age of 8 to 10 years (131). Craniopharyngiomas are the most common tumor of nonglial origin in children (132). Their malignancy is not related to their histologic type but rather to their location, which causes progressive neurologic deterioration and death by involving critical structures. Anesthetic considerations include the following:

- Increased ICP. Hydrocephalus is often associated. The CT scan and MRI film must be reviewed to appropriately plan the anesthetic.
- Full stomach. Delayed gastric emptying occurs in the patient with raised ICP.
- Electrolyte and fluid. Hydration state and electrolyte balance may be altered in the child with intracranial pathology. The syndrome of inappropriate antidiuretic hormone (SIADH) might be present.
- Age-related pathophysiology. Anesthetic considerations are identical with those discussed in earlier sections.
- Positioning. The head should be elevated not more than 10 degrees. Ensure that venous return is not obstructed.

Monitoring

Invasive monitoring should be considered. An arterial line placement for hemodynamic monitoring and blood chemistry sampling is highly recommended. Patients in whom blood loss will be significant, those with expected hemodynamic instability, or those at increased risk for air embolism should receive a central venous catheter. The use of a urinary catheter is mandatory because of the duration of the surgical procedure and the use of diuretic drugs.

Preinduction

Determination of the degree to which ICP is elevated in patients undergoing craniotomy is essential. Patients with large mass lesions, significant tumor edema or obstruction to cerebrospinal fluid outflow will require an anesthetic approach aimed at reducing ICP.

After reviewing the MRI and CT scan, the neuroanesthesiologist may have to discuss with the neurosurgeon whether the use of a ventriculostomy catheter placement first to incise the dura mater incision would be appropriate to assist in the management of raised ICP. No excessive attempt to reduce ICP pharmacologically should be done beyond normal physiologic reserve. This confirms again the importance of reviewing the radiologic information before the induction of anesthesia. The pediatric neuroanesthesiologist must be aware of the clinical condition as well as its related laboratory information to provide an appropriate and rational anesthetic. For instance, these children may show evidence of hypovolemia and low serum osmolality with cerebral edema caused by SIADH which would influence directly the anesthetic management. Furthermore, many of these patients will have already been subjected to an aggressive brain dehydration therapy with the consequence of an important reduction in intravascular volume.

Induction and Intubation

Induction in children with supratentorial lesions, unlike children with normal ICP, should be accomplished with a minimally stimulated, rapidly secured airway, followed immediately by hyperventilation. This sequence of events is of paramount importance in the patient with significantly elevated ICP. Intravenous thiopental (5 to 6 mg/kg), lidocaine (0.5 to 1.0 mg/kg), fentanyl (2 µg/kg), and a nondepolarizing muscle relaxant can be used to prevent sympathetic stimulation during laryngoscopy. It is essential, however, to limit the thiopental dose if aggressive mannitol therapy has been given preoperatively. Cricoid pressure is applied, and the patient is hyperventilated manually with low peak inspiratory pressures to avoid inflation of the stomach. Laryngoscopy should proceed as smoothly as possible. Some anesthesiologists prefer nasotracheal intubation for patients in whom postoperative ventilation is expected or in small infants in whom the tube may be better stabilized.

Maintenance

Following are considerations for maintenance of anesthesia in children with supratentorial lesions.

Ventilation. A $PaCO_2$ between 25 and 30 mm Hg is indicated for patient with increased ICP. Occasionally, a very tight brain with uncontrollable hypertension can require lower levels of $PaCO_2$. However, in this circumstance, caution must be exercised because the vasoconstriction induced by extreme hyperventilation may decrease CPP, leading to ischemia or alternatively shifting blood flow to the hyperemic brain with impaired autoregulation. PEEP is generally avoided to facilitate cerebral venous drainage. The use of PEEP may also decrease MAP in patients with decreased intravascular volume after mannitol therapy, resulting in decreased CPP. However, in patients with impaired oxygenation, small amounts of PEEP may be increased gradually to the minimum necessary to correct hypoxia without affecting venous return.

Positioning. Pediatric patients are usually placed supine for supratentorial procedures with the head elevated slightly to facilitate venous drainage. Extremities should be well padded and the eyes protected from injury. Care must be taken to avoid undue flexion, extension, or rotation of the neck, which could affect venous return and favor cerebral congestion. Prone positioning is discussed in the chapter on posterior fossa surgery.

Anesthetic Agents and Muscle Relaxants. Anesthetic agent selection should be based on the wide body of clinical and laboratory data compiled in this area. To this end, the author selects one of two techniques: either neuroleptanalgesia technique or a balanced inhalational approach. The neuroleptanalgesia technique combines N_2O, a synthetic short-acting narcotic (usually fentanyl citrate), and a nondepolarizing muscle relaxant with either a benzodiazepine, droperidol, or propofol.

With a balanced approach, sub-MAC concentrations of isoflurane are used with N_2O, fentanyl, and a nondepolarizing muscle relaxant. Any nondepolarizing muscle relaxant is likely to be acceptable for the neurosurgical patient; however, agents capable of releasing histamine should be administered with caution. For the infant and small children, the use of pancuronium for its vagolytic properties may be advantageous. Vecuronium for the older children is excellent and predictable.

Fluid Management. Fluid management during craniotomy can be very problematic. Patients with increased ICP usually receive dehydration therapy preoperatively. This increases the possibility of intravascular collapse, especially in light of the substantial blood loss that often accompanies the skin incision and excision of the bone flap. Central venous pressure monitoring can be a valuable aid, and volume expansion is usually effected by colloid solutions such as 5% albumin. Simple craniotomy in patients without significantly increased ICP and in procedures with manageable blood loss frequently use crystalloid replacement only.

Body Temperature. Body temperature should be allowed to decrease passively to 34.5° to 35° C for additional cerebral protection.

Emergence

Anesthetic considerations for emergence include the following:

- Elimination of anesthetic agents
- Reversal of neuromuscular blockade
- Delayed gastric emptying
- Increased ICP

The decision to extubate the trachea at the end of the procedure is made on the basis of the success of the surgical intervention, smoothness of the intraoperative course, normalization of ICP, age of the patient, degree of residual neurologic deficit, and the effect of these factors on respiration and airway protection. Patients without adequate respiratory function will retain CO_2 with the potential for increased ICP and continuous intracerebral vascular bleeding. A gag reflex should be present for airway protection. Children who remain sedated and hyperventilate in the postoperative period should be suspected of having increased ICP. Transfer of the patient to CT scan for an evaluation should be discussed with the neurosurgeon. If this solution is chosen, the anesthetist must accompany the child at all times, and proper monitoring must be used. Neonates with poor pulmonary compliance or an immature respiratory drive may remain intubated postoperatively. In the absence of any adverse complications, the trachea can be extubated when the patient is fully awake and reversal of the neuromuscular blockade and elimination of the anesthetic agents is achieved.

Postoperative Management

Considerations for postoperative management after supratentorial craniotomy include the following:

- Oxygen and respiration
- Temperature homeostasis
- Analgesia
- Neurologic assessment
- Hypertension
- Seizures

As with any postsurgical patient, supplemental oxygen should be administered and the adequacy of respiration assessed. All patients should be admitted to an intensive care unit for monitoring of neurologic and vital signs. Patients requiring postoperative ventilation will require sedation and possibly muscle relaxation to avoid agitation and increased ICP. Body temperature should be maintained at a normal level. Patients with craniotomy are prone to develop neurogenic hyperthermia postoperatively, which would be detrimental. The use of local anesthetic skin infiltration intraoperatively or a cervical superficial plexus blockade at the end of the procedure can reduce the requirement for postoperative intravenous opioid analgesics. A balance between patient comfort and the ability to follow the patient's neurologic status must be sought. An obtunded patient must be investigated for increased ICP or other surgically correctable pathology such as sustained intracranial bleeding.

The most common contributor to postoperative increased ICP is uncontrolled systemic hypertension. When postoperative pain control has been achieved, blood pressure may be controlled with the use of vasodilators. β-blocking drugs have been used successfully, particularly labetalol because of its combined β- and α-blocking properties and because it does not normally cross the blood-brain barrier.

Seizures frequently occur in the immediate postoperative period. Many surgeons place their patients on preoperative anticonvulsant agents and continue them postoperatively. Phenobarbital appears to be the most frequently used drug, and phenytoin or other medications are added for refractory patients.

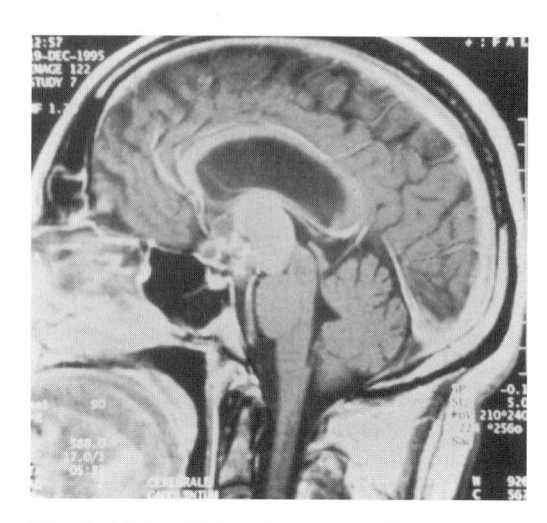

FIG. 7. Midsagittal nuclear magnetic resonance scan showing high-signal mass lesion filling the suprasellar cistern (craniopharyngioma), which is extending from the pituitary fossa to herniate into the third ventricle.

Craniopharyngioma

Craniopharyngioma is the most common intracranial tumor of nonglial origin in the pediatric population (129) (Fig. 7). Although the surgical approach to all craniopharyngioma is to attempt a total removal, it can be achieved in only 65% of patients. The following are special anesthetic considerations for craniopharyngioma surgery.

Positioning. Most often in children, a bitemporal craniotomy is used with a right subfrontal lobe approach. The head is usually positioned in extreme extension. Brain relaxation is essential to limit the effect of excessive brain retractor on the frontal lobe.

Hypopituitarism. Postoperative management should include the administration of gluco- and mineralocorticoid, thyroid, and sex hormones. Insulin-dependent diabetic patients may have reduced insulin requirement. Blood glucose must be monitored carefully.

Diabetes Insipidus. A complication of pituitary surgery is diabetes insipidus. It can be also associated with head trauma. Although usually present in the immediate postoperative period after 4 to 6 hours, it may become clinically evident intraoperatively. A large quantity of dilute urine is associated with a rising serum osmolality and low urine osmolality (<200 mOsm/L). The easiest test for diabetes insipidus is urine specific gravity, which should be <1.002. Hypernatremia and hypovolemia are key features. Fluid management should include 75% of the previous hour's urine output. The patient's electrolyte level will determine the intravenous solution to administer. Therapy consists of fluid replacement with hypotonic solutions such as 50% normal saline with 5% dextrose and replacement of lost electrolytes. Hyperglycemia and superimposed osmotic diuresis may occur if a large volume of 5% dextrose is used.

It is now routine to administer vasopressin or one of its analogues, such as DDAVP (desmopressin acetate) in an early stage. If administered intraoperatively, the aqueous solu-

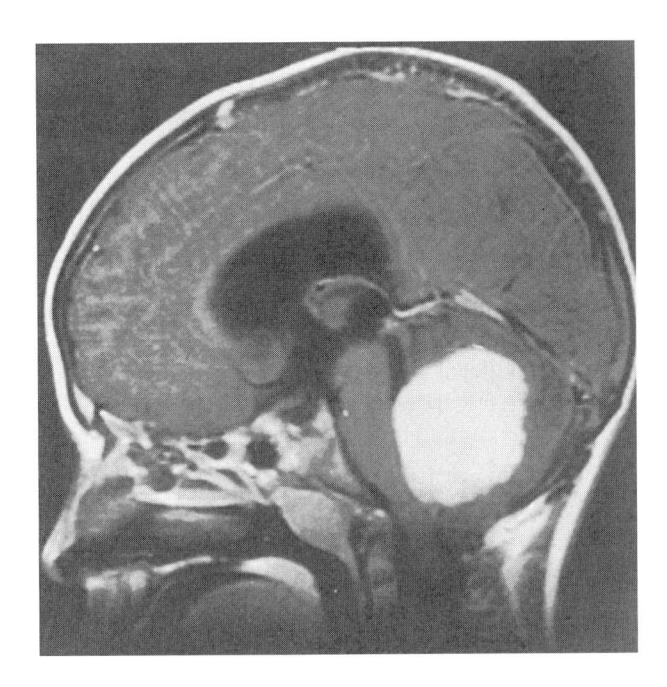

FIG. 8. Hydrocephalus is the result of congenital aqueductal obstruction. The proximal aqueduct and third ventricle are dilated. This astrocytoma *(white mass)* is generating an important increase in the infratentorial compartment pressure. This elevation in pressure is indicated by the bulging of the tentorium, the herniation of the midbrain through the tentoria incisura, and the distortion of the pons against the clivus (bony structure in front of the pons).

tion of DDAVP, although free of cardiovascular side effects, may occasionally produce hypertension. Postoperatively, the intranasal route is often used, and the dose of DDAVP is 0.05 to 0.3 ml/day divided into two doses. If the intravenous route is chosen, the dose should be 10% of the intranasal dose also divided into two doses daily. Vasopressin can also be administered through an infusion and the rate is 0.5 mU/kg per hour. The rate must be adjusted until the desired antidiuresis is achieved.

Hyperthermia. Injury to the hypothalamic thermoregulatory mechanism may result in postoperative neurogenic hyperthermia. Efforts should be made to maintain normothermia.

Seizures. Seizures are seen in the immediate postoperative period in more than 80% of infants and children. Phenytoin should be administered preoperatively or intraoperatively in all patients older than five years old. Patients younger than five years will benefit better with phenobarbitol for seizure control.

Posterior Fossa Surgery

Posterior fossa tumors occur more frequently in children than in adults; 50% to 55% of all pediatric brain tumors are infratentorial (133). The four common types include medulloblastoma (30%), cerebellar astrocytoma (30%), brain-stem glioma (30%), and ependymoma (7%). The remaining 3% include acoustic neuroma, meningioma, ganglioglioma, and so forth. Cerebellar astrocytomas have no sex predilection, but medulloblastomas occur more frequently in males. The common symptoms of a posterior fossa tumor in children are due to hydrocephalus, which is present in 90% of children with medulloblastoma and in almost all children with cerebellar astrocytoma (Fig. 8). The presence on CT scan or MRI of a cyst associated with a lateral white tumor is almost pathognomonic of an astrocytoma. The importance to identify this radiologic sign for the anesthesiologist is related to the vascularization of the tumor. Astrocytomas are rigid, hypoperfused masses, whereas medulloblastomas are highly vascularized. Once again, the anesthetic management is influenced by the information obtained in the review of these radiologic tests.

The most common nontumoral posterior fossa procedure is decompression for Arnold-

Chiari malformation with obex occlusion. The Arnold-Chiari malformation is a complex developmental anomaly characteristically presenting with downward displacement of the inferior cerebellar vermis into the upper cervical spinal canal and elongation of the medulla oblongata and the fourth ventricle (Fig. 9). Preoperatively, the anesthesiologist should pay particular attention to the neurologic symptoms such as cerebellar dysfunction, evidence of upper airway obstruction (inspiratory stridor), cardiovascular instability, and increased ICP.

Anesthetic Considerations

Anesthetic considerations for posterior fossa surgery include the following:

- Age-related pathophysiology.

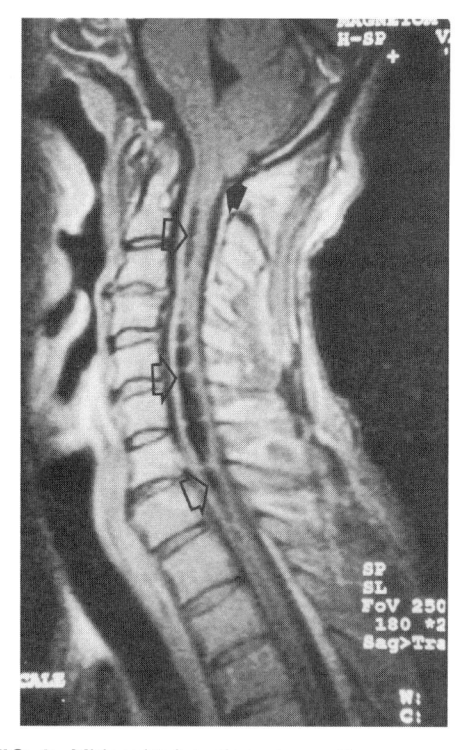

FIG. 9. Midsagittal nuclear magnetic resonance image of an Arnold-Chiari type I malformation showing the cerebellar tonsil engaged through the foramen magnum *(black arrow)* and the association of a cervicospinal syringomyelia *(open arrows)*.

- ICP. Associated symptomatic hydrocephalus, an external ventricular drain is often positioned after induction of anesthesia to facilitate the management of the ICP before opening of the dura mater. The maintenance of cerebral perfusion is essential. In addition, mannitol, furosemide, and corticosteroids may be given. Special attention should be brought to the MRI to determine the importance of the upward engagement. This sign will help in deciding on the administration of diuretic agents. Furthermore, the distance between the pons and the clivus (bony structure in front of the pons) should be >2 mm; if not, it indicates an increased ICP in the infratentorial space.
- Full stomach. Posterior fossa pathology increases gastric emptying time in children and makes the patient prone to regurgitation at induction.
- Associated preexisting problems. *Cardiovascular:* some patients may be hypertensive as a response to brain-stem compression; *pulmonary:* recurrent aspiration pneumonia is a common occurrence; *nervous system;* central sleep apnea occurs and may persist postoperatively.
- Air embolism. See previous discussion on Venous Air Embolism.
- Airway management. Arnold-Chiari malformation or brain-stem compression may cause upper airway dysfunction with inspiratory stridor.
- Fluid and electrolytes. Preoperative attempt to reduce ICP may generate electrolyte imbalance and intravascular volume contraction.
- Premedication.

Preinduction and Induction of Anesthesia

Preinduction. The preinduction assessment is similar to that described for supratentorial procedures. It is important to reinforce that every neuroanesthesiologist should always review the radiologic test available (MRI, CT scan, myelography, and so on) before proceeding with the anesthetic induction. The analysis of this laboratory information is essential to establish a safe anesthetic plan adapted to the patient's needs and to contribute the most favorable outcome for the neurosurgical procedure.

Induction. The induction of anesthesia must be aimed at preserving CPP, avoiding an increase in ICP, and providing an appropriate depth of anesthesia. The choice of anesthetic is not as crucial as the manner in which the medications are administered. A combination of thiopental, atropine, and a nondepolarizing muscle relaxant, associated with a narcotic such as fentanyl, constitute the author's anesthetic preferences. Succinylcholine can be used safely unless the patient shows signs of severe ICP with hemodynamic instability (134). To minimize the possibility of kinking and obstruction of the endotracheal tube, a reinforced armored orotracheal tube may be used. Although many neuroanesthesiologists prefer a nasotracheal tube for better stability and fixation, I use an orotracheal tube with soft bite block to eliminate epistaxis and possible infection.

Patient Positioning

There are three common patient positions for posterior fossa tumor operations. The prone position is used in 55% of all procedures, the sitting position in 30%, and the lateral position in 15%. At the author's institution, all surgical procedures in the posterior cranial fossa or upper cervical spine are performed with the patient in the prone position (135), with the patient lying on a U-bolster or a Relton frame (136) (Fig. 10). The anesthesiologist's responsibility is to apply special care during positioning with regard to ventilation and pressure points and ensuring that flexion of the head does not occlude jugular venous drainage nor displace the endotracheal tube to an endobronchial position. The method of head fixation depends on the age of the patient (i.e., thickness of the skull) and also to the surgeon's needs. Horseshoe headrests are appropriate, but the face of the patient must be padded carefully with special attention paid to the eyes. In a child >3 years of age, the multipin head-holder is often used with 30 to 40 lb of tension per pin. Infiltration of the pin sites with local anesthetic will reduce nociceptive and hemodynamic responses. After pin insertion, the author applies bethadine ointment to limit the possibility of venous air embolism. During maneuver to position the patient, it is important that the depth of anesthesia should be minimal to limit hemodynamic instability and a subsequent decrease in CPP.

Monitoring

Monitoring for posterior fossa surgery is basically the same as in supratentorial craniotomy with the important exception of the precordial Doppler imager for detection of air embolism and the use of somatosensory evoked potentials for monitoring during removal of intramedullary or brain-stem tumor.

Maintenance of Anesthesia

As with induction of anesthesia, no single anesthetic technique has been shown to be superior (137), and the maintenance regimen must be tailored to the need of the patient and the requirement of the surgical procedure. After skin preparation, local anesthetic (bupivacaine 0.125% with epinephrine 1:200,000) should be infiltrated along the incision line (105), and anesthesia depth should be increased before skin incision with fentanyl (3 to 5 µg/kg) or isoflurane or both. The aim is to provide a "slack brain," which will reduce the amount of retractor pressure and allow adequate cerebral perfusion. A nondepolarizing muscle relaxant is given, and the ICP is reduced by mannitol (0.5 g/kg) preceded by furosemide (0.3 mg/kg). During the initial surgical approach, the intermittent positive-pressure ventilation is adjusted to maintain the PaCO$_2$ at 28 to 30 mm Hg.

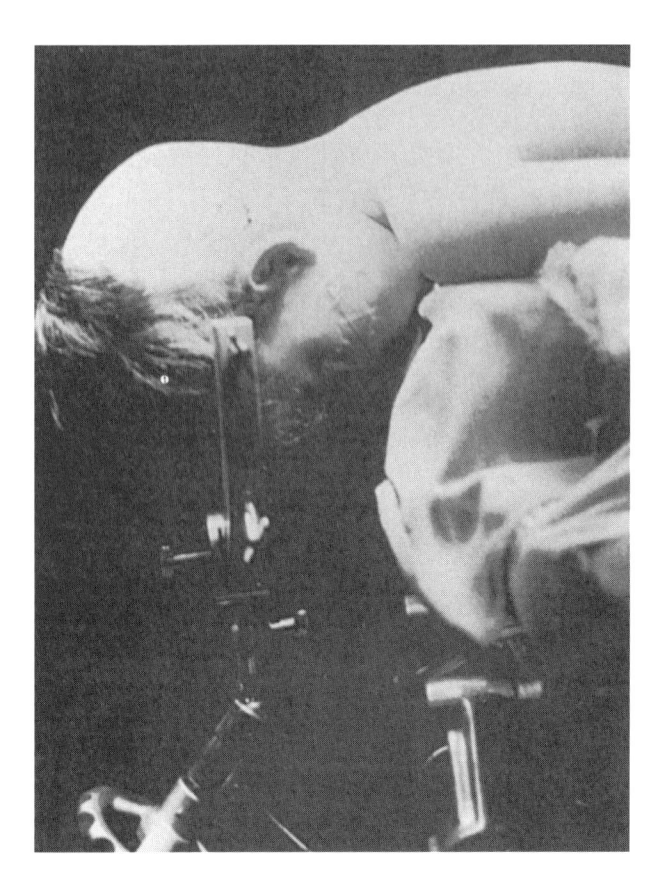

FIG. 10. Intraoperative photograph of a child in prone position for posterior fossa surgery. The patient is positioned on a U-bolster to facilitate pulmonary ventilation preoperatively. This is essential also to limit the increase in intrathoracic pressure, which can lead to a reduction in cerebral venous return. The different pressure points must be carefully padded with special care to the eyes. The anesthesiologist must pay special attention to the flexion of the head to avoid occlusion of jugular venous drainage. Particular care must also be given to the endotracheal tube and accessibility at all times must be planned before beginning the surgical procedure.

Emergence and Recovery

The need for prompt awakening is mandatory but must be combined with the need for a hemodynamically stable and unstimulated patient during extubation. An understanding of the pathologic process will dictate to the neuroanesthesiologist the correct airway management postoperatively. After resection of a midline intrabulbar ependymoma, although patients will show proper respiratory effort in the first hour postoperatively, they will rapidly progress toward respiratory depression because of postsurgical edema. Tracheal intubation with postoperative sedation administered after allowing an immediate postoperative neurologic assessment is advised by the author. Furthermore, tracheal intubation may be essential postoperatively after resection of high intramedullary spinal tumor. In cases in which extubation is appropriate, the preoperative administration of narcotic agents associated with lidocaine, 0.5 to 1.0 mg/kg, in infants and children will facilitate the emergence by reducing coughing and straining, which could otherwise lead to a hypertensive episode and intracerebral bleeding. Postoperative pain management can usually be achieved with intravenous morphine, 50 µg/kg, with acetaminophen, 40 mg/kg rectally. The necessity of avoiding medication that affects the sensorium or the pupil's size is important.

Cerebrovascular Anomalies

Arteriovenous malformations are uncommon congenital or acquired lesions, which provide an important anesthetic challenge mainly in infants and children (11). These malformations consist of large arterial feeding vessels that lead to dilated communicating vessels and finally to veins. These veins are easily identifiable because they carry arterialized blood. Flow of blood through the low-resistance arte-

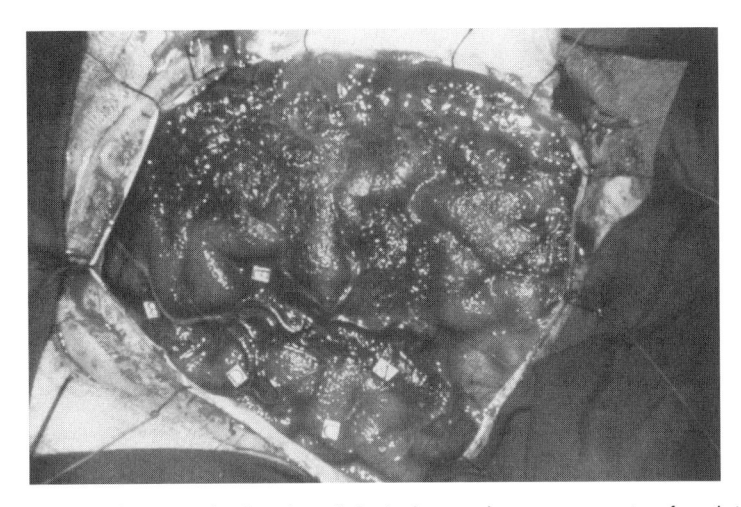

FIG. 11. Intraoperative photograph showing distorted vascular components of an intracranial cortical cerebrovascular malformation.

riocapillary circuitry results in progressive distention and dilatation of the entire venous system of the brain and cranium (Fig. 11). The posterior cerebral artery and the great vein of Galen are examples in the pediatric population (Fig. 12). They usually present clinically in the newborn period with severe congestive heart failure. The saccular dilatation of Galen's vein may be associated with hydrocephalus because of the obstruction of the aqueduct of Sylvius (12). Although most arteriovenous malformations go normally undetected until the fourth or fifth decade of life, 18% of patients present before age 15 years. Cerebral injury may ensue owing to one or more of the following causes:

- Hemorrhage with thrombosis and infarction
- Compression of adjacent neural structures
- Parenchymal ischemia caused by "steal" of blood flow to the low resistance network
- Congestive heart failure (CHF) and hypoperfusion
- Surgical disruption or diversion of the blood flow (Patients with arteriovenous malformations may undergo radiologically controlled embolization. Stereotactic radiosurgery can be used as definitive or adjunctive therapy. Surgical clipping of feeding vessels may be performed as a single- or multiple-stage procedure.)

Anesthetic Considerations

The following are considerations for patients undergoing arteriovenous malformation resection:

- Preexisting pathophysiology. Does the patient present with increased ICP or congestive heart failure? Does the patient have associated congenital defects?
- Age-related pathophysiology. Will organ system immaturity make an impact on the anesthetic technique?
- Blood loss. The possibility of massive blood loss is real. Appropriate precautions must be taken.
- Ventilation pattern. The indication for hyperventilation in the patient with vascular anomalies becomes a contraindication with the moyamoya disease.

Monitoring

Beyond routine monitoring previously discussed, patients undergoing arteriovenous

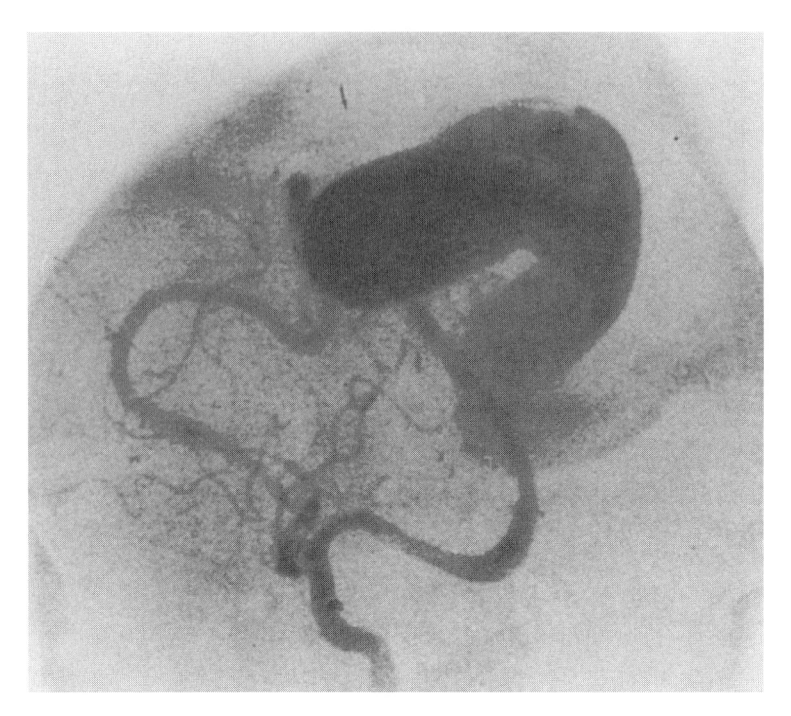

FIG. 12. Vein of Galen varix. A lateral view of an internal carotid artery injection demonstrates emptying of anterior cerebral branches *(upper)* and the middle cerebral *(middle)* into the vein of Galen, which is abnormally expanded to become a varix that drains into the straight sinus and the confluence of sinuses. The effect of this complex congenital arteriovenous connection is the premature dumping of arterial blood into the venous compartment, since there is no capillary resistance bed. Blood flow is preferential through the malformation because of the pressure sump or dump effect, and arterial supply to the surrounding brain, as can be seen from the angiogram, is severely compromised. Cardiac failure is caused by the state of hyperdynamic outflow, which often leads to the death of the patient in the first days of life.

malformation resection should have at least two large-bore intravenous catheters with blood pumps mounted on a blood-warmer device in place before surgery. Intravenous solutions should be warmed from the beginning of the procedure. Arterial line placement is essential. Central venous pressure monitoring is always used on all but the smallest superficial cortical arteriovenous malformations. Urinary catheter placement is mandatory after induction of anesthesia.

Preinduction

Symptomatology varies according to the age at which the disease manifests. Older children most frequently present with evidence of subarachnoid hemorrhage or intraventricular hemorrhage. Over 70% of pediatric patients presenting with spontaneous subarachnoid hemorrhage have arteriovenous malformations as the cause. Seizure is the presenting symptom in approximately 25% of patients. The neonatal presentation of cerebral arteriovenous malformation is the most challenging because it is often associated with congestive heart failure (13). Physical examination shows signs of left or right heart failure such as tachypnea, tachycardia, cyanosis, pulmonary edema, hepatomegaly, and electrocardiographic changes. Laboratory studies provide evidence of severe electrolyte imbalances, which are the inevitable result of aggressive diuretic therapy. Neonates in severe congestive heart failure receive digoxin therapy and may well require tracheal intubation with mechanical ventilation and continuous intravenous inotropic support. Patients with no evidence of congestive heart failure can be premedicated to reduce agitation and hypertension before induction of anesthesia.

Induction and Intubation

Central to induction of anesthesia in children with arteriovenous malformation without congestive heart failure is prevention of an hypertensive response during laryngoscopy. Inhalation or intravenous induction may be performed in the child without evidence of increased ICP. Incremental doses of intravenous induction agent and narcotic are given along with lidocaine before laryngoscopy. A nondepolarizing muscle relaxant without hemodynamic effects such as vecuronium is recommended. Neonates in congestive heart failure will have intravenous access in place before induction. Extreme caution in small infants must be observed, since many anesthetic agents used during induction, including lidocaine, are myocardial depressants and may precipitate cardiovascular collapse (89). Oral or nasal intubation may proceed as the anesthetist prefers.

Maintenance of Anesthesia

Positioning. Positioning for surgery is dependent on the site of the malformation. Arteriovenous malformations most commonly receive their blood supply from the middle meningeal artery distribution and are approached by supratentorial tempoparietal craniotomy.

Ventilation. All patients are mechanically ventilated for control of $PaCO_2$. Patients with hydrocephalus may require some degree of hyperventilation until the pressure is relieved. It is important to maintain normocarbia in children undergoing arteriovenous malformation resection. The importance of maintaining a good CPP in the collateral circulation surrounding the arteriovenous malformation is essential to prevent ischemia of brain parenchyma. However, it is essential to avoid deep hypocapnia, which would decrease CBF in normal vessels and shunt additional blood flow to the low-resistance malformed vessels and increase bleeding from the arteriovenous malformation.

Anesthetic Agents. Anesthetic agents selected for maintenance are similar to those used for any intracranial procedure. In the absence of congestive heart failure, a hypotensive technique may be used at time of ligation of the arteriovenous malformation using drugs such as trimethaphan, nitroprusside, nitroglycerin, or high concentrations of isoflurane. The author has found an infusion of phentolamine to be particularly useful and easily titratable and predictable. Neonates in congestive heart failure are usually on inotropic support and do not tolerate well hypotensive anesthesia. Vasoactive drugs should be infused by central lines if possible.

Fluid Management. Fluid management in patients with arteriovenous malformations is difficult. Neonates may not be able to accommodate fluid loads at all, and children with contracted intravascular compartments resulting from attempts at brain dehydration may experience rapid circulatory collapse after brisk intraoperative bleeding.

Body Temperature. Maintaining body temperature can be difficult in children, especially during massive transfusion (138). It may be beneficial to allow the patient's core temperature to decrease to 34° C to provide the extracerebral protective effect (139). In fact, a study using canine model of transient, complete cerebral ischemia demonstrated that even small, clinically relevant increase in temperature (1° C or 2° C) resulted in significant alterations in both postischemic neurologic function and cerebral histopathology (140). Assuming that these results are transferable to humans, it suggests that, in patients at imminent risk for ischemic neurologic injury, body temperature should be closely monitored and controlled. Furthermore, the clinician should aggressively treat all episodes of hyperthermia until the patient is no longer at risk for ischemic neurologic injury.

Emergence

Anesthetic considerations for emergence include the following:

- Elimination of anesthetic agents
- Reversal of neuromuscular blockade
- Assessment of airway patency and respiration
- Confirmation of thermodynamic stability

Patients with no history of congestive heart failure may be extubated after the elimination of anesthetic agents and reversal of neuromuscular blockade. Patients with a likelihood of significant neurologic deficit, extensive resection, or brain retraction of cerebral edema remain sedated with the trachea intubated into the postoperative period.

Postoperative Management

The basic anesthetic considerations for postoperative care include cerebral edema, congestive heart failure, hypertension, and vasospasm.

Cerebral Edema. Cerebral edema resulting from the lesion or secondary to the surgical procedure may require further therapeutic intervention, such as continuous mechanical ventilatory support and pharmaceutical adjuncts. The transfer to the intensive care unit will be indicated. It is not unusual for the patient with severe arteriovenous malformations to return to full consciousness following surgical removal after only several days. During this period of time, close neurologic observation is required to detect possible clinical deterioration.

Congestive Heart Failure. Although the arteriovenous malformation obliteration reduces the R → L shunt, the patient with preoperative congestive heart failure usually remains in a precarious medical state in the postoperative period and requires transfer to an intensive care unit for observation and continuous therapy. The necessity to maintain adequate CPP but as well reduce the cardiac overload makes the management rather difficult.

Hypertension. In conjunction with analgesics, antihypertensive therapy may be required to avoid sudden increases in blood pressure, which could precipitate rebleeding.

Vasospasm. Vasospasm is not the most common postoperative complication of cerebrovascular surgery but must be considered

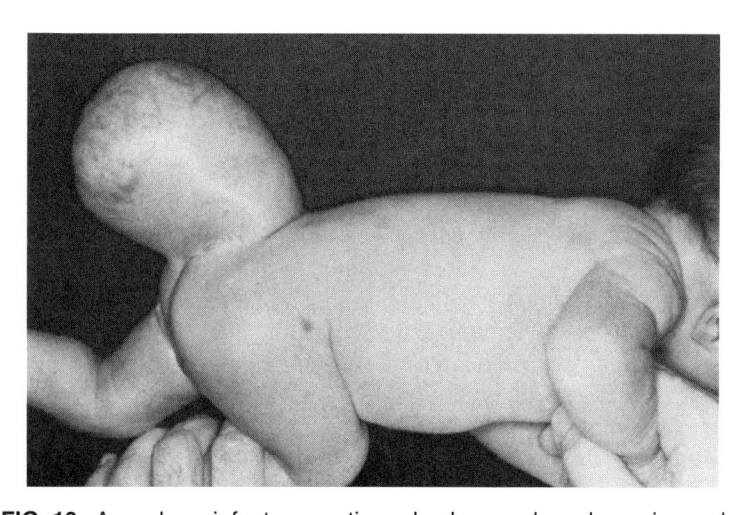

FIG. 13. A newborn infant presenting a lumbosacral myelomeningocele.

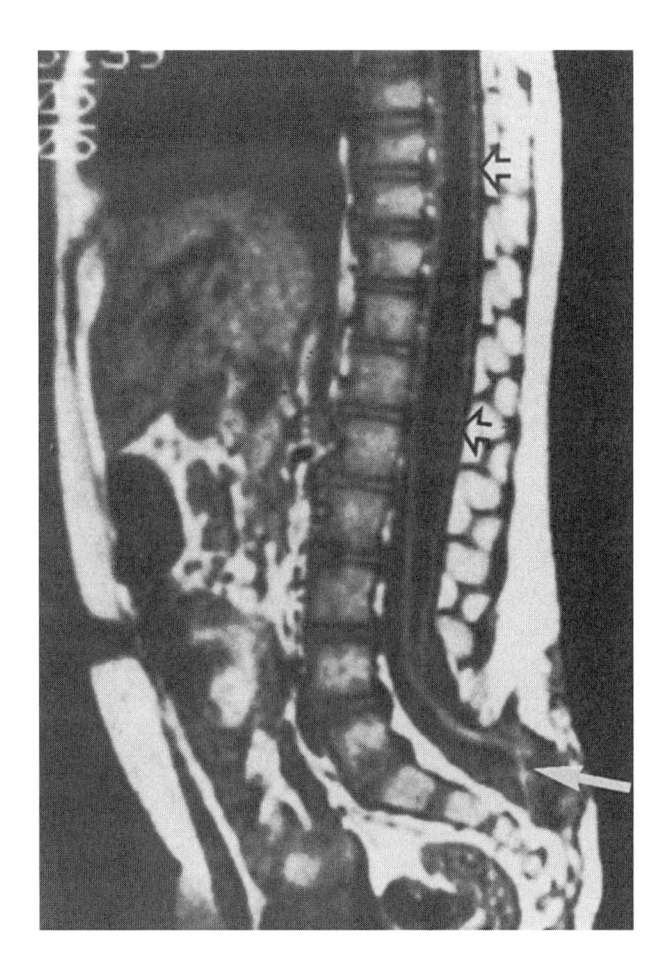

FIG. 14. Midsagittal CT scan of the lumbosacral spine demonstrating a myelomeningocele. The spinal cord lies abnormal and low due to its tethering at the site of the meningocele *(white arrow)*. A large syrinx is seen throughout the length of the cord *(open black arrows)*.

in face of any neurologic deterioration. The pathogenesis of vasospasm is poorly understood, but its early diagnosis is crucial for the future neurologic outcome of the patient. The detection and prevention of vasospasm are essential during postoperative care. The use of transcranial Doppler sonography has become useful in the diagnosis of this complication. The treatment of vasospasm is limited by the use of selective neurologic calcium blocker agents associated with myocardial enhancing-performance drugs. (141).

Myelodysplasia

Hydrocephalus is accompanied by abnormalities in the spinal column and spinal cord in about 70% of hydrocephalic infants (142).

Myelodysplasia refers to an abnormality in the fusion of the embryologic neural groove that normally closes in the first month of gestation. Failure of neural tube closure results in the saclike herniation of meninges (meningocele) or a herniation containing neural elements (myelomeningocele) (Fig. 13). The spinal cord is often tethered caudally by the sacral roots, resulting in orthopedic or urologic symptoms in later childhood if it is not surgically corrected (Fig. 14). Myelomeningoceles most commonly occur in the lumbosacral region, but failure of rostral fusion of the neural groove can result in their formation at any level in the neuraxis. Most children with myelomeningocele also have an associated Arnold-Chiari type I-acquired malformation (see Fig. 9) and therefore, hydrocephalus will develop and become part of the anes-

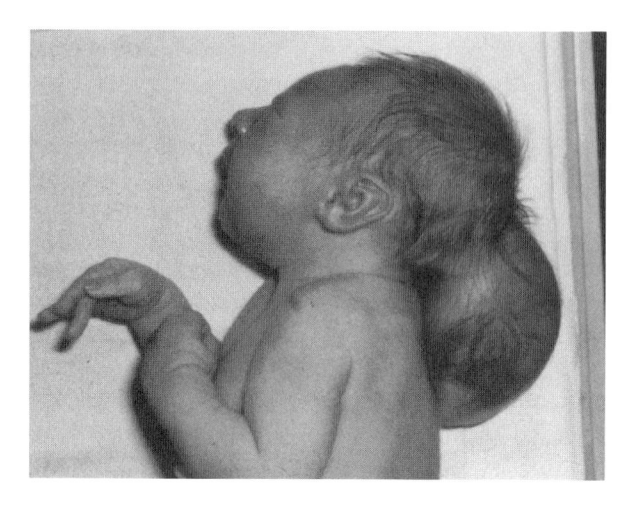

FIG. 15. A newborn infant with a large occipital encephalocele. The encephalocele is covered with atrophic skin and hairs. It contains both CSF and dysgenetic brain tissue. Large encephaloceles such as this one frequently require that the infant be intubated in the lateral position to prevent direct pressure on the sac and its contents.

thetic considerations. An encephalocele is most frequently found in the occipital/suboccipital area or nasally (Fig. 15). Anencephaly represents a defect in anterior closure of the neural groove.

Exposed CNS tissue places the patient at extreme risk of infection, which is the single most common cause of death of myelodysplastic patients (142) (Fig. 16). Patients <1 year old have a greater risk of infection than those >1 year. Patients with myelomeningocele and meningitis have the higher infection rate among those with other etiologies (143). Studies have demonstrated that the incidence of ventriculitis is directly proportional to the speed with which the myelomeningocele is surgically repaired. Ventriculitis occurs in <7% if surgical repair is performed within 48 hours of birth and in 37% of those whose repair is done >48 hours after birth (144). A

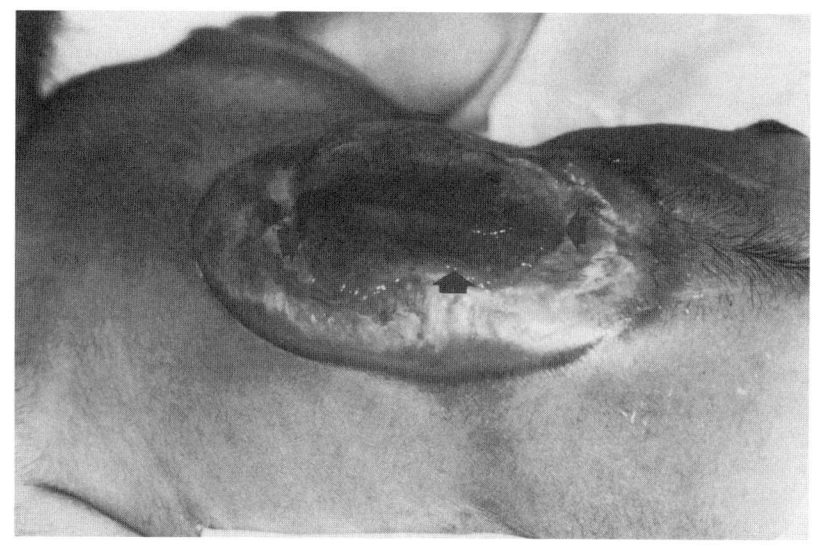

FIG. 16. Myelomeningocele. The central darker unepithelial region represents the neuroplaque (unprotected neural tissue) *(black arrows)*.

further reason to avoid delay in closure is the likelihood of progressive neural damage with eventual decrease in the motor function. For these reasons, myelodysplasia is regarded as a surgical emergency, and most neonates present for closure in the first 24 hours of life.

Anesthetic Considerations

The following are anesthetic considerations for patients with myelodysplasia:

- Coexisting disease. Additional pathology may accompany myelodysplasia (Arnold-Chiari malformation, hydrocephalus).
- Age-related pathophysiology.
- Airway management. Encephaloceles may present particular difficulty in control of the airway.
- Positioning. Protection of the neuroplaque.
- Volume status. High third-space losses from the skin defect.
- Potential for hypothermia. Exposure of large body surface area and loss of third-space fluid.

Preinduction

Infants presenting for repair of myelomeningoceles rarely exhibit increased ICP. Most myelodysplastic patients have an associated Arnold-Chiari malformation (type II) and may have an associated hydrocephalus, which will not always require ventricular shunt placement. Preoperative assessment will show varied neurologic deficits. Seventy-five percent of these deficits are in the lumbosacral region. Lesions above T4 usually result in total paraplegia, and lesions below S1 allow ambulation. The legs and bladder function are severely affected by lesions between L4 and S1 (143,144). Volume status should be assessed in light of the large potential third-space losses from the exposed myelomeningocele.

Monitoring

Routine monitoring is included. Blood loss can be insidious, especially if the sac is large and significant undermining of skin, relaxing incisions, or grafting is required for closure. Blood transfusion may become necessary. Patients with encephaloceles who must undergo craniotomy for repair should have an arterial line placed for blood pressure and hemoglobin measurement. Central venous line may become indicated for nasal encephalocele, which are commonly repaired in a semisitting position.

Induction and Intubation

Patients with lumbosacral or thoracic myelomeningoceles may be induced either in the left lateral position or alternatively supine with the sac protected with a cushioned ring. Most patients can be induced intravenously with thiopental, atropine, and a muscle relaxant before tracheal intubation. Awake laryngoscopy and tracheal intubation after giving intravenous atropine could be an alternative technique in the premature infant. Either a nondepolarizing muscle relaxant or succinylcholine may be used safely (145). Caution should be observed during induction of anesthesia for patients with nasal encephalocele, since airway obstruction is common and poor face-mask fit may be encountered.

Maintenance of Anesthesia

Positioning. After intubation, the patient should be turned to the prone position, avoiding injury to the exposed neural tissue. Chest and hip rolls are then placed to ensure that the abdomen hangs free to facilitate ventilation and reduce intra-abdominal pressure, which may potentially increase bleeding from the epidural plexus. Since most children with myelomeningoceles have an Arnold-Chiari malformation with cervical neurologic considerations, care should be taken to avoid excessive rotation of the neck. Extremities should lie in a relaxed position and be well padded.

Ventilation. Mechanical ventilation is used, but attention must be paid to the risk of barotrauma in the immature lung. Premature infants (especially those <32 weeks and <1500 g) are at increased risk of retinopathy of prematurity (146) and lung injury from prolonged exposure to high oxygen concentrations (147). If possible, F_IO_2 is adjusted in these patients to maintain a PaO_2 of 60 to 70 mm Hg and a saturation of 90% to 95%.

Anesthetic Agents. Anesthesia can be maintained with a variety of agents. Narcotics and ketamine should be avoided because they have been associated with a high incidence of postoperative apnea in neonates. For large repair, the administration of one dose of fentanyl (2 to 3 µg/kg) at the time of skin incision is most indicated. Problems with respiratory depression postoperatively are most frequent when repeated doses have been used. Neurosurgeons may require selective nerve stimulation to identify neural structures which eliminate the use of muscle relaxants.

Fluid Management. As previously noted, blood loss is usually not excessive and fluid management is directed toward replacement of third-space losses. If undermining of skin to allow closure of the wound is extensive and blood loss greater than the usual (>10% of circulating blood volume), adequate intravenous access for transfusion must be in place. Once again, discussion with the neurosurgeon preoperatively will avoid unpleasant intraoperative surprises often associated with important consequences.

Body Temperature. The large area of exposed tissue and the liberal use of surgical preparation solutions increase the risk of hypothermia in patients with myelodysplasia. Active measures to prevent this complication are essential. Care must be taken to prevent

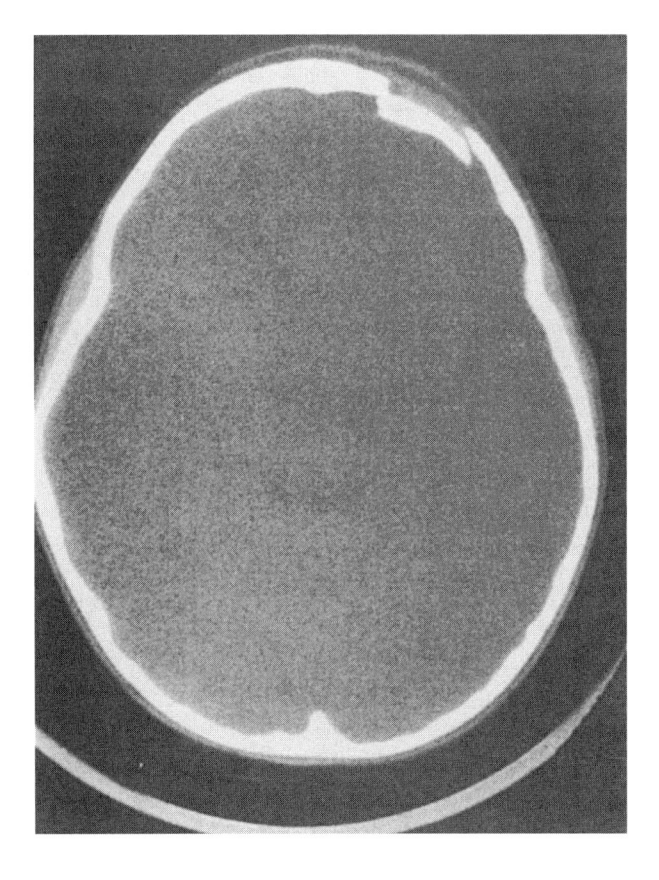

FIG. 17. Axial CT scan of a frontal depressed skull fracture in a 3-year-old boy.

drying or thermal injury to the exposed neural tissue by the use of radiant heat lamps.

Emergence and Postoperative Management

Anesthetic considerations for emergence include (a) elimination of anesthetic agents, (b) reversal of neuromuscular blockade, and (c) assessment of airway patency.

Neonates at risk for apnea after anesthesia, patients with severe central neurologic deficits or those undergoing craniotomy for encephalocele repair should have their tracheas extubated fully awake after elimination of the anesthetic agents and adequate reversal of muscle relaxants. Patients with repair of nasal encephaloceles may have residual obstruction or blood in the oropharynx. It may be necessary to delay extubation in these cases.

Head Injury

Head trauma is a major cause of morbidity and mortality in the pediatric population. Skull fractures are found in >25% of all children who present at hospitals with head injuries (148) and in more than 50% of fatal cases of head trauma in childhood (149) (Fig. 17). Skull fracture classification is provided in Table 3. The incidence of post-traumatic intracranial hematomas varies considerably in children; however, a minority of children with head injuries will become candidates for surgical decompression and treatment (150). Despite this low incidence, failure to recognize the presence of a hematoma may transform an otherwise mild injury into a fatal or permanently disabling one. This medical complication must be recognized early and treated aggressively. Neuroanesthesiologists should remain very attentive to children admitted with head trauma who can talk, since they can progress quickly to sudden death (151,152).

Head injury encompasses many different forms of trauma to the skull and brain; therefore, the pathophysiologic events following head injury are subdivided into intracranial hematomas (epidural, subdural, intracerebral, and brain contusion), brain edema, and systemic effects of head injury. There is a significant difference between adults and children with respect to the pattern of injury sustained. Adults suffer more hematomas than children, whereas the presence of diffuse cerebral edema occurs more often in the pediatric population (153). Children with diffuse brain swelling have a threefold higher mortality rate than those without it (154). Because of the weight and size of the head relative to the rest of the body in infants and small children, cervical spine injury is often associated with head injury in the pediatric population.

Epidural Hematoma

Most frequently caused by arterial bleeding from a middle meningeal artery torn in the course of a deceleration injury, children do not necessarily show an overlying skull fracture. Epidural hematomas make up 25% of all intracranial hematomas and constitute one of the true neurosurgical emergencies (Fig. 18). The clinical presentation in the adult population is described as a period of lucid interval between an initial loss of consciousness and later neurologic deterioration. In children, the initial alteration in the state of consciousness reported in adults is often not seen. When a child is lucid and old enough to complain verbally, increasing

TABLE 3. *Classification of skull fractures in children*

I.	Linear
II.	Depressed
III.	Open (linear or depressed)[a]
IV.	Basal skull fracture[b]

[a]Open skull fractures generally mandate an anesthetic and neurosurgery for irrigation and debridement of involved tissues.

[b]One should not intubate with a nasal tube a patient suspected of having a basal skull fracture involving the anterior cranial fossa floor.

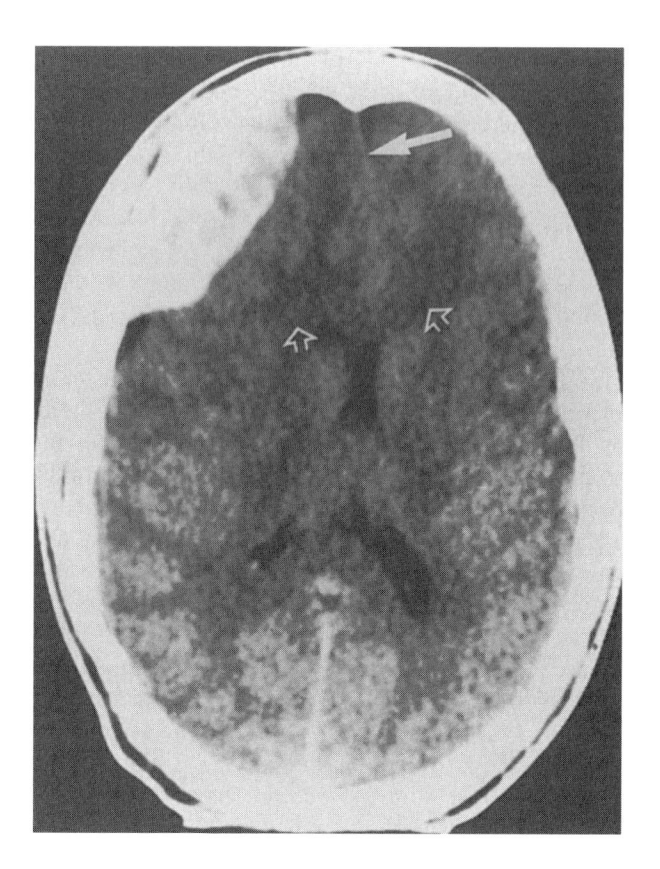

FIG. 18. Axial CT scan of an acute epidural hematoma in 2-year-old boy causing mass effect and shift of brain from right to left *(white arrow)*. The ventricles are pushed across the midline. Intracerebral edema is indicated *(open white arrows)*. Acute epidural hematomas are life-threatening emergencies that demand the swift activation of a skilled team of neuroanesthesiologists and neurosurgeons.

headache will continue until the patient becomes confused or lethargic. However, the rapid development of hemiparesis, posturing, and pupillary dilatation is also typical and may confuse the diagnosis. The pathologic process is explained by a rapid expansion of the hematoma leading to a herniation of the temporal lobe downward through the tentoria incisura impinging on the oculomotor nerve, which is the pupilloconstrictor innervation. The earliest sign will be anisocoria. This herniation eventually leads to a syndrome of rostrocaudal deterioration, which is classically associated with a Cushing triad of bradycardia, slowed and irregular breathing, and widened pulse pressure (155). The relation between the degree of brain shift and the level of consciousness has been confirmed; however, the role of uncal herniation in the syndrome has been questioned (156).

Subdural Hematoma

The subdural hematoma is associated with cortical damage due to parenchymal contusion and blood vessel laceration. The mass effect of the contused and edematous brain may prompt surgical removal of the hematoma if the brain region involved is not functionally important. Recent studies using positron emission tomography have demonstrated that in patients with brain contusion the cerebral metabolism and blood flow were reduced by 50% (157). Severe edema and ICP often lead to persistent neurologic deficits in the postoperative period.

Intracerebral Hematoma

Intracerebral hematoma is a rare type of intracranial hematoma, but carries a poor prognosis. Intraparenchymal hematoma does not require surgery for fear of damaging viable brain tissue.

Anesthetic Considerations

The anesthesiologist usually sees affected children during the early stages of trauma care. There are several anesthetic considerations.

- Resuscitation and stabilization. Airway, breathing, and circulation are the essential components of the initial clinical assessment. The traumatized patient may often have a variety of physiologic disturbances such as acid-base and electrolyte imbalance. Glucose homeostasis and body temperature control may be disturbed.
- Neurologic status. The use of the Glascow Coma Scale provides baseline from which subsequent changes can be evaluated. Symptomatology leading to the presence or not of raised ICP must be evaluated.
- Associated injuries. Pediatric trauma is often associated with high-velocity energy transfer, which leads to associated injuries to the neck, chest, and abdominal organs.
- Full stomach. Evidence of vomiting may suggest pulmonary aspiration and respiratory complications.
- Age-related pathophysiology.

Monitoring

Aside from routine monitoring, an arterial catheter and central venous line placement are indicated. A urinary bladder catheter should be inserted unless contraindicated by an associated post-traumatic bladder neck injury. Central body temperature should be monitored at all times.

Preinduction

Computed tomography scanning remains the procedure of choice in the evaluation of the head injury patient during the first 72 hours. Although the management of an elevated ICP is paramount to a safe anesthetic, adequate airway, ventilation, hemodynamic resuscitation and stabilization must be achieved initially. The maintenance of an adequate CPP and brain tissue oxygenation is the key to brain cell resuscitation and recruitment from the penumbra area.

Induction and Intubation

Providing a patent airway is an essential part of the management of patients with head injury. Although the airway may not be compromised by the injury for patients with affected level of consciousness, it is appropriate to proceed with tracheal intubation to protect the lungs against aspiration of stomach contents or secretions and to provide ventilatory support as part of the management of increased ICP. The association of head injury and neck injury in infants and children is significantly important. Therefore, it is mandatory that induction and ventilation be accomplished with minimal manipulation. Stabilization of the head by an assistant with axial traction is indicated. Until proven otherwise, a cervical spine fracture is always considered in the management of a patient with head injury and should be treated accordingly. Therefore, the use of Sellick maneuver (cricoid pressure) is an absolute contraindication.

Patients not already on ventilatory support but undergoing evacuation of intracranial hematoma should be hemodynamically stable before induction of anesthesia. After a difficult airway has been ruled out and hemodynamic stability obtained, induction of anesthesia should proceed in a rapid-sequence fashion with atropine, thiopental, lidocaine, and either succinylcholine or a nondepolarizing muscle relaxant such as vecuronium. For these patients, ketamine remains contraindicated. In some patients, with extreme intracerebral conditions, the usual clinical presentation includes a Cushing triad, coma, and hemodynamic instability. Tracheal intubation, without evidence of difficult laryngoscopy, should be performed without the assistance of background anesthetic agents other than a muscle relaxant drug such as pancuronium for its sympathetic stimulation. Institution of resuscitation and hemodynamic stabilization associated with manual hyperventilation should be immediately provided. If a surgical evacuation is attempted, the administration of anesthesia should be accomplished progressively according to the patient's needs and hemodynamic responses.

Induction of anesthesia for patients with a suspected difficult airway may require a two-person technique. One must remember that until help becomes available, application of a face mask with 100% oxygen and hyperventilation remains the basis of airway management. Depending on the age of the patient and his or her state of consciousness, the use of volatile anesthetic with assisted ventilation or the use of neuroleptanesthesia with topicalization of the larynx is also recommended. This is not the time to attempt a nonfamiliar technique, with which one is not comfortable or skillful.

Maintenance

The considerations for maintenance of anesthesia are similar to those previously described in **Supratentorial Craniotomy**. Evacuation of intracranial hematoma usually involves a craniotomy for exploration without opening of the dura mater. However, it must be noted that large hematomas may, on evacuation, cause a sudden release of ICP with consequent upward movement of the brain stem through the tentoria incisura. The consequences may be transient hemodynamic instability associated with cardiac arrhythmias.

Emergence and Postoperative Management

Patients with severe head injury will remain intubated for ventilatory support and control of the elevated ICP due to cerebral edema. Transfer to an intensive care unit is indicated for continued care.

Spinal Cord Surgery

The most common diseases that require surgery on the spinal cord are herniated disks, spondylosis, syringomyelia, primary or metastatic tumors, hematomas or abscesses, and trauma. In all cases, compression of the spinal cord may produce ischemia (158), interstitial edema, and venous congestion (159) and interfere with nerve transmission (160). Maintaining spinal cord perfusion pressure and reducing cord compression are the crucial considerations in our clinical management. Despite apparently optimal surgical and anesthetic management devastating neurologic complications still occur during spinal surgery. Intraoperative monitoring of spinal cord function is an essential part of a safe anesthetic. Methods for monitoring the integrity of spinal cord function intraoperatively include (a) the wake-up test, (b) somatosensory evoked potentials, and (c) motor evoked potentials.

The wake-up test remains the traditional method for assessing spinal cord well-being during corrective procedures on the spinal column. Its main advantage is that it assesses anterior spinal cord (i.e., motor) function, but its limitations are that it does so only at one time. The use of somatosensory evoked potential monitors in children, though still not routine, is gaining popularity. It involves the generation of electrical potentials within the neuraxis by stimulation of peripheral nerves such as the median nerve at the wrist or the posterior tibial nerve at the ankle (161). If transmission is intact, a signal is recorded from the scalp or at various sites along the neural pathway. The electrical signals are thought to arise from axonal action potentials and graded postsynaptic potentials during propagation of the impulse from the periphery to the brain. The technique has limitations in that it applies only to the sensory nervous system. The appeal of motor evoked potentials in

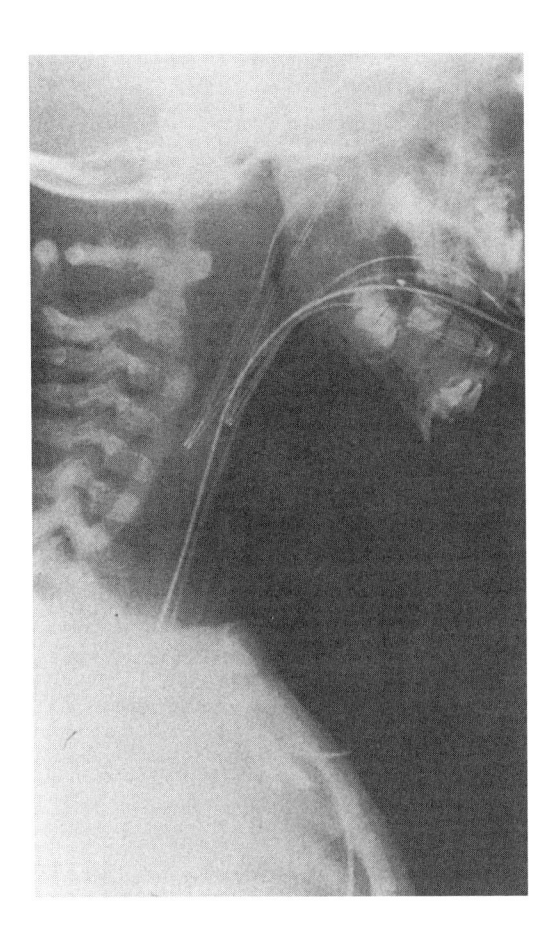

FIG. 19. Lateral cervical radiograph demonstrating the effect of high-velocity cervical spine fracture in a child. There is a total subluxation of the odontoid process and the C1 to C2 junction. All cervical spine precautions must be undertaken before, during, and after intubating patients with these injuries. (From Bissonnette, ref. 162, with permission).

which the motor cortex is stimulated by a transcranial electric current or a pulsed magnetic field generated by a coil placed over the scalp has now increased in anesthesia (161). The anesthetic management should be based on the assurance of proper spinal perfusion pressure and an anesthetic technique allowing neurologic function monitoring.

Cervical Spinal Cord Injury

Because isolated cervical spine injury is rare in the pediatric population compared with their adult counterpart, all children with a severe head injury should be treated as candidates for cervical spine injury until proven otherwise. Their management requires strategies similar to those provided for adults. The mechanism of injury of high cervical cord is associated with high-velocity injuries to the cranium in children (Fig. 19). The classic presentation of cord injury or disruption may be the patient discovered without respiratory efforts and usually in cardiac arrest or profound hypotension, leading subsequently to death from hypoxic/ischemic encephalopathy with or without a serious traumatic brain injury. In this study, all patients with absence of vital signs had confirmation on lateral view x-ray of the neck of the presence of high cervical cord luxation. The physician not aware of this clinical scenario might think that this situation is related only to blood loss due to intraabdominal, pelvic, or thoracic injury or even devastating cerebral injury with loss of brainstem function but not the cervical spine.

The state-of-the-art management of conscious pediatric patients with unstable spinal cord fractures in the operating room now mandates the use of a tracheal intubation performed during constant sedation or neuroleptic anesthesia, ensuring the patient's cooperation during positioning while under continuous somatosensory evoked potential monitoring (if available). The somatosensory evoked potential is recorded immediately before positioning to obtain a baseline recording. After the patient is positioned prone and demonstrates ability to move his or her extremities on command and after the evoked potentials are constant with the prepositioning recording, the patient can be safely anesthetized.

Stabilization of the cervical spine can now be safely performed in the pediatric age group at surgery using bone graft, wires, or titanium plating systems. Intraoperative evoked potentials should be used throughout the procedure until the patient is turned supine and extubated and can follow commands.

ACKNOWLEDGMENTS

The author wants to thank Drs. J.G. Villemure, McGill University, Montreal, Canada, and N. de Tribolet, Lausanne University, Lausanne, Switzerland, for providing several of the figures.

REFERENCES

1. Kleinman S, Bissonnette B: Management of successful pediatric neuroanesthesia. In: Bissonnette B (ed). *Cerebral protection, resuscitation and monitoring: a look into the future of neuroanesthesia.* Philadelphia: WB Saunders, 1992:537–563.
2. Bickler P: Energetics of cerebral metabolism and ion transport. In: Bissonnette B (ed). *Cerebral protection, resuscitation and monitoring: a look into the future of neuroanesthesia.* Philadelphia: WB Saunders, 1992: 563–575.
3. Sokoloff L: Circulation and energy metabolism of the brain. In: Siegel G, Agranoff B, Albers R, Molinoff P (eds). *Basic neurochemistry: molecular, cellular and medical aspects.* New York: Raven Press, 1989: 565–591.
4. Settergren G, Lindblad BS, Persson B: Cerebral blood flow and exchange of oxygen, glucose ketone bodies, lactate, pyruvate and amino acids in anesthetized children. *Acta Paediatr Scand* 1980;69:457–465.
5. Mehta S, Kalsi HK, Nain CK, Menkes JH: Energy metabolism of brain in human protein-calorie malnutrition. *Pediatr Res* 1977;11:290–293.
6. Cross KW, Dear PR, Hathorn MK, et al: An estimation of intracranial blood flow in the new-born infant. *J Physiol (Lond)* 1979;289:329–345.
7. Younkin DP, Reivich M, Jaggi J, et al: Noninvasive method of estimating human newborn regional cerebral blood flow. *J Cereb Blood Flow Metab* 1982;2: 415–420.
8. Rosomoff H, Holaday D: Cerebral blood flow and cerebral oxygen consumption during hypothermia. *Am J Physiol* 1954;179: 85–97.
9. Hernandez MJ, Brennan RW, Bowman GS: Autoregulation of cerebral blood flow in the newborn dog. *Brain Res* 1980;184:199–202.
10. Purves MJ, James IM: Observations on the control of cerebral blood flow in the sheep fetus and newborn lamb. *Circ Res* 1969;25:651–667.
11. Millar C, Bissonnette B, Humphreys RP: Cerebral arteriovenous malformations in children. *Can J Anaesth* 1994;41:321–331.
12. McLeod ME, Creighton RE, Humphreys RP: Anaesthetic management of arteriovenous malformations of the vein of Galen. *Can Anaesth Soc J* 1982;29:307–312.
13. Tweed A, Cote J, Lou H, et al: Impairment of cerebral blood flow autoregulation in the newborn lamb by hypoxia. *Pediatr Res* 1986;20:516–519.
14. Hennes HJ, Jantzen JP: Effects of fenoldopam on intracranial pressure and hemodynamic variables at normal and elevated intracranial pressure in anesthetized pigs. *J Neurosurg Anesthesiol* 1994;6:175–181.
15. Van Aken H: Influence of anesthesia on autoregulation of the cerebral blood flow. *Acta Anaesthesiol Belg* 1976;27:11–19.
16. Gregory G, Ong B, Tweed A: Hyperventilation restores autoregulation in the cerebral circulation in the neonate. *Anesthesiology* 1983;59:427.
17. Lassen NA: Control of cerebral circulation in health and disease. *Circ Res* 1974;34:749–760.
18. Lou HC, Lassen NA, Friis-Hansen B: Impaired autoregulation of cerebral blood flow in the distressed newborn infant. *J Pediatr* 1979;94:118–121.
19. Pilato MA, Bissonnette B, Lerman J: Transcranial Doppler: response of cerebral blood-flow velocity to carbon dioxide in anaesthetized children. *Can J Anaesth* 1991;38:37–42.
20. Cutler RW, Page L, Galicich J, Watters GV: Formation and absorption of cerebrospinal fluid in man. *Brain* 1968;91:707–720.
21. Marcus ML, Heistad DD, Ehrhardt JC, Abboud FM: Regulation of total and regional spinal cord blood flow. *Circ Res* 1977;41:128–134.
22. Hickey R, Albin MS, Bunegin L, Gelineau J: Autoregulation of spinal cord blood flow: is the cord a microcosm of the brain? *Stroke* 1986;17:1183–1189.
23. Goto T, Crosby G: Anesthesia and the spinal cord. In: Bissonnette B (ed). *Cerebral protection, resuscitation and monitoring: a look into the future of neuroanesthesia.* Philadelphia: WB Saunders, 1992:493–521.
24. Rubinstein A, Arbit E: Spinal cord blood flow in the rat under normal physiological conditions. *Neurosurgery* 1990;27:882–886.
25. Guha A, Tator CH, Rochon J: Spinal cord blood flow and systemic blood pressure after experimental spinal cord injury in rats. *Stroke* 1989;20:372–377.

26. Griffiths IR: Spinal cord blood flow in dogs: The effect of blood pressure. *J Neurol Neurosurg Psychiatry* 1973;36:914–920.
27. Griffiths IR: Spinal cord blood flow in dogs. 2. The effect of the blood gases. *J Neurol Neurosurg Psychiatry* 1973;36:42–49.
28. Pelligrino DA, Miletich DJ, Hoffman WE, Albrecht RF: Nitrous oxide markedly increases cerebral cortical metabolic rate and blood flow in the goat. *Anesthesiology* 1984;60:405–412.
29. Leon JE, Bissonnette B: Transcranial Doppler sonography: nitrous oxide and cerebral blood flow velocity in children [published erratum appears in *Can J Anaesth* 1992;39:409]. *Can J Anaesth* 1991;38:974–979.
30. Hoffman WE, Miletich DJ, Albrecht RF: The effects of midazolam on cerebral blood flow and oxygen consumption and its interaction with nitrous oxide. *Anesth Analg* 1986;65:729–733.
31. Phirman JR, Shapiro HM: Modification of nitrous oxide-induced intracranial hypertension by prior induction of anesthesia. *Anesthesiology* 1977;46:150–151.
32. Sakabe T, Kuramoto T, Kumagae S, Takeshita H: Cerebral responses to the addition of nitrous oxide to halothane in man. *Br J Anaesth* 1976;48:957–962.
33. Todd MM, Drummond JC: A comparison of the cerebrovascular and metabolic effects of halothane and isoflurane in the cat. *Anesthesiology* 1984;60:276–282.
34. Manohar M, Goetz TE: Cerebral, renal, adrenal, intestinal, and pancreatic circulation in conscious ponies and during 1.0, 1.5, and 2.0 minimal alveolar concentrations of halothane-O_2 anesthesia. *Am J Vet Res* 1985;46:2492–2497.
35. Lazzell V, Bissonnette B, Lerman J: Effect of halothane on the cerebral blood flow in infants and children. A hysteresis phenomenon. *Anesthesiology* 1989;71:A327.
36. Lazzell V, Bissonnette B: Transcranial Doppler: Effect of halothane on cerebral hemodynamics in children. *Anesthesiology* 1989;71:A332.
37. Madsen JB, Cold GE, Hansen ES, Bardrum B: Cerebral blood flow, cerebral metabolic rate of oxygen and relative CO_2-reactivity during craniotomy for supratentorial cerebral tumours in halothane anaesthesia. A dose-response study. *Acta Anaesthesiol Scand* 1987;31:454–457.
38. Wollman H, Alexander S, Cohen P: Cerebral circulation of man during halothane anesthesia: effects of hypocarbia and of d-tubocurarine. *Anesthesiology* 1964;25:180–188.
39. Christensen MS, Hoedt-Rasmussen K, Lassen NA: Cerebral vasodilatation by halothane anaesthesia in man and its potentiation by hypotension and hypercapnia. *Br J Anaesth* 1967;39:927–934.
40. Adams RW, Gronert GA, Sundt TM Jr, Michenfelder JD: Halothane, hypocapnia, and cerebrospinal fluid pressure in neurosurgery. *Anesthesiology* 1972;37:510–517.
41. Leon JE, Bissonnette B: Cerebrovascular responses to carbon dioxide in children anaesthetized with halothane and isoflurane. *Can J Anaesth* 1991;38:817–825.
42. Newberg LA, Michenfelder JD: Cerebral protection by isoflurane during hypoxemia or ischemia. *Anesthesiology* 1983;59:29–35.
43. Leon J, Bissonnette B: Does cerebrovascular hysteresis exist under isoflurane anesthesia. *Can J Anaesth* 1991;72:S160.
44. Bissonnette B, Leon JE: Cerebrovascular stability during isoflurane anaesthesia in children. *Can J Anaesth* 1992;39:128–134.
45. Archer DP, Labrecque P, Tyler JL, et al: Cerebral blood volume is increased in dogs during administration of nitrous oxide or isoflurane. *Anesthesiology* 1987;67:642–628.
46. Scheller MS, Todd MM, Drummond JC, Zornow MH: The intracranial pressure effects of isoflurane and halothane administered following cryogenic brain injury in rabbits. *Anesthesiology* 1987;67:507–512.
47. Artru AA, Nugent M, Michenfelder JD: Enflurane causes a prolonged and reversible increase in the rate of CSF production in the dog. *Anesthesiology* 1982;57:255–260.
48. Scheller MS, Tateishi A, Drummond JC, Zornow MH: The effects of sevoflurane on cerebral blood flow, cerebral metabolic rate for oxygen, intracranial pressure, and the electroencephalogram are similar to those of isoflurane in the rabbit. *Anesthesiology* 1988;68:548–551.
49. Lu G, Gibson J, Frost E: Cerebral vasodilating effect of sevoflurane vs. isoflurane. *Anesthesiology* 1990;73:A625.
50. Werner C, Kochs E, Hoffman W: The effects of sevoflurane on neurological outcome from incomplete ischemia in rats. *J Neurosurg Anesthesiol* 1991;3:237.
51. Lutz LJ, Milde JH, Milde LN: The cerebral functional, metabolic, and hemodynamic effects of desflurane in dogs. *Anesthesiology* 1990;73:125–131.
52. Muzzi DA, Losasso TJ, Dietz NM, et al: The effect of desflurane and isoflurane on cerebrospinal fluid pressure in humans with supratentorial mass lesions. *Anesthesiology* 1992;76:720–724.
53. Pierce E, Lambertson C, Deutsch S: Cerebral circulation and metabolism during thiopental anesthesia and hyperventilation in man. *J Clin Invest* 1962;41:1664–1669.
54. Michenfelder JD: The interdependency of cerebral functional and metabolic effects following massive doses of thiopental in the dog. *Anesthesiology* 1974;41:231–236.
55. Shapiro HM, Galindo A, Wyte SR, Harris AB: Rapid intraoperative reduction of intracranial pressure with thiopentone. *Br J Anaesth* 1973;45:1057–1062.
56. Rockoff MA, Goudsouzian NG: Seizures induced by methohexital. *Anesthesiology* 1981;54:333–335.
57. Renou AM, Vernhiet J, Macrez P, et al: Cerebral blood flow and metabolism during etomidate anaesthesia in man. *Br J Anaesth* 1978;50:1047–1051.
58. Milde LN, Milde JH, Michenfelder JD: Cerebral functional, metabolic, and hemodynamic effects of etomidate in dogs. *Anesthesiology* 1985;63:371–377.
59. Fragen RJ, Shanks CA, Molteni A, Avram MJ: Effects of etomidate on hormonal responses to surgical stress. *Anesthesiology* 1984;61:652–656.
60. Laughlin TP, Newberg LA: Prolonged myoclonus after etomidate anesthesia. *Anesth Analg* 1985;64:80–82.
61. Michenfelder JD, Theye RA: Effects of fentanyl, droperidol, and innovar on canine cerebral metabolism and blood flow. *Br J Anaesth* 1971;43:630–636.
62. Van Hemelrijck J, Fitch W, Mattheussen M, et al: Ef-

fect of propofol on cerebral circulation and autoregulation in the baboon. *Anesth Analg* 1990;71:49–54.
63. Pinaud M, Lelausque JN, Chetanneau A, et al: Effects of propofol on cerebral hemodynamics and metabolism in patients with brain trauma. *Anesthesiology* 1990;73:404–409.
64. Fleischer JE, Milde JH, Moyer TP, Michenfelder JD: Cerebral effects of high-dose midazolam and subsequent reversal with Ro 15-1788 in dogs. *Anesthesiology* 1988;68:234–242.
65. Nugent M, Artru AA, Michenfelder JD: Cerebral metabolic, vascular and protective effects of midazolam maleate: comparison to diazepam. *Anesthesiology* 1982;56:172–176.
66. Jobes DR, Kennell EM, Bush GL, et al: Cerebral blood flow and metabolism during morphine: nitrous oxide anesthesia in man. *Anesthesiology* 1977;47:16–18.
67. Yaster M, Koehler RC, Traystman RJ: Effects of fentanyl on peripheral and cerebral hemodynamics in neonatal lambs. *Anesthesiology* 1987;66:524–530.
68. Takeshita H, Okuda Y, Sari A: The effects of ketamine on cerebral circulation and metabolism in man. *Anesthesiology* 1972;36:69–75.
69. Shapiro H, Wyte S, Harris A: Ketamine anaesthesia in patients with intracranial pathology. *Br J Anaesth* 1972;44:1200–1204.
70. Cottrell JE, Hartung J, Giffin JP, Shwiry B: Intracranial and hemodynamic changes after succinylcholine administration in cats. *Anesth Analg* 1983;62:1006–1009.
71. Millar C, Bissonnette B: Awake intubation increases intracranial pressure without affecting cerebral blood flow velocity in infants. *Can J Anaesth* 1994;41:281–287.
72. Minton MD, Grosslight K, Stirt JA, Bedford RF: Increases in intracranial pressure from succinylcholine: prevention by prior nondepolarizing blockade. *Anesthesiology* 1986;65:165–169.
73. Lanier WL, Milde JH, Michenfelder JD: The cerebral effects of pancuronium and atracurium in halothane-anesthetized dogs. *Anesthesiology* 1985;63:589–597.
74. Vesely R, Hoffman WE, Gil KS, et al: The cerebrovascular effects of curare and histamine in the rat. *Anesthesiology* 1987;66:519–523.
75. Rosa G, Sanfilippo M, Vilardi V, et al: Effects of vecuronium bromide on intracranial pressure and cerebral perfusion pressure. A preliminary report. *Br J Anaesth* 1986;58:437–440.
76. Welch K: The intracranial pressure in infants. *J Neurosurg* 1980;52:693–699.
77. Raju TN, Vidyasagar D, Papazafiratou C: Intracranial pressure monitoring in the neonatal ICU. *Crit Care Med* 1980;8:575–581.
78. Bekemeyer WB, Pinstein ML: Neurogenic pulmonary edema: new concepts of an old disorder. (Review). *South Med J* 1989;82:380–383.
79. Milley JR, Nugent SK, Rogers MC: Neurogenic pulmonary edema in childhood. *J Pediatr* 1979;94:706–709.
80. Colice GL: Neurogenic pulmonary edema. *Clin Chest Med* 1985;6:473–489.
81. Malik AB: Mechanisms of neurogenic pulmonary edema. *Circ Res* 1985;57:1–18.
82. Carlson RW, Schaeffer RC Jr, Michaels SG, Weil MH: Pulmonary edema following intracranial hemorrhage. *Chest* 1979;75:731–734.
83. Ciongoli AK, Poser CM: Pulmonary edema secondary to subarachnoid hemorrhage. *Neurology* 1972;22:867–870.
84. Baigelman W, O'Brien JC: Pulmonary effects of head trauma (Review). *Neurosurgery* 1981;9:729–740.
85. Terrence CF, Rao GR, Perper JA: Neurogenic pulmonary edema in unexpected, unexplained death of epileptic patients. *Ann Neurol* 1981;9:458–464.
86. Hodges FI: Pathology of the skull. In: Tavaras J (ed). *Radiology diagnosis—imaging—intervention: Neuroradiology and radiology of the head and neck.* Philadelphia: JB Lippincott, 1989:123.
87. Grant E, Richardson J: Infant and neonatal neurosonography technique and normal anatomy, radiology diagnosis—imaging—intervention. In: Tavaras J (ed). *Neuroradiology and radiology of the head and neck.* Philadelphia: JB Lippincott, 1989:453.
88. Wilder-Smith OH, Ravussin P, Bissonnette B: [Neuromonitoring in anesthesia]. [French]. *Ann Fr Anesth Reanim* 1995;14:95–102.
89. Garner L, Stirt JA, Finholt DA: Heart block after intravenous lidocaine in an infant. *Can Anaesth Soc J* 1985;32:425–428.
90. Salem MR: Cricoid pressure for preventing gastric insufflation in infants and children. (Letter; comment). *Anesthesiology* 1994;80:1182–1183.
91. Moynihan RJ, Brock-Utne JG, Archer JH, et al: The effect of cricoid pressure on preventing gastric insufflation in infants and children. *Anesthesiology* 1993;78:652–656.
92. Rosenberg H, Gronert GA: Intractable cardiac arrest in children given succinylcholine. (Letter). *Anesthesiology* 1992;77:1054.
93. Lerman J, Berdock SE, Bissonnette B, et al: Succinylcholine warning. (Letter). *Can J Anaesth* 1994;41:165.
94. Lazzell VA, Carr AS, Lerman J, et al: The incidence of masseter muscle rigidity after succinylcholine in infants and children [see comments]. *Can J Anaesth* 1994;41:475–479.
95. Frankville DD, Drummond JC: Hyperkalemia after succinylcholine administration in a patient with closed head injury without paresis. *Anesthesiology* 1987;67:264–266.
96. Tong TK: Succinylcholine-induced hyperkalemia in near-drowning. (Letter). *Anesthesiology* 1987;66:720.
97. Iwatsuki N, Kuroda N, Amaha K, Iwatsuki K: Succinylcholine-induced hyperkalemia in patients with ruptured cerebral aneurysms. *Anesthesiology* 1980;53:64–67.
98. John DA, Tobey RE, Homer LD, Rice CL: Onset of succinylcholine-induced hyperkalemia following denervation. *Anesthesiology* 1976;45:294–299.
99. Sloan MH, Lerman J, Bissonnette B: Pharmacodynamics of high-dose vecuronium in children during balanced anesthesia. *Anesthesiology* 1991;74:656–659.
100. Bissonnette B: Fluid therapy. In:Hughes DG, Mather SJ, Wolf A. London (eds). *Handbook of neonatal anaesthesia.* WB Saunders, 1995:110–132.
101. Korosue K, Heros RC, Ogilvy CS, et al: Comparison of crystalloids and colloids for hemodilution in a model of focal cerebral ischemia. *J Neurosurg* 1990;73:576–584.
102. Ravussin P, Archer DP, Meyer E, et al: The effects of rapid infusions of saline and mannitol on cerebral blood volume and intracranial pressure in dogs. *Can Anaesth Soc J* 1985;32:506–515.
103. Albin MS, Bunegin L, Dujovny M, et al: Brain retrac-

tion pressure during intracranial procedures. *Surg Forum* 1975;26:499–500.
104. Araki T, Kato H, Kogure K: Neuronal damage and calcium accumulation following repeated brief cerebral ischemia in the gerbil. *Brain Res* 1990;528:114–122.
105. Hartley E, Bissonnette B, St. Louis P, et al: Scalp infiltration with bupivacaine in paediatric brain surgery. *Can J Anaesth* 1991;73:29–32.
106. St. Louis P, Das I, Rybczynski J, et al: Determination of bupivacaine in plasma by high-performance liquid chromatography. Levels after scalp infiltration in children. *Clin Biochem* 1991;24:463–467.
107. Lanier WL, Stangland KJ, Scheithauer BW, et al: The effects of dextrose infusion and head position on neurologic outcome after complete cerebral ischemia in primates: examination of a model. *Anesthesiology* 1987;66:39–48.
108. Pulsinelli WA, Levy DE, Sigsbee B, et al: Increased damage after ischemic stroke in patients with hyperglycemia with or without established diabetes mellitus. *Am J Med* 1983;74:540–544.
109. Marshall LF, Smith RW, Rauscher LA, Shapiro HM: Mannitol dose requirements in brain-injured patients. *J Neurosurg* 1978;48:169–172.
110. Ravussin P, Abou-Madi M, Archer D, et al: Changes in CSF pressure after mannitol in patients with and without elevated CSF pressure [published erratum appears in *J Neurosurg* 1989;70(4):662]. *J Neurosurg* 1988;69:869–876.
111. Cote CJ, Greenhow DE, Marshall BE: The hypotensive response to rapid intravenous administration of hypertonic solutions in man and in the rabbit. *Anesthesiology* 1979;50:30–35.
112. Schettini A, Stahurski B, Young HF: Osmotic and osmotic-loop diuresis in brain surgery. Effects on plasma and CSF electrolytes and ion excretion. *J Neurosurg* 1982;56:679–684.
113. Cottrell JE, Robustelli A, Post K, Turndorf H: Furosemide- and mannitol-induced changes in intracranial pressure and serum osmolality and electrolytes. *Anesthesiology* 1977;47:28–30.
114. Bissonnette B, Davis P: Thermal regulation—physiology and perioperative management in infants and children. In: Motoyama E, Davis P (eds). *Smith's anesthesia for infants and children*. St. Louis: Mosby-Year Book, 1996:5.1–5.20.
115. Bissonnette B, Sessler DI, LaFlamme P: Passive and active inspired gas humidification in infants and children. *Anesthesiology* 1989;71:350–354.
116. Bissonnette B, Sessler DI: Passive or active inspired gas humidification increases thermal steady-state temperatures in anesthetized infants. *Anesth Analg* 1989;69:783–787.
117. Bissonnette B: Temperature monitoring in pediatric anesthesia. In: Pullerits J, Holtzman R (eds). *Anesthesia equipment for infants and children*. Boston, Little, Brown, 1992:63–81.
118. Bissonnette B, Sessler DI, LaFlamme P: Intraoperative temperature monitoring sites in infants and children and the effect of inspired gas warming on esophageal temperature. *Anesth Analg* 1989;69:192–196.
119. Harris MM, Strafford MA, Rowe RW, et al: Venous air embolism and cardiac arrest during craniectomy in a supine infant. *Anesthesiology* 1986;65:547–550.
120. Harris MM, Yemen TA, Davidson A, et al: Venous embolism during craniectomy in supine infants. *Anesthesiology* 1987;67:816–819.
121. Meridy HW, Creighton RE, Humphreys RP: Complications during neurosurgery in the prone position in children. *Can Anaesth Soc J* 1974;21:445–453.
122. Marshall WK, Bedford RF: Use of a pulmonary-artery catheter for detection and treatment of venous air embolism: a prospective study in man. *Anesthesiology* 1980;52:131–134.
123. Cucchiara RF, Bowers B: Air embolism in children undergoing suboccipital craniotomy. *Anesthesiology* 1982;57:338–339.
124. Lasjaunias P: Interventional neuroradiology in children. *Child Nerv Syst* 1995;11:33–37.
125. Thompson D, Malcolm G, Jones B, et al: Intracranial pressure in single-suture craniosynostosis. *Pediatr Neurosurg* 1995;22:235–240.
126. Diaz JH, Lockhart CH: Hypotensive anaesthesia for craniectomy in infancy. *Br J Anaesth* 1979;51:233–235.
127. Duffner PK, Cohen ME, Freeman AI: Pediatric brain tumors: an overview. *Ca Cancer J Clin* 1985;35:287–301.
128. Gold E: Epidemiology of brain tumors. *Rev Cancer Epidemiol* 1982;1:245–278.
129. Farwell JR, Dohrmann GJ, Flannery JT: Central nervous system tumors in children. *Cancer* 1977;40:3123–3132.
130. Farwell JR, Dohrmann GJ, Flannery JT: Intracranial neoplasms in infants. *Arch Neurol* 1978;35:533–537.
131. Anonymous: A study of childhood brain tumors based on surgical biopsies from ten North American institutions: sample description. Childhood Brain Tumor Consortium. *J Neurooncol* 1988;6:9–23.
132. Anonymous: The epidemiology of headache among children with brain tumor. Headache in children with brain tumors. The Childhood Brain Tumor Consortium. *J Neurooncol* 1991;10:31–46.
133. Rorke L, Schut L: Introductory survey of pediatric brain tumors. In: McLaurin R, Schut L, Venes J, Epstein F (eds). Pediatric Neurosurgery. Survey of the developing nervous system. Section of pediatric neurosurgery of the American Society of Neurological Surgeons. Philadelphia: WB Saunders, 1989:335–337.
134. Stirt JA, Grosslight KR, Bedford RF, Vollmer D: "Defasciculation" with metocurine prevents succinylcholine-induced increases in intracranial pressure. *Anesthesiology* 1987;67:50–53.
135. Humphreys RP, Creighton RE, Hendrick EB, Hoffman HJ: Advantages of the prone position for neurosurgical procedures on the upper cervical spine and posterior cranial fossa in children. *Childs Brain* 1975;1:325–336.
136. Relton JE, Hall JE: An operation frame for spinal fusion. A new apparatus designed to reduce haemorrhage during operation. *J Bone Joint Surg (B)* 1967;49:327–332.
137. Todd MM, Warner DS, Sokoll MD, et al: A prospective, comparative trial of three anesthetics for elective supratentorial craniotomy. Propofol/fentanyl, isoflurane/nitrous oxide, and fentanyl/nitrous oxide [see comments]. *Anesthesiology* 1993;78:1005–1020.
138. Bissonnette B: Temperature monitoring in pediatric anesthesia. *Int Anesthesiol Clin* 1992;30:63–76.
139. Busto R, Globus MY, Dietrich WD, et al: Effect of mild hypothermia on ischemia-induced release of neurotransmitters and free fatty acids in rat brain. *Stroke* 1989;20:904–910.

140. Wass CT, Lanier WL, Hofer RE, et al: Temperature changes of < OR 1 degree C alter functional neurologic outcome and histopathology in a canine model of complete cerebral ischemia. *Anesthesiology* 1995;83: 325–335.
141. Archer D, Bissonnette B, Ravussin P: Cardiac performance enhancement for the prevention and treatment of delayed cerebral ischemia due to vasospasm. *Ann Fr Anesth Reanim* 1996;1996;15:328–338.
142. Ersahin Y, Mutluer S, Guzelbag E: Cerebrospinal fluid shunt infections. *J Neurosurg Sci* 1994;38:161–165.
143. Lorber J: Results of treatment of myelomeningocele. An analysis of 524 unselected cases, with special reference to possible selection for treatment. *Dev Med Child Neurol* 1971;13:279–303.
144. Lorber J: Some paediatric aspects of myelomeningocele. *Acta Orthop Scand* 1975;46:350–355.
145. Dierdorf SF, McNiece WL, Rao CC, et al: Failure of succinylcholine to alter plasma potassium in children with myelomeningocoele. *Anesthesiology* 1986;64:272–273.
146. Flynn J: Retinopathy of prematurity. In: Martyn L (ed). *Pediatric ophthalmology.* Philadelphia: WB Saunders, 1987:1487–1516.
147. Bryan MH, Hardie MJ, Reilly BJ, Swyer PR: Pulmonary function studies during the first year of life in infants recovering from the respiratory distress syndrome. *Pediatrics* 1973;52:169–178.
148. Harwood-Nash DC: Fractures of the petrous and tympanic parts of the temporal bone in children: a tomographic study of 35 cases. *Am J Roentgenol Radium Ther Nucl Med* 1970;110:598–607.
149. Freytag E: Autopsy findings in head injuries from blunt forces. Statistical evaluation of 1,367 cases. *Arch Pathol* 1963;75:402–408.
150. Hendrick E, Harwood-Nash D, Hudson A: Head injuries in children: a survey of 4465 consecutive cases at the Hospital for Sick Children, Toronto, Ontario, Canada. *Clin Neurosurg* 1964;11:46–54.
151. Humphreys RP, Hendrick EB, Hoffman HJ: The head-injured child who "talks and dies." A report of 4 cases. *Childs Nerv Syst* 1990;6:139–142.
152. Sharples PM, Storey A, Aynsley-Green A, Eyre JA: Avoidable factors contributing to death of children with head injury. *Br Med J* 1990;300:87–91.
153. Bruce DA, Alavi A, Bilaniuk L, et al: Diffuse cerebral swelling following head injuries in children: the syndrome of "malignant brain edema." *J Neurosurg* 1981; 54:170–178.
154. Aldrich EF, Eisenberg HM, Saydjari C, et al: Diffuse brain swelling in severely head-injured children: a report from the NIH Traumatic Coma Data Bank. *J Neurosurg* 1992;76:450–454.
155. Cushing H: Some experimental and clinical observations concerning the states of increased intracranial pressure. *Am J Med Sci* 1902;124:375–382.
156. Ross DA, Olsen WL, Ross AM, et al: Brain shift, level of consciousness, and restoration of consciousness in patients with acute intracranial hematoma. *J Neurosurg* 1989;71:498–502.
157. Langfitt TW, Obrist WD, Alavi A, et al: Computerized tomography, magnetic resonance imaging, and positron emission tomography in the study of brain trauma. Preliminary observations. *J Neurosurg* 1986; 64:760–767.
158. Sandler AN, Tator CH: Effect of acute spinal cord compression injury on regional spinal cord blood flow in primates. *J Neurosurg* 1976;45:660–676.
159. Kato A: Disturbance of the circulation in the spinal cord with epidural neoplasm. *Med J Osaka Univ* 1985; 35:63–71.
160. Griffiths IR, Trench JG, Crawford RA: Spinal cord blood flow and conduction during experimental cord compression in normotensive and hypotensive dogs. *J Neurosurg* 1979;50:353–360.
161. Lam A: Do evoked potentials have any value in anesthesia? In: Bissonnette B (ed). *Cerebral protection, resuscitation and monitoring: a look into the future of neuroanesthesia.* Philadelphia, WB Saunders, 1992: 657–683.
162. Bissonnette B. Anesthesia for neurosurgical procedures. In:Gregory GA (ed). *Pediatric anesthesia.* New York, Churchill Livingstone, 1994:375–421.

14

Common and Uncommon Coexisting Diseases That Complicate Pediatric Anesthesia

Ann G. Bailey and J. Michael Badgwell

Even diseases have lost their prestige, there aren't so many of them left....Think it over...no more syphilis, no more clap, no more typhoid...antibiotics have taken half the tragedy out of medicine."

—Louise-Ferdinand Celine (1960)

Isn't it always the case that the simple surgical procedure turns out to be scheduled for a not-so-simple pediatric patient? Come to think of it, if kids were healthy, there would be very little need for surgery in childhood with the exception of trauma and congenital disorders. By understanding the underlying diseases with which many children present, a safe and effective anesthetic can be delivered.

PULMONARY SYSTEM

UPPER RESPIRATORY INFECTION

Pathophysiology

The child with a runny nose who presents for surgery seems to be the most common clinical scenario we as clinicians see.[a] It may be important to differentiate a viral upper respiratory tract infection from other causes of a runny nose (Table 1). The other causes of rhinorrhea may have different anesthetic implications.

Why is a URI such a problem? Most young children average 6 to 9 URIs per year. Children who attend day care and who live in crowded conditions or with a mother who smokes may have a higher incidence of URIs. The mean duration of a URI is 7 to 9 days; reactive airways may persist for up to 6 weeks. Therefore, the logistical implications of trying to schedule elective surgery around a URI can be mind-boggling for parents and clinicians.

Viruses may affect any portion of the respiratory tract (Table 2). A URI may affect the lower respiratory tract to some degree, but may not be clinically evident. With lower tract involvement, there is airway hyperresponsiveness, which may lead to laryngospasm, coughing, and bronchospasm.

The increased production and decreased clearance of mucus in the lower airways increases the potential for atelectasis and pneumonia. Collapse of lobes or entire lungs may occur intraoperatively in children with recent URIs. Furthermore, there may be an increase in the incidence of postintubation croup among children with URI compared with healthy children in those <1 year of age. Overall, a child with a URI and endotracheal anesthesia has a significant increase in risk of respiratory complication compared with that of the healthy child having surgery and anesthesia.

Anesthetic Management

Preoperative Assessment

If surgery is nonelective (e.g., appendectomy, surgery for incarcerated hernia), one should proceed with anesthesia. If the surgery

---

[a]Ed. Note (JMB): For another viewpoint of management of the child with upper respiratory infection (URI), see Chapter 1.

TABLE 1. Differential diagnosis of runny nose

Runny nose diagnoses
Allergic rhinitis
Vasomotor rhinitis—crying
Prodromal stages of systemic viral illness (varicella, rubeola influenza)
Prodromal stages of bacterial illness (epiglottitis, adenotonsillitis)
Sinusitis

TABLE 2. Pathophysiologic effects of upper respiratory infection (URI)

Symptoms of URI	Effects
Increased nasal secretions	Laryngospasm
Increased lower airway secretions	Atelectasis/pneumonia
Increased airway edema and inflammation	Postintubation croup
Increased tachykinins	Airway reactivity
Decreased M_2 receptor function	Airway reactivity

is elective, the decision of whether to proceed with surgery can usually be based on the history and physical findings. Table 3 contains guidelines to help in making the decision.

Laboratory Data. Laboratory tests are costly and usually a waste of time. Complete blood counts (CBCs) and chest radiographs may not demonstrate anything unusual with a URI.[b] Do not order these tests unless there is a clear-cut indication of a serious condition (e.g., you want to diagnose pneumonia preoperatively in a child with rales, rhonchi, and a hot appendix).

Anesthetic Technique

Anticholinergic agents (atropine or glycopyrrolate) should be given to dry secretions and to block the increased cholinergic responses. Whether to intubate is a cost/benefit analysis. Children with colds have reactive airways and are prone to the "spasm" family of disasters (e.g., laryngospasm, bronchospasm). Therefore, many of us are more comfortable with a tracheal tube in these children to protect their airways. Others prefer not to manipulate the airway in the first place. Inhalation agents all promote bronchodilation; they are a good base anesthetic. Make sure that your anesthetic depth is sufficient, especially during intubation. Ensure that there is a leak around the endotracheal tube in young children to minimize postintubation croup. If the anesthetic will be long-lasting, use a humidifier to decrease drying effects on the airway. Although there is a theoretical advantage to a deep extubation, if this is not the clinician's usual practice, this is not the time to learn. Supplemental oxygen en route to the postanesthesia care unit and until the child is fully awake will minimize the hypoxemia that these children are prone to develop in the immediate postoperative period. Regional techniques are fine if the child, the surgeon, and the operative procedure all allow. For example, a 1-month-old infant with an incarcerated hernia may be a candidate for a caudal or spinal anesthetic in experienced hands.

ASTHMA

Pathophysiology

Asthma is a reactive airway disorder that affects many different age groups. It is difficult to describe the clinical state for asthma for each population, but there are three defining characteristics for all ages:

- Airway obstruction that is reversible or partially reversible either spontaneously or with treatment
- Airway inflammation
- Increased airway responsiveness to a variety of stimuli (5)

All that wheezes is *not* asthma (Table 4). The prevalence of asthma, however, has increased over the past 10 years, particularly in children. Airway obstruction in asthma is initiated by an inflammatory response, triggered

---

[b]Ed. Note (JMB): A negative chest x-ray may be counterproductive in postponing a case when factors other than the chest x-ray mitigate toward postponement. For example, a pushy surgeon may look at you and the really sick kid and say, "Let's go ahead, the x-ray is normal."

TABLE 3. Historical, physical, and other factors for determining whether to proceed with elective surgery in the child with URI*

Pro	Con
History	
Child "always keeps a cold, and this is as good as he gets."	A recent or ongoing fever
"Cold was much worse last week. Just a little runny nose now."	Acting sick
"Just a runny nose for the last several days; no other symptoms."	Poor appetite
	Has been coughing (not a chronic cough)
	Just developed symptoms last night (might develop into full-blown systemic illness)
Physical examination	
Clear lungs	Thick, green purulent nasal discharge
Active cheerful-looking child	Lethargic or ill-appearing child
Clear rhinorrhea	Wheezing, rales, or rhonchi
Other factors	
Older child	Child <1 year of age
Short, noninvasive operation	History of reactive airway disease
Social issues (parents drove 12 hours in the snow to get to hospital; family came from out of town; parents lost wages to be at hospital today; insurance will run out or deductible will expire in less than 1 month)	Major operation
	Endotracheal intubation required

*All factors must be considered "on-balance"; no *one* factor "swings" the decision.

by the release of inflammatory mediators from bronchial mast cells, macrophages, and epithelial cells. Therefore, therapeutic intervention is aimed at reducing bronchial inflammation (e.g., corticosteroid therapy).

Anesthetic Management

Preoperative Assessment

The following are helpful questions to ask when taking the patient history:

TABLE 4. Differential diagnosis of wheezing in children

Large obstruction	Large and small obstruction
Vascular ring	Asthma
Laryngotracheomalacia	Viral bronchiolitis
Enlarged lymph nodes or tumor	Cystic fibrosis
Laryngeal web	Bronchopulmonary dysplasia
Tracheostenosis or bronchostenosis	Aspiration
Obstructed endotracheal tube	Vascular engorgement
	Pulmonary edema
	Carinal or main-stem intubation
	α_1-antitrypsin deficiency

- How often does the child have asthma attacks? This question seeks an answer of how severe the condition is.

- What precipitates them? If stress and activity are factors, sedative premedication may be indicated. If the child only wheezes with colds, he or she should be asymptomatic for URI symptoms (for at least 4 to 6 weeks after a recent episode, if possible).

- What makes wheezing episodes go away? Knowing how easily the episodes resolve will be helpful if the child develops bronchospasm in the operating room.

- Is the child on chronic medication? What medication? How often? By what route? It is important to continue these medications throughout the perioperative period. Therefore, parents should be told to continue this regimen until the child comes to the operating room.

- Has the child taken corticosteroids in the last 6 months? Ever? Oral or inhaled? Chronic or frequent corticosteroid use indicates severe asthma. Use of systemic corticosteroids in the last 6 months is an indication for stress dose coverage (Table 5). For children with severe asthma, pretreatment with oral corticosteroids 1 to 2 days preoperatively may be indicated.

- Is the child followed up by a pediatrician or pulmonologist? There is likely to be reasonable control of the asthma if routine care is provided, rather than just emergency room visits.

Physical Examination. Active wheezing or markedly decreased breath sounds are ominous signs and should be corrected before surgery, if possible. Ideally, the chest should be clear unless the parents state that "the chest never clears."

Laboratory Data. Unless there is a specific indication (e.g., rales or rhonchi), no laboratory tests or pulmonary functions should be "routinely" ordered. The most valuable pulmonary function test is peak expiratory flow rate, a test that correlates well with forced expiration volume in 1 second (FEV_1) but is difficult to get in children <5 years of age.

Anesthetic Technique

Premedication. If indicated, premedication (e.g., oral midazolam, 0.5 to 0.75 mg/kg) may be given 15 to 20 minutes before induction. If the child routinely uses an inhaler and has it, a preoperative dose is helpful.

Induction. Induction can be accomplished by any route. Thiopental is fine, as long as the child is not actively wheezing. A dose of thiopental is given to provide sufficient anesthetic depth to attenuate airway reflexes at intubation (5 to 6 mg/kg). Propofol, because of its lesser histamine-releasing capacity, may be better than etomidate or thiopental in children with asthma. Ketamine is a bronchodilator and may be the drug of choice in an acute episode in which the patient is actively wheezing. Halothane and sevoflurane are both good inhalation agents for induction, and both promote bronchodilation.

Maintenance. A maintenance technique using primarily volatile agents will promote bronchodilation. Agents that are known to cause histamine release (e.g., atracurium or morphine) are avoided in the severe asthmatic. If the patient is intubated and is actively wheezing, a β_2-agonist via the endotracheal tube may be considered (Table 5). Aminophylline is no longer a first-line drug, but may prove useful if initial therapy with corticosteroids and β_2-agonists fails to control bronchospasm.

TABLE 5. *Drugs in asthma*

Drugs	Dose/Route	Notes
Steroids		
Prednisone or prednisolone	1–2 mg/kg/d in single or divided doses orally	No need to taper if <3 d
Hydrocortisone	5–7 mg/kg/dose IV every 4–6 h	More mineralocorticoid activity than methylprednisolone
Methylprednisolone	2 mg/kg IV load; 0.5–1 mg/kg every 6 h postoperatively	Clinical effects begin within 1–3 hours; maximum at 4–8 hours
β_2-agonists		
Albuterol (salbutamol)	4–8 puffs through endotracheal tube (ETT); 1–2 puffs orally; metered dose inhaler 0.01 ml/kg of 0.5% solution nebulized	Only 2.5–12% of delivered dose reaches end of ETT when aerosolized at connector of ETT (sizes 3.0–6.0)
Metaproterenol	2 puffs orally; 0.0 1 ml/kg of 5% solution nebulized	Not as long in duration as albuterol
Xanthines		
Aminophylline	5 mg/kg IV load over 15 minutes; then 0.5–1.2 mg/kg/h for 1 mo–16 y	Watch for toxicity; not a first-line drug

TABLE 6. Cystic fibrosis implications

Organ	Problems	Treatment	Anesthetic Implications
Lungs	Viscous secretions and defective transport lead to plugging and infections. Hypoxemia occurs earlier than hypercarbia.	Vigorous and frequent chest physiotherapy; nutritional supplements; antibiotics; pulmonary lavage; lung transplantation	Optimize lung function preoperatively. Endotracheal tube may need frequent suctioning. Higher FIO_2 may be needed. Hydration prevents inspissated secretions. Preoperative status and type of surgery dictate postoperative intubation status.
Intestinal tract	Exocrine pancreatic insufficiency results in malabsorption and malnutrition. Meconium ileus may present in the neonatal period. Rectal prolapse can occur in 20–30%.	Pancreatic enzyme replacement; vitamin supplement; nutritional supplement	Coagulopathy from vitamin K deficiency may contraindicate regional anesthetic.
Biliary tract	Obstruction of bile canaliculi can cause biliary cirrhosis and portal hypertension.	Treatment for liver failure; rarely liver transplantation	Coagulopathy may be present.
Pancreas	After 10 years, hyperglycemia and ketoacidosis may occur.	With marked elevation and polyuria, insulin is required.	In older children, check glucose.
Nose	Nasal polyposis is common.	Surgical removal	Extreme care if nasal intubation is required for a procedure.

Emergence. Two schools of thought regarding tracheal extubation exist—deep and awake. The patient with asthma may not be the one on which you wish to practice your first deep extubation. If you are comfortable with it, however, and particularly if the patient has reacted to the endotracheal tube during periods of light anesthesia, removing the tube while the patient is deeply anesthetized (e.g., spontaneously breathing sufficient concentrations of volatile agent)[c] may help to provide a smooth wake-up. Alternatively, an awake extubation may be performed. Adding opioid agents (e.g., fentanyl, 1 to 2 µg/kg) or intravenous (IV) lidocaine (1 mg/kg) or both as the child emerges will help to smooth the awake extubation. Another high-yield, low-risk maneuver would be to give a β_2-agonist via the endotracheal tube before extubation.

---

[c]Ed. Note (JMB): For a complete discussion of awake versus deep tracheal extubation, the reader is referred to Chapter 6.

CYSTIC FIBROSIS

Pathophysiology

Cystic fibrosis is a recessive disorder that occurs in 1 in 2000 caucasian births. Obstruction of exocrine glands with abnormal mucus and electrolyte secretion can lead to problems in several organs, particularly the lungs and the digestive tract. The disease can vary from very mild with only malabsorptive symptoms to very severe with end-stage cardiopulmonary failure. The degree of organ involvement determines the anesthetic implications (Table 6).

Anesthetic Management

Preoperative Assessment

History. Because clinical manifestations may vary from mild (e.g., asymptomatic) to severe (e.g., cardiopulmonary failure), information regarding severity of illness and current therapy determine the anesthetic risk. The following are questions to ask:

- How old was the child when symptoms began?
- What is the pulmonary status? How often is chest physiotherapy given? How often and when was the most recent pulmonary "clean-out?" What are the usual oxygen-hemoglobin saturations? (Most parents can give this information.)
- What medication is the child taking? (This often indicates which organs are involved.)
- Who routinely follows up the child for care? (Routine care by a pediatrician or pulmonologist usually implies optimal status has been achieved).

Physical Examination. The most important physical finding in cystic fibrosis is the overall appearance of the patient. Patients may look entirely normal, or they may be malnourished with variable degrees of respiratory distress. Evidence of hypoxemia (e.g., cyanosis, clubbing) respiratory failure, and clinical evidence of right heart failure may be present. Lung auscultation may reveal rhonchi and wheezes. Rarely, abdominal examination will reveal hepatomegaly.

Laboratory Data. No routine laboratory tests or radiographs are needed. If the organ system involvement or the surgical procedure dictates, arterial blood gases, chest radiographs, pulmonary function tests, electrocardiogram (ECG), liver function tests, and clotting studies may be indicated.

Anesthetic Technique

There is no absolute contraindication to premedication of children with cystic fibrosis. One must be careful, however, to monitor the patient after sedation and not to overly sedate the patient. Atropine or glycopyrrolate can be given if clinically indicated. Good hydration should be maintained perioperatively to prevent inspissation of secretions.

A tracheal tube allows suctioning of the airway, and controlled ventilation is indicated in most situations. In fact, pulmonary lavage intraoperatively usually helps the patient. Nitrous oxide should be avoided in patients with evidence of bullae, pneumothorax, or bowel obstruction. A good general anesthetic that allows the patient to awaken readily with full neuromuscular function would be the optimal technique. No specific agent can be recommended as the best.

If coagulopathy is ruled out, regional techniques may be appropriate, including continuous epidural anesthesia. High-level spinal or epidural motor block, however, may decrease the child's ability to cough. A combined regional and general anesthetic technique will help to provide a rapid recovery with good analgesia and may help to improve pulmonary function postoperatively.

MUSCULOSKELETAL SYSTEM AND SKIN

CEREBRAL PALSY

Pathophysiology

Cerebral palsy (CP) is defined as any nonprogressive central motor deficit dating to events in the prenatal or perinatal period. It is not a specific disease, but rather a group of disorders of varied causes. Clinically, the children can be divided into groups:

- Spastic CP (quadriplegia, paraplegia, hemiplegia, monoplegia)—the most common type. Spasticity and rigidity become more evident as the child grows older. Pseudobulbar palsy is often present if spasticity is bilateral, and this accounts for drooling and swallowing difficulties. Seizures may be present.
- Extrapyramidal CP. Hypotonia will be manifested in infancy and choreoathetoid movements later in childhood. This is rare and usually secondary to kernicterus.

- Atonic CP. This is a descriptive term for hypotonia due to central nervous system damage. Mental function may be severely impaired. Spasticity develops later in childhood.
- Mixed types. These are combinations of the above.

Many children with CP have normal or borderline intelligence; the inability to communicate clearly often gives an erroneous impression of mental retardation. The long-term outlook is often determined by the child's intellectual capacity. Motor disabilities are treated with (a) physical therapy to prevent contractures, (b) surgical therapy to improve mobility and decrease spasticity (e.g., dorsal rhizotomy), and (c) medical therapy to control spasticity (e.g., baclofen, dantrolene, benzodiazepines).

Anesthetic Management

Preoperative Assessment

History. Because the variation in severity of CP is great, only a thorough history and physical examination will provide the information needed. Questions to ask include the following:

- Does your child have difficulties with swallowing? (Some may choke on pills and solids; only liquid pain medications can be ordered orally.)
- Does your child have a history of gastroesophageal reflux?
- Does your child drool or obstruct easily?
- Does your child have seizures and, if so, how often?
- Does your child have painful muscle spasms?
- Is your child on medication for spasms?
- How much does your child understand?
- Does your child have frequent pneumonias?

Physical Examination. Some children with CP look entirely normal, whereas others have severe contractures. Many of these children are much smaller than predicted age. The severely contracted child may present airway difficulties if neck mobility is limited. Positioning for surgery will also be problematic. The presence of upper airway noises preoperatively indicate potential for airway obstruction in the postoperative period. Rhonchi in the lower airways may indicate a tendency to aspirate secretions or to poorly mobilize them. Some children develop a significant restrictive lung disease from scoliosis. Venous access may be problematic if severe contractures are present.

Laboratory Data. Some children with CP are chronically malnourished and anemic. A CBC may be helpful, particularly if blood loss is anticipated. Other tests are indicated by the individual child's condition and the surgery.

Anesthetic Technique

Preoperative. Sedative premedication may be given, particularly in children who have had previous procedures and are very anxious. Children with poor pharyngeal coordination are not good candidates for preoperative sedation. An antisialagogue is helpful in children with drooling.

Induction. If gastroesophageal reflux is present, a rapid-sequence induction is indicated. Succinylcholine does not cause exaggerated increase in potassium in children with CP. If there is no contraindication, a mask induction is fine, but it must be realized that oral secretions may precipitate laryngospasm and airway obstruction. Although children with cerebral palsy usually react normally to nondepolarizing relaxants, some children, particularly those on anticonvulsants, may have resistance to nondepolarizing muscle relaxants. Placement of the nerve stimulator on the affected spastic extremities may falsely lead one to give more relaxant than is indicated because of muscle wasting.

Maintenance. Children with severe CP often have increased sensitivity to opioids. Therefore, titration of analgesics to effect is important. These children are at high risk for developing hypothermia intraoperatively, particularly malnourished children with little subcutaneous fat. Therefore, the room should be made warm and a forced-air warmer used for anything other than minor short procedures.

Postoperative. Painful muscle spasms are commonly seen postoperatively, particularly with orthopedic procedures involving tendon and muscle manipulations. Opioids are often ineffective in treating these muscle spasms, but local anesthetics via the caudal or epidural route may be very effective. If a regional technique is not an option, benzodiazepines should be considered in the postoperative period when the patient is in pain from muscle spasm.

MUSCULAR DYSTROPHY

The muscular dystrophies are a group of familial disorders characterized by progressive weakness and loss of striated musculature. Classification is based on onset, rate of progression, distribution of muscle involvement, and mode of inheritance. The most common form of muscular dystrophy is Duchenne's muscular dystrophy (DMD), also known as childhood or pseudohypertrophic muscular dystrophy.

Duchenne's muscular dystrophy is inherited as an X-linked recessive trait, occurring in 1 in 3600 live-born males. It occurs in females, but only in females with Turner's syndrome. Approximately 25% of cases occur as a genetic mutation. Therefore, a family history of this disorder may be lacking.

Duchenne's muscular dystrophy begins in some subtle ways. These children are not as well coordinated as their peers and may have a slight delay in reaching milestones. Most children will develop coordination problems by 2 to 3 years of age and will develop classic symptoms of DMD by the time they are 3 to 5 years of age. Typically, children with DMD become wheelchair-bound in early adolescence, and death occurs before age 20 in 75% of the patients.

The basic problem in DMD is the deficiency of dystrophin, an encoded protein. Cardiomyopathy is a constant feature of this disease, and its severity is not related to the severity of the neuromuscular disease. Also, dystrophin is missing within the conduction system of the heart, which may explain why some of these children with DMD have dysrhythmias and are difficult to resuscitate if they have a cardiac arrest. Intellectual impairment occurs in most of these patients, since dystrophin is also absent from the brain. Duchenne's muscular dystrophy should be suspected in any child who, as an infant, has an unexplained cardiac arrest under anesthesia, particularly with succinylcholine.

Organ system involvement and age of the patient influence the anesthetic management (Table 7).

Anesthetic Management

Preoperative Assessment

History. It is important to determine the level of intellectual and motor function of the child. Many children with DMD will be followed by specialists. If cardiac evaluation or pulmonary evaluation has been recently performed, the results should be reviewed before anesthetizing the child for elective surgery.

Physical Examination. Many children with CP exhibit a tachycardia, which may indicate

TABLE 7. *Muscular dystrophy*

Musculoskeletal
 Hypertrophied muscle mass is due to fatty infiltrates. Profound atrophy occurs in late stages and leads to progressive kyphoscoliosis.
Pulmonary
 Pulmonary function plateaus at 10–12 y and subsequently decreases as a result of restrictive component. Vital capacity <30% of that predicted will increase postoperative complications.
Cardiac
 Most older children have a cardiomyopathy, which leads to decreased left ventricular function and congestive heart failure; papillary muscle dysfunction causes mitral regurgitation. Dysrhythmias are common.
Central nervous system
 The mean IQ is 85; up to 25% have a frank mental defect.
Gastrointestinal
 There is poor esophageal motility; delayed gastric emptying.

underlying cardiac disease. Overall appearance will give an indication as to the degree and severity of the disease. An older child who is wheelchair-bound is obviously more prone to complications than a young child with few manifestations.

Laboratory Data. An ECG and chest x-ray are useful in older children. It is not clear whether all children in their adolescence need cardiology evaluation preoperatively. Unless the child is symptomatic, it is difficult to predict which children have a significant cardiomyopathy. For major procedures such as spinal fusion for scoliosis, a preoperative echocardiogram may help define the anesthetic and surgical risks relative to the cardiac status. Pulmonary function studies are indicated for major procedures in older children who are wheelchair-bound, since vital capacity <30% of predicted value increases the likelihood of postoperative ventilation.

Anesthetic Technique

Preoperative. If the child is severely debilitated and unable to manage secretions, glycopyrrolate (0.01 mg/kg IV) before or at induction will help to decrease the volume of oral secretions.

Induction. Avoid succinylcholine![d] Many cases of acute hyperkalemic arrest have been reported with DMD and other forms of myopathy (7,8). In patients with either recognized or unrecognized neuromuscular disease, there is an up-regulation of the acetylcholine receptors with an increase in the number of acetylcholine receptors that are extrajunctional (10). This up-regulation is the reason for hyperkalemia of various degrees after succinylcholine administration. After succinylcholine, hyperkalemia usually occurs within 2 to 3 minutes. Unfortunately, this is the same time that the clinician is busy with intubation, taping in the endotracheal tube, checking the breath sounds, and so on, and may or may not be watching the ECG, which by this time may show peaked T-waves. In fact, the T-wave becomes so large that it is read as a QRS complex, and the ECG may report a rate that has "doubled" compared with the baseline heart rate. It is important not to treat this "pseudotachycardia," but recognize it as a problem with the T-wave and as an indicator of hyperkalemia. It will be obvious from the precordial stethoscope and pulse oximeter that the true rate has not doubled. The pseudotachycardia of hyperkalemia may rapidly progress to a more chaotic and life-threatening rhythm disturbance, including cardiac arrest. When hyperkalemia is suspected, treatment should begin. Calcium chloride (10 mg/kg) will help to reverse the effects of hyperkalemia.

In addition, sodium bicarbonate, 1 to 2 mg/kg, may be required if lab data indicates. If the circulation becomes unstable and the patient develops bradycardia or hypotension, epinephrine, 5 to 10 µg/kg, may be administered. Epinephrine will enhance the movement of potassium into the cell as well as help stabilize the circulation. The use of glucose and insulin should be reserved until the child has a stable circulation.

Maintenance. Whether to use volatile anesthetic agents in children with DMD is very controversial. Rhabdomyolysis may occur after both halothane and isoflurane anesthetics when no succinylcholine is given. Furthermore, the association of malignant hyperthermia (MH) susceptibility and DMD is also controversial, since many children with DMD who have received volatile anesthetics have had reactions that resemble MH. Are all

---

[d] Ed. Note (JMB): The decision by the Food and Drug Administration (FDA) to contraindicate the use of succinylcholine in infants, children, and adolescents for routine intubation caused an immense uproar in the pediatric anesthesia world (1–6). Recently, however, the FDA has changed the contraindication to a box warning. This revision may help us ever so slightly in a medicolegal sense but does not change the clinical implications. As clinicians, the distinction of contraindication versus box warning matters little. It is more important that we recognize implications made evident by the package insert admonitions. The rare but often fatal outcome of cardiac arrest after administration of succinylcholine to children with either recognized or unrecognized DMD is well known (7,8). Although the estimated incidence of this problem is 1 in 500,000 anesthetics, there have been 20 or 30 case reports over the past 5 to 10 years that document this problem. Therefore, clinicians should be able to recognize hyperkalemia and to treat it (9).

patients with DMD susceptible to MH? Probably not. A relation between MH and DMD, however, does exist. Muscular dystrophy causes muscle membrane instability that is aggravated by MH-triggering agents. Children with diagnosed muscular dystrophy, however, may have normal halothane contracture studies, an observation that supports the theory that MH and DMD are independent disorders. In addition, volatile agents have been used successfully in DMD for spinal fusion surgery. In the final analysis, there is no definitive answer regarding whether to avoid volatile agents in all cases of DMD. If one does choose to use a volatile agent in a child with DMD, monitoring for signs of MH should be extensive, and dantrolene should be readily available **(see Malignant Hyperthermia Treatment)**.

When cardiac involvement is known to exist in a patient with DMD, appropriate anesthetic agents should be used to minimize cardiac depression. Neuromuscular function is monitored carefully, because full reversal will be necessary to successfully extubate. Smaller doses of nondepolarizing agents may be indicated. The need for postoperative ventilation is anticipated if preoperative vital capacity is <30% of predicted value. The risks associated with delayed gastric emptying and poor esophageal motility are also considered.

MALIGNANT HYPERTHERMIA

"The world...was created by neither Gods nor men, but was, is, and will be eternally living fire, regularly becoming ignited and regularly becoming extinguished."
—Heraclitus (c. 535–475 BC)

Pathophysiology

Malignant hyperthermia (MH) is a pharmacogenetic disorder primarily affecting skeletal muscle. It is an autosomal dominant trait with variable penetrance. The incidence is variously reported as 1 in 15,000 children and 1 in 40,000 adults (11) to 1 in 200,000 (in Denmark) (12). Since this is not a disorder that one can "outgrow," the difference in incidence in children and adults presumably reflects a greater exposure to halothane and succinylcholine in childhood, both of which are potent triggers of MH.

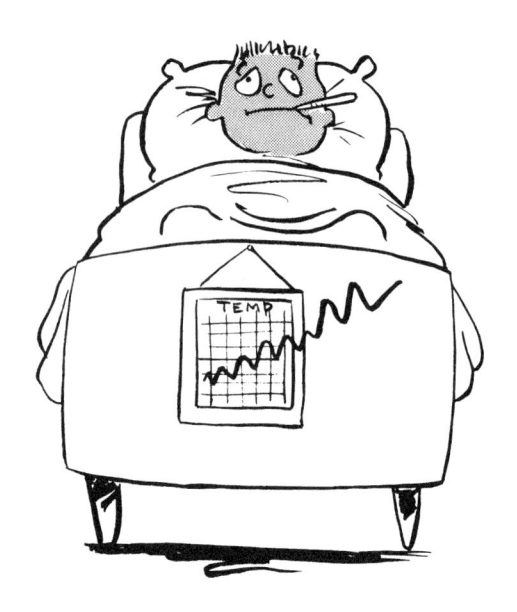

MH-susceptible persons have enhanced release and ineffectual reuptake of calcium from the sarcoplasmic reticulum. The result is increased myoplasmic calcium that initiates a hypermetabolic state, as evidenced by increased CO_2 production and increased O_2 consumption. MH is diagnosed initially when mixed venous O_2 decreases and the CO_2 of venous blood rises. Onset of MH is also heralded by an increased end-tidal CO_2 on capnography, assuming that there is no increased compensatory ventilation. A patient who is spontaneously breathing may exhibit tachypnea. A patient on a low inspired concentration of oxygen may have unexplained arterial desaturation owing to increased O_2 consumption. Tachycardia is an early sign of hypermetabolism. Dysrhythmias can occur secondary to fever, acidosis, hyperkalemia, and hypoxemia. Fever is usually a late sign, occurring after mechanisms of heat dissipation are overwhelmed and peripheral vasoconstriction ceases. Other signs of MH include rigidity (either masseter muscle rigidity or full-blown body rigidity), coagulopathy, renal failure, myoglobinuria, and ultimately cardiac arrest.

Many musculoskeletal syndromes are associated with MH. It is controversial whether all patients with DMD are MH-susceptible, but patients with muscular dystrophies are to be considered at high risk for development of MH. One of the factors leading to the confusion in the diagnosis of MH is that patients with DMD, when given succinylcholine, may also develop hyperkalemia. In some cases, this hyperkalemia is fatal. In addition, patients with other unrecognized myopathies who are given succinylcholine may develop hyperkalemia, possibly with fatal outcome. These episodes may be mislabeled as MH. We know now that not all cases of hyperkalemia under anesthesia are due to MH.

Other hereditary musculoskeletal diseases with a possible association with MH include central core disease and the King-Denborough syndrome. Many patients with muscular abnormalities such as strabismus and idiopathic kyphoscoliosis have been associated with a higher than usual incidence of MH. Patients with these conditions do not necessarily require unusual precautions, just a heightened awareness on the part of the anesthesiologist. Otolaryngologic procedures tend to be associated with a higher than usual incidence of MH.

Anesthetic Management

Preoperative Assessment

History. One should always ask about a family history of reactions to an anesthetic. Although most answers will be nebulous ("Uncle Joe took 2 days to wake up from his anesthesia"), some will be very direct ("My aunt got very hot while under anesthesia and they told her to let all of her family know"). Patients who have been diagnosed may have a medical alert bracelet or carry a letter from their physician. All reports of misadventures with previous anesthetics should be looked into, ideally by review of the anesthetic record. A national registry for MH-susceptible patients now exists, and there may be information there that can help you (717-531-6936). The fact that the child has been previously anesthetized with triggering agents without a problem does not prove that he or she is free of MH susceptibility. Children and adults may have had previous uneventful surgeries. Always be suspicious if things don't seem to be going right.

Physical Examination. There is no physical finding that will delineate which patients are MH-susceptible. One should evaluate every patient for evidence of neuromuscular disease.

Laboratory Data. There are no noninvasive studies that document the presence of MH susceptibility. Creatine phosphokinase (CPK) levels may be elevated, but have not proved reliable as a screening tool. The gold standard test for diagnosis remains the muscle biopsy for halothane-caffeine contracture studies. This test can be performed only at one of a few sites. The patient must weigh ~20 kg to have sufficient muscle removed for the test, which is performed under regional anesthesia or under a general anesthetic without triggering agents. In some situations, it may be appropriate to define MH susceptibility with a muscle biopsy before elective surgery. In most cases, it will be impractical or impossible to have that information, and a nontriggering technique should be performed.

Anesthetic Technique

The child who presents with a history of MH susceptibility for elective surgery should not be a major disruptive event for the anesthesiologist. Cool, calm, and rational planning will help to make the anesthetic experience more enjoyable for all involved.

Machine Preparation. Most hospitals have abandoned the concept of a "vapor-free" anesthetic machine dedicated to only the MH-susceptible population. Rather, running 10 L/min of oxygen flows through a fresh circuit with new soda lime for 20 minutes will effectively rid the system of trace inhalation agent. If the fresh gas outlet hose can be changed, 10 minutes is sufficient.

Avoid the "Bad Drugs." This is easy in the 90s. Drugs that trigger MH include the inhalation agents (desflurane, sevoflurane, halothane, isoflurane, and enflurane) and succinylcholine. By contrast, local anesthetics, narcotics, propofol, nondepolarizing muscle relaxants, and benzodiazepines all appear to be safe. Nitrous oxide is also considered a nontriggering agent.

Dantrolene Prophylaxis. Most MH-susceptible individuals do not require prophylactic treatment with dantrolene. The side effects (weakness, nausea, and vomiting) do not warrant treating susceptible patients (except in rare circumstances) before surgery. In fact, in children with preexisting muscle weakness secondary to myopathy, the resultant weakness from the dantrolene may precipitate respiratory insufficiency. In the rare situation, one may consider giving IV dantrolene 2.5 mg/kg just before induction in someone who truly is at high risk (e.g., in an MH-susceptible patient prior to a case where extreme hemodynamic instability is expected).

Monitors. Appropriate monitors include ECG, core temperature (e.g., rectal or tympanic membrane), blood pressure, pulse oximeter, stethoscope, and capnography.

Dantrolene Availability. Dantrolene and sterile water for reconstitution should be immediately available.

Postoperative. Can the MH-susceptible patient be discharged home after an uneventful nontriggering anesthetic? This is controversial, but MH-susceptible patients may undergo nontriggering anesthetics without any sequelae related to MH. Therefore, postoperative admission solely on the basis of MH susceptibility label is usually not warranted. An appropriate policy is to watch the child for 4 hours postoperatively. If there are no signs or symptoms of MH and if the parents appear to understand a discussion of the disease process and what we have been looking for, the child is allowed to go home.

Treatment

Treatment of the MH crisis has been nicely outlined by the Malignant Hyperthermia Association of the United States (MHAUS) (Table 8).

Aftercare. Afterward, you will have the responsibility of educating the family and pro-

---

TABLE 8. Treatment of malignant hyperthermia (MH)

1. Stop triggering anesthetic agents immediately and conclude surgery as soon as possible.
2. Hyperventilate with 100% O$_2$ at high flow rates.
3. Administer:
   a. Dantrolene: 2–3 mg/kg initial bolus with increments up to 10 mg/kg total. Continue dantrolene until symptoms are controlled. Occasionally, a dose greater than 10 mg/kg may be needed.
   b. Sodium bicarbonate: 1–2 meq/kg increments guided by arterial pH and PCO$_2$. Bicarbonate will combat hyperkalemia by driving potassium into cells.
4. Actively cool patient:
   a. If needed, IV iced saline (not lactated Ringer's solution) 15 ml/kg every 10 minutes × 3. Monitor closely.
   b. Lavage stomach, bladder, rectum, and peritoneal and thoracic cavities with iced saline.
   c. Cool body surface with ice and hypothermia blanket.
5. Maintain urine output. If needed, mannitol 0.25 g/kg IV, furosemide 1 mg/kg IV (up to four doses each). Urine output greater than 2 ml/kg/h may help prevent subsequent renal failure.
6. Calcium channel blockers should not be given when dantrolene is administered because hyperkalemia and myocardial depression may occur.
7. Insulin for hyperkalemia. Add 10 U regular insulin to 50 ml of 50% glucose and titrate to control hyperkalemia. Monitor blood glucose and K+ levels.
8. Postoperatively, continue dantrolene, 1 mg/kg IV every 6 h for 72 h to prevent recurrence. Lethal recurrence of MH may happen. Observe in an intensive care unit.
9. Call the MHAUS MH Hotline Consultant for expert medical advice and further medical evaluation (209) 634-4917 and ask for Index Zero.
10. Report MH events to The North American Malignant Hyperthermia Registry (717) 531-6936.

viding information for all involved. It is important to get the family involved with MHAUS and to consider whether other family members need referral for testing. A letter documenting the events that occurred, which is given to the family after the dust settles, will certainly be helpful for other care providers in the future.

MASSETER MUSCLE RIGIDITY

Masseter muscle rigidity, or masseter spasm, is an intense contraction of the masseter muscle occurring after induction of anesthesia with halothane and the administration of succinylcholine. Perhaps one of the major changes in the perception of MH is the belief among many experienced clinicians that masseter spasm as a clinical entity does not exist. We cannot, however, become overly cavalier. Masseter spasm as a clinical sign is still one of the early indicators of MH, especially when it occurs as part of a *generalized* myotonic contracture in MH-susceptible persons (13). It is also appreciated, however, that isolated masseter spasm is actually a part of a continuum of degrees of masseter contracture and occurs (to some degree) in all patients who are given succinylcholine (14–16). In other words, masseter muscle tone increases in children after succinylcholine before generalized muscle relaxation. Sometimes, this normal tightening is intense.

After the administration of succinylcholine, the masseter muscle is most intensely contracted at the end of fasciculations, a time when the nerve stimulator would indicate paralysis of the neuromuscular junction (15). Most of us have been taught to intubate the child's trachea at the end of fasciculations. However, if the child has been anesthetized with halothane, given succinylcholine, and then develops masseter muscle rigidity, intubation may be difficult. The intense masseter muscle contraction has nothing to do with the neuromuscular junction. Rather, the masseter muscle contraction is an intramyocellular contracture—the same type of contracture found in eye muscles after succinylcholine.

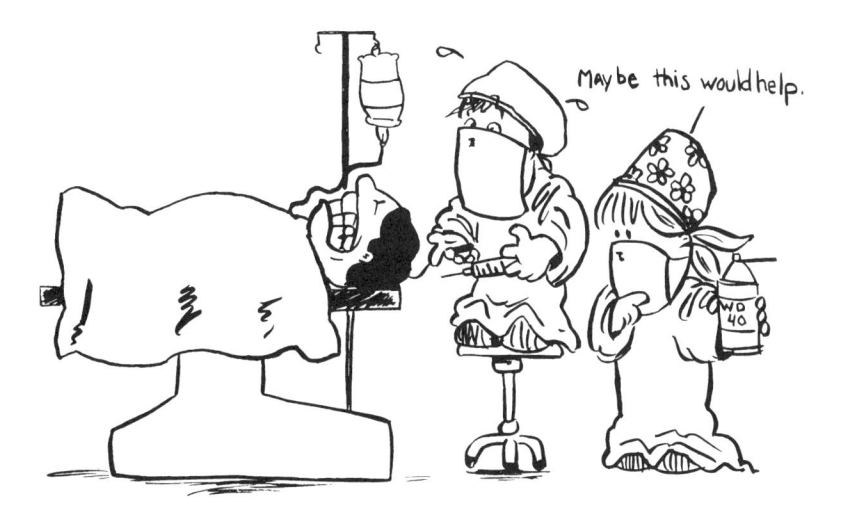

So, what to do when a child has a masseter spasm? The best way to deal with masseter spasm is to avoid it. Therefore, many pediatric anesthesiologists have discontinued the routine use of succinylcholine after halothane. Succinylcholine is still the drug of choice for laryngospasm and for rapid-sequence induction. But what if you get called in to help a colleague who has anesthetized a child with halothane, given succinylcholine, and now has a child with masseter spasm? It is time to ventilate and wait. The masseter spasm will usually resolve promptly. If it does not or if the patient can't wait (i.e., if oxygen-hemoglobin desaturation or bradycardia occurs), one can usually manage tracheal intubation; although it may be with some difficulty. What to do after the child survives masseter spasm? What do you tell the parents? Do you get a muscle biopsy? You are presented with a clinical conundrum.

The next diagnostic step after resolution of masseter spasm may be somewhat controversial, but most experts would agree on one simple and informative test—testing the urine for myoglobin. If the urine is negative for myoglobin, benign neglect may be the most beneficial, least harmful, thing to do. If positive, the child should be referred to a neurologist for evaluation of a possible myotonic disorder.

At this point after masseter spasm, many (if not most) anesthesiologists will continue the anesthetic using non-triggering agents, while monitoring for signs of MH. Others will continue the case using volatile agents (17,18). If one chooses to continue with a volatile anesthetic in a child after masseter spasm, one must carefully observe for signs of MH. In patients who are breathing spontaneously, increasing ventilation may balance increased production of CO_2. Therefore, if a patient is at risk for developing MH, he or she should be paralyzed and ventilated. If CO_2 increases in the presence of constant minute ventilation, one should think of MH. If this and other signs point to MH, it is appropriate to proceed with the full-blown treatment for MH (see above) All volatile anesthetics are immediately stopped, fresh gas flow is turned up to a very high rate (about 15 to 20 L/min; enough to wash the volatile anesthetics out of the patient and the machine), dantrolene, 2 to 3 mg/kg, is given, and a large fluid bolus of 15 ml/kg of balanced salt solution is given. If muscle rigidity is present, it will decrease after successful therapy. If tachycardia and rigidity persist, more dantrolene is given (up to 10 mg/kg). If urine output cannot be increased with fluid load, diuretics should be given. Hyperkalemia is a late finding in MH. There will be an enormous increase in CPK, since these patients undergo rhabdomyolysis.

Patients who are suspected of having MH should be followed up for recrudescence in an intensive care unit for 24 hours.

EPIDERMOLYSIS BULLOSA

Pathophysiology

Epidermolysis bullosa is a genetically determined disorder of the skin characterized by blister formation. Depending on the level of blistering, the over 20 different subtypes are classified into three major groups: simplex, junctional, and dystrophic. Dystrophic epidermolysis bullosa, the most clinically significant form, can be autosomal dominant or recessive, with an incidence of 1 in 50,000 to 1 in 300,000. In this subtype, injury occurs because of separation of the epidermis from the dermis by shearing forces.

Repeated bullae formation and healing lead to scarring of the mouth, esophagus, tongue, eyelids, fingers (leading to digital fusion and mitten deformity), and trunk. Malnutrition and anemia are common. Unfortunately, as these children become older, they may develop squamous cell carcinoma.

Anesthetic Management

Preoperative Assessment

History. Families with epidermolysis bullosa are usually able to tell you what causes blistering, where most of the injuries occur, and what they can and cannot do. Patients may have a recent history of corticosteroid intake and have adrenal suppression. Patients should be asked about previous surgery and whether any problems developed. Scarring of the mouth and oropharynx is progressive; an easy airway management in the past does not guarantee the same in the future.

Physical Examination. Children with epidermolysis bullosa often are small for their age, as a result of malnutrition. Particular attention should be aimed at examination of the extremities for IV access sites. The child's hands may be very deformed. Attention to the size of the mouth opening is also important.

Laboratory Data. Because anemia is often severe, a preoperative hemoglobin is recommended for all but the most minor of procedures. Other laboratory tests are indicated by the type of surgery and the clinical condition of the patient.

Anesthetic Technique

Monitors. In children with epidermolysis bullosa, monitors need to be modified for placement. In placing adhesive monitors, remember that it is not pressure, but shearing forces that cause problems. For the ECG, one may cut off the sticky portion of the pads and place the central portion with only the gel under the patient's back. Alternatively, needle electrodes may be inserted after the child is asleep. For the blood pressure cuff, one may use web roll or some type of padding under the cuff. In all but the most severe cases, pressure cycling of the cuff doesn't cause blistering. For pulse oximetry, the reusable probes are fine to gently place on a digit or extremity. If the digits are mitted, a disposable probe with the clear plastic backing left on, or the adhesive cut off, can be used over the end of the extremity or ear. For the precordial stethoscope, no adhesive backing is allowed. Esophageal stethoscopes are not recommended because of esophageal involvement in many patients. A skin or esophageal temperature probe is placed under the patient's back .

Intravenous Lines. Padding is used under the tourniquet to prevent shear forces. A catheter is placed wherever you can find a vein and tied in place with thin strips of gauze (e.g., Kerlex) or umbilical tape. For major procedures (or when the IV line took forever to secure), you may suture the IV line in place after the child is asleep.

Airway Management

If the airway looks challenging on examination, you may need to do a fiberoptic intubation. If the airway looks "do-able" and the case requires intubation, one may proceed, but with these caveats:

- Pressure of the mask against the face won't blister, but friction will. Therefore, 0.5% to 1% hydrocortisone cream is smeared over the contact surface of the mask and on the patient's chin.
- Oral airways shouldn't be used unless needed, because they can cause blisters.
- A laryngeal mask airway can be used if it is well lubricated and inserted with great care and expertise; otherwise it might be better to intubate.
- Endotracheal intubation may be accomplished without laryngeal bullae formation. Children with epidermolysis bullosa may, however, have an increased risk of laryngospasm. The endotracheal tube and blade should be well lubricated to minimize trauma.

Induction

Inhalation induction is fine for children, unless a history of reflux exists. Thiopental may also be used in these patients without adverse effects. Previously, epidermolysis bullosa patients were thought to be at risk for porphyria, but this was probably due to errors in diagnosis.

Maintenance

All anesthetic agents have been found to be safe in children with epidermolysis bullosa. Succinylcholine does not appear problematic, although a theoretic consideration exists in those patients with severe muscle atrophy.

Regional Anesthesia

Brachial plexus, subarachnoid, and epidural blocks have been used successfully. Subcutaneous injection of local anesthesia, however, should be avoided.

HEMOGLOBINOPATHIES

SICKLE CELL ANEMIA

"When is a crisis reached? When questions arise that can't be answered."
—Ryszard Kapusckinsky

Pathophysiology

Hemoglobin S (HbS) results from substitution of an amino acid on the beta chain of the hemoglobin molecule. Under deoxygenated conditions, the erythrocytes change form and irreversibly sickle. With an abundance of sickling erythrocytes, sickle cell crises develop. A sickled erythrocyte is fragile and prone to hemolysis, resulting in a lifespan of only 10 to 20 days. Sickled erythrocytes also form aggregates that cause vaso-occlusive problems in microvasculature. It is primarily the vaso-occlusive propensity that affects various organ systems (Table 9).

Sickle Trait

Children who are heterozygous rarely present with clinical problems related to sickling. They may show isosthenuria (inability to concentrate urine) as they grow older. Approximately 30% to 50% of the hemoglobin in the erythrocytes is HbS. With extreme hypoxemia (PaO_2 < 20 to 30 torr), sickling may occur. No extraordinary measures are needed with sickle trait, just good anesthesia.

Sickle C Disease

After homozygous SS disease, sickle C disease (SC) is the most severe hemoglobinopathy. Many of the complications seen in SS disease are also seen in SC. Unlike SS disease, the children with SC disease often have higher hemoglobin levels (9 to 11 g/dl). This may make simple transfusion somewhat tricky, since the balance between hemoglobin A and viscosity will need to be weighed. A partial exchange transfusion is sometimes indicated (38). The anesthetic management is identical with that of SS patients.

Sickle-β-Thalassemia

Sickle-β-thalassemia (S-B thal) usually has much milder manifestations than SS disease. Often, the anemia associated with this state is not as severe as with SS. Some institutions will treat S-B thal with exchange transfusions preoperatively, whereas others may take a more conservative approach.

TABLE 9. Sickle cell anemia

Central nervous system
  Transient ischemic attacks and strokes can occur in childhood; adults tend to have hemorrhagic infarcts; treatment is chronic transfusions, often monthly.
Spleen
  Repeated microinfarctions usually render the patient functionally asplenic by 4–5 years old; chronic antibiotic therapy is indicated for prophylaxis against *Streptococcus pneumoniae*; occasionally may develop splenic sequestration crisis in which spleen suddenly traps RBCs and profound anemia results.
Kidney
  Microinfarcts of the medulla lead to isosthenuria, the inability to concentrate urine. Occasionally, hematuria and renal failure develop.
Hepatobiliary
  Because of hemolysis, bile stones are common; cholecystectomy is often required.
Bones/extremities
  Vaso-occlusive sickling within the bones cause painful extremities; hydration and analgesia are usually sufficient to treat. Leg ulcers are common in adolescence; aplastic crises can occur with profound anemia.
Lungs
  Microinfarctions cause progressive restrictive pattern. Acute infarctions cause acute chest syndrome, which leads to consolidation on chest x-ray, hypoxia, and possibly death. Treatment is RBC transfusion and perhaps epidural local anesthetics.
Cardiovascular
  Left ventricular hypertrophy and cardiomegaly are common by age 20. Right ventricular hypertrophy results from chronic hypoxia.
Others
  Priapism and delayed growth are typical.

Anesthetic Management

Preoperative Assessment

History. Of particular importance is the number and frequency of crises that the patient has experienced in the past. A child who has frequent crises and has required transfusions for complications is probably at higher risk than the child who is relatively asymptomatic. A previous history of acute chest syndrome should also be a "red flag."

In addition, it is important to find out who follows the patient on a routine basis. If the child sees a hematologist regularly, information about baseline hemoglobins and percentage of HbS will be available.

Laboratory Data. At the very least, hemoglobin/hematocrit values are required. A recent hemoglobin electrophoresis is important to learn the percentage of abnormal hemoglobin that is present. Other tests are indicated by the patient's clinical status.

Anesthetic Technique

Preoperative Transfusion. This is one of those areas in which large controversy and little science are available. There are *three schools of thought about transfusion preoperatively:*

- *Everyone gets an exchange transfusion* to lower the HbS to <30% and to elevate the Hb to >10 g/dl. (This was actually the practice of most pediatric anesthesiologists polled at a recent national gathering of pediatric anesthesiologists.)
- *Everyone receives a simple transfusion* to raise the total hemoglobin to a level of 10 g/dl without consideration for the percentage of HbS. This is done with sequential transfusions over the preceding few weeks or as a single transfusion of 15 to 20 ml/kg immediately before surgery.
- *Only children who are "high risk" receive a transfusion* preoperatively. High risk is determined by their history of frequent crises or acute chest syndrome and by the type of procedure to be done. When transfusions are not routinely performed, the highest incidence of perioperative complications occur in patients having thoracotomies, laparotomies, and tonsillectomies.

The question of simple transfusion to Hb ≥ 10 versus exchange transfusion to Hb ≥ 10 and HbS <30% is still unanswered. The incidence of serious complications is similar in the two groups. Both groups may develop acute chest syndrome. Those who receive a preoperative exchange transfusion may have a higher incidence of transfusion-related complications compared with the conservative transfusion group. Further recommendations are awaiting studies that may indicate an advantage of one technique over the others.

The issue of preoperative transfusion is as clear as mud, and most transfusion policies are institutionally determined (i.e., "that's the way we've always done it"). To be safe, one should consult with his or her hematologist before anesthetizing any patient with SS disease. A rational discussion with the hematologist and the surgeon will allow for a plan that is mutually agreed upon, taking all factors into account.

Premedication. In children with SS disease, heavy premedication that may depress respirations is not a good idea in an unmonitored setting without supplemental oxygen. An anxiolytic agent such as oral midazolam is reasonable if it is indicated and can be given 15 to 20 minutes before surgery **(see Chapter 16)**.

Induction and Maintenance. Although there is no ideal anesthetic technique for children with SS disease, complications may be minimized by following these recommendations:

- Avoid hypotension.
- Avoid hypoxemia.
- Avoid hypothermia.
- Avoid hypovolemia.

Inpatients may be hydrated preoperatively. Since more of these patients come in on the day of surgery, however, preoperative IV hydration is usually not an option. Surgery for these patients should be done early in the day to avoid a long fast, and they (like other children scheduled for surgery) may have clear liquids up until 2 to 3 hours before surgery. After an IV is started, a fluid bolus of 10 to 15 ml/kg will help to avoid potential early problems with hypovolemia. At least 40% to 50% oxygen should be delivered intraoperatively. Oxygen (100%) should be delivered before extubation, and the patient should be transported to the postanesthesia care unit with oxygen by face mask. If the patient is to be admitted postoperatively, oxygen by face mask or nasal cannula should be continued for 24 hours. The operating room should be warmed, and usual methods for heat conservation should be undertaken.

Use of Tourniquets

The issue of whether tourniquets may be used on extremities is controversial. Patients with SS disease who have limb tourniquets applied intraoperatively may experience complications or crisis but this is not so in every case.

Regional Anesthesia

Some textbooks discourage the use of spinal anesthesia because of the potential for hypotension and decreased tissue perfusion. By contrast, other experts are now reporting success with epidural blockade to improve oxygenation and perfusion in children experiencing crises. In addition, it is important for children with SS disease to have adequate analgesia postoperatively; therefore, regional analgesia with neuraxial narcotics or local anesthetics may be beneficial. In the final analysis, if the aforementioned recommendations are followed, regional anesthesia may be useful for perioperative analgesia.

Monitoring Volume Status

Urine output may not be a reliable indicator of volume status, because the kidney cannot concentrate. For major operations with large blood and fluid requirements, a central venous catheter to monitor filling pressure may be indicated.

Outpatient Management

Outpatient management of patients with SS disease is becoming common practice. When surgery has been minimally invasive, patients may be discharged after the patient appears fully recovered, is adequately hydrated, has no nausea or vomiting, and has oxygen-hemoglobin saturation >95% on room air (or is back to baseline values). If the patient requires large quantities of analgesics to control pain, overnight observation with supplemental oxygen may be indicated.

HEMOPHILIA

Pathophysiology

Hemophilia is caused by hereditary factor VIII (hemophilia A) or factor IX (hemophilia B) deficiency. Both are X-linked recessive traits and therefore affect only males. There is, however, *marked variability in the severity* of the disease.

- Patients with less than 1% of normal factor activity are considered to have *severe* disease.
- Patients with 1% to 5% activity have *moderate* disease.
- Patients with 5% to 25% activity have *mild* disease.

Patients with severe involvement often present early in life, perhaps with excessive bleeding associated with circumcision. Toddlers present with oral bleeding, superficial hemarthroses, and intramuscular hemorrhages. When the child with hemophilia is 4 to 5 years of age, hemarthroses are the predominant presentations. Intracranial hemorrhage is the leading cause of death among those with hemophilia, with a mortality rate of 50%. Surgery and dental extractions can cause significant bleeding even in those with mild involvement.

Anesthetic Management

Preoperative Assessment

History. Usually, the family knows how severe the disease is, how often bleeds occur, what type of factor replacement and how much is needed for usual "bleeds," and where venous access is usually obtained. Some children have central venous access such as Portacaths for frequent transfusion therapy. There is a high incidence of HIV infection in hemophiliacs who were transfused in the early 1980s before the routine screening of blood. Most families know the HIV status of their children.

Physical Examination. There is generally nothing unusual about the physical examination unless major bleeds have recently occurred. The usual good evaluation should be performed, paying close attention to venous access sites.

Laboratory Studies. Although the partial thromboplastin time (PTT) may be elevated, this is not particularly helpful information. More importantly, one must know the factor VIII (or in the case of hemophilia B, factor IX) activity preoperatively. About 10% of hemophiliacs develop inhibitors. Therefore, an assay should be performed if there has been a previous history of inhibitor deficiency.

Factor Replacement. The hematologist should be consulted regarding factor replacement before you proceed. Factor activity should be at least 50% and ideally 100% before surgery begins. Requirements differ for factors VIII and IX (Table 10).

Often patients are given a bolus of factor to increase activity to a desired level preoperatively, and a continuous infusion may be used intra- and postoperatively. Factor replacement may continue for several days after the surgical procedure.

Anesthetic Technique

To prevent hematoma formation, no intramuscular injections are allowed. Also to prevent bleeding complications, nasal intubations and manipulations are avoided, even after factor has been given unless absolutely necessary. Severe nosebleeds can be precipitated. Analgesics other than acetylsalicylic acid (aspirin) or nonsteroidal anti-inflammatory drugs (NSAIDs) should be used to control postoperative pain.

Regional Anesthesia

Although successful axillary blocks without complications have been reported and although peripheral blocks are unlikely to cause problems after correction of factor deficiencies, central blocks such as caudals, spinals, and epidurals would have more serious sequelae if bleeding occurred. Therefore, their use is controversial, even after factor replacement.

TRISOMY 21: DOWN'S SYNDROME

Children with trisomy 21 (Down's syndrome) have abnormalities of multiple organ systems and can present for a multitude of surgical procedures. Knowing the potential for problems can potentially avert major disasters (Table 11).

Respiratory Tract/Airway

Because of a relative immunodeficiency, children with Down's syndrome have a

TABLE 10. *Factor replacement requirements*

Factor	Half-life	% increase/U[a]/kg
VIII	8–12 h	2
IX	24 h	0.5–1

[a]Ed. Note (JMB): A unit of activity is defined as the activity of 1 ml of plasma. Recombinant factor therapy given rather than pooled donor factor or FFP has significantly decreased infectious complications related to repeated transfusions. Newer still are agents being developed to counteract the inhibitors.

TABLE 11. *Anesthetic Implications of Down's syndrome*

Systemic findings	Implications
Respiratory: large tongue, frequent upper respiratory infections, subglottic stenosis or small trachea, big tonsil, obstructive sleep apnea	Difficult intubation; prone to airway obstruction; several endotracheal tube sizes should be available
Cardiac: congenital defects; prone to pulmonary hypertension	SBE prophylaxis; cardiology consultation if disease is present, but not adequately assessed and treated
Endocrine: hypothyroidism; low circulating catecholamine levels	Older patients may need thyroid replacement.
Gastrointestinal: duodenal atresia and Hirschprung's disease common	Rapid-sequence induction if bowel obstruction is present.
Central nervous system: various degrees of mental retardation	Often pleasant and cooperative, especially younger patients; intramuscular ketamine in less cooperative patients
Musculoskeletal: lax muscles and ligaments; atlantoaxial instability possible	Less muscle relaxant needed; stabilize neck during anesthesia; inform surgeons of issue during positioning

SBE, subacute bacterial endocarditis.

propensity for URIs. In addition, they may have airway obstruction secondary to lax pharyngeal tone, large tongue, adenotonsillar hypertrophy, and crowding of the midfacial structures. These children may also have subglottic stenosis and therefore may require smaller endotracheal tubes.

Cardiovascular System

Approximately 40% to 60% of children with Down's syndrome have associated cardiac anomalies (Table 12)

Endocrine System

Children with Down's syndrome have an increased incidence of congenital hypothyroidism that may or may not be detectable by history and physical examination.

TABLE 12. *Cardiovascular defects in children with Down's syndrome*

Cardiac defects	Percentage
Endocardial cushion defects	40
Ventricular septal defect	27
Patent ductus arteriosus	12
Tetrology of Fallot	8
Atrial septal defect/pulmonary hypertension/others	13

Gastrointestinal System

Duodenal atresia and Hirschsprung's disease are frequently seen in children with Down's syndrome and often are the cause of surgery in the neonatal period.

Central Nervous System

Although some degree of mental retardation is present in all children with Down's syndrome, the degree is extremely variable. As a general rule, these children are very friendly and cooperative.

Musculoskeletal System

Muscle and ligament tone is extremely lax and contributes to strabismus and atlantoaxial instability. Approximately 15% of Down's children <21 years of age will have atlantoaxial instability, although almost all are asymptomatic. Therefore, these children, with or without symptomatic instability of the cervical spine, require careful airway management **(see also page 276).**

Anesthetic Management

Preoperative Assessment

History. Associated anomalies should be identified. In noncardiac cases, one should ask about cardiac disease and, if present, ask what has been done and who follows the child on a routine basis. It should be ascertained whether the child snores loudly, has trouble breathing at night, or has gait problems. The parents should be asked about the results of the most recent cervical spine radiographs. Many of the older children compete in the Special Olympics and are required to have cervical spine films to participate.

Physical Examination. The airway is carefully examined. Is the tongue very large? Is the neck very short? Is there a murmur that no one has recognized? The extremities are examined for possible venous and arterial access problems. Because of the laxity of tissues, IV lines in these children can be a real challenge.

Laboratory Data. There are no routine laboratory tests for children with Down's syndrome. Laboratory tests are ordered according to what is needed for the procedure and the patient's condition. *Routine flexion and extension neck films are not necessary unless neurologic signs or symptoms are present.* Unfortunately, radiographic data is not very reliable in definition or prediction of problems in these children.

Anesthetic Technique

Children should not be heavily sedated in an unmonitored setting, because they may develop airway obstruction. If the airway looks as if it might be problematic, atropine or glycopyrrolate may be given early (as soon as the IV goes in, or intramuscularly, if needed). Prophylaxis against subacute bacterial endocarditis is given to children with congenital heart defects, when indicated **(see Chapter 12)**. Many pediatric anesthesiologists administer the required antibiotics after induction when the IV is placed. There is no optimal induction technique. On one hand, venous access may prove difficult; on the other hand, an inhalation technique might lead to airway obstruction. Therefore, one does what one does best! An appropriate endotracheal tube for the size of the patient is chosen. If the child is particularly small for age, scale down a half-size from the usual (usual = age in years divided by 4 + 4 for toddlers and up). As long as there is a leak around the endotracheal tube at <30 cm H_2O, postintubation croup should not be a problem. If the child has atlanto-occipital instability, manipulation of the neck becomes an issue. Some clinicians perform a fiberoptic intubation, and some perform an awake intubation in this clinical scenario. Realistically, either of these may not be feasible in an uncooperative child. Common sense dictates that even in the asymptomatic patient, neck stability should be maintained during intubation, and abnormal head positions should be avoided during surgery. Hypersensitivity to atropine in children with Down's syndrome is a myth; give it when indicated in the usual doses.

LATEX ALLERGY

Latex allergy is a reaction to latex exposure that varies from contact dermatitis to full-blown anaphylaxis. The following are clinical signs of latex allergy:

- Increased vascular permeability (urticaria and laryngeal edema)
- Contraction of smooth muscle (bronchospasm)
- Vasodilatation (flushing and hypotension)
- Stimulation of sensory nerve endings (pruritus)
- Cardiac histamine receptor stimulation (tachycardia and arrhythmias)

The following groups are at risk for developing latex allergy:

1. Children with neural tube defects (e.g., meningomyelocele, spina bifida, and congenital urologic anomalies).
2. Patients with a history of atopy. Children with a banana, chestnut, or avocado allergy suggest a protein cross-reactivity with latex.
3. Health care workers.

Most health care workers and those with occupational exposure exhibit a type 4, T-cell–mediated, delayed hypersensitivity allergic reaction. Although this sounds complex, it usually means only *contact dermatitis* and is often related to the additives in latex products.

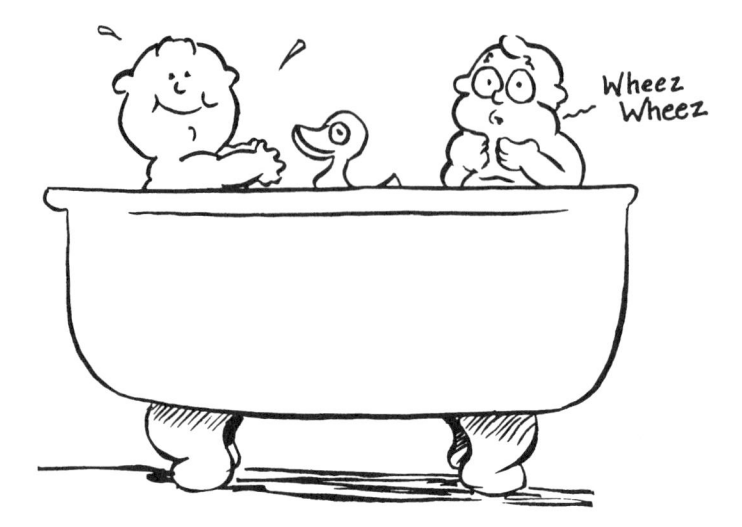

The more worrisome reaction is a type 1 IgE-mediated anaphylactic reaction. This reaction requires previous antigen exposure, as many children with congenital anomalies have had. After latex exposure in susceptible children, the symptoms of latex anaphylaxis present typically within 30 minutes following induction of anesthesia, but the onset of symptoms has been reported from 5 to 290 minutes. The manifestations of a latex allergic reaction can vary from mild flushing to cardiovascular collapse.

Anesthetic Management

Preoperative Assessment

History. Preoperative diagnosis usually is made by a history of balloon or glove intolerance or allergies to medical products (e.g,. urinary catheters). Other factors associated with latex allergy include the following:

- History of asthma
- Allergy to rubber
- Allergy to food products (especially bananas and avocados)
- Rash caused by adhesive tape
- Daily rectal disimpaction
- Nine or more previous surgeries
- Elevated total IgE levels

Children with spina bifida are routinely tested for latex allergy. If a child tests negative for latex allergy, it does not necessarily mean that he or she will not develop an allergy during subsequent procedures. By contrast, a positive result will help the clinician to know when to avoid latex.

Physical Examination. There are very few physical findings that will help in the detection of latex allergy. Signs or symptoms of an allergic reaction after application of a latex containing tourniquet may be an early "tip-off."

Laboratory Data. If latex allergy is suspected and testing is indicated, three tests can be done:

- The *skin prick test* is sensitive, cheap, and fast. It involves putting a piece of latex glove in sterile saline for up to 24 hours and placing a drop of solution on the patient's arm to make a skin patch. The disadvantage of this test is that it can precipitate an anaphylactic reaction in someone who is extremely sensitive.
- The RAST (radioallergosorbent test) is less sensitive and may take 2 to 8 weeks

to obtain. However, it is safe for the patient.
- The LAST (latex allergosorbent test) avoids radioisotopes and can be performed in less than 6 hours.

Anesthetic Technique

Preoperative Preparation. Although there is controversy about pretreating patients with histamine (H_1 and H_2) blockers and corticosteroids if the patient has a previous history of anaphylaxis, the following premedication may be indicated:

- IV premedication
  - Diphenhydramine (Benadryl) 1 mg/kg
  - Methylprednisolone (Solumedrol) 1 mg/kg
  - Ranitidine (Zantac) 0.5–1 mg/kg
- Oral premedication
  - Diphenhydramine (Benadryl) 1 mg/kg
  - Prednisone 1 mg/kg
  - Ranitidine 1 to 2 mg/kg

For patients at high risk for latex allergy who have no previous history of allergic reaction, there is no consensus on how aggressively to avoid latex in the operating room. Clearly, the most antigenic substance in the operating room is powdered latex gloves. Other sources of latex allergens are less likely to be problematic in patients with no history of allergic responses. The decision to make the operating room latex-free for those with no history of an allergic reaction is institutionally determined at this time.

For those with a history suggestive of latex allergy, full latex precautions (e.g., avoid latex products) must be taken. The biggest problem is knowing which products are latex-free. Nonlatex alternatives for the operative setting, however, are readily available. *Safe* products in the operating room include the following:

- Vinyl and neoprene gloves
- Tape—Microfoam, Durapore
- Dressings—Tegaderm and Steri-Strips
- Catheters—Malecot catheters
  - Silicone Foley catheters
- Jelco and Deseret IV catheters
- Steridrapes
- Nellcore sensors
- Silicone IV sets
- Red dot ECG electrodes

Nonsafe products for the latex allergy patient include the following:

- Latex gloves
- Catheters—red rubber
- Tape—Band-Aids, paper tape, cloth adhesive
- Dressings—Micropore

Latex precautions in the operating room include the following:

- Use nonlatex gloves (most important).
- If latex-free IV tubing is unavailable, use stopcocks and tape over latex ports.
- Avoid multidose vials; remove top or draw up through 22-µ filter; use glass vials whenever possible.
- Wrap blood pressure connecting tube with webril.
- Use Velcro tourniquets.
- Avoid histamine-releasing drugs.
- Use neoprene bellows for the Ohmeda ventilator; if not available, use gas flows <10 l/min and consider washing ventilator bellows bag or using circuit filter.
- Place sign on operating room door that patient is allergic to latex.
- A latex allergy cart can be very helpful, which should include:
  - Glass syringes
  - Drugs in glass ampules

- IV tubing without latex injection ports
- Neoprene reservoir bags
- Webril
- Neoprene gloves
- Ambu bags with silicone valves
- Neoprene bellows for ventilator

Diagnosis of Latex Anaphylaxis

Onset of latex anaphylaxis is generally 20 to 60 minutes after exposure to the antigen (range 5 to 290 minutes). It usually presents as a clinical triad: (a) hypotension (most common), (b) rash, and (c) bronchospasm.

Treatment of Intraoperative Anaphylaxis

The following are recommendations for treatment of anaphylaxis:

- Think of it! (i.e., keep an open mind as to the possibility of anaphylaxis)
- Use 100% O_2.
- Discontinue anesthetics, blood, and antibiotic infusions.
- Withdraw antigen.
- Give epinephrine, 0.5 to 5 µg/kg IV bolus; infusion of 1 to 4 µg/kg/min may be required.
- Carry out volume resuscitation 10 to 20 ml/kg.
- Give diphenhydramine, 0.5 to 1 mg/kg IV bolus.
- Give ranitidine 1 mg/kg IV.
- Administer corticosteroids: methylprednisolone 1 to 2 mg/kg up to 1 to 2 g.
- Give albuterol if needed to treat wheezing.
- Give sodium bicarbonate, 0.5 to 1 mg/kg, for persistent hypotension and acidosis.
- Inspect airway before extubation; check for air leak.

Watch out for red herrings!

Note that antibiotic or muscle relaxant allergies can be present in the latex-allergic patient.

NEUROBLASTOMA

Neuroblastomas are the most common solid tumor in infancy and the third most common malignancy in children. Patients with these tumors often present before 2 years of age; 25% of the tumors are congenital. Because neuroblastomas are derived from embryonic tissue of neural crest origin, they may occur anywhere along the sympathetic nervous system. Although most frequently in the retroperitoneal space, neuroblastomas are also found in the neck, mediastinum, pelvis, and along the paraspinal sympathetic ganglia. The most common presentation consists of signs or symptoms related to a mass effect. Very few children present with symptoms of increased catecholamine secretion, although most have elevated levels in urine or serum. Neuroblastomas tend to metastasize early and are found in lymph nodes, bone marrow, liver, and skin. Metastatic disease is managed primarily with chemotherapy, followed by surgical resection of the primary tumor. The best outcomes occur with complete surgical removal of the tumor. Intraoperative hypertension and tachycardia are rare (<3%), but tachycardia alone may be seen with tumor manipulation in these patients. In addition, about 50% of children with neuroblastoma experience hypotension after removal of the tumor, which will resolve with blood and fluid therapy.

Anesthetic Management

Preoperative Assessment

History. The type of presentation largely determines what questions to ask. For example, in the case of a thoracic tumor, one should ask if the child has a history of respiratory distress. (This is uncommon, since neuroblastomas are usually in the posterior mediastinum.) Is there a history of flushing, diarrhea, diaphoresis, or hypertension? Affirmative answers to these questions indicate increased catecholamine secretion. One should ask about bone pain and gait disturbance. These symptoms suggest lower extremity involvement or spinal canal involvement.

Physical Examination. The child may have hepatomegaly if metastatic liver involvement has occurred. Petechiae can be an indication of bone marrow involvement. There may be skin involvement appearing as blue subcutaneous nodules ("blueberry muffins"). In addition to a thorough physical examination, one must note the vital signs; tachycardia and hypertension herald the potential for hemodynamic instability intraoperatively. Significant hypertension that is present preoperatively should be treated before surgery.

Laboratory Data. A 24-hour collection of urine for catecholamine levels will assist in making the diagnosis of neuroblastoma. A preoperative CBC is indicated because anemia, leukopenia, and thrombocytopenia all may be present as a result of bone marrow involvement. Preoperative evaluation usually includes CT scan or MRI of the chest or abdomen to document the extent of the tumor. These should be reviewed preoperatively to understand the site of the surgical procedure and how involved it will be. Depending on the extent of the procedure, cross-matched blood should be available.

Anesthetic Technique

If an IV line is present, an IV induction with pentothal or propofol is appropriate. In the absence of an IV, an inhalation induction may be done if it is not contraindicated (e.g., in the presence of large abdominal mass with risk for regurgitation). Maintenance is most easily accomplished with a volatile anesthetic that does not sensitize the myocardium to dysrhythmias. Although isoflurane has historically been the agent of choice, sevoflurane with its hemodynamic stability, lack of sensitization, and low solubility allowing rapid changes in concentration may be a better choice. Halothane with its dysrhythmogenic potential and desflurane with its tendency to cause hypertension and tachycardia at higher concentrations would not be the best choices.

Depending on the surgical site, regional analgesia for postoperative pain control is certainly an option. If abdominal or thoracic surgery is planned, continuous epidural analgesia would provide good pain control. Monitors for the procedure should include the usual noninvasive monitors. In addition, if the tumor is large or there is reason to suspect hemodynamic instability, an arterial line should be placed. A second IV line is indicated for potentially big operations; the IVs should be in the upper extremities if the inferior vena cava will be compressed during the operation. Although it is uncommon, the potential for hypertension and tachycardia exists, and one should be prepared to use esmolol and nitroprusside if it occurs. After the tumor is removed, one should be prepared to administer fluid volume. If hypotension continues, a vasopressor such as phenylephrine or dopamine may be needed.

WILMS' TUMOR/NEPHROBLASTOMA

Wilms' tumor is the most common childhood abdominal malignancy. The incidence is about 1 in 15,000 live births. It may be associated with aniridia, hemihypertrophy, genitourinary anomalies, neurofibromatosis, and Beckwith-Wiedemann syndrome. Affected children usually present with an abdominal mass before the age of 5 years.

Once the abdominal tumor is identified, further workup to include chest CT, MRI of the abdomen and pelvis, and renal ultrasonography is performed. This confirms the kidney as the site of origin, demonstrates renal vein and inferior vena cava involvement, scans for pulmonary metastases, and determines whether the contralateral kidney is involved. When surgical excision is complete and there is only regional extension or no extension of the tumor, 4-year survival rate after surgery and chemotherapy is greater than 90%. Some children with more extensive nephroblastomas may also require radiation therapy.

Anesthetic Management

"My veins are filled, once a week with a neopolitan carpet cleaner distilled from the Adriatic and I am bald as an egg. However, I still get around and am mean to cats."
—John Cheever
(1982, concerning his cancer treatment)

Preoperative Assessment

History. Most children with Wilms' tumor are otherwise fairly healthy, and routine questions should be asked of the parents. Sometimes diagnosis is delayed until the tumor is large, and gastrointestinal symptoms of fullness or obstruction may be present. History of chemotherapy or radiation therapy should be ascertained. Doxorubicin (Adriamycin) is often used and can cause cardiac toxicity when the total dose exceeds 300 mg/m^2. A child who has received cardiotoxic chemotherapy has usually had follow-up echocardiograms to evaluate function. The parents can often tell you when the last echocardiogram was done and what the results were.

Physical Examination. The child with a large abdominal mass should be examined in the usual fashion. It is critically important that no one palpates the child's abdomen with great zest and fervor, since there is the potential for rupture of a tense tumor. If preexcision rupture occurs, the prognosis worsens considerably.

Laboratory Data. It is important for the anesthesiologist to know the results of the preoperative workup. The location and extent of tumor involvement should give an indication of the magnitude of the operation. The abdominal MRI should be checked to see whether inferior vena cava extension exists. If present, the case may be fraught with major blood loss. The chest CT will indicate whether pulmonary metastases are present, which might (although not usually) become clinically significant. A CBC and a type and cross-match for packed red blood cells should be performed preoperatively.

Anesthetic Technique

The child with a very large abdominal mass may be a candidate for a rapid-sequence induction if some degree of stomach or bowel compression exists. After the child is anesthetized and intubated, one should secure good venous access, ideally in the upper extremities when the inferior vena cava is involved. Many of these children will receive Broviac catheters or other types of central lines for long-term chemotherapy during the initial anesthetic procedure. If these are done before tumor resection, they provide valuable vascular access for the major procedure. A continuous epidural for postoperative analgesia can be placed after induction or before emergence in children having major abdominal procedures. This is optional. The maintenance technique should be tailored to the child's medical condition. It is the rare case in which the patient would not be extubated at the end of surgery.

PRUNE-BELLY SYNDROME

Although the name "prune-belly syndrome" has been given to this constellation of congenital anomalies, the deficient abdominal musculature that gives the prune-belly appearance is only one manifestation of the primary abnormality: *in utero* urethral obstruction. Urethral obstruction malformation complex is a more appropriate name to describe the cause and pathophysiology of prune-belly syndrome (19–27). Urethral obstruction may cause two significant derangements *in utero:* bladder distention and the oligohydramnios deformation complex. Bladder distention interferes mechanically with the development of surrounding tissues, producing the other characteristic alterations of prune-belly syndrome that may be present in varying degrees: bladder wall hypertrophy, hydroureter and associated renal dysplasia, abdominal distention leading to abdominal muscle deficiency, and excess skin, cryptorchidism, persistent urachus, chest deformity, lack of accessory muscles of respiration, colon malrotation, and iliac vessel compression leading to a lower limb deficiency (19,20).

Because amniotic fluid is essential for pulmonary development (21), inadequate fetal urinary output secondary to urethral obstruction and the resultant oligohydramnios can lead to congenital pulmonary hypoplasia (19). Oligohydramnios may also result in fetal compression causing limb defects and Potter facies, characterized by micrognathia and malformed ears and nose (19).

Prune-belly syndrome is rare; the incidence is estimated to be 1 in 50,000 births. The mortality rate may approach 50% before age 2 years, depending on the type and severity of abnormalities. Males are affected 20 times more often than females owing to transmission by superficial X-linkage mimicry (22). Distinguishing features of *in utero* diagnosis by ultrasonography include the presence of fetal ascites, distended bladder, and cystic masses, as well as maternal oligohydramnios (23,24). Fetal surgical decompression of urinary tract obstruction has been attempted (25). Although this procedure prevented abdominal wall laxity, it apparently was too late to prevent severe pulmonary and renal involvement (25).

Preoperative Evaluation

The anesthetic considerations for children with prune-belly syndrome must focus on the renal and pulmonary systems (26). The weak or absent abdominal muscles, chest deformity, outward flaring of the ribs, and lack of accessory muscles of respiration may lead to atelectasis, recurrent respiratory infection, and reduced expiratory effort. The infant with prune-belly syndrome may have little or no ability to cough. Although elective surgery should be rescheduled if the child has a significant pulmonary infection, many of these children are never totally free of respiratory disease. Preoperative antibiotic treatment and chest physiotherapy may be indicated if surgery cannot be delayed.

Evaluation of the child's pulmonary status includes a careful history, physical examination, and chest radiographs. Pulmonary function test would be of limited accuracy and value in this child. The history and physical examination may reveal cyanosis, respiratory distress, fever, nasal flaring, cough, difficulty feeding, and wheezing. The chest radiographs may reveal poor inspiratory effort, changes consistent with a chronic disease such as peribronchiolar thickening, and acute changes indicative of an infectious process.

Preoperative evaluation of renal function will dictate NPO orders (nothing by mouth) and intraoperative fluid and electrolyte management. The blood urea nitrogen (BUN) concentration of 50 mg/dl may reflect either dehydration or chronic renal insufficiency. Further evaluation of renal function including determination of serum electrolytes, creatinine, and urine specific gravity is indicated. With chronic obstructive nephropathy, the outer cortical nephrons are relatively spared and maintain their glomerular filtration rate, whereas juxtamedullary nephrons are markedly impaired (27). As a result, the ability to concentrate urine may be lost and obligate urine flow results.

The clinical implications of this type of renal tubular dysfunction and failure to reabsorb water and electrolytes may affect the anesthetic management. A history of polydipsia ("he drinks a lot"), constant voiding ("his diapers are always wet"), and dilute urine suggest that tubular reabsorption is deficient. If so, the child may be dehydrated and at risk for further dehydration during the NPO interval. If the child is dehydrated, the case should be postponed until appropriate fluid replacement is administered. If the child's state of hydration is adequate, oral intake of clear fluids such as water, apple juice, or electrolyte glucose solution (e.g., Pedialyte) should be encouraged until 3 hours before the scheduled surgery (28). If the child has renal tubular dysfunction, characterized by obligate urinary loss, IV fluids should be administered during the NPO interval to replace urinary loss and minimize dehydration. A maintenance fluid such as 5% dextrose in 0.25 normal saline should be administered at a rate of 4 ml/kg/hour. In the absence of renal disease, administration of IV fluids is not needed unless surgery is delayed or IV access is required for antibiotic administration.

A hemoglobin concentration of 11 g/dl with a hematocrit of 33% in a 10-month-old infant may indicate mild anemia, presumably due to renal disease. If the child is dehydrated, he or she may be hemoconcentrated and more anemic than these values indicate.

Preoperative sedation has been discouraged by previous authors for fear of respiratory depression (29). Recently, the use of oral midazolam as a preoperative sedative has gained wide acceptance and is not associated with prolonged recovery or respiratory depression (30). If this child were a few months older, separation anxiety might be a factor and midazolam, 0.5 mg/kg, could be given orally despite pulmonary sedation. Anticholinergic agents can be administered intravenously at the time of induction. If urodynamic studies were planned, anticholinergic agents would be contraindicated because they can interfere with smooth muscle contraction.

Anesthetic Technique

Anesthesia may be induced intravenously with a butterfly technique if an IV cannula is not in place; or, an inhalation induction can be performed (see Chapter 2). Anesthesia may be maintained with 65% nitrous oxide with 35% oxygen and isoflurane, 0.5% to 2%, using controlled ventilation. Intraoperative monitoring of airway pressure, tidal volume, end-tidal CO_2, and pulse oximetry are indicated. Muscle relaxants are not required because the abdominal musculature is lax. Avoiding muscle relaxants eliminates one of the possibilities of postoperative hypoventilation. For the same reason, opioid agents should not be administered.

Intraoperative fluid management is dependent on fluid and electrolyte status and renal function. In the absence of renal disease or electrolyte imbalance, maintenance fluids can be continued at 4 ml/kg/hour and fluid deficits from the NPO interval replaced in the first hour of surgery. Fluid loss related to surgery should be negligible in this case.

If a combined regional technique and general anesthesia is the clinician's preferred procedure for management of postoperative pain, it should not be withheld in these patients.

If the child has no or minimal pulmonary involvement, he or she may be extubated at the end of the procedure in the operating room. However, if significant pulmonary pathology was present preoperatively or if signs of pulmonary disease such as copious secretions, oxyhemoglobin desaturation, or poor compliance were evident intraoperatively, extubation should be delayed until the patient is vigorous and demonstrates adequate ventilatory exchange, both clinically and with pulse oximetry. After extubation, the child should be placed in a humidified hood or croup tent for 24 to 36 hours. If pulmonary involvement is significant, chest physical therapy may be indicated.

OSTEOGENESIS IMPERFECTA

Osteogenesis imperfecta is a rare, hereditary disease of bone that occurs in about 1 in 30,000 live births. It was originally classified on the basis of presentation at birth or early infancy as osteogenesis imperfecta congenita, or as osteogenesis imperfecta tarda when patients presented later in childhood. The current classification includes four major classes based on the clinical profile (31). Because the common underlying defect appears to be a quantitative or qualitative defect of collagen formation, there is a burgeoning literature attempting to correlate the four clinical classes and specific genetic defects (32).

Clinical Manifestations

Children with type I osteogenesis imperfecta, the most common type, present with bone fragility, hearing loss, blue sclerae, and autosomal dominant inheritance. Type II is characterized by severe, life-threatening fractures, is possibly autosomal recessive, and is usually associated with fetal or early neonatal demise. Type III is also marked by severe skeletal deformities, autosomal recessive inheritance, and poor prognosis, although not as severe as type II. Children with type IV osteogenesis imperfecta present with bone fragility of variable severity, rare hearing loss, and autosomal dominant inheritance. These subtypes are broad guidelines to symptomatology, and there is wide individual variation in clinical presentation, even within families.

The principal characteristic of osteogenesis imperfecta is osteoporotic bones that fracture easily, sometimes with trivial trauma. The fractures classically are transverse and subperiosteal, often without much displacement. Because weight-bearing, by itself, can cause the fractures, the long bones often show evidence of repeated fractures and consequent bowing. Kyphoscoliosis is common and may be severe enough to inhibit ventilation enough to cause cor pulmonale. Rib fractures can also contribute to restrictive chest wall defects. Because of the long bone and spinal abnormalities, these patients have a shortened stature. Fractures of the skull and face are also distinctive, with mandibular fractures being common and facial bone fractures rare. The skull is often a mosaic of bone islands, with frontal bossing and an overhanging occiput. This "helmet head" deformity functionally acts to flex the neck at rest.

Other aspects of connective tissue are also involved in osteogenesis imperfecta. There can be considerable laxity of the joints, thin skin, and fragility of the tendons. Umbilical and inguinal hernias are relatively common in patients with osteogenesis imperfecta. Of particular interest during airway maneuvers is the teeth. Teeth in affected patients tend to be discolored, misshapen, and very brittle, fracturing easily with minor trauma. Patients can also have cardiac lesions such as atrial or ventricular septal defects, mitral insufficiency, and aortic insufficiency. There have also been reports of a higher incidence of cleft palate, hydrocephalus, and premature arteriosclerosis.

Another area of interest to anesthesiologists is the potential for bleeding disorders. In some patients with osteogenesis imperfecta, there is platelet dysfunction secondary to decreased release of platelet factor 3. Although the platelet count is normal, platelet adhesiveness is diminished.

Hyperthermia in children with osteogenesis imperfecta has raised concern about malignant hyperthermia (MH) in these patients. Some patients with osteogenesis imperfecta appear to have hyperthermia and hyperhidrosis during general anesthesia that is not the same as in MH syndrome (33). The signs disappear with discontinuation of the anesthetic and surface cooling. Both abnormal central nervous system control of temperature and abnormal cellular metabolism have been suggested. Some investigators have found elevated serum thyroxine levels, increased oxygen consumption, and elevated temperatures in these patients and have postulated that there is a generalized metabolic disturbance in some children with osteogenesis imperfecta (34). Several patients have had severe metabolic acidosis on induction, although not the classic picture of MH (35). Patients with both osteogenesis imperfecta and MH, or a clinical event that could be interpreted as such, have also been reported (36). This has led to controversy about the potential for MH in patients with osteogenesis imperfecta; others feel that the evidence is not adequate to support this and that the occurrence of both osteogenesis imperfecta and MH in the same patient is coincidental (37,38). There is not a large body of evidence supporting a strong relation between osteogenesis imperfecta and MH, although future studies may change this.

Orthopedic management of osteogenesis imperfecta has become aggressive (31). In the past, simple splinting was the primary treatment for fractures. Currently, a balanced approach of casting, bracing, physical therapy, and surgery is used for treatment of fractures, straightening of limbs, and strengthening of muscle mass to prevent fractures. Patients now come to the operating room for a variety of both elective and urgent procedures to stabilize long bones. There has been great interest in a variety of hormonal and pharmacologic modalities to strengthen bone and minimize fractures. Agents have included fluoride, vitamin D, calcitonin, and various gonadal hormones. However, there has yet to appear a pharmacologic agent that successfully improves these patients and their defects.

Anesthetic Management

Preoperative Assessment

History. A careful history is oriented toward the patient's skeletal system and past fractures. The amount of trauma necessary to cause a fracture is useful information when handling the child since there is wide individual variation. Also, a history of vertebral fractures will encourage obtaining preoperative cervical films to evaluate stability and the presence of deformities. A history of ventilatory problems or recurrent pneumonia may be an indication of significant rib cage and spinal deformities. Exercise tolerance in the older child may give useful information about the progression of the child's disability and cardiopulmonary reserve.

Physical Examination. Physical examination is also oriented to the skeletal system. Special attention is placed on examination of the head and neck. It is important to note the normal, comfortable position of the head at rest, the ability to open the mouth, any instability of the mandible, and the flexibility and range of motion of the cervical spine. During the chest examination, it is important to detect any evidence of pulmonary or cardiac disease. Previously undiagnosed murmurs should be evaluated before elective surgery. If there are signs of ventilatory impairment from kyphoscoliosis, rib fractures, or other thoracic cage deformities, pulmonary function testing is indicated.

Laboratory Data. Testing is largely determined by the history and physical examination. As already mentioned, pulmonary function testing is indicated if there is a history of recurrent respiratory difficulties or if the physical examination reveals severe bony abnormalities. Chest radiography is performed if there is a question of an acute pulmonic process versus chronic changes. If there is a history of easy bruisability or bleeding, obtaining a bleeding time and coagulation profile is indicated.

Anesthetic Technique

Premedication. There is no specific indication or contraindication for premedicants in these patients outside of the normal precautions for chronically ill children. Older literature suggests avoidance of atropine because of a tendency to decrease heat dissipation, but this has never been clearly demonstrated. Children with osteogenesis imperfecta are usually not retarded and are appropriate in their reactions and fears. Older children are aware of their deformities and the various reactions these provoke in people. A calm, understanding approach to these children is necessary to reassure them and help them through the perioperative period. If sedation is indicated, it should be given.

Positioning. Extreme care must be taken in positioning the patient. In particularly severe cases, movements as benign as changing a diaper have resulted in femoral fractures. Therefore, great care must be taken in moving and positioning the patient and all pressure points generously padded. In some cases, the patient's kyphoscoliosis or hydrocephalus may result in abnormal postures requiring support on the operating table in the form of blankets or towels. Tourniquets for facilitating vascular access or preventing blood loss must be applied carefully, if at all. There is a single case report of central retinal artery occlusion in a prone patient with the confounding variable of deliberate hypotension (39). Care should be taken to avoid external pressure on the eyes if the patient is in the prone position.

Monitoring. Children with osteogenesis imperfecta are monitored in the same fashion as other children for anesthesia and surgery. Careful padding under the blood pressure cuff and anywhere else there is pressure on the patient's body will decrease the risk of fractures or abrasion of the thin skin. Although some have suggested eschewing the use of a blood pressure cuff to avoid the possibility of fracture, there is little evidence that this is necessary.

Induction. There are no specific contraindications to anesthetic agents, with one possible exception (33). It is usually recommended that succinylcholine be avoided, if possible, to eliminate the risk of fasciculation-induced fractures. Although there have not been a large number of reported incidents demonstrating the danger of succinylcholine, it is reasonable to substitute a nondepolarizing relaxant, if clinically applicable.

There are many reasonable methods of anesthetic management for patients with osteogenesis imperfecta. If there are questions about the airway, inhalation induction with halothane and nitrous oxide-oxygen will allow evaluation of the patency of the airway during spontaneous ventilation. Ketamine has been used in patients with osteogenesis imperfecta to provide general anesthesia for minor procedures without airway manipulation. If the airway is not in question, IV induction with thiopental followed by a nondepolarizing muscle relaxant is a reasonable induction technique. Various combinations of nitrous oxide-oxygen, volatile agents, and narcotics have been used successfully for maintenance of anesthesia in affected patients, with little to recommend one technique over the other.

Probably the most important factor is the technique that produces the least upset in the child while ensuring controlled induction. IV, inhalation, rectal, or intramuscular inductions are all possibilities. Regional anesthesia can be used in these patients, but the presence of vertebral fractures, a bleeding tendency, or long bone fractures with minimal trauma such as turning to place the block increase the risk of these techniques.

Airway Management. Airway management can be one of the most challenging aspects of anesthetic care. Pressure from the face mask can cause mandibular or facial fractures, whereas teeth are easily broken during laryngoscopy. Extension of the head conveys some risk for cervical spine fracture.

Patients with osteogenesis imperfecta often have increased frontal-occipital diameters, short necks, and barrel chests that make placement of a laryngoscope difficult. Fiberoptic laryngoscopy is a reasonable alternative to standard laryngoscopy.

Complications. Probably the most disturbing intraoperative complication that is unique to patients with osteogenesis imperfecta is the appearance of hyperthermia, tachycardia, and tachypnea from increased metabolism, as discussed previously. This reaction is associated with normocarbia and easily controlled by surface cooling. If there is no response to cooling measures, an arterial blood gas measurement can be obtained to rule out the mixed metabolic/respiratory acidosis of MH.

Ventilation-perfusion abnormalities are not uncommon in children with osteogenesis imperfecta. Kyphoscoliosis, thoracic cage deformities, and recurrent infections contribute to varying degrees of abnormality. Humidified gases, tracheobronchial toilet, and positive end-expiratory pressure are useful in minimizing the abnormalities.

Extubation. Children with osteogenesis imperfecta usually have the normal range of responses to anesthetic and analgesic medications. However, they often have relatively weak respiratory muscles, kyphoscoliosis, and thoracic cage abnormalities, which decrease the margin of safety for ventilation. Because of this, extubation is prudent only when the patient is fully awake. Postoperative analgesia can be provided in a variety of ways, but the titration of small doses of narcotic is especially efficacious in providing pain relief with minimal depression.

REFERENCES

1. Rosenberg H, Gronert GA: Intractable cardiac arrest in children given succinylcholine. *Anesthesiology* 1992; 77:1054.
2. Package Insert: Anectine (succinylcholine chloride) Injection, USP. Burroughs Wellcome Company, June 1993.
3. Badgwell JM, Hall SC, Lockhart C: Revised label regarding use of succinylcholine in children and adolescents: II. (Letter). *Anesthesiology* 1994;80:243–245.
4. Morell RC, Berman JM, Royster RI, et al: Revised label regarding use of succinylcholine in children and adolescents: I. (Letter). *Anesthesiology* 1994;80:242–245.
5. Kent RS: Revised label regarding use of succinylcholine in children and adolescents: I and II (reply). *Anesthesiology* 1994;80:244–245.
6. Lerman J, Berdock SE, Bissonnette B, et al. Succinylcholine warning. (Letter). *Can J Anaesth* 1994;41:165.
7. Sethna NF, Rockoff MA: Cardiac arrest following inhalation induction of anaesthesia in a child with Duchenne's muscular dystrophy. *Can Anaesth Soc J* 1986;33:799–802.
8. Smith CL, Bush GH: Anaesthesia and progressive muscular dystrophy. *Br J Anaesth* 1985;57:1113–1118.
9. Gronert GA, Theye RA: Pathophysiology of hyperkalemia induced by succinylcholine. *Anesthesiology* 1975;43:89–99.
10. Martyn JA, White DA, Gronert GA, et al: Up-and-down regulation of skeletal muscle acetylcholine receptors: effects on neuromuscular blockers. *Anesthesiology* 1992;76:822–843.
11. Kalow W, Britt BA, Chan FY: Epidemiology and inheritance of malignant hyperthermia. *Int Anesthesiol Clin* 1979;17:119–139.
12. Ording H: Incidence of malignant hyperthermia in Denmark. *Anesth Analg* 1985;64:700–704.
13. O Flynn RP, Shutack JG, Rosenberg H, Fletcher JE: Masseter muscle rigidity and malignant hyperthermia susceptibility in pediatric patients: an update on management and diagnosis. *Anesthesiology* 1994;80:1228–1233.
14. Vanderspek AF: Triggering agents continued after masseter spasm: there is proof in this pudding! *Anesth Analg* 1991;73:364–365.
15. Vanderspek AF, Fang WB, Ashton-Miller JA, et al: Increased masticatory muscle stiffness during limb muscle flaccidity associated with succinylcholine administration. *Anesthesiology* 1988;69:11–16.
16. Leary NP, Ellis FR: Masseteric muscle spasm as a normal response to suxamethonium. *Br J Anaesth* 1990;64:448–492.
17. Littleford JA, Patel LR, Bose D, et al: Masseter muscle spasm in children: implications of continuing the triggering anesthetic. *Anesth Analg* 1991;72:151–160.
18. Berry FA: Masseter spasm in perspective. (Editorial). *Paediatr Anaesth* 1991;1:61–63.
19. Pagon RA, Smith DW, Shepard TH: Urethral obstruction malformation complex: a cause of abdominal muscle deficiency and the prune belly. *J Pediatr* 1979;94: 900–906.
20. Pramanik AK, Altshuler G, Light IJ, Sutherland JM: Prune-belly syndrome associated with Potter (renal nonfunction) syndrome. *Am J Dis Child* 1977;131:672–674.
21. Inselman LS, Mellins RB: Growth and development of the lung. *J Pediatr* 1981;98:1–15.
22. Riccardi VM, Grum CM: The prune belly anomaly: heterogeneity and superficial X-linkage mimicry. *J Med Genet* 1977;14:266–270.
23. Garrett WJ, Kossoff G, Osborn RA: The diagnosis of fetal hydronephrosis, megaureter, and urethral obstruction by ultrasonic echocardiography. *Br J Obstet Gynaecol* 1975;82:115–120.
24. Bovicelli L, Rizzo N, Orsini LF, Michelacci L: Prenatal diagnosis of the prune belly syndrome. *Clin Genet* 1980;18:79–82.
25. Nakayama DK, Harrison MR, Chinn DH, de Lorimier AA: The pathogenesis of prune belly. *Am J Dis Child* 1984;138:834–836.
26. Cramolini CM: Diseases of the renal system. In: Katz J, Steward DJ (eds). *Anesthesia and uncommon pediatric diseases*. Philadelphia: WB Saunders, 1987.
27. Wilson DR: Micropuncture study of chronic obstructive nephropathy before and after release of obstruction. *Kidney Int* 1972;2:119–130.
28. Splinter WM, Schaefer JD, Zunder IH: Clear fluids three hours before surgery do not affect the gastric fluid contents of children. *Can J Anaesth* 1990;37:498–501.
29. Hannington-Kiff JG: Prune-belly syndrome and general anesthesia. *Br J Anaesth* 1970;42:649–652.
30. Feld LH, Negus JB, White PF: Oral midazolam preanesthetic medication in pediatric outpatients. *Anesthesiology* 1990;73: 831–834.
31. Gertner JM, Root L: Osteogenesis imperfecta. *Orthop Clin North Am* 1990;21:151–162.
32. Edwards MJ, Graham JM Jr: Studies of type 1 collagen in osteogenesis imperfecta. *J Pediatr* 1990;117:67–72.
33. Libman RH: Anesthetic considerations for the patient with osteogenesis imperfecta. *Clin Orthop* 1981;159: 123–125.
34. Cropp GJ, Myers DN: Physiological evidence of hypermetabolism in osteogenesis imperfecta. *Pediatrics* 1972; 49:375–391.
35. Sadat-Ali M, Sankaran-Kutty M, Adu-Gyamfi Y: Metabolic acidosis in osteogenesis imperfecta *Eur J Pediatr* 1986;145:582–583.
36. Rampton AJ, Kelly DA, Shanahan EC, Ingram GS: Occurrence of malignant hyperpyrexia in a patient with osteogenesis imperfecta. *Br J Anaesth* 1984;56: 1443–1446.
37. Ryan CA, Al-Ghamdi AS, Gayle M, Finer NN: Osteogenesis imperfecta and hyperthermia. *Anesth Analg* 1989;68:811–814.
38. Brownell AK: Malignant hyperthermia: relationship to other diseases. *Br J Anaesth* 1988;60:303–308.
39. Bradish CF, Flowers M: Central retinal artery occlusion in association with osteogenesis imperfecta. *Spine* 1987;12:193–194.

15

Management of the Child with Major Trauma

Aleksandra J. Mazurek and J. Michael Badgwell

"The paper tells that twenty-two thousand met their death last year by auto, and that we are well on our way to beat that record. Fourteen billion dollars we paid...about $635,000 a piece with no charge at all for the wounded."
—Will Rogers (1926)

Trauma is the number one cause of death in children between the ages of 1 and 14 years. Because the appropriate management of traumatized children by all health care providers significantly affects morbidity and survival, it is important to review the care of these children at all stages after the traumatic incident, beginning with a discussion of the initial resuscitative care of the traumatized child.

EQUIPMENT

The challenges intrinsic to the care of the injured child often have to do with the lack of availability of suitable equipment. For example, equipment to keep the child warm may not be available. Pediatric body proportions and shape make children more vulnerable to heat loss. Low body temperature on admission is considered a predictor of poor outcome (1). The ability to rewarm or maintain body temperature has increased considerably during the last years with the invention of convective heating devices **(see Prevention of Hypothermia)**.

In addition to patient warming devices, rapid transfusion devices are needed when the likelihood of massive blood transfusion is high. Caution has to be exercised with such devices so that air is not introduced when the fluid or blood units are spiked. In rapid heating and fluid delivery, there is also a possibility of introducing microbubbles of gas released in the heating process (2,3).

ROOM PREPARATION IN THE EMERGENCY DEPARTMENT

In most instances, the anesthesiologist is responsible for the victim's airway management, but the role of the trauma team leader belongs either to the surgeon or the emergency physician. Regardless of who it is, the team leader should be designated in advance. Tasks should be rehearsed, execution of tasks should be exact, and the location of necessary equipment and whom to call for backup assistance must be known. A special larger room within the emergency department ought to be assigned as the trauma room (Fig. 1). It should contain all the needed equipment (Fig. 2) and should be easily accessible to the transporting team.

Along with the prominently displayed Glasgow Coma Scale, useful tools like Broselow's tape ought to be within reach. Broselow's tape is a yardstick that allows for quick approximation of the child's weight and has resuscitation medication dosages and equipment size printed for that weight (Fig. 3). Airway equipment such as endotracheal tubes, oral airways, and masks of various sizes should be clearly displayed and easy to reach (Fig. 4). The treatment room should be sufficiently large to convert to an operating room if the need for an emergency thoracotomy arises. Surgical trays (thoracotomy, vascular, cardiac) should be stored nearby for such an occasion. In this

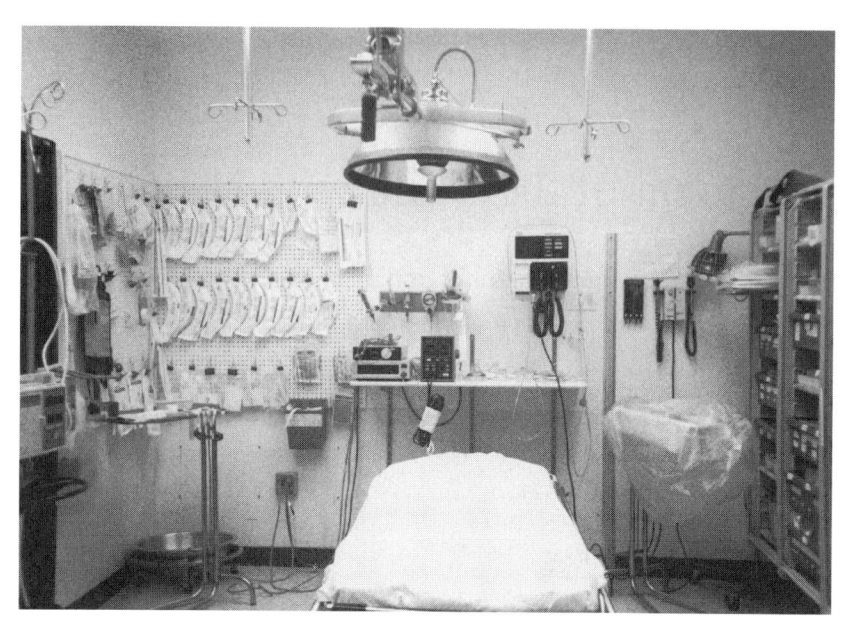

FIG. 1. A special, larger room within the emergency department is assigned as the trauma room. This room should be specially reserved for pediatric trauma and equipped accordingly, if space and resources allow.

way, the trauma room in an emergency department may also be useful in disaster management. The following equipment is needed: an electrocardiograph (ECG) monitor, a device for noninvasive blood pressure measurement, transducers for arterial tracing and central venous pressure (CVP), a pulse oximeter, a device to measure temperature, a capnograph (an end-tidal CO_2 monitor [$ETCO_2$]) or, at the very least, a CO_2 detector (Fig. 5). Both $ETCO_2$ detectors are useful tools to confirm endotracheal tube placement. The capnograph allows for consistent hyperventilation immediately after endotracheal intubation. A portable capnograph is used in transport.

Keeping an operating room available for trauma patients in a pediatric hospital may be costly and unnecessary. In most hospitals, room turnover is frequent enough that during working hours a room can be made available within a half-hour. During off hours, a designated trauma room is set up and ready for potential patients. The anesthesiologist on call refers to a checklist of equipment while preparing the room. The list serves not only as a reminder of the equipment needed, but also forces the physician to locate and check the pieces of equipment that are not used frequently.

Every morning the person on call prepares for storage in a refrigerator a set of drugs or syringes to be used during emergency interventions. Also available in all units are various sets of transport monitors and gas sources. In our operating rooms, we use a transport trolley containing an oxygen/air blender, a portable monitor capable of recording SaO_2 and ECG, an $ETCO_2$ monitor, and monitors for measuring pressures invasively.

Even the best-prepared medical system will not succeed unless personnel are educated about how it is supposed to function and updated whenever system changes are made. There is a continuous need for refresher courses as well as quality improvement through analysis of procedures and correction of mistakes.

INITIAL RESUSCITATION AND CARE

"I don't want to achieve immortality through my work. . . . I want to achieve it through not dying."

—Woody Allen

Hypothermia

Although extreme hypothermia (e.g., such as that which would occur in a child who falls into an ice-covered lake) may actually preserve central nervous system and myocardial function, hypothermia that is less than extreme is detrimental to the traumatized child. By depressing hemodynamic function and prolonging acidosis, hypothermia decreases the child's response to cardiopulmonary resuscitation. Furthermore, hypothermia increases oxygen consumption while decreasing oxygen delivery (release) to tissues. Perhaps more important is the fact that hypothermia impairs platelet function and may lead to prolonged bleeding. In addition, the postoperative consequences (rewarming, hypotension, shivering, and discomfort) can significantly contribute to perioperative morbidity. Hypothermia assumes greater importance in the traumatized pediatric patient compared with the adult because of the child's larger surface-to-body weight ratio and higher metabolic rate. Therefore, it is important in the course of management to promote the preservation of body heat in traumatized children.

Prevention of Hypothermia

No single method or device used alone will reliably prevent inadvertent hypothermia. Results are best when several methods are combined. If possible, patients kept in a holding area should be well covered with warmed blankets. The ambient operating room temperature should be maintained at 22° to 24° C for the incoming trauma patient. Intraoperatively, skin preparations and irrigation fluid should be heated and warm saline pads placed on exposed surfaces when possible.

Intravenous (IV) fluids should be warmed for traumatized children, especially when large fluid shifts and rapid replacement are anticipated. The infusion of heated (37° to 42° C) IV fluids using simple conductive fluid warmers helps to provide core normothermia. Rapid-infusion devices are now available that can fully warm blood to 37° C at flow rates as high as 750 ml/min for each 8F IV catheter. (Note: Always monitor CVP if using these high flow rates in children.) Cold blood is viscous and difficult to infuse, and it worsens peripheral vasoconstriction. Furthermore, rapid infusion of cold blood via a central line may cause dysrhythmias. At 4° C, the oxygen-hemoglobin association curve is shifted so far to the left that even at venous oxygen tension, hemoglobin is still 100% saturated. Therefore, cold blood is unable to provide oxygen to tissues and acts only as an inert volume expander.

Active airway heaters and humidifiers used in the operating room (but not much anymore) are impractical in the acute situation in the emergency room (4). If available, however, a high-surface-area hygroscopic membrane filter (heat and moisture exchanger [HME]) may be placed in the airway to provide adequate heat and moisture in both children (5) and adults.

Heated mattresses containing water are cumbersome and not very efficient (6). A more effective approach is to use a forced-air convective exchange blanket, which consists of an extremely light air mattress through which heated air is forced by a compressor **(see Figure 3, Chapter 2)**. By providing both insulation and active cutaneous warming, the forced-air exchange blanket is a very effective method of preventing intraoperative hypothermia (7). In fact, the incidence of surgical wound infection and the duration of hospital stay are decreased in patients kept warm intraoperatively (8).

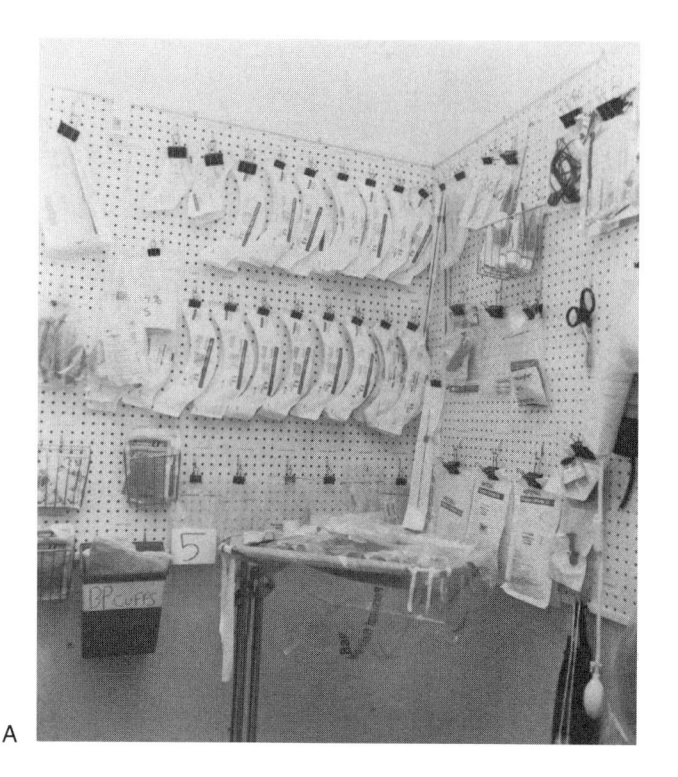

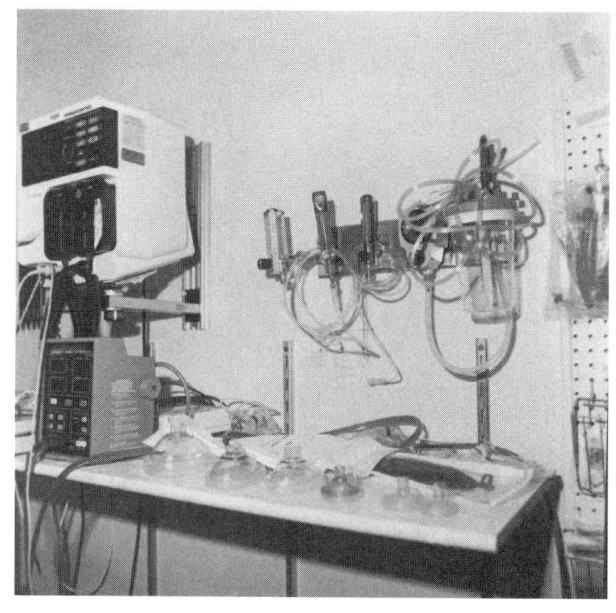

FIG. 2. In the pediatric trauma room, equipment should be readily available for endotracheal intubation **(A)**, suction **(B)**, and administration of medication **(C** and **D)**.

C

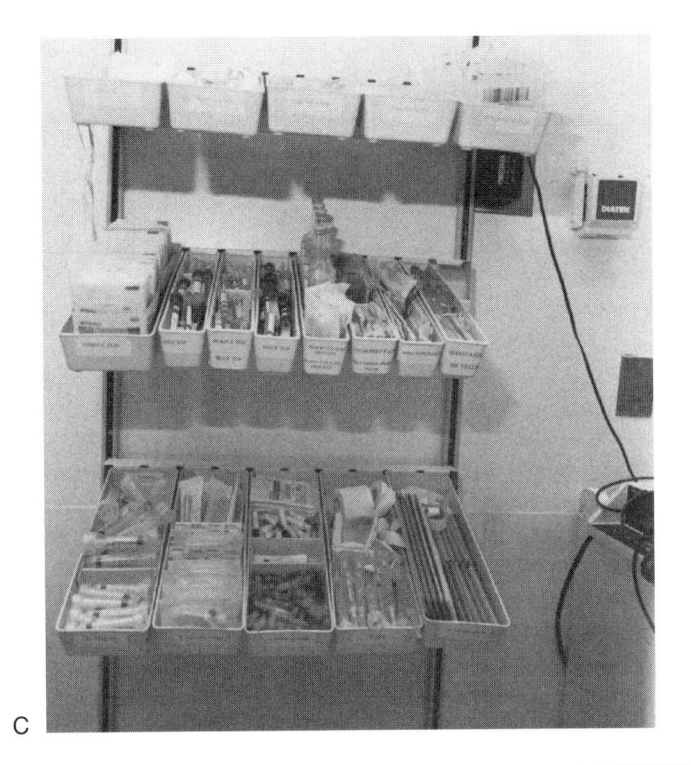

D

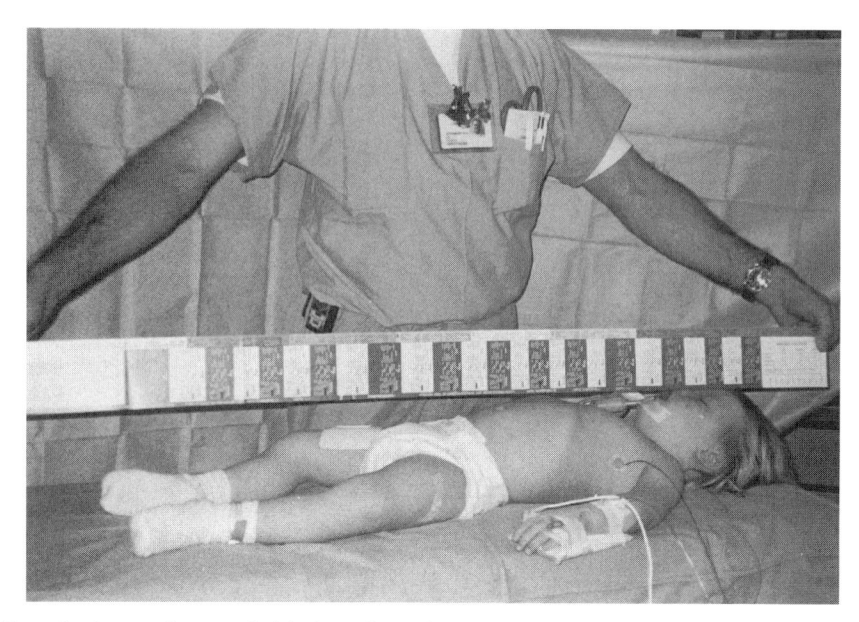

FIG. 3. Broselow's tape is a yardstick that allows for quick approximation of the child's weight, medication dosage, and equipment size.

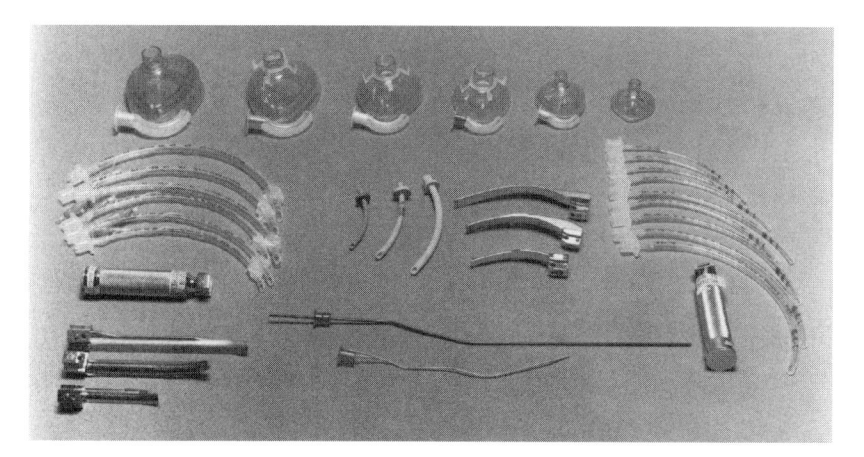

FIG. 4. Airway equipment for any emergency should be available in the trauma room.

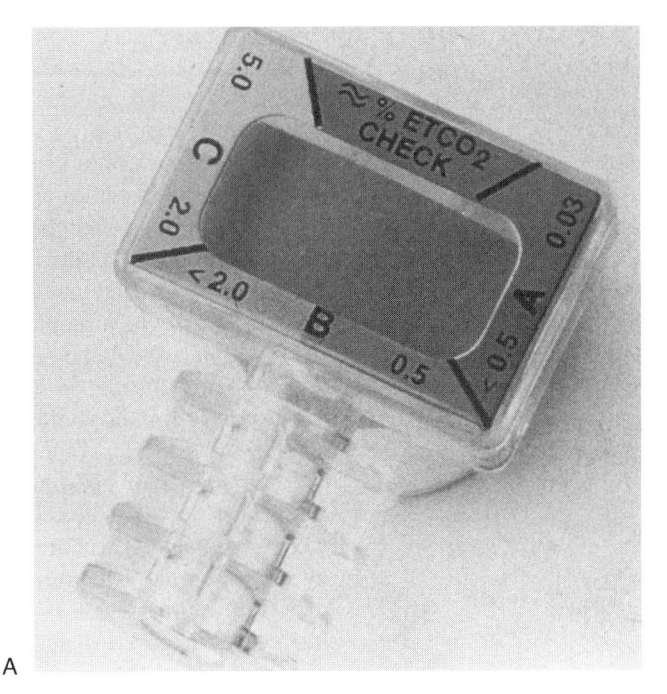

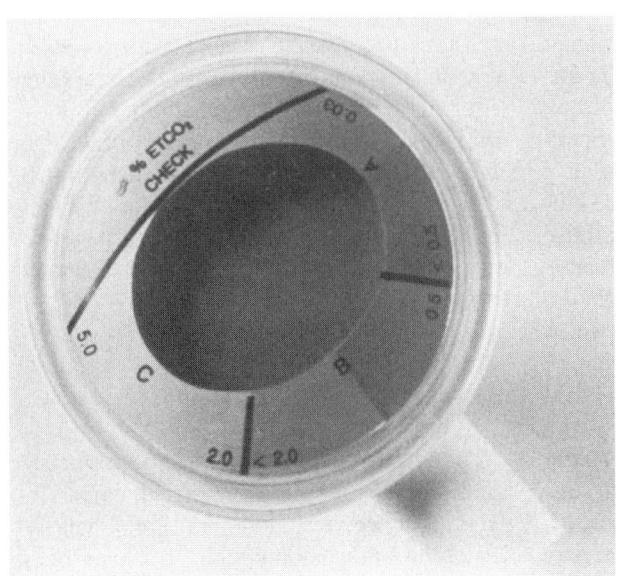

FIG. 5. Portable, accurate end-tidal CO$_2$ detectors are available in several different models **(A** and **B)**.

INITIAL ASSESSMENT AND TREATMENT

The systematic approach to an injured child who requires life support measures is no different from the approach to an adult requiring such measures and follows the familiar ABC steps:

- Airway
- Breathing
- Circulation, IV access
- Disability (i.e., abbreviated neurologic examination)
- Exposure (clothes must be removed to expose the entire body)

A = Airway

Swelling, secretions, and bleeding from trauma, and collapse of soft tissue as the child loses consciousness, may cause obstruction of the airway. If obstruction is present, the airway should be opened by head-tilt/chin-lift or, with neck injury, by gentle suction (9). Spontaneously breathing children should receive supplemental oxygen, either by face mask or by nasal cannula. If respiratory compromise persists, positive-pressure ventilation, using bag and mask and endotracheal intubation, may be required. In a child with suspected neck injury, endotracheal intubation may be particularly troublesome **(see Endotracheal Intubation and Chapter 4)**.

Adequacy of ventilation and patency of the airway is confirmed by the absence of subcostal and intercostal retractions, equal breath sounds, coordinated chest and abdominal rise, pulse oximetry readings, and arterial blood gas determinations. Gastric dilation that occurs as a result of crying or positive-pressure ventilation may compromise ventilation. If this occurs, the stomach should be decompressed using a suction catheter. A portable anesthesia breathing circuit is preferred to a self-inflating resuscitation bag, since the former allows spontaneous respiration but the latter requires positive-pressure ventilation that may cause gastric dilation. Traumatized children are usually better off if they are allowed to breath spontaneously if they can, with added support as necessary.

Generally speaking, if a traumatized child can tolerate a plastic artificial oral airway, he or she is obtunded enough to require an endotracheal tube. This is also true for nasal airways, but an artificial nasal airway may produce epistaxis or nasopharyngeal bleeding (especially in the hypothermic child with a coagulopathy disorder). Therefore, artificial airways have limited usefulness in the trauma situation.

Head injury in children may result in a fluctuating level of consciousness that may worsen airway obstruction, hypoxemia, and hypoventilation. Depressed consciousness may, in turn, aggravate or cause further central nervous system damage. Fear of central nervous system damage is the reason behind aggressive airway management. Temporary measures (e.g., jaw thrust, oral airway insertion, and suctioning oral secretions) are often required to provide oxygenation, but these measures may not be relied on over time when level of consciousness may be changing. In addition, a high F_IO_2 should be administered and the cervical spine immobilized **(see Airway Management in Suspected Cervical Injury)**.

B = Breathing

The evaluation of breathing pattern, auscultation for symmetric air entry, diagnosis of pneumothorax or hemothorax, immediate insertion of thoracostomy tube, or closure of an open chest wound should take care of life-threatening lung and chest problems.

C = Circulation

The most significant pathophysiologic defect in traumatized children is usually hemorrhagic shock. The earliest manifestations of shock are delayed capillary refill, mottled skin, and cool extremities. Tachycardia also occurs early in shock and indicates a loss of circulating blood volume. In the unanesthetized patient, systolic blood pressure remains relatively constant because of peripheral vasoconstriction. Systolic blood pressure may be maintained until there is a 30% to 40% loss of circulating blood volume. Diastolic blood pressure also may be maintained because of vasoconstriction and , therefore, the hypovolemic patient may have a narrowed pulse pressure. By contrast, in the anesthetized child, diastolic blood pressure is a good indicator of filling pressure and decreases in the hypovolemic child, often precipitously after the induction of anesthesia. Peripheral pulses may be absent, depending on the intensity of vasoconstriction. Absent or narrowed peripheral pulses and tachycardia should alert the clinician that cardiovascular collapse is imminent.

Arterial pH is a good indicator of circulatory status. If pH is low in the presence of normal or low carbon dioxide, it should be assumed that circulating blood volume is inadequate, until proved otherwise. Metabolic acidosis, secondary to low perfusion state in hypovolemic children is corrected with adequate fluid resuscitation. If the pH falls below 7.2 in a child with adequate ventilation, sodium bicarbonate may be added to fluid replacement (dose = body weight in kg × 0.15 meq × base deficit, given as an IV bolus, followed by reassessment of the pH) (10).

Initial treatment of hemorrhagic shock is intravascular resuscitation with crystalloid solutions. Therefore, establishing vascular access with large-bore cannulas has top priority. Percutaneous cannulation of internal jugular or subclavian veins is hazardous during initial resuscitation because of the risk of pneumothorax or hemothorax (11). If the clinician is proficient with cannulation of these large central veins, this procedure is recommended in life-threatening situations in which no other access is available. Furthermore, if abdominal or thoracic bleeding is suspected, at least one IV site should be in the neck or upper extremity. In addition, a CVP is essential if use of a rapid mechanical infusion system is planned. Internal jugular or subclavian veins may be cannulated using techniques that require only slight modifications from those used in adults.

From its introduction in the 1950s, the timely revival of the intraosseous infusion technique has made obtaining vascular access easier (12). We are now reminded that the technique can save lives (13). In the 1994 edition of the Pediatric Advanced Life Support (PALS) course, a strong recommendation is made that intraosseous access should be established if reliable venous access cannot be achieved within three attempts or 90 seconds, whichever comes first (14). (For a description of this technique, **see Chapter 3.**)

D = Disability

The word disability is a reminder to assess neurologic baseline status at the time of admission. The child's brain is poorly protected, and its response to an insult is different from that of an adult. Children develop malignant brain edema within hours after an injury, which may often escalate in spite of aggressive therapeutic measures. Malignant brain edema may occur even in patients who were lucid on admission to the hospital. The level of consciousness is often a good predictor of outcome. Since a significant number of patients are intubated, sedated, and often paralyzed for a prolonged period of time, it is essential to perform a short neurologic examination before administration of any drugs. The acronym AVPU (*a*wareness, response to *v*erbal stimuli, response to *p*ainful stimuli, and *u*nresponsive) serves as a reminder to conduct the basic assessment of consciousness and pupillary size. AVPU is easy to remember as a guideline for treatment. By contrast, the Glasgow Coma Scale is easily forgotten if not used routinely to assess patient status **(see The Child with Head Injury)**. The scale may be displayed on the wall in the trauma room, however, for easy visibility and access (Table 1).

TABLE 1. *Glascow Coma Scale for Infants and Children*

Score	Variable
	Best motor response
6	Obeys commands
5	Localizes pain
4	Withdraws from pain
3	Abnormal flexion
2	Abnormal extension
1	Flaccidity
	Best verbal response (modified for children)
5	Appropriate words or social smiles, fixes and follows
4	Cries but consolable
3	Persistently irritable
2	Restless, agitated (moans only)
1	None
	Eye opening
4	Spontaneous
3	Opens to voices
2	Opens to pain
1	None

E = Exposure

The word "exposure" serves as a reminder to completely undress the patient without regard for the cost of the garments to ensure that no other injuries are missed. Attention should be paid to the ease with which children become hypothermic. When the child is stabilized, the patient is log-rolled for examination of the posterior aspect of the body.

SECONDARY SURVEY

When the initial assessment is finished and the life-threatening conditions (airway obstruction, pneumothorax, hemorrhage) are resolved, the patient must undergo a systematic head-to-toe examination. At the same time, radiographs are taken of the head, cervical spine, chest, abdomen, or limbs. If appropriate, a computed tomography (CT) scan (of the whole body), an ultrasound examination, or an IV pyelogram may be performed. Peritoneal lavage is not considered a sensitive test in children and has been replaced by the latter modalities in the last decade. In case of blunt trauma, a patient's condition can usually be stabilized for diagnostic investigations. Only 20% of these patients require surgical intervention. Gunshot wound victims, on the other hand, especially those with entrance wounds below the nipple line, require operation emergently 90% of the time.

When medical facilities lack the staff or equipment to manage pediatric care, patients require expeditious transfer to a level I facility (15). A level I pediatric trauma center is equipped and staffed to handle the care of a child with multiple-organ injury. Interhospital transfer of a critically ill child has to be agreed on by two physicians who have been in communication about a patient's status and who agree on the arrangements for transport of the patient and the patient's escort.

ENDOTRACHEAL INTUBATION

Protocols for endotracheal intubation of the child with multiple trauma are aimed at making the task simple, organized, and successful **(see also Chapter 4)**. The goals of intubation in the traumatized patient are (a) to maintain and protect the airway; (b) to provide the ventilatory support and, if appropriate, hyperventilate; (c) to minimize the risk of further cervical injury; and (d) to prevent cardiovascular decompensation. Management of the airway is presented as steps:

- Quickly assess the airway and breathing status of the patient.

- Establish adequate ventilation and oxygenation by face mask or endotracheal intubation.

- Anesthetic agents are frequently required for endotracheal intubation in the traumatized pediatric patient. The choice of a full- or reduced-dose hypnotic agent or sedative depends on the patient's hemodynamic stability.

- Medications useful for intubation include the following:
  - Atropine, 10 μg/kg IV before intubation
  - A sedative/hypnotic/analgesic, depending on cardiovascular/central nervous system status.

Ketamine	1 to 2 mg/kg
Thiopental	1 to 5 mg/kg
Midazolam	0.05 to 0.1 mg/kg
Lidocaine	1 to 1.5 mg/kg
Fentanyl	1 to 2 μg/kg

  - Muscle relaxants

Succinylcholine	2 mg/kg
Rocuronium	1.2 mg/kg
Pancuronium	0.1 to 0.2 mg/kg

- In addition to an assistant watching monitors and reporting vital sign changes to the anesthesiologist, other assistants may be needed during intubation, such as the following:
  - One person to apply cricoid pressure and hand the physician the endotracheal tube
  - One person to apply in-line stabilization (without traction) in patients at risk for cervical spine instability **(see Airway Management in Suspected Cervical Injury)**
  - One person to inject and flush medications
- After intubation, one should carry out the following:
  - Check for bilateral breath sounds personally.
  - Check for sounds over the epigastrium (indicating esophageal intubation).
  - Check for the presence of exhaled carbon dioxide.
  - Observe for bilateral chest expansion.
  - Note the length marker of the endotracheal tube at the gum line.
  - Recheck above items after taping the endotracheal tube in place.

Premedication

In general, children with multiple-system trauma or head injury should not receive sedative premedication. In the child with pain who is awake, responsive, and has a stable circulatory status, the IV administration of morphine sulfate (0.05 to 0.1 mg/kg) or fentanyl (2 to 4 μg/kg) may be appropriate to provide analgesia. Remember, however, that agitation in a traumatized child may be caused by hypoxia or increased intracranial pressure (ICP). Therefore, these conditions should be ruled out, or treated if appropriate, before sedative analgesic medications are given. Atropine (0.02 mg/kg) may be given IV at the time of induction to prevent the bradycardia associated with laryngoscopy and with the administration of succinylcholine or fentanyl.

Monitors

Along with the usual monitors, an arterial catheter is essential. A CVP catheter is not essential in the initial phase of resuscitation and may be inserted after the patient has been stabilized. Volume status may be monitored using diastolic blood pressure, capillary refill time, and urine output as a further measure of volume depletion, a decreasing end-tidal CO_2 value (when ventilation is constant) indicates decreasing pulmonary perfusion (16).

Induction of Anesthesia

Hypovolemia and a full stomach put traumatized children at risk for both hypotension and pulmonary aspiration during induction of anesthesia. Therefore, a rapid-sequence induction with an IV agent, preoxygenation, and cricoid pressure is indicated in most cases. In the child in whom neck injury is suspected, struggling may have dire consequences; in these cases, preoxygenation may be avoided if it causes the child to struggle more vigorously. Cricoid pressure should be avoided in cases of known or suspected fractured larynx (child in respiratory distress with history of neck trauma, absence of cry or phonation, anterior neck soft tissue swelling, and subcutaneous crepitus).

Intravenous Agents

The requirements for IV anesthetics are decreased after trauma and hemorrhage because (a) the volume of distribution is decreased; (b) dilution of serum proteins (especially after crystalloid resuscitation) occurs, and, thus, less drug is bound and more free, active drug is available; and (c) blood flow to the brain and heart is well maintained despite poor perfusion to other organs. The IV anesthetic agent that is chosen should cause minimal depression of the heart and dilation of the peripheral vasculature. It is well known that ketamine supports blood pressure when the sympathetic nervous system is intact. There are data indicating that ketamine causes myocardial depression and hypotension in animals with severe hypovolemia (17). Therefore, as an induction agent in traumatized children, ketamine should be given slowly (1 to 2 mg/kg) to those with moderate hypovolemia and probably not at all to those with severe hypovolemia. Ketamine increases ICP and is contraindicated in children with head trauma.

Initially, in severely hypovolemic and obtunded children who require immediate surgery, oxygen and a muscle relaxant may be all that are required. In less severe cases with moderate hypovolemia, fentanyl (0.5 to 2 µg/kg), followed by a rapid-acting muscle relaxant, provides stable hemodynamics during anesthetic induction. The possibility of awareness exists with these regimens but may be a small price to pay for keeping a child alive. Judicious monitoring and the use of adjuvant drugs as needed based on clinical signs will minimize the risk of awareness. In children who receive no anesthetic agent or only fentanyl for induction or in patients for whom only fentanyl is used as the sole maintenance anesthetic agent, midazolam (0.05 to 0.2 mg/kg) may be given after hemodynamic stability is achieved to provide amnesia.

Because it decreases cerebral oxygen consumption, ICP, and cerebral blood flow, thiopental is the drug of choice in children with head injury and stable volume and hemodynamic status. To minimize myocardial depression and venodilation in these children, thiopental should be given slowly. The hemodynamic effects of midazolam are similar to the effects of thiopental in hypovolemic children, and midazolam is less reliable in inducing anesthesia. Propofol is similar to the effects of thiopental as a myocardial depressant and may cause hypotension. As in adults, etomidate may be useful in hypovolemic patients, but experience in children is limited.

Muscle Relaxants

In the trauma situation, the ideal muscle relaxant should have a rapid onset of paralysis and minimal hemodynamic effect; also, it should not increase ICP or intraocular pressure. Although succinylcholine is not an ideal drug, the administration of 2 mg/kg is a rapid and effective aid in gaining control of the airway. The effects of this drug dissipate quickly, allowing revision of the airway management plan, if necessary. Hyperkalemia, secondary to the administration of succinylcholine, is not of concern in the early burn and trauma situation. Although succinylcholine causes a transient increase in ICP, this effect has not been shown to adversely affect outcome in head-injured patients. The advantages of promptly gaining control of the airway (i.e., the favorable effect on ICP of improved oxygenation and ventilation) outweigh the possibility of the minor effect of a transient increase in ICP secondary to succinylcholine.

Vecuronium and rocuronium are other useful muscle relaxants in the trauma situation. The administration of these agents (vecuronium, 0.15 to 0.4 mg/kg; rocuronium, 1.0 to 1.5 mg/kg) provide intubating conditions in 0.5 to 1 minute and is not associated with significant hemodynamic side effects or increased ICP. Priming techniques should be avoided because even a small dose of vecuronium may produce apnea or airway obstruction in the hypovolemic child. Atracurium and mivacurium have histamine-releasing properties that may cause hypotension. The tachycardia that may result from the vagolytic effects of pancuronium is undesirable in situations of acute trauma, in which the heart rate is being used as an indicator of cardiovascular status. Pancuronium, however, may be a useful drug when bradycardia is anticipated as a result of the vagotonic effect of fentanyl.

MAINTENANCE OF ANESTHESIA

Anesthetic Agents

Children with marginal volume restoration are probably best managed with an opioid/oxygen/muscle relaxant technique. Morphine, because of its vagal stimulation, histamine release, and α-adrenergic blocking effect, is not a good drug for these children. Likewise, meperidine should be avoided because of its histamine-releasing properties. Fentanyl provides good analgesia and provides hemodynamic stability in children with tenuous cardiovascular status. Because there is some venodilation with fentanyl, the initial doses should be small (2 to 10 µg/kg). If the child tolerates a small dose, incremental doses (up to 25 to 50 µg/kg) may be given. Sufentanil and alfentanil do not appear to have any significant pharmacodynamic advantage over fentanyl. Likewise, propofol has limited usefulness in hypovolemic pediatric patients, because it may depress cardiac output in a dose-dependent fashion in normovolemic children (18). These adverse hemodynamic effects are likely to be exaggerated in the hypovolemic child; however, isoflurane, in appropriate inspired concentrations, is a useful drug in traumatized pediatric patients after stable cardiovascular and hemodynamic status are achieved. Isoflurane may be useful to promote vasodilation in the child who has been volume-restored, but who is still vasoconstricted.

Nitrous oxide is a myocardial depressant, reduces the concentration of oxygen that can be delivered, and may fill air-containing spaces that may be present in traumatized patients (e.g., pneumothorax and bowel obstruction). Therefore, it is rarely useful in the trauma setting.

VOLUME REPLACEMENT

Crystalloid

The goal of fluid management during maintenance of anesthesia for surgical repair of trauma is to replenish vascular and interstitial fluid volumes. As in adults, trauma and hypovolemic shock in children are associated with a decrease in functional extracellular fluid volume and an increase in intracellular volume (19). Therefore, additional resuscitative fluid should mimic that of extracellular fluid (sodium concentration = 140 to 150 meq/L) (20). Effective resuscitation (i.e., that which is associated with survival) requires the administration of red blood cells (RBCs) and crystalloid in excess of the amount of blood that is lost (21). Therefore, effective resuscitation after massive hemorrhage causes edema, swelling, and obligatory weight gain (22). It is not the goal of resuscitation to prevent this edema. It should be emphasized that the administration of hypotonic solutions (e.g., 5% dextrose in water or 5% dextrose in 0.2 normal saline) causes intracellular edema without the beneficial effects of intravascular and interstitial repletion. Children, like adults, need balanced salt solutions to replace traumatic and surgical losses **(see Chapter 9)**.

It is recommended that dextrose-containing solutions be avoided in the trauma situation unless, based on the patient's history, hypoglycemia is documented or strongly suspected. The hormonal stress response to trauma produces hyperglycemia in children. The administration of dextrose-containing solutions may cause further hyperglycemia, which has the potential to worsen cellular injury in partially ischemic brain tissue (through the mechanism of increased lactic acid production). Therefore, dextrose-containing solutions should not be used as a routine fluid for use in the volume restoration of hypovolemic children.

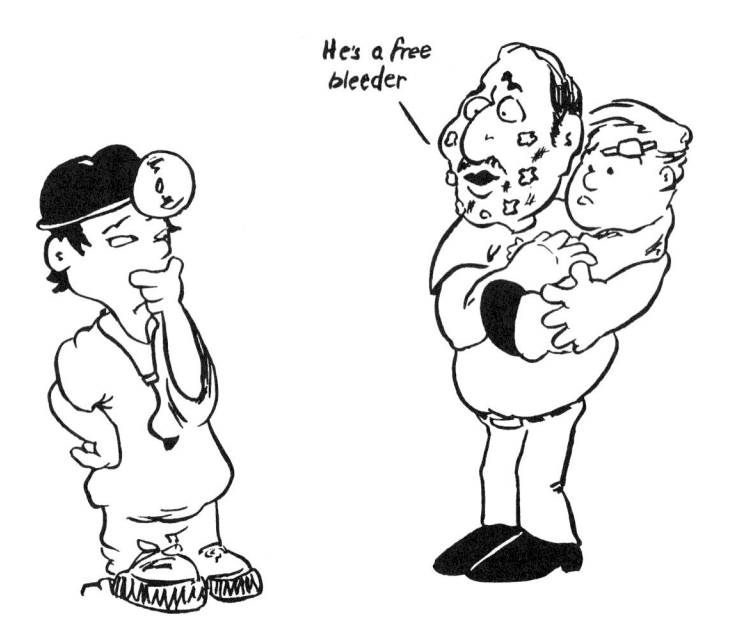

Blood Component Therapy

Although measurements of ongoing blood loss during surgery in the traumatized child may be attempted, these measurements are usually unreliable and may unnecessarily consume the time of ancillary personnel, who could be doing other more important things for the critically ill child. Rather, one can rely on clinical signs, such as capillary refill, temperature gradient (e.g., between core and skin), urine output, CVP, and diastolic blood pressure, as guides for estimating blood loss and volume status. Remember that the hematocrit is merely a reflection of the ratio of RBCs to everything else that has been given (e.g., crystalloid and colloid); therefore, it is not a reflection *per se* of volume status. The hematocrit is, however, a useful guide for further therapy (i.e., more RBCs versus more fluid). Specific blood components (e.g., RBCs, platelets) are discussed in **Chapter 9.**

THORACOABDOMINAL TRAUMA

Abdominal Trauma

"Everybody that hasn't got a gun is being shot by somebody. A flask and a gun are now considered standard equipment and are supposed to accompany every tough kid when he steps into long pants."
—Will Rogers (1925)

Abdominal trauma is very common in the pediatric population and can be a source of significant difficulty, including failure to resuscitate. Most trauma involving the abdomen is blunt in origin; penetrating trauma is relatively rare. The relatively large liver and spleen in children make them especially vulnerable to injury and are the most commonly injured organs in the abdomen. Fracture and laceration injuries of liver and spleen are common and can be accompanied by significant blood loss. Until recently, patients who presented with an acute abdomen after trauma were brought immediately to the operating room for exploratory laparotomy, resulting all too often in an unstable intraoperative course. Because of tamponade of open vessels by hematoma, a fractured spleen or lacerated liver may temporarily cease to bleed. After the abdomen is opened, however, the tamponade will be released, and massive bleeding may ensure. Unfortunately, massive bleeding is frequently difficult to control and may result in hypotension, a need for transfusion, and cardiac arrest. The spleen and liver are difficult to repair during the best of conditions, and when massive bleeding occurs, the surgical procedure becomes very challenging. Furthermore, patients who have had a splenectomy have decreased ability to phagocytize bacteria and may develop overwhelming sepsis.

For these reasons, many trauma centers now treat blunt abdominal trauma in children with nonsurgical evaluation and management if at all possible. The patient with suspected intra-abdominal pathology is initially evaluated with either CT or ultrasound imaging of the abdomen. If injury of the liver or spleen is detected, the patient may be treated medically (22). Blood is administered to maintain adequate intravascular volume and perfusion (23). If it is not possible to maintain adequate hemodynamic stability with blood and fluid administration, surgery is then considered. The liver and spleen are preserved if at all possible, with removal done only as a last resort.

With the increased use of seatbelts, there is an increased incidence of jejunal and ileal injury (24). This injury is detected by the presence of free air on radiologic films, by the appearance of acute abdominal signs, or by peritoneal tap and lavage. Closure of the bowel perforation is performed surgically.

Thoracic Trauma

"The more unsteady the nerve of the pistol holder, the better the shooting he can do, because he takes in a bigger radius. There has never been a case where the attempted killer missed everybody with an automatic pistol; but on the other hand, there have been very few cases where only the original shot at has been hit."

—Will Rogers (1925)

Thoracic trauma in children is frequently the result of either a fall or a motor vehicle accident (25,26). Penetrating trauma from a knife or firearm may be seen in adolescents, but is rare in younger children. Types of chest injuries are significantly different in children than in adults; the anatomy of children produces a different pattern of injury (27). Children have less bone and more cartilage in the rib cage and therefore a more elastic chest wall. As a result of these factors, there are fewer rib fractures in children than in the adult population, and in contrast to adults, first rib fractures are not associated with significant mortality in children.

After blunt chest trauma, lung contusion, and hemothorax or pneumothorax are the most common injuries in children (28,29). Diagnosis of hemothorax and pneumothorax is similar to that in adults. After lung contusion, there may an initial period of adequate gas exchange followed by progressive impairment. There may be progressive deterioration of pulmonary function and the added risk of secondary injury from hypoxemia and acidosis. Therefore, prospective evaluation by both medical and nursing staff is important to detect and minimize the potential detrimental effects of lung contusion. Although supplemental oxygen may be the only management needed, tracheal intubation and mechanical ventilation with positive end-expiratory pressure are occasionally necessary.

Flail chest is less common in children because of the elasticity of the chest wall. If flail chest occurs, management is the same in children as in adults. Although traumatic aortic rupture is very unusual in children, the most common presenting sign is cardiac arrest; mortality is high because recognition is late. Diaphragmatic rupture is also rare and difficult to document. Diagnosis is made only during laparotomy or thoracotomy.

Myocardial contusion is increasingly recognized in children and occurs when the heart is compressed between the sternum and the spine (30). Electrocardiographic currents are useful in this situation, which appears within the first 24 hours of injury in most children with significant injury. Cardiac enzymes have been used for diagnosis in some instances but are not particularly reliable. Echocardiography is useful and is a noninvasive method of determining whether there is significant wall motion abnormality or depression of stroke volume. Patients with a significant contusion respond as if they have decreased myocardial contractility. Therefore, compromised myocardial contractility should be considered when administering both fluids and anesthetics. Pulmonary artery catheterization with cardiac output determinations may be useful in patients with symptoms of contusion. Other problems that can occur with cardiac contusion include valve dysfunction, traumatic septal defect, pericardial tamponade, and cardiac dysrhythmias.

THE CHILD WITH HEAD INJURY

Of children suffering from multiple organ injuries, 75% suffer head trauma. In many cases, the head injury may not be severe. When injuries are severe, they are often debilitating or fatal (31). The predominance of head injuries in pediatric trauma victims can be explained by a child's anatomy. Until late childhood, the head is a large, heavy organ. It is poorly protected by thin cranial bones, which fuse only after 18 months of life. The head is supported by a proportionally thin neck with weak musculature and an immature cervical spine whose ligaments are lax in early life. Its joint facets are almost horizontal. The neck structure offers poor restraint to the head which, if propelled, acts very much like a missile. In the face of obvious head injury, cervical spine injury should be assumed until it is ruled out.

The mortality of children increases dramatically if multiple trauma is associated with closed head injury. Injury secondary to hypoxia, hypotension, edema, increasing ICP, and increased metabolic demand (e.g., seizures or fever) may be attenuated with appropriate care. In hypotensive children with closed head injury, hypotension is usually caused by something other than the head injury (e.g., abdominal injury). Infants occasionally become hypotensive, however, from a head injury because of blood loss into either the subgaleal or epidural space. The infant with an open fontanelle and mobile sutures is more tolerant of an expanding intracranial mass. Therefore, a bulging fontanelle in an infant who is not in coma should be treated as a severe injury.

Neurologic evaluation focuses on the presence of increased ICP. Increased ICP is common in children with head injury and occurs most often without a mass lesion. The Glasgow Coma Scale provides a fairly accurate estimate of ICP. The verbal portion of this test has been modified for the preverbal child (Table 1). In general, an infant or child who can cry is given a full verbal score, and a child who can wiggle, open, and answer (i.e., a child who can wiggle fingers and toes, open the eyes, and answer simple questions) has a Glasgow Coma Score of about 12 to 15 and probably does not have a raised ICP. On the other hand, a child with a Glasgow Coma Score of ≤8 probably has significantly increased ICP, and the child with a score of ≤6 has increased ICP that demands immediate and aggressive intervention to prevent uncal herniation. Although children often vomit after head injury without increased ICP, persistent vomiting and recurring seizures indicate an increase in ICP.

Airway Management in Suspected Cervical Injury

The incidence of cervical spine injury in children is between 0.7% and 36% (32,33). Cervical spine injury is often seen in the patient with head trauma and is further complicated by the difficulty of identifying the injury on radiograph when the person reading the film is not a pediatric radiologist. Furthermore, children can suffer spinal cord injury, yet show no abnormality on the radiograph. One may suspect this situation if there is a history of transient neurologic deficit. Therefore, many children with closed head injury are treated as if they have unstable cervical spines (see following text) (Fig. 6). Guide-

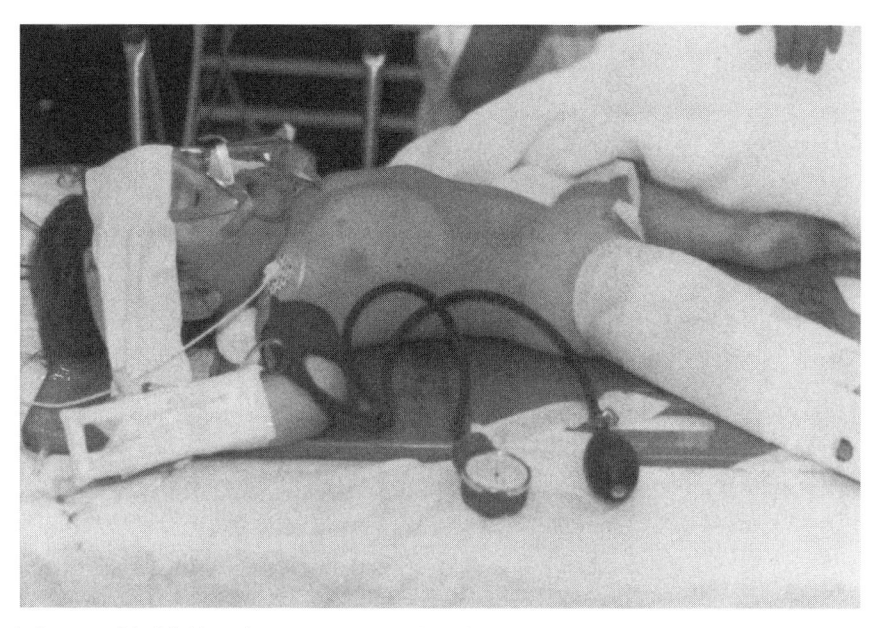

FIG. 6. A 3-year-old child has been transported to the trauma center for care. Note that she is on a backboard with a neck roll, and her head and neck are secured. A warmed blanket has been placed on her to prevent heat loss, but this blanket has been turned back for the examination.

lines for identifying and treating cervical spine injury include:

- Suspicion for injury is less in responsive patients ≥12 years old without neck pain or tenderness and with a negative lateral cervical spine radiograph.
- Suspicion for injury is greater in patients with history of neurologic deficit or those who complain of neck pain (or are too young to complain), who have neck tenderness, or who are comatose. These patients may require flexion-extension films under the supervision of the neurosurgery service in addition to a lateral cervical spine film before the injury is ruled out. The child's cervical spine is considered unstable until all evidence confirms the absence of injury.

In many cases, evidence for the absence of injury remains equivocal. If so, further evaluation over time may be needed to ensure that the child is free of cervical spine injury. Until then, the patient may need to remain in a rigid cervical collar and needs to be treated as having cervical instability (Fig. 7).

Unless these children are severely obtunded, intubation without anesthetic agents (awake intubation) is usually impractical. In addition, laryngoscopy in the awake child is a potent stimulator of intracranial hypertension. Because of the acute nasal-pharyngeal-laryngeal angles in children <8 years old, blind nasotracheal intubation is rarely successful and may result in inadvertent intracranial insertion if basilar skull fracture is present. Fiberoptic intubation requires a prerequisite level of skill and, even in the best of hands and static conditions, it is time-consuming. Therefore, it has limited use in acute trauma.

In the anesthetized child whose neck is being held in neutral position by in-line stabilization, oral laryngoscopy under direct vision usually allows successful endotracheal intubation (Fig. 8). When using this technique, the head and neck are maintained in anatomic alignment with the body by the insertion of the assistant's fingertips under the child's mastoid processes and holding the neck and head in a straight

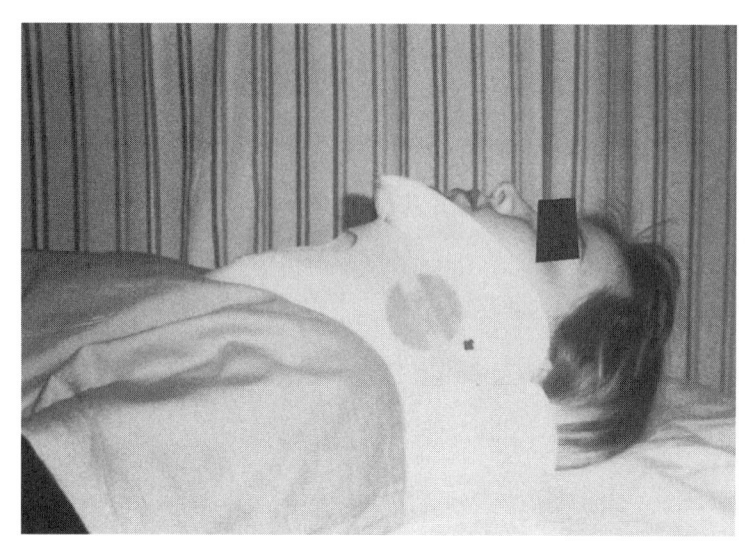

FIG. 7. In children with suspected cervical spine injury, a rigid collar is worn until it is determined that no injury exists.

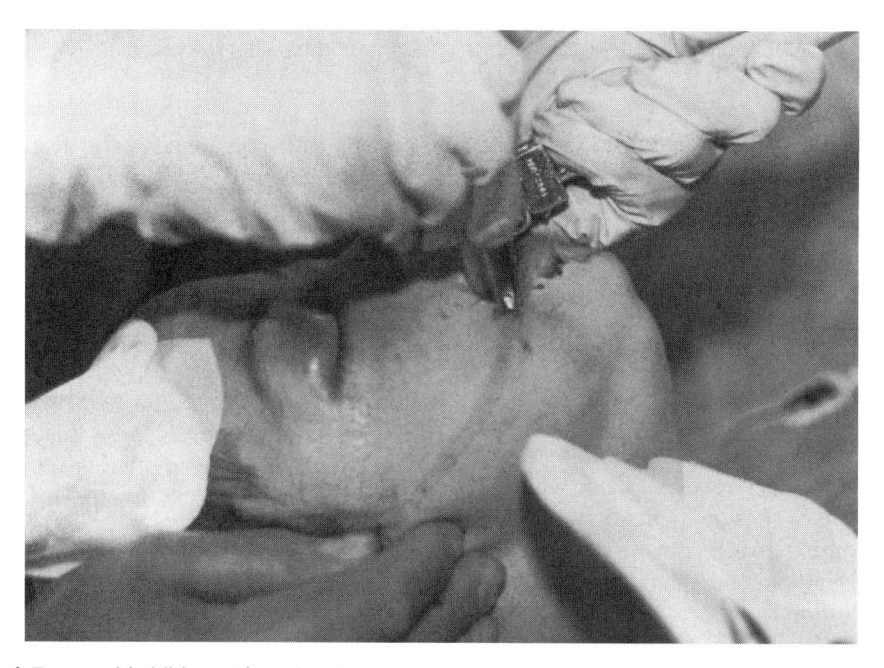

FIG. 8. A 7-year-old child transferred to the trauma center 24 hours after head and neck injury. When this child needed reintubation, the cervical collar was briefly removed and the trachea was intubated while we held in-line cervical stabilization. Note the presence of a dressing covering a subdural drainage bolt.

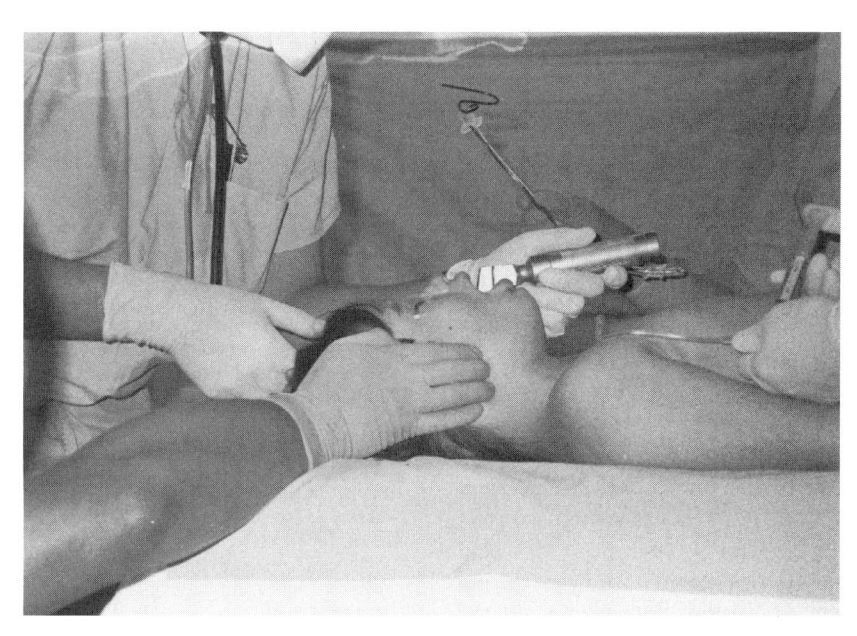

FIG. 9. It often takes four persons to perform tracheal intubation in a child with suspected cervical spine injury: one to intubate, one to apply in-line stabilization, one to apply cricoid pressure (if indicated), and one to administer drugs.

cephalad line (Fig. 9). During in-line stabilization, no axial traction is applied. Axial traction may cause further disruption of the cervical spine and should be avoided. In-line stabilization prevents the endoscopist from putting the child's head into extreme flexion or extension. A second assistant should apply cricoid pressure. If the child arrives with a cervical stabilization device in place, it may be easily removed (while maintaining in-line stabilization) to gain access to the child's larynx. If a younger child's relatively large occiput causes undue neck flexion that prevents adequate laryngoscopy, it is safe to cautiously place (while maintaining in-line stabilization) a small towel under the shoulders.

Fluid Management in Head-Injured Patients

Restoration of volume in hypovolemic children with closed head injury almost always takes priority over considerations of raised ICP. To maintain perfusion to the brain and other vital organs, it is of paramount importance to maintain the child's circulatory status. In children with head injury, as in those without head injury, any isotonic crystalloid may be used for fluid resuscitation. Colloid provides no clinical advantages and is more expensive. Although Ringer's lactate (RL) is not isotonic (RL = 273 mOsm/L compared with normal saline = 308 Osm/L), it may be used to resuscitate the child in large amounts before arrival in the emergency department or operating room. In addition, the serum osmolality and hematocrit should be determined, both initially and at intervals, and further fluid should be replaced with either RL, normal saline, or RBCs. The administration of mannitol for diuresis may be followed by a triphasic response consisting of (a) increased blood volume, increased blood pressure, and possibly increased ICP; (b) return to normal blood pressure; and (c) hypotension. Therefore, the administration of mannitol should be delayed until children are hemodynamically stable. When the patient is hemodynamically stable, loop diuretics may be given to augment the effect of mannitol.

AIRWAY TRAUMA

External Trauma (Cricothyroid Separation)

Although protected from fracture by its pliability, the pediatric larynx can sustain cricothyroid separation. Because external damage may be minimal, cricoid separation is suspected in the injured child who presents with dysphonia, dysphagia, stidor, hemoptysis, or subcutaneous emphysema. Evaluation of the child includes cervical films (soft tissue and spine), chest radiographs, barium swallow, and CT scan of the neck. Because cervical spine injury may be present, laryngoscopy is performed in the neutral position. If the vocal cords and subglottic area are visualized during laryngoscopy, intubation is performed. If the vocal cords and the subglottis are obscured, tracheostomy is performed. Blind endotracheal intubation is contraindicated.

SUMMARY

"If cholera or small pox, or some disease killed and left affected that many [as trauma], Congress would be working and appropriating money and doing every mortal thing necessary to do something about it."

—Will Rogers (1926)

The traumatized pediatric patient may be aided by prevention, intervention, and legislation (e.g., laws requiring air bags safe for infants and children in automobiles). Although prevention of trauma is the concern of everyone, intervention primarily concerns the well-prepared health care provider, who strives to effect a positive outcome.

REFERENCES

1. Jurkovich GJ, Greiser WB, Luterman A, Curreri PW: Hypothermia in trauma victims: an ominous predictor of survival. *J Trauma* 1987;27:1019–1024.
2. Stevenson GW, Tobin M, Hall SC: Fluid warmer as a potential source of air bubble emboli. (Letter). *Anesth Analg* 1995;80:1061.
3. Wolin J, Vasdev GM: Potential for air embolism using Hotline Model HL90 fluid warmer. (Letter). *J Clin Anesth* 1996;8:81–82.
4. Chalon J, Patel C, Ali M, et al: Humidity and the anesthetized patient. *Anesthesiology* 1979;50:195–198.
5. Bissonnette B, Sessler DI: Passive or active inspired gas humidification increases thermal steady-state temperatures in anesthetized infants. *Anesth Analg* 1989;69:783–787.
6. Joacchimsson PO, Hedstrand U, Tabow F, Hansson B: Prevention of intraoperative hypothermia during abdominal surgery. *Acta Anaesthesiol Scand* 1987;31:330–337.
7. Kurz A, Kurz M, Poeschl G, et al: Forced-air warming maintains intraoperative normothermia better than circulating-water mattresses. *Anesth Analg* 1993;77:89–95.
8. Kurz A, Sessler DI, Lenhardt R: Perioperative normothermia to reduce the incidence of surgical-wound infection and shorten hospitalization. Study of Wound Infection and Temperature Group. *N Engl J Med* 1996;334:1209–1215.
9. Seidel JS, Burkett DL: *Instructors Manual for Pediatric Advanced Life Support.* Dallas: American Heart Association, 1987.
10. American College of Surgeons: *Advanced Trauma Life Support Student Manual.* Chicago: American College of Surgeons, 1989:222.
11. Ferguson M, Max MH, Marshall W: Emergency department infraclavicular subclavian vein catheterization in patients with multiple injuries and burns. *South Med J* 1988;81:433–435.
12. McNamara RM, Spivey WH, Unger HD, Malone DR: Emergency applications of intraosseous infusion. *J Emerg Med* 1987;5:97–101.
13. La Fleche FR, Slepin MJ, Vargas J, Milzman DP: Iatrogenic bilateral tibial fractures after intraosseous infusion attempts in a 3-month-old infant. *Ann Emerg Med* 1989;18:1099–1101.
14. American Heart Association: *Pediatric Advanced Life Support.* Elk Grove Village, IL: American Academy of Pediatrics, 1994.
15. Cales RH, Anderson PG, Heilig RW Jr: Utilization of medical care in Orange County: the effect of implementation of a regional trauma system. *Ann Emerg Med* 1985;14:853–858.
16. Badgwell JM, McLeod ME, Lerman J, Creighton RE: End-tidal PCO$_2$ measurements sampled at the distal and proximal ends of the endotracheal tube in infants and children. *Anesth Analg* 1987;66:959–664.
17. Weiskopf RB, Bogetz MS, Roizen MF, Reid IA: Cardiovascular and metabolic sequelae of inducing anesthesia with ketamine or thiopental in hypovolemic swine. *Anesthesiology* 1984;60:214–219.
18. Murray DJ, Forbes RB, Mahoney LT: Comparative hemodynamic depression of halothane versus isoflurane in neonates and infants: an echocardiographic study. *Anesth Analg* 1992;74:329–337.
19. Shires GT, Cunningham JN, Baker CR, et al: Alterations in cellular membrane function during hemorrhagic shock in primates. *Ann Surg* 1972;176:288–295.
20. Shires GT, Coln D, Carrico J: Fluid therapy in hemorrhagic shock. *Arch Surg* 1964;88:688–693.
21. Shires GT, Canizaro PC, Carico CJ: Shock. In: Schwartz SI (ed). *Principles of surgery,* ed 3. New York: McGraw-Hill, 1979:139–144.
22. Cogbill TH, Moore EE, Jurkovich GJ, et al: Nonopera-

tive management of blunt splenic trauma: a multicenter experience. *J Trauma* 1989;29:1312–1317.
23. Consentino CM, Luck SR, Barthel MJ, et al: Transfusion requirements in conservative nonoperative management of blunt splenic and hepatic injuries during childhood. *J Pediatr Surg* 1990;25:950–954.
24. Newman KD, Bowman LM, Eichelberger MR, et al: The lap belt complex: intestinal and lumbar spine injury in children. *J Trauma* 1990;30:1133–1138.
25. LoCicero J III, Mattox KL: Epidemiology of chest trauma. *Surg Clin North Am* 1989;69:15–19.
26. Peclet MH, Newman KD, Eichelberger MR, et al: Thoracic trauma in children: an indicator of increased mortality. *J Pediatr Surg* 1990;25: 961–965.
27. Snyder CL, Jain VN, Saltzman DA, et al: Blunt trauma in adults and children: a comparative analysis. *J Trauma* 1990;30:1239–1245.
28. Colombani PM, Buck JR, Dudgeon DL, et al: One-year experience in a regional pediatric trauma center. *J Pediatr Surg* 1985;20:8–13.
29. Peclet MH, Newman KD, Eichelberger MR, et al: Patterns of injury in children. *J Pediatr Surg* 1990;25: 85–91.
30. Langer JC, Winthrop AL, Wesson DE, et al: Diagnosis and incidence of cardiac injury in children with blunt thoracic trauma. *J Pediatr Surg* 1989;24:1091–1094.
31. Luerssen TG, Klauber MR, Marshall LF: Outcome from head injury related to patient s age: a longitudinal prospective study of adult and pediatric head injury. *J Neurosurg* 1988;68:409–416.
32. Pang D, Wilberger JE, Jr: Spinal cord injury without radiographic abnormalities in children. *J Neurosurg* 1982; 57:114–129.
33. Hastings RH, Marks JD: Airway management for trauma patients with potential cervical spine injuries. *Anesth Analg* 1991;73:471–482.

16

Sedation, Analgesia, and Anesthesia for Painful or Frightening Procedures Outside the Operating Room

Lawrence Roy

"When we turn to one another for counsel we reduce the number of our enemies."
—Kahlil Gibran

Anesthesia departments are frequently confronted by requests from medical and surgical colleagues for advice regarding conscious and deep sedation for procedures relegated to locations other than the operating room. Pediatric anesthesiologists are acknowledged authorities in the use of sedative and anesthetic drugs in infants and children. However, anesthesiologists are, for the most part, unfamiliar with the location and problems associated with these procedures and the drugs that have traditionally been prescribed by their medical colleagues. When anesthesiologists are consulted about conscious sedation issues, the advice is generally supported with anesthetic principles and approved guidelines (1). Although this advice may lead to improved patient safety, it may also lead to misunderstanding. Not all specialists accept such directives since they feel that their needs are unique. Therefore, they often generate their own protocols, which may allow substandard care (2).

CONSCIOUS SEDATION CONTROVERSIES

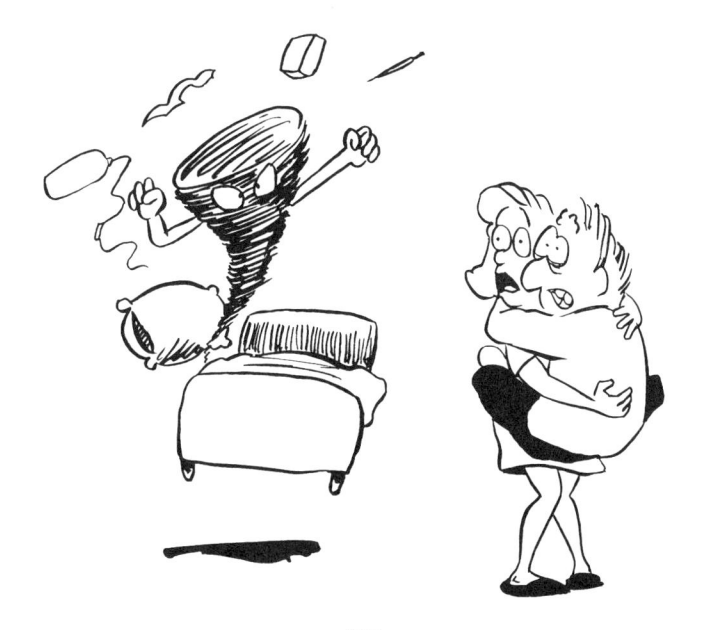

In principle, relegating the sedation of children with more complicated sedation issues to a qualified anesthesiologist is the optimal choice for sedation safety (3). This practice, however, may be impractical. In fact, the provider of conscious sedation is rarely an anesthesiologist. Usually, it is a medical colleague who may possess various resuscitative skills. The goal of drug administration is a state known as conscious sedation. It is becoming apparent that nonanesthetic sedation providers increasingly require guidance regarding the nature and complications of the drugs they are using, presedation assessment and preparation, appropriate monitoring during and after the procedure, and discharge guidelines (2). Most important, the personnel involved in sedation must come to an understanding of what is meant by the term "conscious sedation."

What Is Conscious Sedation?

Conscious sedation is defined in the most recent Guidelines for Monitoring and Management of Pediatric Patients During and After Sedation for Diagnostic and Therapeutic Procedures (1) as "a medically controlled state of depressed consciousness that (1) allows protective reflexes to be maintained; (2) retains the patient's ability to maintain a patent airway independently and continuously, and (3) permits an appropriate response by the patient to physical stimulation or verbal command, e.g., 'open your eyes.'"

Who Should Provide and Supervise Conscious Sedation?

The American Academy of Pediatrics (AAP) Committee on Drugs states that the person who provides sedation must be competent to use conscious sedation techniques and capable of managing complications associated with such techniques (1). Guidelines issued by the Department of Anesthesia, The Hospital for Sick Children (HSC)—Toronto state:

> ...personnel administering the sedation should be experienced in this technique and must have some training in pediatric advanced life support. A responsible physician should be available for both preoperative assessment and post sedation management. Airway management expertise is essential. Personnel must be able to identify signs of early and late airway complications and be competent in airway management (abilities should include the maintenance of an airway during spontaneous ventilation, intermittent positive pressure ventilation with a mask and a self inflating resuscitation bag and previous exposure to methods required to secure the airway).

Some centers have chosen to write their own guidelines rather than adopt those of the AAP (1,2). Although most directives are based on the AAP guidelines,[a] some of these new protocols may set out lenient directives with regard to fasting, monitoring, and appropriate personnel. If such guidelines are followed, a greater burden of responsibility is placed on knowledge of airway and resuscitative skills. The HSC document, shows a realization of this and includes the following warning: "Note: Those physicians utilizing these drugs alone or in combination should be familiar with these agents and aware of their potential respiratory complications."

PRESEDATION ASSESSMENT AND PREPARATION

"Alas! Regardless of their doom,
the little victims play!
No sense have they of ills to come
Nor care beyond today."
—Thomas Gray

There is general accord that sedation is appropriate for American Society of Anesthesiologists (ASA) classification I and II patients. Many nonanesthesia personnel, however, may find the ASA classifications to be confusing

---

[a]Ed. Note (JMB): The Harvard Medical School, Department of Anesthesia Sedation Guidelines (internal document) note "the minimum number of personnel shall be two—the operator and the monitor (an assistant trained to monitor appropriate physiologic parameters and to assist in any supportive or resuscitation measures required). Such personnel will be available to the patient from the time of administration of sedative medication until the recovery is judged adequate, or the care of the patient is transferred to personnel performing recovery care."

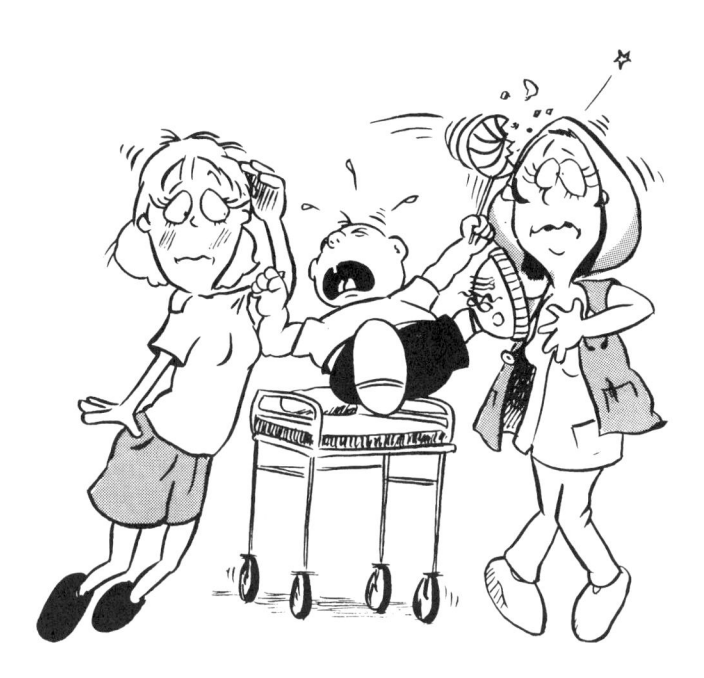

and worrisome. Therefore, the HSC document has included examples of the ASA types of pediatric patients.

Class I patients are normal healthy patients.
Class II patients have mild systemic disease, that is, patients with significant disease now well controlled as a result of medical treatment.

Examples of class II patients include those with the following conditions:

- Renal disease with controlled hypertension
- Cardiac disease with surgically corrected cardiac lesions (ventricular septal defect, atrial septal defect, transposition of the great arteries, patent ductus arteriosus)
- Neurologic disease—hydrocephalus controlled with functioning ventriculoperitoneal shunt, seizures controlled with medication
- Pulmonary disease—ex-premature with bronchopulmonary dysplasia, mild asthma managed at home with bronchodilators and presently asymptomatic
- Syndromes not involving the cardiovascular or respiratory systems including the upper airway

Vade and colleagues (3) infer that the safety of sedation practice may be ensured by limiting conscious sedation to ASA I and II patients. An accompanying editorial, however, notes that ASA I and II patients do not represent all patients who may need sedation (4). Older children with neurologic disorders, chronically ill children in pain, trauma patients, intensive care patients, patients with significant cardiovascular and pulmonary disease are examples of ASA III children requiring sedation for painful or frightening procedures. We recommend that ASA III patients be evaluated by an anesthesiologist before sedation. Furthermore, patients who have airway anomalies or who have experienced airway complications during past anesthetics or sedations should be thoroughly assessed before any sedative agent is administered.

Fasting Controversies

"You cannot reason with a hungry belly; it has no ears."

—Greek Proverb

Patients at HSC were rarely required to fast prior to publication of sedation guidelines. After the guidelines were introduced, however, there has been remarkable compliance with the recommended NPO (nothing by mouth) intervals. The current fasting directive states: "All patients should be kept NPO from solid food from midnight but may drink clear fluids up to two hours prior to the procedure."

A major factor in preventing aspiration is the maintenance of reflexes (i.e., cough and gag). Deeper levels of sedation may occur, which may be associated with loss of these critical protective reflexes. Therefore, fasting before the procedure is essential (5–7). An inconsistent situation arises from time to time, in which infants who have been deprived of their timely nourishment remain awake and crying during an investigation following high doses of chloral hydrate. The procedure is abandoned, the infant is fed and subsequently sleeps soundly—perhaps too soundly. Reports of adverse events (e.g., aspiration) occurring in the automobile while returning home suggest that these infants and children should remain NPO following discharge (8). The issues that remain unresolved are whether these patients should be fed before sedation or whether they should be fed once the procedure has been discontinued, in the hope of securing some cooperation and completion of the study or procedure.

A more difficult issue is that of the emergency patient. Children awaiting emergency surgery are at high risk for pulmonary aspiration, and this risk may be reduced by preanesthetic fasting (9,10). The AAP guidelines note that, if possible, such patients benefit from delaying the procedure and administering appropriate therapy to reduce gastric volume and increase the gastric pH (1). The duration of fasting may not influence gastric acidity in emergency patients but does reduce gastric volume significantly (10). When proper fasting is not ensured, the increased risks of sedation must be carefully weighed against its benefits and the lightest effective sedation used. Schurizek and associates (10) recommended a 4-hour fasting period for emergency patients when appropriate. However, the authors noted that even after 4 hours of fasting, 50% of the children admitted for emergency surgery were at risk for developing pulmonary aspiration. Perhaps the soundest approach, since a safe interval cannot be predicted (9), is to secure the airway in any child who presents for anesthesia following trauma.

What Is Deep Sedation?

Anesthesiologists are rarely involved in the delivery of conscious sedation. Let's face it. We usually provide deep sedation or general anesthesia. Anesthesiologists are usually uncomfortable with a patient who is reacting to painful stimuli and thus will administer additional medication rendering the patient unconscious. Moreover, our medical colleagues often have unrealistic expectations. Because an anesthesiologist is present, the "conscious sedation" should be dramatic; that is, the patient will not move to painful stimuli. Coté (8) has eloquently summarized the issue when referring to conscious sedation.

> "This phrase [conscious sedation] is an oxymoron that should be removed from the medical literature. When caring for children, particularly when they have to remain quiet for any length of time, one must induce pharmacologic coma; let us be honest and call deep sedation exactly what it is and take proper care of these deeply sedated patients."
> —Charlie Coté, MD

The definition of deep sedation—a medically controlled state of depressed consciousness or unconsciousness from which a patient may not be aroused—describes the condition of most "consciously sedated" children. Furthermore, deep sedation may be accompanied by a partial or complete loss of protective reflexes, and includes the inability to maintain a patent airway independently and respond purposely to physical stimulation or verbal command (1).

DRUGS COMMONLY USED BY NONANESTHESIA PERSONNEL

Chloral Hydrate

Chloral hydrate has been used for rendering children immobile during painless procedures for many years. At HSC, indications for its use include ophthalmologic procedures, radiology, computed tomography (CT) and magnetic resonance imaging (MRI) scans, echocardiogram, and electroencephalograph (EEG) examinations.

Dose response and physiologic changes after chloral hydrate have been studied in children (11–14). Increasing doses of chloral hydrate (25, 50, and 70 mg/kg) in children undergoing dental procedures significantly affected the diastolic pressure and end-tidal CO_2 in children aged 21 to 42 months of age (11). In another dental study, doses of 50 to 75 mg/kg of chloral hydrate were not associated with changes in vital signs or other adverse effects during the sedation interval (12). A prospective study examining the safety of high-dose chloral hydrate (80 to 100 mg/kg) suggested that high-dose chloral hydrate provides safe and effective sedation for children undergoing CT; however, vomiting, hyperactivity, and respiratory complications were observed (13). Sedation lasting longer than 2 hours was not observed (13). After the administration of triclofos sodium (note: 1 g triclofos sodium = 600 mg of chloral hydrate) to infants, there was no reduction in SaO_2, but respiratory rate increased.

Controversies

Monitoring Requirements. Despite the safe record and absence of respiratory depression in sedated children, there are reports of death following unrecognized overdose of chloral hydrate (15). Therefore, our sedation committee recommends the use of respiratory monitors when using this drug. Constant monitoring of blood pressure is to be avoided because this maneuver may awaken a sedated infant or child. Continuous pulse oximetry will provide an indication of perfusion.

Fasting and Sleep Deprivation. Some argue that fasting may be unnecessary and may increase the dose requirements of chloral hydrate. To date, this controversy remains unresolved. Until it is resolved, we recommend following the NPO guidelines whenever possible. It follows that chloral hydrate may not be the perfect drug in an urgent investigation when the child is not fasting. In this situation, unwarranted delay or cancellation may occur owing to the reluctance of anesthesiologists to provide further care in nonfasted children.

Sleep deprivation has been used as a means of guaranteeing a successful sedation. However, Canet and associates (16) demonstrated an increased incidence of respiratory difficulties even with minor degrees of sleep deprivation in healthy infants.

Other Controversies. Chloral hydrate in high doses will arrest cells in mitosis and alter the number of chromosomes in a cell; furthermore, the metabolite of chloral hydrate trichloroacetic acid induces liver tumors in rodents. These findings follow long-term administration. Steinberg (17) noted that he was unaware of any epidemiologic studies of humans who chronically ingested chloral hydrate. He concluded that risk to humans from exposure to chloral hydrate in doses up to 100 mg/kg cannot be predicted directly from rodent data, particularly when the animal model was given an excessively high dosage for a long period of time compared with the intermittent dosage in the human experience. Steinberg further concluded that chloral hydrate should not be withdrawn on the basis of available data. Replacing chloral hydrate with another drug may carry greater risks. Steinberg (17) also recommended limiting the dose of chloral hydrate administered to newborns and avoiding prolonged periods of sedation because they cannot clear the metabolites.

Recommendations

The dose recommendations are as follows: 50 to 100 mg/kg up to a maximum dose of 2 g by mouth. The duration of significant sedation is generally 90 to 120 minutes. A designated recovery area is essential. Premature discharge of infants who have been heavily sedated with chloral hydrate has resulted in severe consequences (18).

Meperidine/Phenergan/Thorazine

The combination of meperidine 2 mg/kg, promethazine 1 mg/kg, and chlorpromazine 1 mg/kg, called DPT for the commercial names of these drugs (Demerol, Phenergan, and Thorazine) has also been referred to as CM3 or cardiac mixture 3. Despite problems with this mixture of drugs, the cocktail still remains one of the most popular means of sedating children (18).

Controversies

Significant episodes of hypotension, apnea, and prolonged recovery have been reported with DPT (19,20). Furthermore, no antagonist is available to reverse adverse effects of chlorpromazine and promethazine. The children are often awake and crying during the procedure and unconscious for many hours thereafter. Yaster and associates (21) describe this combination as a dangerous approach to sedation. Coté (18) designates this combination of drugs as inappropriate. Complications related to DPT administration include the following (18–20):

- Dystonic reactions
- Orthostatic hypotension
- Pulmonary aspiration
- Prolonged sedation (>7 hours)
- Respiratory depression
- Seizures resulting in death
- Ventilatory arrest

"It makes little sense to administer two phenothiazines which are long acting drugs with a long acting narcotic, especially when phenothiazines have been demonstrated to have antianalgesic properties and potentiate the respiratory depression produced by narcotics."
—Charles Coté

DPT has been removed from the HSC formulary principally because of the prolonged period of recovery after administration and the high incidence of complications as previously listed.

Recommendations

At the Hospital for Sick Children, DTP is not a recommended combination.

"Every human being has like Socrates, an attendant spirit; and wise are they who obey its signals. If it does not always tell us what to do, it always cautions us what not to do."
—Lydia M. Child

Ketamine

Ketamine has been administered orally in doses of 6 to 10 mg/kg. In such doses, purposeless movement may occur, which may limit its usefulness in specific situations such as in radiation therapy (18,22). Because it is associated with copious oral secretions, the concomitant administration of atropine or glycopyrrolate may be helpful (23). However, atropine pretreatment may be unnecessary when ketamine is administered as a preanesthetic medication. Nystagmus may occur in patients receiving ketamine (6 mg/kg orally) (24).

Controversies

Oral ketamine can occasionally produce airway obstruction. Strict adherence to the AAP guidelines is therefore essential (1). The use of ketamine is limited to anesthesiologists in many institutions. Some support the view that the oral administration of ketamine in the appropriate dose is not associated with significant complications and does not require the attendance of an anesthesiologist (25).

Recommendations

Ketamine may be given orally, 6 to 10 mg/kg. Consider a reduced dosage in combination with oral midazolam. Intravenous (IV) administration must be supervised by an anesthesiologist.

Pentobarbital

Pentobarbital is perhaps the most commonly used sedative for diagnostic imaging. However, problems include insufficient duration of action, respiratory depression, and other side effects such as ataxia, irritability, and lethargy (26).

Controversies

Radiologists prefer IV pentobarbital because of its rapid onset of action and low incidence of complications (27). However, pentobarbital may render patients somewhat hypersensitive to painful stimulation (23,28). This precludes its use for painful procedures unless accompanied by a narcotic (e.g., fentanyl). Pentobarbital in combination with other sedatives or narcotics, however, significantly increases the risk of respiratory obstruction (18). In fact, severe or prolonged oxygen hemoglobin desaturation may occur within 5 minutes after IV administration (29).

Recommendations

The following are guidelines for pentobarbital administration:

1. Draw up pentobarbital 5 mg/kg in a 3-ml syringe.
2. In a 10-ml syringe, dilute pentobarbital with normal saline (NS) to make a total volume of solution of 10 ml.
3. Clean the port of the saline lock with alcohol.
4. Inject 5 ml (2.5 mg/kg) of the pentobarbital solution over 20 seconds.
5. Observe the patient for drowsiness, and wait 30 seconds to 1 minute.
6. Give the next 2.5 ml (1.25 mg/kg) pentobarbital solution over 20 seconds. Assess the patient for 1 minute, repeat the 2.5 ml (1.25 mg/kg) dose over 30 seconds, if necessary.
7. If 5 minutes after the complete dose (10 ml = 5 mg/kg) has been given, the patient remains awake and moving, a supplemental dose of 1 mg/kg in 5 ml NS may be given over 30 seconds.

The maximum dosage of pentobarbital regardless of weight is 150 mg.

Midazolam

Midazolam is a short-acting water-soluble anxiolytic with no analgesic properties. It inhibits the stress response through a reduction in available catecholamines. Such effects do not appear to be a significant problem in healthy children. Midazolam, because of its short duration, predictable onset, and lack of active metabolites may be superior to other sedative agents when used for conscious sedation. The popular routes of administration are IV, oral, and intranasal. Respiratory depression may be significant, and apnea may occur with higher doses and rapid rates of administration (30). Clinical investigators stress the importance of slow IV administration of midazolam (31). "Midazolam should only be used in closely monitored situations such as routinely apply when general anesthesia is administered" (32).

Controversies

Fentanyl potentiates the effects of midazolam. Over 80 deaths had been reported to the FDA by 1988 after the administration of combinations of midazolam and fentanyl (33). The package insert warns of respiratory problems and the need for skilled personnel and equipment to provide an adequate airway and appropriate ventilation (30). Some have discouraged this combination outside an operating room setting (21). Dysphoria has been observed after the administration of oral midazolam (34); thus, patient and case selection are important considerations when using the oral route.

Recommended Dosage and Route of Administration

The following are commonly used dosages for midazolam (34,35):

Oral	0.5 to 0.75 mg/kg
Intranasal	0.2 to 0.3 mg/kg
Intravenous	0.05 to 0.1 mg/kg

After intranasal midazolam administration, onset time ranges from 8 to 10 minutes, whereas with oral administration onset may be 12 to 15 minutes (35). Although the intranasal route may seem more advantageous, it has been associated with significant respiratory depression and an objectionable burning sensation (35,36).

In the event that a combination of IV midazolam and narcotic are contemplated, a maximum of two midazolam doses of 0.05 mg/kg should be set with a maximum fentanyl dosage of 3.0 µg/kg or maximum morphine dosage of 0.15 mg/kg, administered cautiously in three divided doses. Following the occurrence of respiratory depression in a 14-month-old toddler after fentanyl (6 µg/kg) and midazolam (0.11 mg/kg), it was concluded that "fentanyl and midazolam must be individualized and administered by titration to effect rather than by a fixed dosage schedule" (37). It is also recommended that sedative drugs be diluted when treating children to avoid inadvertent overdose. Naloxone (a narcotic antagonist) and flumazenil (a specific benzodiazepine antagonist) must be immediately available to reverse significant respiratory depression (21).

Flumazenil

Flumazenil is a reversal agent that is a competitive antagonist at the benzodiazepine receptor. Studies indicate the mean plasma half-life to be 0.7 to 1.3 hours, and its duration of action has varied from 15 to 140 minutes. Flumazenil should be immediately available when the parenteral administration of a benzodiazepine is contemplated (37).

Controversies

Some clinicians have advocated the routine use of flumazenil after administration of midazolam for conscious sedation (38). This practice seems inadvisable since resedation, though infrequent, is always a possibility. Therefore, after flumazenil administration, SaO_2 must still be monitored until the effect of midazolam has dissipated (37).

Recommended Dosage and Route of Administration

Flumazenil may be given by intravenous injection, at a dose of 10 µg/kg IV over 15 seconds followed by a waiting period of 1 to 3 minutes. If necessary, the dose may be repeated up to four times at 1 to 3 minute intervals to a total dose of 50 µg/kg. If resedation occurs, doses may be repeated every 20 minutes, or the effective dose may be given hourly as infusion.

Nitrous Oxide

When administered alone, nitrous oxide has minimal cardiovascular and respiratory effects and has been used for many years in combination with oral or IV sedation in pediatric dental procedures. Combinations of chloral hydrate, 25 mg/kg, and hydroxyzine, 1 mg/kg, with nitrous oxide 30% to 50% result in analgesia and sedation without loss of consciousness and airway reflexes (23).

Controversies

Litman and associates (39) determined that children age 1 to 3 years when sedated with midazolam, 0.5 mg/kg, and nitrous oxide in varying concentrations (15% to 60%) did not develop any respiratory complications. However, as the nitrous oxide was increased beyond 15%, there was a progression toward deep sedation. The authors concluded that such combinations should be administered by trained and experienced personnel with appropriate monitoring and observation of the patient. Such a view was supported by other clinicians who are concerned about the potential for administration of hypoxic mixtures by unfamiliar health personnel (23).

The administration of nitrous oxide is further complicated by the unresolved potential for occupational hazards (40). Thus, efficient scavenging devices must be used to limit nitrous oxide levels to <25 ppm (parts per million) in the United States (NIOSH standards) and <30 ppm (Canadian Standards Association). Guidelines to the Practice of Anaesthesia (49) recommend the dilution of waste anesthetic gases through increased room ventilation at 20 changes per hour (CSA standard Z317.2).

Concern as to whether administration of nitrous oxide leads to depression of laryngeal reflexes has been allayed (42). The investigators administered radiopaque dye orally to children after administration of nitrous oxide/oxygen in a concentration of 20% to 65%. No children demonstrated depression of laryngeal reflexes.

Recommended Dosages

The use of nitrous oxide and oxygen in a 50:50 concentration for the reduction of uncomplicated fractures in the emergency room is safe and effective. This method, however, requires patient cooperation. The agent must be self-administered to avoid profound sedation (43). When increased levels of nitrous oxide or the addition of other sedative agents are contemplated, the administration should be supervised by responsible, trained personnel. Nitrous oxide/oxygen is provided in some centers for oncology patients requiring bone marrow aspirations and lumbar punctures, for burn patients requiring dressing changes, and for patients with lacerations requiring suture closure in the emergency room (personal communication).

Conscious Sedation Drug Dosages

The following is the HSC Sedation Protocol 1995—Department of Anesthesia:

Drug	Dose
Chloral hydrate	50 to 100 mg/kg orally or rectally to a maximum dose of 2 g
Diazemuls	0.1 mg/kg IV
Diazepam	0.2 mg/kg orally
Midazolam	0.05 mg/kg IV dose may be repeated once as needed; maximum dose 1.5 mg/kg IV
Midazolam	0.5 to 0.75 mg/kg orally for children < 20 kg
	0.3 to 0.5 mg/kg orally for children > 20 kg
Flumazenil	Injection: 0.1 mg/ml 10 µg/kg IV over 15 seconds. Wait 1 to 3 minutes. If necessary, dose may be repeated up to four times at 1- to 3-minute intervals to total dose of 50 µg/kg. If resedation occurs, doses may be repeated every 20 minutes, or the effective dose may be given hourly as infusion.
Morphine	0.05 to 0.1 mg/kg IV; dose may be repeated once at a 15 minute interval; 0.3 mg/kg orally
Naloxone	0.01 to 0.10 mg/kg IV; should be reserved for emergency use—severe obtundation and respiratory depression. After administration of naloxone, patients must be cared for in a constant care setting and discharged only when they are fully awake and a minimum time of 3 hours has elapsed.
Pentobarbital	4.0 to 5.0 mg/kg IV to a maximum of 100 mg
	6.0 mg/kg IM for children ≤15 kg
	5.0 mg/kg IM for children ≥15 kg

Nitrous oxide/oxygen — Administration of nitrous oxide, especially in combination with other drugs, should comply with AAP guidelines (1).

Remote Sedation Locations

In the Emergency Room

Management of sedation for children in the emergency department (ED) is hampered by the customary chaotic environment. Most procedures are associated with significant discomfort (e.g., laceration repair, fracture reduction, lumbar puncture, and bone marrow aspiration). A busy ED is not an ideal location for monitoring and managing sedated patients, particularly for extended intervals (43). The sedation guidelines developed by the AAP are difficult to adhere to in a busy ED setting (1). Indeed, a US survey (44) revealed as of 1991 that most pediatric EDs do not comply with these guidelines.

Emergency department patients are at increased risk for aspirating stomach contents (9,10). Procedures in the ED are by definition nonelective and thus have not been preceded by a significant fasting interval. The absorption of drugs administered orally may be delayed owing to coincidental pain. Thus, parenteral administration may be the preferred route of administration. An ideal ED sedative would be administered orally or intramuscularly, have a rapid onset, short duration, and rapid recovery (43). It should be potentially reversible, produce a predictable degree of sedation, and would not affect ventilation and airway reflexes. Such a drug does not exist at this time. However, clinicians remain hopeful for a future pharmacologic breakthrough in this search for a perfect sedative.

Chloral hydrate, diazepam, midazolam, morphine, fentanyl, and ketamine have been used successfully by the ED physician. Chloral hydrate with its wide margin of safety appears particularly well suited to ED requirements. It is administered in a dose of 25 to 50 mg/kg and with the time to sedation (20 to 60 minutes) and recovery (20 to 60 minutes) appropriate for procedures such as wound repair, foreign body removal, and abscess drainage (43). Major criticisms of the drug are variability in clinical response and the absence of analgesic properties. Ketamine, 2.0 mg/kg, combined with midazolam, 0.1 mg/kg, and atropine, 0.01 mg/kg, given intramuscularly for laceration repair has recently been introduced in the ED at Children's Memorial Hospital Chicago (personal communication).

Midazolam recently has been popularized for use in the ED when administered orally or nasally. A study compared oral and nasal routes of administration and concluded that single doses of midazolam, 0.5 mg/kg orally or 0.25 mg/kg nasally, are safe and effective when administered for laceration repair to anxious children in the ED. The onset time was judged to be roughly 15 minutes after oral administration and 10 minutes for the nasal route. The nasal route was associated with increased difficulty of administration (45). Emergence delirium is a potential complication resulting from the oral administration of midazolam (46). Doses greater than 0.5 mg/kg have been associated with an increased incidence of unpleasant dysphoria (34).

Intranasal midazolam, 0.2 mg/kg, in combination with sufentanil, 0.75 µg/kg, was administered to children for laceration repair and compared with a similar group receiving im meperidine, promethazine, and chlorpromazine. The authors found this combination of nasal sufentanil/midazolam to be an appealing alternative to the conventional combination DPT (47).

Management of pain and sedation during closed reduction of forearm fractures has long been an ED issue. A commonly used method of IV sedation with narcotic and benzodiazepine was recently reexamined (48). Meperidine, 2.0 mg/kg, and midazolam, 0.1 mg/kg, were administered intravenously to children. Most patients cried out briefly during the reduction maneuver but resumed sleeping following the reduction. In fact, the authors write "we have come to expect and prefer this typical reaction as it appears to demonstrate the desired level of sedation" (48). Although no patients experienced apnea, two patients received a narcotic antagonist to treat progressive respiratory depression.

The investigators recommended that IV sedation should be performed only with proper observation and physiologic monitoring of blood pressure, pulse rate, and oxygen saturation levels. Most of these patients were sedated for 30 to 60 minutes. Recovery consisted of drowsiness and ataxia, which lasted an additional 30 to 60 minutes. A combination of sedation and IV regional anesthesia may be the most desirable approach to the forearm fracture (49). Although preparation and administration of an IV regional block may be tedious, the diminished need for sedation combined with the profound analgesia of an IV block leads to impressive results. Indeed, patients may require only a brief period of observation after reduction because of the reduced sedation/narcotic dosages. Some clinicians have suggested the use of self-administered 50% nitrous oxide and 50% oxygen for providing pain relief during manipulation of closed forearm fractures. Pain relief is reasonable, complications rare, and ease of administration remarkable. The provision of monitoring, moment-to-moment observation, and avoidance of other sedatives and narcotics are essential measures when using this technique (50).

For Cardiology Procedures

Cardiologists use sedation in infants and small children for transthoracic cardiac echocardiography, diagnostic cardiac catheterization, and transesophageal echocardiography. More intense sedation and anesthesia methods are required in the interventional cardiac catheterization laboratory.

Young patients scheduled for cardiac echocardiography at HSC are usually sedated with an oral preparation of chloral hydrate (50 to 100 mg/kg). Onset of sedation with this agent can be somewhat protracted. The administration of intranasal midazolam (0.4 mg/kg in two divided doses at 5- to 10-minute intervals) has been advocated. Investigators concluded that intranasal midazolam is safe and effective for echocardiographic studies in uncooperative infants. The advantages of this method were its rapid onset (5 to 15 minutes), short duration of action (25 to 45 minutes), few complications, and ease of administration (51).

Patients undergoing diagnostic cardiac catheterization at HSC are managed with morphine, 0.05 mg/kg, and midazolam, 0.05 mg/kg IV. Javorski and colleagues (52) describe the administration of DPT (see earlier description) in advance of the morphine/midazolam combination. At HSC, the DPT formulation has been removed from the formulary in the interest of safety. However, this measure has hampered the ability of cardiologists to adequately sedate their patients. Requests for advice regarding alternate sedation methods have increased owing to the elimination of this drug combination. Javorski and colleagues (52) note that when infants and children are difficult to sedate or require high doses of standard medication, ketamine, 0.2 to 0.5 mg/kg, is administered by intermittent bolus or by continuous infusion (1 mg/kg/hour). The authors note that in noninterventional procedures general anesthesia is reserved for uncooperative patients when sedation techniques prove inadequate.

For Diagnostic Imaging

Radiologists are often confronted with the dilemma of sedating an infant or child. The very nature of their task (high-quality imaging) dictates the need for a motionless child (seconds to hours). Most investigations are painless procedures but may be associated with an element of terror (from the patient's perspective).

With the introduction of CT for children, sedatives were used increasingly by radiologists. The demand for sedation continues to increase and therefore the potential for severe complications does as well. In 1982, Mitchell and associates (53) noted that the incidence of life-threatening reactions were unusually frequent (4%)—four times the expected rate. The risk of an adverse reaction in this group was increased in subjects who received high doses of drugs and in those who received four or more sedative agents. Life-threatening reactions were identified only in infants <3 months of age. Eight years later, Cohen (54) wrote of his concerns in an editorial regarding the management of pediatric sedation by radiologists. He stated that patient evaluation, patient monitoring criteria for discharge, and staff training and certification were not high priorities within radiology departments. In fact, the pediatric radiologist may have the greatest potential to do harm to his or her patients through the administration of sedative agents than by any other radiologic procedure. The editorial alludes to one survey wherein 129 pediatric radiologists reported a total of 9 deaths and 18 cases of respiratory arrest occurring as complications of pediatric sedation. These remarks were in response to an article that examined sedation practices in 1990 in the United States (55). At that time, adherence to AAP guidelines (1) was limited, fasting guidelines were often overlooked, and monitoring during deep sedation fell short in a sizable number of hospitals. Chloral hydrate was the first-line drug for sedation for CT.

Since 1990, an increased awareness has led to significant changes at HSC (Toronto). After the formation of a Diagnostic Imaging Sedation Committee, new protocols, fasting guidelines, sedation formulary, monitoring guidelines, sedation record, and discharge guidelines have been introduced. Vade and colleagues (3) recently examined the value of adopting the AAP guidelines (1). They emphasized the value of medical screening and patient selection and endorsed the adherence to AAP guidelines for monitoring and management of pediatric sedations.

Sedative agents used by radiologists for sedation during painless imaging include pentobarbital, chloral hydrate (29) and midazolam (56). Pereira and associates (29) determined that IV pentobarbital provided faster and superior quality sedation for CT scan than intramuscular pentobarbital or orally administered chloral hydrate. IV pentobarbital provided adequate sedation within 7 minutes, whereas the intramuscular route took an average of 44 minutes to achieve an adequate level. The incidence of patient desaturation was increased in patients receiving IV pentobarbital and chloral hydrate. Patients in the chloral hydrate group were much younger. Severe and prolonged desaturations were associated only with IV pentobarbital. The authors concluded that IV pentobarbital provided superior quality sedation. However, this method may be inappropriate for departments unfamiliar with sedation routines or those lacking adequate resuscitation facilities. The risk of hypoxia and thus the increased need for monitoring and possible interventions were noted.

Table 1 lists the sedatives used in the Department of Medical Imaging (HSC) for MRI and CT.

Pediatric interventional radiology has seen a steady growth in recent years, and the need for significant sedation or general anesthesia is essential. Procedures undertaken by interventional radiologists are not painless. Although sedation is commonly used, general anesthesia is requested when the procedure is lengthy, when past sedation has been ineffective, for particularly painful procedures, or when the procedure is complex. When sedation is the selected method, combinations of chloral hydrate, fentanyl, and pentobarbital are used (28). Table 2 lists the protocols for drug dosages and

TABLE 1. *Current sedative dosages used in the Department of Medical Imaging (HSC)*

Drug	Dose	Range	Route
Chloral hydrate	50 mg/kg	50–100 mg/kg	Oral
Pentobarbital	2 mg/kg	2–6 mg/kg	IV

TABLE 2. *Drug dosages for sedation of children according to weight at HSC*

Drug	Dose	Maximum dose	Route
	Sedation Protocol for Children >10 kg		
Meperidine	1.0/kg	2 mg/kg	IV
Morphine	0.05 mg/kg	0.1 mg/kg	IV
Diazemuls	0.1 mg/kg	10 mg	IV
Midazolam	0.05 mg/kg	0.1 mg/kg	IV
	Sedation Protocol for Children <10 kg		
Pentobarbital	3 mg/kg	6 mg/kg	IV
Demerol	1 mg/kg	2 mg/kg	IV
	Sedation Protocol for Children <5 kg		
Chloral hydrate	50–100 mg/kg	100 mg/kg	Oral

routes of administration set by the Division of Interventional Radiology—Department of Medical Imaging (HSC). To date, the use of fentanyl has been restricted to members of the Department of Anesthesia (HSC).

For Hematology and Oncology Procedures

Painful diagnostic and therapeutic procedures are often required for pediatric cancer patients. Patients' anxiety and pain may be managed with behavioral techniques, local anesthesia, conscious sedation, deep sedation, and finally general anesthesia (56). Many hospitals do not have an organized approach for children's procedural pain. Some centers avoid the administration of conscious sedation because of concerns regarding safety, time, and prolonged recovery (57). Others rely on DPT or chloral hydrate and diazepam; the former plagued with undesirable complications and the latter lacking in analgesic properties. Pain remedies are often haphazard and introduced only after the child becomes unmanageable. Indeed, the initial experiences of the child may well alter the perception of treatment and its associated pain. Some advocate delaying the initial bone marrow until general anesthesia or deep sedation can be provided (57,58).

Commonly used medications for sedation before bone marrow aspirations, biopsies, and lumbar punctures are narcotics, benzodiazepines, barbiturates, DPT, and occasionally nitrous oxide (58). After the administration of oral ketamine (10 mg/kg), pediatric oncology patients experienced very little procedural distress and no cardiorespiratory difficulties. However, the authors noted that 30 minutes after administration 47% of patients were completely unresponsive. Recovery generally took 2 to 4 hours (25). Ketamine in doses of 6 mg/kg has been noted to be effective as a premedication to facilitate parental separation and induction of anesthesia (24). Perhaps in this dosage fewer patients would be completely unresponsive at 20 to 30 minutes.

Midazolam has been shown to be safe and effective for the management of patients scheduled for lumbar puncture and bone marrow aspiration. The major risk of midazolam administration is hypoventilation and hypoxemia. Episodes of desaturation generally occur within 10 minutes of IV administration (0.05 mg/kg). Thus a person skilled in pediatric airway management should be available and clinicians performing procedures under conscious sedation should be aware of potential need for assisted ventilation. Clinically significant episodes of hypoxemia (<90%) occurred in 13% of children receiving midazolam (58). Midazolam (0.2 mg/kg IV) when combined with local anesthesia was preferred to fentanyl (0.004 mg/kg IV) for managing bone marrow or lumbar puncture (59).

The administration of nitrous oxide alone is effective in alleviating anxiety and discomfort in cooperative children (60). Some centers have managed these procedures (lumbar puncture and bone marrow) with nitrous oxide alone or in combination with IV or oral midazolam (personal communication). The issue as to whether this method requires the presence of an anesthesiologist remains unclear (61).

MONITORING CHILDREN IN REMOTE LOCATIONS

Monitoring children in remote locations always presents unique challenges. The differing capabilities of monitors to accurately access vital signs in very small infants and children, the indeterminate medical status of a child in the midst of an evaluation, and all the aggravations of administering anesthesia on foreign ground are combined. The gravity of this situation continues, with ongoing reports of cardiac and respiratory arrest, deaths, or neurologic injury in children who were sedated and improperly monitored. Anesthetic-related cardiac arrests are three times more likely to occur in children than adults, and perianesthetic morbidity is significantly increased in infants <1 month of age. Many of our nonanesthesia colleagues believe that the intensity of monitoring required by our discipline is excessive. Indeed, the application of the ASA Monitoring Standards in certain remote locations can be frustrating. Considering the risk-benefit ratio (assuming one benefits from 1 or 2 hours of pharmacologic coma), however, the absolute necessity of appropriate monitoring is clear.

Traveling to Radiology

All the currently available monitors have no physical properties that prevent their use in any standard radiologic suite. New small portable monitors with multiple functions are ideal for traveling. ECG, noninvasive blood pressure, two pressure transducers, temperature, oximetry, and even capnometry all are available in one small box. These units can be observed through leaded windows or on a video monitor if there are environmental hazards to care providers if they were to remain at the bedside. Many anesthesia machines now incorporate integrated monitoring and can function for both anesthesia delivery and physiologic monitoring.

Traveling to the MRI Department

In the standard radiologic suite, monitoring problems typically derive from the physical limitations of the facility and access to the patient. On entering the MRI suite, one must also consider the interaction of monitoring devices with the intense magnetic and radiofrequency (RF) emissions from the scanner. These interactions can include interference with the function of the monitor, attraction of ferrous devices into the magnet, and patient injury from objects attracted to the magnet or from induced electrical currents. Wave guides (copper pipes in the walls) can be used to pass cables and tubing through walls while maintaining RF shielding. Magnetic saturation of electronic transformers can be avoided by locating monitors outside the magnet room and passing cables and other equipment through the wave guides. Copper or aluminum housings can be used to shield devices in the scanning room from RF. A clear understanding of the manner in which signals are derived for each monitoring modality can be used to successfully monitor pediatric patients in the MRI suite.

Electrocardiography

Despite installation of ECG monitoring in currently manufactured GE or Siemens 1.5 T magnets, ECG signals remain distorted. The flow of blood (which is itself an electrical conductor) within a magnetic field creates small eddy currents which change the ECG vector. Braiding of the ECG cables is recommended to minimize the antennae effect and degradation of the ECG signal. Cables should not be coiled because this increases the likelihood that an induced current may injure the patient.

Blood Pressure

Automated oscillometry has been shown to be accurate in even small premature infants and is slowly becoming a standard. The pneumatic principles used do not interfere with MRI imaging (as long as the electronic unit is either shielded or outside of the room). Many people commonly lengthen the hose or put two hoses together without altering pressure determination. Problems of artifact due to patient movement or rhythm disturbances apply to children as they do in adults.

Oximetry

Most commercially available oximeters work in the MRI, although the cable and probe must be shielded with aluminum foil or attached to a distal site with the cable led away from the magnet.

Capnometry

Some states mandate CO_2 monitoring during all general anesthetics. Aspirating systems are much easier for traveling than in-line systems because they are less cumbersome and lighter. There is also less risk of extubating a child with an aspirating system, and they are compatible with MRI. Aspirating systems do not require aluminum foil shielding as a flow-through infrared system would. Endotracheal tubes with side ports for more accurate monitoring of CO_2 at a distal site in the tube are recommended.

Temperature

Temperature monitoring in children is imperative in most radiology suites because the room is kept cool for the computer systems. Heating blankets and radiant lights cannot be used because they interfere with imaging. In the MRI suite, RF causes a rise in body temperature. Thermistors have been associated with burns and should be used with care. Liquid crystal thermometers are less likely to burn the patient, but are not as easily observed or monitored.

Anesthesia Machines

The Ohmeda Excel-210 MRI (Madison, WI) is a standard anesthesia machine model that has been manufactured using nonferrous material. It consists of 99.8% stainless steel, brass, aluminum, and plastic, and it can be placed directly in the MRI scanning room. Non-MRI–specific anesthesia machines have been used successfully in the scanning room without any problems by keeping the machines 20 to 30 feet away from the core of the magnet.

ANESTHESIA OUTSIDE THE OPERATING ROOM

Providing anesthesia for infants and children for procedures outside the operating room is a challenging task for anesthesiologists. The experience occurs in an unfamiliar setting not designed for the purpose of providing anesthesia, while working with individuals who may not be accustomed to the unique needs of the anesthesiologist. In addition, the anesthetic requirements vary from simple sedation to general anesthesia, which may have to be repeated daily on an outpatient basis for up to several weeks.

Propofol

The introduction of the IV agent propofol has liberated the anesthesiologist from the operating room. This agent is well suited for deep sedation for painful or frightening procedures in remote locations. This drug provides rapid onset and emergence from anesthesia with minimal residual hangover (62). Patients may be discharged with minimal recovery time (63). Propofol is an effective induction agent in unpremedicated children (64); a dose range of 2.5 to 3.0 mg/kg is recommended to induce sleep. Maintenance can be accomplished through repeated doses or a constant infusion (63). Pain on injection can be alleviated with the concomitant administration of IV lidocaine. This agent is associated with some drawbacks, such as hypotension, apnea, pain on injection, and involuntary movements (65). Apnea, however, may be the most significant negative characteristic. Nevertheless, when it is suggested that this agent may be administered by nonanesthesia personnel, pediatric anesthesiologists question the merit of such statements (65). Delay in managing apnea in a pediatric patient may lead to severe adverse consequences (63). The latest generation of lightweight and compact transport monitors have also expedited travel for the anesthesiologist.

There are many remote locations where anesthesiologists may now provide care. The following locations represent situations in which the provision of anesthetic presence has truly made a difference.

Deep Sedation/Anesthesia for Hematology and Oncology Patients

"True kindness presupposes the faculty of imagining as one's own the suffering and joys of others."
—André Gide

As of 1990, it was the accepted standard of care at the Memorial Sloan-Kettering Cancer Cancer in New York to perform diagnostic procedures with the patient under general anesthesia (57). This experience is similar to that at HSC Toronto, where the administration of deep sedation or general anesthesia is judged to be preferable to conventional methods of sedation and analgesia.

Parents, patients, and physicians all recognize the superiority of deep sedation managed by a department of anesthesia. The need for a well-equipped treatment room with an anesthesia machine, monitors, piped anesthetic gases, and appropriate scavenging expedites the quality of care and the rate at which patients can be managed.

Patients with IV access *in situ* (many patients have a central venous line) receive propofol (bolus administration, 2 to 3 mg/kg) and nitrous oxide/oxygen, whereas those patients without IV access often request anesthesia by mask with incremental concentrations of halo-

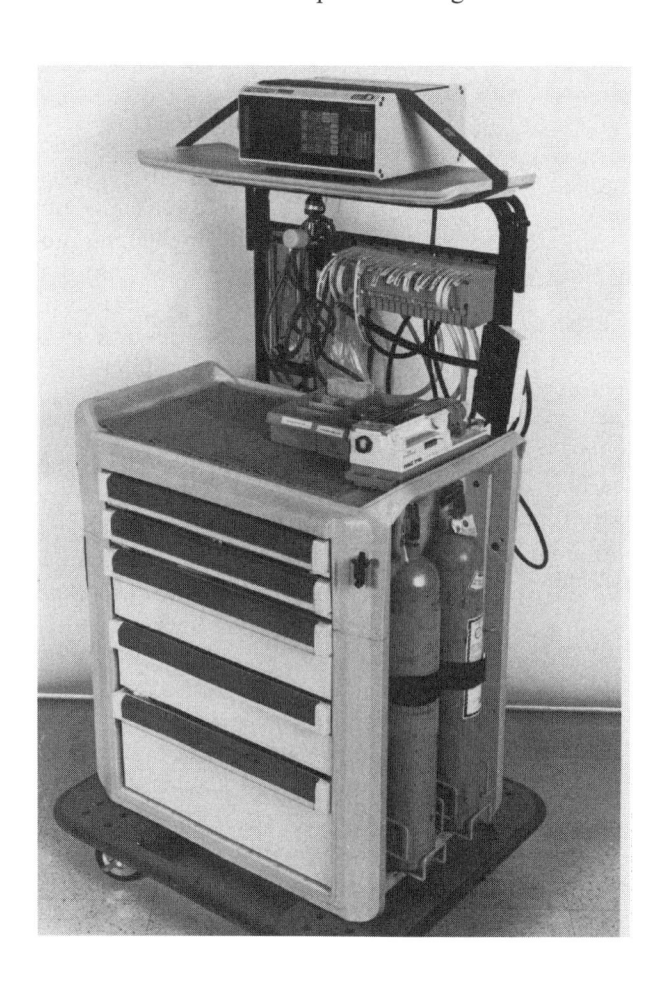

FIG. 1. The transportable sedation/anesthesia vehicle.

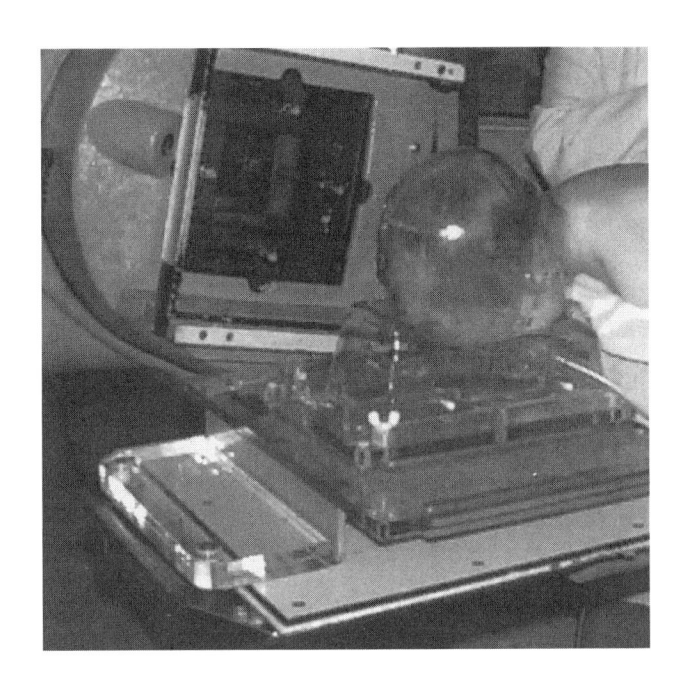

FIG. 2. An 18-month-old child in the prone position for radiation of brainstem. The patient is anesthetized with intravenous propofol infusion and is breathing spontaneously without airway support.

thane and nitrous oxide/oxygen. These patients are recovered in a step-down area adjacent to the anesthetic treatment room and generally discharged after they have recovered from the effects of anesthesia and chemotherapy.

Patients who have had bone marrow transplantation and who continue to require strict isolation present a unique set of circumstances. A portable sedation/anesthesia vehicle has been assembled at HSC Toronto (Fig. 1). This device allows the delivery of deep sedation at the bedside of these isolated patients.

Recently, word of anesthetic mobility has reached the offices of the radiation oncologist (62). Although failed sedation for radiation therapy is an uncommon occurrence (personal communication), anesthetic input is requested with increasing frequency. These children may require radiation treatment daily for up to 6 weeks; thus, the anesthetic technique must be simple and unassociated with significant morbidity. Tracheal intubation should be avoided where possible, since airway instrumentation over a 6-week course may well lead to increased respiratory complications. The laryngeal mask airway may be a preferable alternative (66).

Radiation sites were constructed without consideration for the provision of anesthesia; thus, the absence of medical gases, wall suction, and adequate scavenging capability create a formidable task for the anesthesiologist (62) (Fig. 2). Radiation hazard necessitates complete isolation of the patient for 5 to 10 minute intervals. The patient is monitored by means of two video cameras—one that transmits images of the patient and the other that relays images of the non-invasive blood pressure (NIBP), ECG, away gas machine (AGM), and saturation monitors. The anesthetic of choice at HSC is a propofol bolus (2 to 3 mg/kg) followed by an infusion (100 µg/kg/min IV). This dosage schedule is similar to that established for sedating children in an MRI unit (67).

Hematology and Oncology Issues

The following are considerations for hematology and oncology patients:

• Accommodation of newly diagnosed children on admission is preferable (generally with acute lymphatic leukemia requiring lumbar punctures, and bone marrow aspirations and biopsies) because initial experiences of the child may well alter the perception of treatment and its associated pain (4,6).

- IV access provokes significant anxiety in hematology/oncology patients. Some present with an accessed central venous line; however, those without established IV access require special care. Application of EMLA cream to the dorsum of the patients' hands, nitrous oxide administration, or halothane/N$_2$O/O$_2$ by mask without IV access all are measures worthy of consideration.

- Parental presence is almost always requested and in most instances beneficial (68–71).

Deep Sedation/Anesthesia for Gastroenterology Patients

Gastrointestinal endoscopists frequently use a combination of diazepam and meperidine to sedate patients, but there is always concern regarding the complications of profound sedation, that is, respiratory depression, prolonged sedation, and delayed discharge (72,73). Such concerns have prompted the examination of propofol anesthesia as an alternative to traditional sedation techniques. The administration of propofol for procedural sedation in lieu of narcotics and benzodiazepines has been investigated (72). Adequacy of sedation, no respiratory depression, reduced nausea and vomiting, and reduced time to discharge all are characteristics of a propofol anesthetic supervised by an anesthesiologist. There is universal support of the administration of supplemental oxygen because in many of these studies alarming levels of oxygen desaturation were observed in as many as 20% of study patients, regardless of the method of sedation (73,74). These observations support the view that such techniques should be supervised by an anesthesiologist.

Children anesthetized with propofol and breathing spontaneously without airway support are at greater risk for aspiration. The insertion of a gastroscope is stimulating. Often patients retch, swallow, or hiccup. All patients must be fasting, and appropriate airway equipment (endotracheal tubes, laryngoscope, and wall suction) should be readily available.

"Colonoscopy can be a painful procedure due to stimulation of sensitive viscera" (74). Recently, the administration of propofol/fentanyl, and midazolam/fentanyl has been compared with more conventional methods of sedation (diazepam/meperidine). The authors were unable to recommend one method as being more advantageous than the others (74). They concluded that although propofol/fentanyl may allow for earlier discharge, such an advantage may be offset by the high incidence of desaturation with this technique. The anesthetic technique (HSC) for colonoscopy consists of propofol/fentanyl/O$_2$. The profound sedation/anesthesia and the rapid rate of recovery have provided for high patient and parent satisfaction. Our experience is supported by those who compared midazolam and meperidine with propofol alone for endoscopic procedures in children (72). The use of propofol improved the adequacy of sedation, reduced the incidence of respiratory depression requiring intervention, and reduced the mean length of stay after the procedure (77 minutes for propofol compared with 143 minutes for diazepam and meperidine). Propofol (administered by an anesthesiologist) resulted in better operating conditions, decreased side effects, improved safety, and improved bed utilization and nursing requirements.

Deep sedation/general anesthesia at HSC is generally available in the gastroenterology unit. Such a unit is more often child- and parent-friendly (61). The added costs of providing an anesthetic treatment room may be offset by increased efficiency and improved utilization of nursing time.

Gastroenterology Issues

Before the introduction of deep sedation/anesthesia, significant time was allocated to the establishment of adequate and safe conscious sedation. In the presence of a deeply sedated comfortable child, the gastroenterology consultant may probe beyond a reasonable time interval. Procedure duration should be scheduled for less than 1 hour. All remote location procedures are viewed as minor and of short duration, not requiring airway instrumentation or controlled ventilation.

Some patients scheduled for gastroscopy are being investigated for esophageal disease. Achalasia, esophageal stricture, and severe erosive gastritis related to grade 3 or 4 reflux are lesions that dictate the need for protection of the airway. Upper endoscopy procedures for these patients are performed in the operating room where patients are routinely paralyzed, intubated, and ventilated. Although the actual procedure might very well be undertaken in the gastroenterology suite, patients would ultimately have to be transferred to the post-anesthesia recovery unit, which is adjacent to the operating room.

Deep Sedation/Anesthesia and Diagnostic Imaging

Anesthesiologists are frequently called to manage uncooperative children for MRI and CT scan. General anesthesia is an obvious option. However, deep sedation provided by an anesthesiologist may be a more desirable alternative. The optimal sedation/anesthesia technique for radiologic procedures should have rapid onset, allow dosage flexibility, provide a motionless state, and allow for rapid awakening minimizing the need for a recovery room (75). Studies examining the benefits of propofol in such situations have clearly demonstrated its superiority. Rapid onset, spontaneous ventilation without airway support, absence of vomiting, and rapid predictable emergence are features of propofol induced deep sedation/anesthesia (67, 76,77).

Patients at HSC are routinely managed with propofol infusions for MRI and CT scans as described by Frankville and associates (67). A loading dose of propofol of 2 mg/kg/, followed by an infusion of propofol at a rate of 100 µg/kg/min, generally provides a satisfactory outcome. None of the patients who received propofol in the study required intubation. However, several patients became apneic after the induction dose. This has been our experience; that is, patients frequently require manual ventilation until the bolus effect has dispersed. Most patients emerge almost immediately upon discontinuation of the infusion. Moreover, most do not require transport to the recovery room, and most are ready for discharge within 30 minutes of completion of the procedure. Patients who require sedation or anesthesia for MRI occasionally encounter mild partial upper airway obstruction. Elevation of the shoulders or insertion of a "sniff position pillow" will likely guarantee airway patency (78) (Fig. 3).

Older patients also encounter mild airway obstruction accompanied by increased respiratory effort, which in turn diminishes the quality of the image. These patients have been managed with a laryngeal airway mask, N_2O/O_2, and a propofol infusion,

Diagnostic Imaging Issues

The following issues need to be considered in taking a child for diagnostic imaging:

Consent. Occasionally consent is not secured by the radiologist because no intervention is contemplated. Preanesthetic assessment must include confirmation of verbal or written consent for sedation/anesthesia.

Need for deep sedation/anesthesia. Anesthesia is occasionally requested without the benefit of prior assessment as many of these patients are transferred from distant locations. Often the child may cooperate fully with the addition of parental presence or conscious sedation.

Request for assistance following failed conscious sedation. In the past, patients had not fasted; thus, the option of elective deep sedation/anesthesia was unavailable. Since many diagnostic imaging departments now adhere to published sedation guidelines, this group of patients (who have failed con-

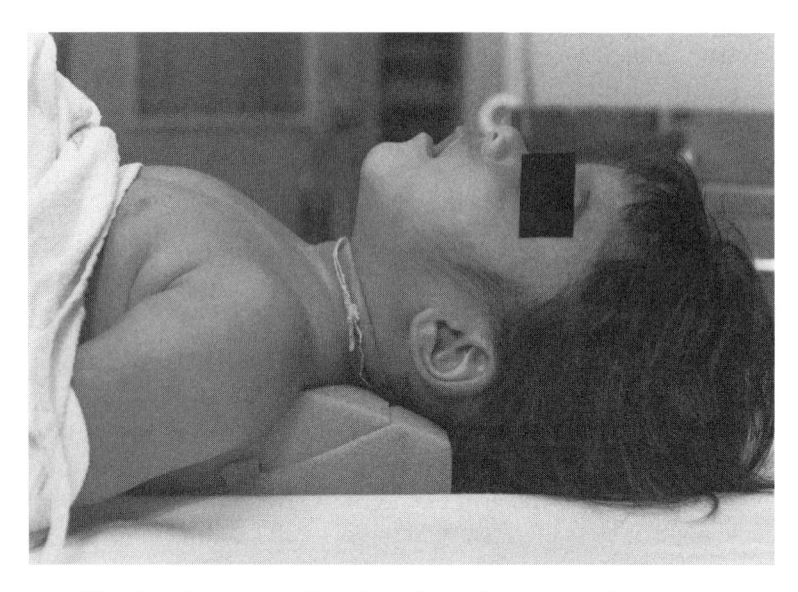

FIG. 3. Elevation of the shoulders or insertion of a sniff position pillow helps to maintain airway patency.

scious sedation) are at least fasting when assistance is requested (1). The dilemma is whether to defer until another date, recommend additional sedation, or provide anesthetic support.

Deep Sedation/Anesthesia and Other Medical Specialties

With the expansion of the sphere of anesthesia, medical colleagues as noted previously have requested anesthesia assistance. Muscle and nerve biopsy, laser treatment of port wine stains, echocardiography, and multiple joint injections in young children—procedures often managed in the recent past with sedation and local anesthesia now are complemented with the addition of deep sedation supervised by an anesthesiologist. The administration of propofol, with N_2O/O_2, is well suited for such procedures.

Concern exists regarding the incendiary potential of the laser and enriched atmospheres during treatment of port wine stain. Propofol infusion/oxygen in combination with fentanyl, 1 µg/kg, has been used at HSC, whereas other centers have opted for a laryngeal airway mask and a combination of propofol or vapor and N_2O/O_2. The laryngeal airway mask reduces the risk of an enriched atmosphere at the operative site (usually the face) (79).

Young patients requiring transthoracic echocardiography are generally sedated with chloral hydrate orally (50 to 100 mg/kg). Some authors have advocated the use of intranasal midazolam (0.2 mg/kg repeated in 5 to 10 minutes, if necessary, to a total dose of 0.4 mg/kg) (51), noting that oral agents have a slow and variable onset and may have an unnecessarily prolonged effect. Occasionally, such sedation regimens are ineffective, and these patients are managed with a propofol infusion supervised by an anesthesiologist. Propofol anesthesia administered without endotracheal intubation for outpatient transesophageal echocardiography has been demonstrated as a safe and effective technique in selected children (80). Initial experiences at HSC with this procedure in a remote location were discouraging. These patients were generally afflicted with significant disease (many severely cyanotic), and thus the combination of repeated doses of propofol and apnea in combination with esophageal instrumentation led to significant episodes of desaturation. Esophageal echocardiography at HSC is now undertaken in an operating room suite because of these earlier experiences.

Deep Sedation/Anesthesia for Burn Dressing Changes

"Of all the needs (there are none imaginary) a lonely child has, the one that must be satisfied . . . if there is going to be hope and a hope for wholeness, is the unshaking need for an unshakable God."

—Maya Angelou

Perhaps one of the most exciting sedation initiatives at HSC has been the introduction of deep sedation and general anesthesia for burn dressing changes (Fig. 4). Burn wound management now consists of frequent (sometimes daily) debridement and dressing changes. The sessions can be extremely uncomfortable, and traditionally burn patients have been sedated with a combination of IV diazepam/morphine. Patients are now managed with combinations of N_2O/O_2, propofol, narcotic, and midazolam. Such an initiative is not unique to this hospital, since others have also identified the advantages of providing care outside the operating room (81).

Observations that conventional pain management may be inadequate for major burn dressing changes, more efficient use of operating room and nursing time, and a positive impact on the morale of patients, parents, and nurses have prompted the establishment of anesthesia treatment facilities in burn treatment units at HSC and elsewhere.

Burn Unit Issues

The following are issues to be considered when administering sedation or anesthesia for a child with burns:

Fasting. Because of the high caloric requirements of young burn patients, traditional fasting stipulations have been waved for patients receiving continuous gastrojejunal tube feeds. Patients now receive their continuous gastrojejunal feeds until just before induction of deep sedation/anesthesia. Such an alteration in care has not been associated with increased morbidity, and recent investigations suggest that there may

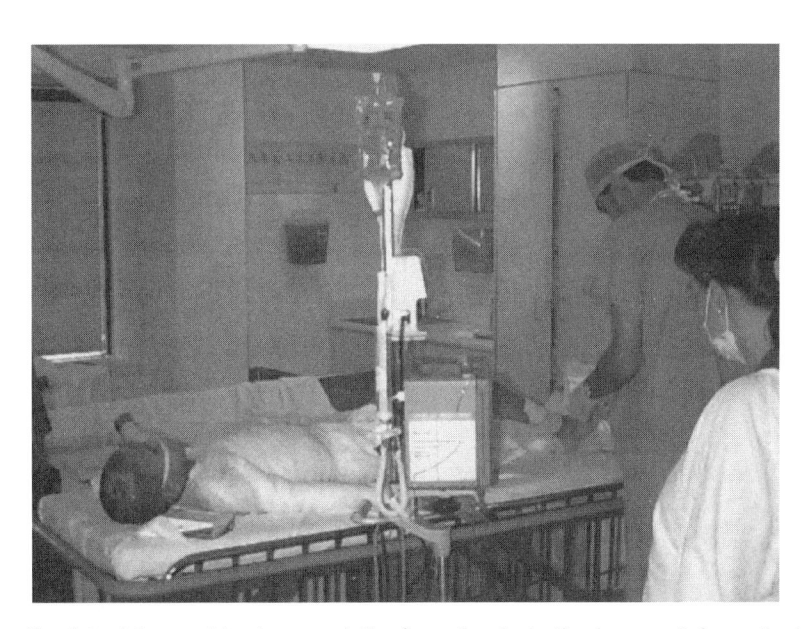

FIG. 4. Anesthesiologists provide deep sedation/anesthesia in the burn unit for patients requiring burn dressings or wound debridement.

not be an increased risk of aspiration in these patients (82).

Consent. An initial consent is secured for ongoing burn care. The parents are asked to review information brochure from the Department of Anesthesia before each procedure.

Procedure duration <1 hour. All non–operating room procedures are viewed as minor and of short duration not requiring airway instrumentation or controlled ventilation. The dispatch of these burn dressing cases has been expedited through the allocation of additional nursing personnel for these procedures.

Recovery. All patients managed in a non–operating room setting undergo recovery in designated recovery locations. In the event that the procedure or patient status is of a complex nature requiring intensive postoperative monitoring, an operating room time and location are secured.

Oral Transmucosal Fentanyl Citrate

Although of limited use as a surgical premedication **(see Chapter 2)**, oral transmucosal fentanyl citrate (Fentanyl Oralet) has a unique indication in the child without an IV who is to undergo a painful procedure such as a burn dressing change (Fig. 5). Experienced clinicians in large pediatric burn centers have found oral transmucosal fentanyl citrate to be very useful in this situation. Nausea and vomiting, associated with oral transmucosal fentanyl citrate (15 µg/kg) during other applications, has not been a problem in patients undergoing burn dressing changes.

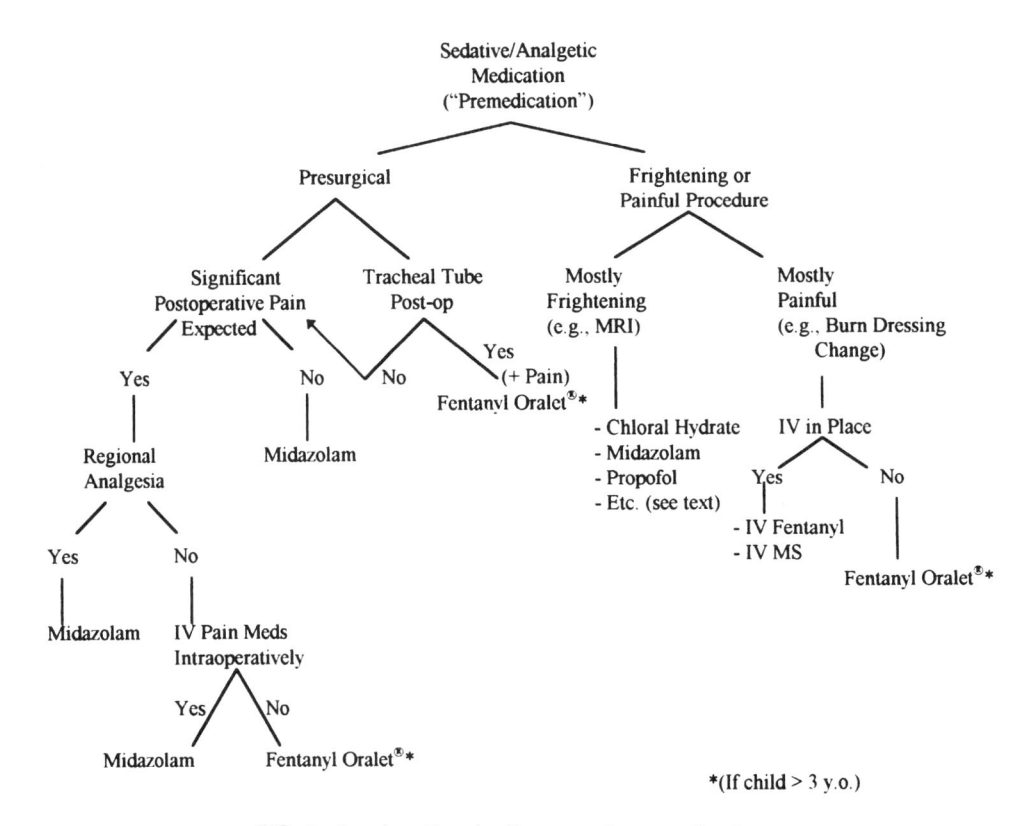

FIG. 5. An algorithm for the use of premedications.

SUMMARY

"OK, OK anesthesia" (61) is no longer an acceptable mode of care for children during painful minor procedures. Anesthesiologists are now capable of providing care beyond the limits of the operating room suite. This anesthetic presence benefits patients, parents, and attending medical colleagues.

"It were better for him that a millstone were hanged about his neck, and he cast into the sea, than that he should offend one of these little ones."

—Bible *(Luke 17:2)*

ACKNOWLEDGMENTS

The author would like to acknowledge the help of Dr. J.E.S. Relton and Ms. S.L. Loo in the preparation of this chapter.

REFERENCES

1. American Academy of Pediatrics Committee on Drugs: guidelines for monitoring and management of pediatric patients during and after sedation for diagnostic and therapeutic procedures. *Pediatrics* 1992;89:1110–1115.
2. Coté CJ: Sedation protocols: why so many variations? *Pediatrics* 1994;94:281–283.
3. Vade A, Sukhani R, Dolenga M, Habisohn-Schuck C: Chloral hydrate sedation of children undergoing CT and MR imaging: safety as judged by American Academy of Pediatrics guidelines. *AJR* 1995;165:905–909.
4. Frush DP, Bisset GS III: Sedation of children in radiology: time to wake up. *AJR* 1995;165:913–914.
5. Splinter WM, Stewart JA, Muir JG: Large volumes of apple juice preoperatively do not affect gastric pH and volume in children. *Can J Anaesth* 1990;37:36–39.
6. Coté C: NPO after midnight for children: a reappraisal. *Anesthesiology* 1990;72:589.
7. Sievers TD, Yee JD, Foley ME, et al: Midazolam for conscious sedation during pediatric oncology procedures: safety and recovery parameters. *Pediatrics* 1991;88:1172–1179.
8. Coté CJ: Monitoring guidelines: do they make a difference? *AJR* 1995;165:910–912.
9. Bricker SR, McLuckie A, Nightingale DA: Gastric aspirates after trauma in children. *Anaesthesia* 1989;44:721–724.
10. Schurizek BA, Rybro L, Boggild-Madsen NB, Juhl B: Gastric volume and pH in children for emergency surgery. *Acta Anaesthesiol Scand* 1986;30:404–408.
11. Wilson S: Chloral hydrate and its effects on multiple physiological parameters in young children: a dose-response study. *Pediatr Dent* 1992;14:171–177.
12. Houpt MI, Sheskin RB, Koenigsberg SR, et al: Assessing chloral hydrate dosage for young children. *J Dent Child* 1985;52:364–369.
13. Greenberg SB, Faerber EN, Aspinall CL: High dose chloral hydrate sedation for children undergoing CT. *J Comput Assist Tomogr* 1991;15:467–469.
14. Jackson EA, Rabbette PS, Dezateux C, et al: The effect of triclofos sodium sedation on respiratory rate, oxygen saturation, and heart rate in infants and young children. *Pediatr Pulmonol* 1991;10:40–45.
15. Cohen MR: Chloral hydrate overdoses implicated in deaths. *Nursing* 1993;23:25.
16. Canet E, Gaultier L, D'Allest AM, Dehan M: Effects of sleep deprivation on respiratory events during sleep in healthy infants. *J Appl Physiol* 1989;66:1158–1163.
17. Steinberg AD: Should chloral hydrate be banned? *Pediatrics* 1993;92:442–446.
18. Coté CJ: Sedation for the pediatric patient. *Pediatr Clin North Am* 1994;41:31–58.
19. Snodgrass WR, Dodge WF: Lytic/"DPT" cocktail: time for rational and safe alternatives. *Pediatr Clin North Am* 1989;36:1285–1291.
20. Obrien JF, Falk JL, Carey BE, Malone LC: Rectal thiopentone compared with intramuscular meperidine, promethazine, and chloropromazine for pediatric sedation. *Ann Emerg Med* 1991;20:644–647.
21. Yaster M, Nichols DG, Deshpande JK, Wetzel RC: Midazolam-fentanyl intravenous sedation in children: case report of respiratory arrest. *Pediatrics* 1990;86:463–467.
22. Hollister GR, Burn JM: Side effects of ketamine in pediatric anesthesia. *Anesth Analg* 1974;53:264–267.
23. Zeltzer LK, Jay SM, Fisher DM: The management of pain associated with pediatric procedures. *Pediatr Clin North Am* 1989;36:941–964.
24. Gutstein HB, Johnson KL, Heard MB, Gregory GA: Oral ketamine preanesthetic medication in children. *Anesthesiology* 1992;76:28–33.
25. Tobias JD, Phipps S, Smith B, Mulhern RK: Oral ketamine premedication to alleviate the distress of invasive procedures in pediatric oncology patients. *Pediatrics* 1992;90:537–541.
26. Bloomfield EL, Masaryk TJ, Caplin A, et al: Intravenous sedation for MR imaging of the brain and spine in children: pentobarbital versus propofol. *Radiology* 1993;186:93–97.
27. Strain JD, Harvey LA, Foley LC, Campbell JB: Intravenously administered pentobarbital sodium for sedation in pediatric CT. *Radiology* 1986;161:105–108.
28. Towbin RB, Ball WS Jr: Pediatric interventional radiology. *Radiol Clin North Am* 1988;26:419–440.
29. Pereira JK, Burrows PE, Richards HM, et al: Comparison of sedation regimens for pediatric outpatient CT. *Pediatr Radiol* 1993;23:341–344.
30. Anderson CTM, Zeltzer LK, Fanurik D: Procedural pain. In: Schechter, Berde, Yaster (eds). *Pain in infants, children & adolescents*. Baltimore, Williams and Wilkins, 1993.
31. Diament MJ, Stanley P: The use of midazolam for sedation of infants and children. *AJR* 1988;150:377–378.
32. Schwartz S, Bevan JC, Roberts G, Dean DM: Midazolam sedation and local anaesthesia compared with general anaesthesia for paediatric outpatient dental surgery. *Paediatr Anaesth* 1992;2:309–315.
33. Bailey PL, Pace NL, Ashburn MA, et al: Frequent hypoxemia and apnea after sedation with midazolam and fentanyl. *Anesthesiology* 1990;73:826–830.

34. McMillan CO, Spahr-Schopfer IA, Sikich N, et al: Premedication of children with oral midazolam. *Can J Anaesth* 1992;39:545–550.
35. Malinovsky JM, Populaire C, Cozian A, et al: Premedication with midazolam in children: effect of intranasal, rectal and oral routes on plasma midazolam concentrations. *Anaesthesia* 1995;50:351–354.
36. Karl HW, Rosenberg JL, Larach MG, Ruffle JM: Transmucosal administration of midazolam for premedication of pediatric patients: comparison of the nasal and sublingual routes. *Anesthesiology* 1993;78:885–891.
37. Bailey PL, Pace NL, Ashburn MA, et al: Frequent hypoxemia and apnea after sedation with midazolam and fentanyl. *Anesthesiology* 1990;73:826–830.
38. Rodrigo MR, Chan L, Hui E: Flumazenil reversal of conscious sedation for minor oral surgery. *Anaesth Intensive Care* 1992;20:174–176.
39. Litman RS, Berkowitz RJ, Ward DS: Levels of consciousness and ventilatory parameters in young children during sedation with oral midazolam and increasing concentrations of nitrous oxide. (Abstract). *Anesthesiology* 1995;83:A1182.
40. Young ER, DelCastilho R, Patell M, Kestenberg SH: Scavenging system developed for the Magill anesthetic circuit for use in the dental office. *Anesth Prog* 1990;37:252–257.
41. Canadian Anaesthetists' Society: Guidelines to the practice of anaesthesia. *Can J Anaesth* 1994;41:7.
42. Roberts GJ, Wignall BK: Efficacy of the laryngeal reflex during oxygen-nitrous oxide sedation (relative analgesia). *Br J Anaesth* 1982;54:1277–1281.
43. Wattenmaker I, Kasser JR, McGravey A: Self-administered nitrous oxide for fracture reduction in children in an emergency room setting. *J Orthop Trauma* 1990;4:35–38.
43 Binder LS, Leake LA: Chloral hydrate for emergent pediatric procedural sedation: a new look at an old drug. *Am J Emerg Med* 1991;9:530–534.
44. Hawk W, Crockett RK, Ochsenschlager DW, Klein BL: Conscious sedation of the pediatric patient for suturing: a survey. *Pediatr Emerg Care* 1990;6:84–88.
45. Connors K, Terndrup TE: Nasal versus oral midazolam for sedation of anxious children undergoing laceration repair. *Ann Emerg Med* 1994;24:1074–1079.
46. Doyle WL, Perrin L: Emergence delirium in a child given oral midazolam for conscious sedation. *Ann Emerg Med* 1994;24:1173–1175.
47. Bates BA, Schutzman SA, Fleisher GR: A comparison of intranasal sufentanil and midazolam to intramuscular meperidine, promethazine, and chlorpromazine for conscious sedation in children. *Ann Emerg Med* 1994;24:646–651.
48. Varela CD, Lorfing KC, Schmidt TL: Intravenous sedation for the closed reduction of fractures in children. *J Bone Joint Surg* 1995;77:340–345.
49. Olney BW, Lugg PC, Turner PL, et al: Outpatient treatment of upper extremety injuries in childhood using intravenous regional anaesthesia. *J Pediatr Orthop* 1988;8:576–579.
50. Selbst SM, Henretig FM: The treatment of pain in the emergency department. *Pediatr Clin North Am* 1989;36:965–978.
51. Latson LA, Cheatham JP, Gumbiner CH, et al: Midazolam nose drops for outpatient echocardiography sedation in infants. *Am Heart J* 1991;121:209–210.

52. Javorski JJ, Hansen DD, Laussen PC, et al: Paediatric cardiac catheterization: innovations. (Review). *Can J Anaesth* 1995;42:310–329.
53. Mitchell AA, Louik C, Lacouture P, et al: Risks to children from computed tomographic scan premedication. *JAMA* 1982;247:2385–2388.
54. Cohen MD: Pediatric sedation. *Radiology* 1990;175:611–612.
55. Keeter S, Benator RM, Weinberg SM, Hartenberg MA: Sedation in pediatric CT: national survey of current practice. *Radiology* 1990;175:745–752.
56. Harcke HT, Grissom LE, Meister MA: Sedation in pediatric imaging using intranasal midazolam. *Pediatr Radiol* 1995;25:341–343.
57. Ferrari L, Barst S, Pratila M, Bedford RF: Anesthesia for diagnostic and therapeutic procedures in pediatric outpatients. *Am J Pediatr Hematol Oncol* 1990;12:310–313.
58. Sievers TD, Yee JD, Foley ME, et al: Midazolam for conscious sedation during pediatric oncology procedures: safety and recovery parameters. *Pediatrics* 1991;88:1172–1179.
59. Sandler ES, Weyman C, Conner K, et al: Midazolam versus fentanyl as premedication for painful procedures in children with cancer. *Pediatrics* 1992;89:631–634.
60. Henderson JM, Spence DG, Komocar LM, et al: Administration of nitrous oxide to pediatric patients provides analgesia for venous cannulation. *Anesthesiology* 1990;72:269–271.
61. Hassall E: Should pediatric gastroenterologists be I.V. drug users? *J Pediatr Gastroenterol Nutr* 1993;16:370–372.
62. Martin LD, Pasternak LR, Pudimat MA: Total intravenous anesthesia with propofol in pediatric patients outside the operating room. *Anesth Analg* 1992;74:609–612.
63. Bloomfield EL, Masaryk TJ, Caplin A, et al: Intravenous sedation for MR imaging of the brain and spine in children: pentobarbital versus propofol. *Radiology* 1993;186:93–97.
64. Hannallah RS, Baker SB, Casey W, et al: Propofol: effective dose and induction characteristics in unpremedicated children. *Anesthesiology* 1991;74:217–219.
65. Cauldwell CB, Fisher DM: Sedating pediatric patients: is propofol a panacea? *Radiology* 1993;186:9–10.
66. Grebenik CR, Ferguson C, White A: The laryngeal mask airway in pediatric radiotherapy. *Anesthesiology* 1990;72:474–477.
67. Frankville DD, Spear RM, Dyck JB: The dose of propofol required to prevent children from moving during magnetic resonance imaging. *Anesthesiology* 1993;79:953–958.
68. Schulman JL, Foley JM, Vernon DT, Allan D: A study of the effect of the mother's presence during anesthesia induction. *Pediatrics* 1967;39:111–114.
69. Baines D, Overton JH: Parental presence at induction of anaesthesia: a survey of N.S.W. hospitals and tertiary paediatric hospitals in Australia. *Anaesth Intens Care* 1995;23:191–195.
70. Hannallah RS, Rosales JK: Experience with parents' presence during anaesthesia induction in children. *Can Anaesth Soc J* 1983;30:286–289.
71. Bevan JC, Johnston C, Haig MJ, et al: Preoperative parental anxiety predicts behavioural and emotional responses to induction of anaesthesia in children. *Can J Anaesth* 1990;37:177–182.

72. Nadwidny LA, Smith LJ, Jones AB, Seal RF: The use of propofol vs diazepam/meperidine for pediatric GI endoscopic procedures. (Abstract 7). North American Society for Pediatric Gastroenterology and Nutrition 7th Annual Meeting, 1993.
73. Freeman ML, Hennessy JT, Cass OW, Pheley AM: Carbon dioxide retention and oxygen desaturation during gastrointestinal endoscopy. *Gastroenterology* 1993;105: 331–339.
74. Kostash MA, Johnston R, Bailey RJ, et al: Sedation for colonoscopy: A double-blind comparison of diazepam/meperidine, midazolam/fentanyl and propofol/fentanyl combinations. *Can J Gastroenterol* 1994;8:27.
75. Spear RM: Deep sedation for radiological procedures in children: enough is enough. *Paediatr Anaesth* 1993; 3:325.
76. Valtonen M: Anaesthesia for computerised tomography of the brain in children: a comparison of propofol and thiopentone. *Acta Anaesthesiol Scand* 1989;33:170–173.
77. Barst SM, Merola CM, Markowitz AE, et al: A comparison of propofol and chloral hydrate for sedation of young children during magnetic resonance imaging scans. *Pediatr Anaesth* 1994;4:243.
78. Shorten GD, Armstrong DC, Roy WI, Brown L: Assessment of the effect of head and neck position on upper airway anatomy in sedated paediatric patients using magnetic resonance imaging. *Pediatr Anaesth* 1995;5: 243–248.
79. Garbin GS, Bogetz MD, Grekin RC, Frieden IJ: The laryngeal mask an airway during laser treatment of port wine stains. (Abstract). *Anesthesiology* 1991;75:A953.
80. Marcus B, Steward DJ, Khan NR, et al. Outpatient transesophageal echocardiography with intravenous propofol anesthesia in children and adolescents. *J Am Soc Echocard* 1993;6:205–209.
81. Dimick P, Helvig E, Heimbach D, et al: Anesthesia-assisted procedures in a burn intensive care unit procedure room: benefits and complications. *J Burn Care Rehabil* 1993;14:446–449.
82. Fischer C, Jenkins M, Gottschlich M: Perioperative enteral nutrition in pediatric burn patient. (Abstract). *Anesthesiology* 1995;83:A1164.

17

Postanesthesia Care Issues

Robert D. Valley

"Even a minor event in the life of a child is an event of that child's world and thus a world event."
—Gaston Bachelard

The initial recovery from surgery and anesthesia is a critical period during a child's perioperative course. Adverse events are reported to occur in up to 13% of all pediatric patients during their stay in the postanesthesia care unit (PACU) (1). Optimal perioperative care of children requires a dedicated unit that is equipped and staffed to provide routine care and has the ability to detect and manage problems that may occur in the immediate postoperative period. PACU issues that will be discussed in this chapter include recovery from anesthesia and surgery, routine care in the PACU, and specific problems in the PACU.

RECOVERY FROM ANESTHESIA AND SURGERY

Goals of Recovery

"What angel wakes me from my flow'ry bed?"
—William Shakespeare

To assess recovery it is important to know the preoperative baseline status of the patient. A child with central nervous system (CNS) dysfunction (e.g., cerebral palsy) or cardiorespiratory disease (e.g., bronchopulmonary dysplasia or cyanotic heart disease) can be expected to return to a different baseline than that of an otherwise healthy child. Another baseline assessment is a recovery score given the patient on admission to the PACU, the well-known "PAR" score (Table

TABLE 1. Aldrete postanesthesia recovery score

Criterion	Score
Activity	
Able to move four extremities voluntarily or on command	2
Able to move two extremities voluntarily or on command	1
Able to move 0 extremity voluntarily or on command	0
Respiration	
Able to deep breathe and cough freely	2
Dyspnea or limited breathing	1
Apneic	0
Circulation	
BP ± 20% of preanesthetic level	2
BP ± 20%–50% of preanesthetic level	1
BP ± 50% of preanesthetic level	0
Consciousness	
Fully awake	2
Arousable on calling	1
Not responding	0
Color	
Pink	2
Pale, dusky, blotchy, jaundiced, other	1
Cyanotic	0

Reprinted with permission from Williams & Wilkins. Aldrete JA, Kroulik D: A postanesthetic recovery score. *Anesthesia and Analgesia* 49:924–934, 1970.

1).[a] The goals of recovery vary, depending on the planned disposition of the patient. It may be safe to discharge a semiconscious patient to the intensive care unit, but certainly not to the patient's home. A definition

---

[a] Ed. Note (JMB): I have modified the traditional PAR score to one that reflects the type of child the PACU nurses love to have delivered to them. The Badgwell PAR Score: pink = 5; asleep = 5. Hence, the perfect score of 10 is a spontaneously breathing "unobstructed" child after deep extubation who is still asleep. A pink awake infant who is calm and not crying (e.g., an infant with a good regional anesthetic on board), however, also qualifies for a 10.

TABLE 2. Pediatric PACU discharge criteria

Inpatient and outpatient	Outpatient
Return of protective airway and respiratory reflexes to level of adequate gas exchange	CNS recovery to near baseline level of consciousness
Cardiovascular stability	BP, HR, RR, and temperature at normal levels for age
Neurologic status appropriate for current level of sedation or postsurgical condition	Pain under control such that oral analgesics will suffice for further pain management
Adequate duration of observation after administration of potent medications (e.g., narcotics, naloxone, flumazenil, vasoactive drugs), usually 30 to 60 minutes	Hydration status adequate to allow discharge even if oral intake is minimal for the next 6 to 8 h
	Nausea and vomiting not intractable
Pain and vomiting under reasonable control	Ability to ambulate as appropriate for age (for young children ambulation is not necessary as long as parents are instructed about risk of injury)
Absence of surgical complications (e.g., excessive bleeding)	

BP, blood pressure; HR, heart rate; RR, respiration rate.

of the goals of recovery can be drawn from commonly accepted PACU discharge criteria (Tables 2 and 3).

Rate of Recovery

Numerous factors affect the rate of recovery from anesthesia and surgery, including the duration and depth of anesthesia, the type of anesthetic agents used, the use of preoperative sedatives and other adjunctive medications, and the adequacy of pain control. The rate of return to baseline is also affected by the physiologic status of the patient.

TABLE 3. Steward's postanesthesia scoring system

Criterion	Score
Consciousness	
Awake	2
Responding to stimuli	1
Not responding	0
Airway	
Coughing on command or crying	2
Maintaining good airway	1
Airway requires maintenance	0
Movement	
Moving limbs purposefully	2
Nonpurposeful movements	1
Not moving	0

From Steward, ref. 13, with permission.

Recovery from Inhalation Anesthesia

The recovery rate from inhalation anesthesia depends on the agent's alveolar partial pressure, potency, saturation of body tissues, and the blood and tissue solubilities of the agent or agents used. Also important is the adequacy of postoperative ventilation. The MAC-awake (i.e, minimum alveolar concentration at which 50% of patients respond to a simple command) of most inhalation agents is 0.3 to 0.6 of standard MAC (2–4). A child who arrives in the recovery room immediately after a deep extubation requires a longer period to recover than a child arriving after an awake extubation performed after spontaneous eye opening and an ability to follow commands. The effects of inhalation anesthetic solubility on recovery time are most easily understood by comparing blood/gas partition coefficients (at equilibrium, the ratio of the concentration of agent in blood to the concentration in the gas phase). The greater the blood gas solubility coefficient, the longer it will take to "wash out" the agent, assuming equivalent degrees of alveolar ventilation (5). The duration and depth of anesthesia are more important determinants of the rate of recovery when more soluble anesthetic agents are used and tissue compartments have become saturated with anesthetic agent (Fig. 1). Because the primary route of elimination for all inhaled anesthetic agents is through the lungs,

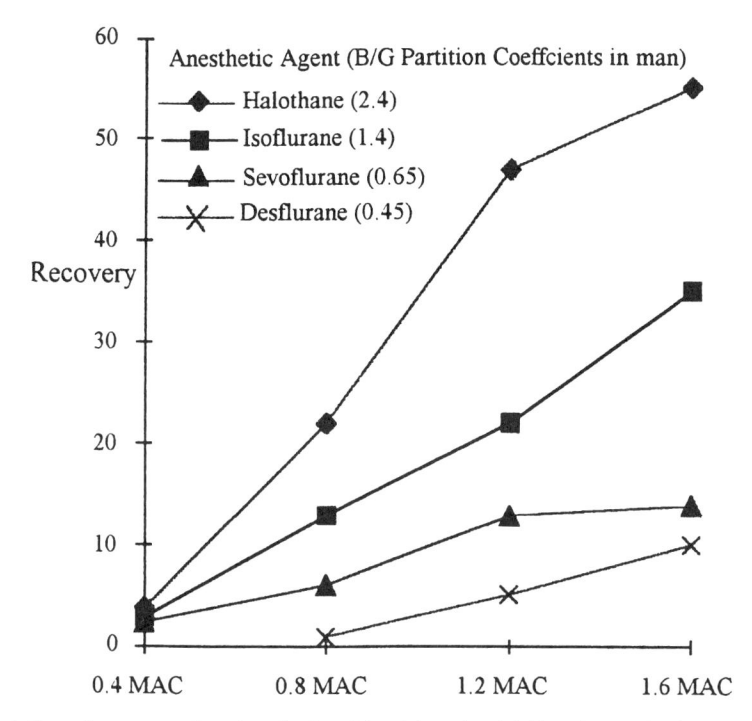

FIG. 1. The relation of recovery time in minutes (Y axis) and solubility of anesthetic agents. The greater the solubility (i.e., the greater the blood/gas coefficient), the longer it will take to "wash out" the agent (assuming equivalent levels of alveolar ventilation). (Reprinted in modified form with permission from Eger EL, Johnson BH, Rates of awakening from anesthesia with I-653 isoflurane, and sevoflurane: a test of the effect of anestheia concentration and dose. *Anesthesia and Analgesia:* 1987,66:977.)

hypoventilation and increased dead-space ventilation will prolong awakening.

"Of all ebriosity, who does not prefer to be intoxicated by the air he breathes?"
—Henry David Thoreau

Recovery from Intravenous Agents

Recovery from intravenous (IV) anesthetic agents depends on type, potency, and amount of agent used, its distribution in the body and its rate of elimination and metabolism. Unlike inhalation anesthetics, rapid onset does not necessarily mean rapid offset. Many hypnotic agents (e.g., thiopentothal, propofol) have a short duration of action after a single large-bolus dose because of their rapid redistribution to body compartments other than the brain. As these peripheral sites become saturated, offset of action becomes a function of elimination or metabolism. Thus, duration and quantity of agent used are important considerations affecting recovery times. This is a more important consideration for agents with long elimination half-lives such as barbiturates, diazepam, and morphine than for more rapidly metabolized agents such as propofol, midazolam, or fentanyl. Many factors can affect the elimination rate of IV drugs including volume of distribution, hepatic metabolic capacity, renal function, and relative blood flow to the kidneys and liver. Because of this, the recovery rate from IV agents is frequently less predictable than the recovery rate from inhalation agents, especially in neonatal patients with immature hepatic and renal function.

Although all inhalation agents probably work through a similar mechanism of action, this is not the case for IV agents. Variations in mechanism of action significantly affect the rate and type of recovery. For example, narcotic agents are generally more potent respiratory than CNS depressants. A patient waking from a narcotic-based anesthetic may open his or her eyes on command but remain apneic unless asked to breathe. High doses of ketamine often result in a patient presenting to the PACU with adequate respiratory effort but a prolonged time to awakening. A final word about the choice of anesthetic agent and recovery. Frequently, the choice of an anesthetic agent or agents is not as important as is the skilled use of the agent for an individual patient and a given procedure.

Central Nervous System and Cardiovascular Recovery

It is impossible to separate cardiorespiratory recovery from CNS recovery because of the central control of many essential physiologic functions. At MAC-awake levels of anesthesia, adult patients usually maintain an otherwise normal unprotected airway. In infants, MAC-awake has not been well defined, but adequacy of CNS recovery is frequently equated with spontaneous eye opening, purposeful movements and the ability to follow commands. Infants and small children cannot be expected to follow commands, but spontaneous eye opening and purposeful movements such as reaching for an endotracheal tube are good indicators of an improving level of consciousness. It is important to remember that the level of arousal is frequently a balance between the amount of residual anesthetic (inhalation agent, narcotic, or sedative) and the degree of noxious or painful stimuli. Sudden elimination of painful stimuli by narcotic administration or dosing of an epidural can be expected to result in a more pronounced effect of residual anesthetic/sedative agents.

"A baby is God's opinion that life should go on."
—Carl Sandberg

Remember that all inhalation agents, narcotics, benzodiazepines, barbiturates, and propofol cause a dose-dependent depression of ventilatory drive. Tidal volume or respiratory rate or both may be reduced. Sighing or maximal inspiratory efforts may occur only on command or following noxious stimuli. Despite this, most children will have sustained ventilatory effort and an adequate, though depressed, response to carbon dioxide (CO_2) early in their recovery following an inhalation anesthetic. Higher levels of CNS arousal may be achieved before adequate spontaneous ventilatory effort returns following high doses of narcotics.

Many factors may predispose the postoperative patient to hypoxia including airway obstruction, atelectasis, increased closing capacity, reduced sighing, or splinting from inspiratory pain and central hypoventilation with a diminished tidal volume or respiratory rate increase in response to CO_2. Although recent evidence has shown that the hypoxic ventilatory response may be maintained in the presence of residual inhalation anesthetic (if normal ventilatory response changes in CO_2 are allowed to occur), recovering patients may fail to respond to hypoxia with an increase in tidal volume, predisposing them to further atelectasis (6). Neonatal patients have a diminished response to hypoxia and hypercarbia even in the absence of anesthetic agents (7–10). Standard measures of wakefulness used in the PACU have not been found to correlate with oxygenation (Tables 2 and 3) (11). This underscores the importance of supplemental oxygenation and continuous pulse oximetry for all patients. For premature infants considered at risk for retinopathy of prematurity, oxygen should be used judiciously and rapidly weaned to avoid prolonged periods of hyperoxia.

Recovery of Neuromuscular Function

Reversal of neuromuscular blockade usually takes place in the operating room before extubation. Occasionally, a patient will be brought to the PACU with significant residual neuromuscular blockade. This may be due to an inadequate dose of reversal agent or may occur after an attempt to reverse a block that is too dense to permit pharmacologic reversal. Neuromuscular weakness may be enhanced by residual inhalation anesthetic, hypothermia, some antibiotics (e.g., aminoglycosides), preexisting myopathies and drugs (e.g., dantrolene).

Whenever significant hypoventilation or inability to maintain an airway occurs in the PACU, residual neuromuscular blockade should be considered as a cause. Train of four or tetanic electrical stimulation is uncomfortable in the awake patient. In this situation, sustained head lift, vigorous cry, or forceful hip flexion can be used as indices of adequate neuromuscular function (12,13). It is of interest to note that recent studies have demonstrated a pronounced depression of the ventilatory response to hypoxia (but not to hypercarbia) with subparalytic doses of nondepolarizing muscle relaxants (14,15). This implies that even when return of neuromuscular function is judged adequate by conventional criteria, patients may still be at increased risk of developing hypoxia as a result of depression of the normal hypoxic ventilatory response. Residual neuromuscular blockade may be treated with additional reversal agent if not already given or if given in inadequate amounts. Occasionally, calcium chloride may improve neuromuscular function if weakness is due to antibiotic administration (16). Pharmacologic reversal of residual nondepolarizing neuromuscular blocking agent may not be possible if significant paralysis remains despite adequate doses of reversal agent. In this situation, airway protection, ventilatory support and sedation will be necessary until neuromuscular function returns.

When Is It Appropriate to Extubate?

Although most children are extubated in the operating room, some children arrive in the PACU with an endotracheal tube in place. Children may be extubated in two ways—either under deep inhalation anesthesia or after a return to wakefulness as demonstrated by spontaneous eye opening, grimacing, and purposeful movements. Most clinicians would agree that the worst time to extubate children is during a light plane of general anesthesia at which time they seem particularly prone to laryngospasm. Regardless of the depth of anesthesia, return of adequate neuromuscular function is vital before extubation.

Deep extubation may be advantageous when coughing and bucking on the endotracheal tube may disrupt surgical repairs, increase bleeding, or cause bronchospasm on emergence of a child with reactive airway disease.

"The bravest sight in the world is to see a great man struggle against adversity."
—Seneca

Nevertheless, if you want to avoid the scrutiny of others watching you struggle with adversity, you may want to avoid deep extubation in the presence of a known difficult airway (e.g., Treacher-Collins, Pierre Robin, history of obstructive sleep apnea), a suspected difficult postoperative airway (e.g., following creation of a velopharyngeal flap), a full stomach, or a history of prematurity **(see Chapter 8)**. Children who are extubated deep should have their stomach suctioned and their oropharynx cleared of blood or secretions. If appropriate, an oral or nasal airway can be inserted. Extubation is then accomplished after a spontaneous inspiration with the patient at a surgical plane of anesthesia. Patients should be given supplemental oxygen and kept on their side with the bed in a neutral or head down position until awake. They require close observation as airway obstruction and laryngospasm may still occur.

Awake extubation is the preferred method of extubation by most clinicians **(see Chapter 6)**. The oropharynx is cleared. After a return to wakefulness, a positive-pressure breath with 100% oxygen is given and the endotracheal tube removed. Supplemental oxygen is given initially and then weaned as tolerated.

ROUTINE CARE IN THE PACU

Transport to the PACU

Safe transport of the child from the operating room to the PACU requires observance of the following practices:

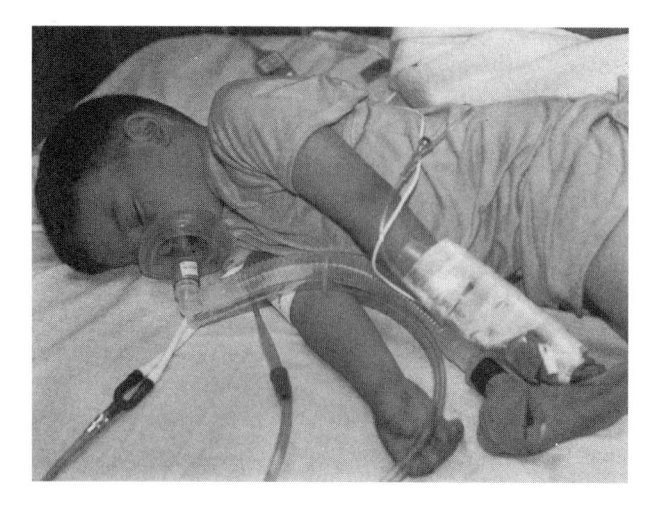

FIG. 2. A child just before transport to the PACU. Note that the child is on his side (the time-honored "tonsil position"), has suction available, has a secure intravenous line, and is receiving supplemental oxygen through a pillow face mask and Jackson-Rees breathing circuit.

- Constant monitoring of the patient's airway (a hand on the chin will support the airway as well as monitor for exhaled breath), chest movement, and color.

- Positioning of the sedated patient with the head turned to the side to minimize the chances of aspiration of secretions, blood, or gastric contents (Fig. 2). Care must be taken to prevent self-injury by the disoriented, flailing child.

- Recognition of the common occurrence of hypoxemia during transport has led many clinicians to routinely administer supplemental oxygen during transport (17,18) (Fig. 2).

- For transport from remote locations or if the child has been unstable or is receiving vasoactive infusions, a higher level of monitoring may be indicated, including pulse oximetry, electrocardiography (ECG), and arterial blood pressure.

Stage 1 and Stage 2 Recovery

Many recovery facilities must deal with a large mix of patients, including adults as well as children, outpatients, and inpatients. To accomplish this, most facilities provide at least two areas for recovery. The first stage of recovery, stage 1, receives all patients directly from the operating room or remote anesthetizing location. Here an intensive care unit (ICU) level of care is provided. Although not absolutely necessary, it is desirable to have some separation of children from adult patients in stage 1 recovery. This allows for the creation of an environment that is less frightening to the recovering child, where there are cartoon characters on the walls, where a crying child won't disturb adult patients, and where nurses will feel comfortable allowing parents to be with their children (see below).

Stage 2 recovery is reserved for outpatients after they have met basic discharge criteria from stage 1. Occasionally, children will come directly to stage 2 recovery if they have received only conscious sedation after minor procedures. Ideally, a separate area for children will provide the same advantages as for stage 1 recovery. A play area that allows children the opportunity to return to normal activities provides the staff with a useful tool for deciding suitability for discharge home. In this area, patients are allowed to sit up and eventually ambulate, if appropriate. IV lines are discontinued after adequate hydration is ensured and vomiting reasonably controlled. Patients are frequently offered clear liquids but children should not be required to drink before discharge. Forced oral fluids may only increase the incidence of postoperative vomiting (19). Patients are then allowed to dress and a final assessment is made by the anesthesiologist and nursing staff.

Before discharge home, an important function of the nursing and physician staff is to give instructions to the parent or responsible adult accompanying the patient about activity restrictions, wound care, medications to be taken, follow-up appointments, and whom to call for problems such as excessive vomiting, uncontrolled pain, inability to void, or surgical bleeding.

Monitoring

Routine monitoring in the PACU (stage 1) includes respiratory rate, blood pressure, pulse oximetry, ECG, fluid balance, and temperature. Other than continuous pulse oximetry and ECG, how frequently other physiologic parameters are measured is dictated by the observed status of the patient and the procedure from which the patient is recovering. In addition to the above, nursing staff should provide an intermittent evaluation of mental status, sedation level, and pain.

A stage 1 PACU that must care for inpatients as well as outpatients should be equipped to monitor any physiologic parameter necessary at an ICU level of care, including intracranial pressure, intravascular pressures, cardiac output, and end-tidal CO_2. Rapid access to blood gas analysis and measurement of hematocrit, electrolytes, and blood glucose should be considered standard of care for any stage 1 recovery area.

Monitoring in stage 2 recovery is usually restricted to intermittent measures of routine vital signs and occasionally pulse oximetry. Alert, stable patients may have no further vital signs measured following transfer from stage 1 recovery.

Nursing Care

Skilled nursing care is vital to the smooth functioning of a pediatric PACU. PACU nurses must be able to provide an ICU level of care from arterial-line management to assisting in a full resuscitation. They must also be skilled in airway assessment and the provision of basic airway support measures such as the jaw-thrust/chin-lift maneuver, in the use of oral and nasal airways, bag/mask ventilation, and in assisting with intubation and extubation. For the routine patient, nursing staff must be comfortable dealing with emergence delirium, providing comfort and reassurance to the frightened child, and assessing and treating pain. In addition, nursing staff should provide an objective assessment of the recovery from anesthesia. This is often accomplished by using a standardized recovery score such as the Aldrete Postanesthesia Recovery Score or Steward's Postanesthesia Scoring System (Tables 1 and 3). Nursing care in a stage 2 recovery area is explained in the section on **Stage 1 and Stage 2 Recovery.**

Parents in the PACU

After children are awake enough to appreciate their surroundings, allowing parents to be in the PACU with them can help alleviate much fear and anxiety. Concerned parents will be able to see that their child is all right and can resume participation in their child's care. This is not to say that parents should always be brought into the PACU. If a child is unstable or there are excessive nursing demands, parents should remain in the waiting area. The benefits to the child's care may be undermined if parents are overly protective, anxious, or hostile.

Discharge

Discharge criteria from the PACU are listed in Table 2. Nursing staff should regularly assess the patient for suitability for discharge. Some institutions have a minimum required length of stay. Practice trends and the use of shorter-acting agents frequently allow patients to meet discharge criteria from stage 1 PACU within 30 minutes. The length of stay should not be dictated by protocol. Instead, it should be determined by the individual needs of each patient. For outpatients, nursing staff will usually make the decision when a patient is ready for transfer to a stage 2 recovery area. The final responsibility for discharge home or to any inpatient unit belongs to the anesthesiologist.

SELECTED PROBLEMS IN THE PACU

Respiratory Problems

Persistent agitation, a depressed level of consciousness, hypoxemia, or unexplained hypercarbia all may be symptoms related to respiratory compromise. Respiratory distress may be the result of upper or lower airway obstruction, aspiration pneumonitis, pneumothorax, or pulmonary edema. Adequate respiratory effort may be impaired by central respiratory depression, uncontrolled pain with splinting, or mechanical factors such as a distended abdomen or a body cast that is too tight.

Upper Airway Obstruction

"Never confuse movement with action."
—Ernest Hemingway

Transient upper airway obstruction is relatively common in the immediate recovery period. The child's vigorous attempt to inhale through an obstructed airway leads to a respiratory pattern in which the chest caves in as the stomach goes up. This respiratory pattern has been variously termed *paradoxical respiration* or rocker-bottom breathing (it is paradoxical because the chest and stomach usually rise together during normal inspiration). This type of obstruction is not to be confused with effective ventilation.

The sedated child may have pharyngeal hypotonia with a posteriorly displaced tongue, which results in inspiratory obstruction. Arousing the patient or a chin-lift or jaw-thrust maneuver is usually adequate to restore patency. If these measures are inadequate, placement of an oral or nasal airway and suctioning of the oropharynx may be necessary. Care should be taken when airway adjuncts are used. A child with an intact gag reflex will not tolerate an oral airway, and its improper placement may make the airway worse. Nasal airways should be placed cautiously or not at all in patients following oronasal procedures. Excessive bleeding or disruption of the surgical repair may occur.

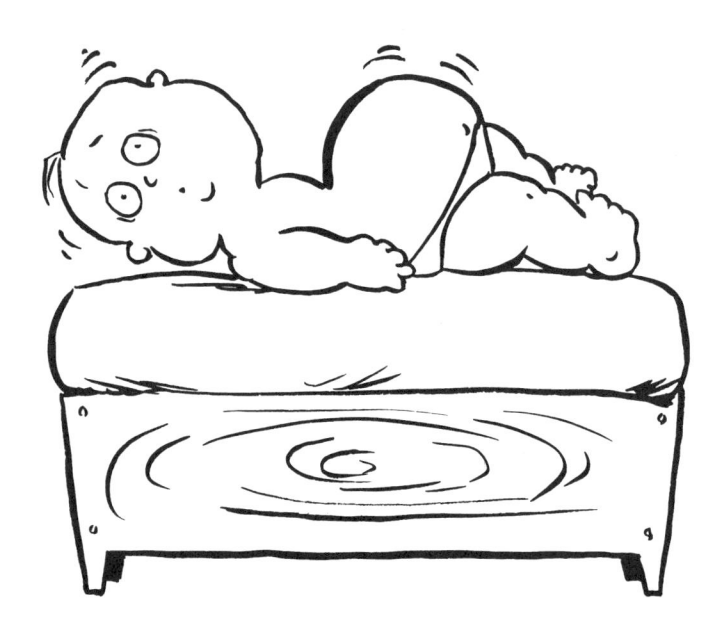

If airway obstruction persists despite the previously mentioned measures or if it is accompanied by high-pitched inspiratory stridor, laryngospasm or subglottic edema may be present. Laryngospasm usually responds to positive pressure by mask with 100% oxygen and time. Persistent laryngospasm may require the administration of succinylcholine, 0.5 to 1.0 mg/kg, to relax the vocal cords. Blood or secretions may be irritating the laryngeal inlet and should be cleared.

Postintubation Croup

Postintubation croup is secondary to subglottic edema. It is most common in children over the age of 3 months and younger than 4 years of age. Early reports note an incidence of postextubation croup as high as 6%, whereas more recent studies report an incidence of 1% (20–22). The lower incidence may be attributable to better airway management with careful attention to the use of appropriately sized endotracheal tubes and the use of endotracheal tubes made of less reactive (implant tested) materials. Postextubation croup or stridor may be more likely when an oversized tube has been used (no leak by 20 to 40 cm H2O of airway pressure) and when the intubation was traumatic or repeated attempts were required to place the tube. A history of bucking (coughing) while the tube is in place or a change in positioning after intubation may predispose to postextubation croup.

In most situations, postextubation croup or stridor can be managed expectantly with reassurance and the administration of cool mist. More severe stridor may improve with the administration of nebulized racemic epinephrine (0.25 to 0.5 ml of a 2.25% solution in 2 to 3 ml of normal saline). Such patients require close observation because rebound hyperemia and a return of symptoms may occur. Some clinicians prophylactically administer corticosteroids (dexamethasone, 0.2 to 0.5 mg/kg IV) before extubation of patients considered at high risk of developing subglottic edema.

Other Causes of Airway Obstruction

Upper airway obstruction that is persistent may be due to one or more factors such as excessive soft tissue swelling (e.g., tongue swelling following ischemic injury by a lingual retractor), uncontrolled bleeding, or a narrowed postoperative oropharynx as following cleft palate repair or creation of a velopharyngeal flap. Some patients improve after upright positioning (if awake) and assistance with clearing of blood or secretions. Moderate sedation and pain control may be beneficial when agitation is making bleeding worse or is resulting in excessive inspiratory effort and dynamic airway obstruction. The clinician should always be prepared to reintubate these difficult patients if they deteriorate or fail to improve with the aforementioned measures.

Lower Respiratory Problems

Lower Airway Obstruction

Lower airway obstruction should be suspected in an agitated child with tachypnea, retractions, a prolonged expiratory phase, and wheezing or faint breath sounds on auscultation. Excessive lower airway secretions, aspirated material, or bronchospasm may be the cause. Oxygen should always be administered as dictated by peripheral saturations. Coughing may clear secretions, and bronchospasm usually responds to the administration of a bronchodilator such as albuterol (0.01 to 0.03 ml/kg of a 0.5% solution in 2 to 3 ml of nebulized saline or two to four puffs from a metered-dose inhaler). Refractory bronchospasm may require additional treatment with corticosteroids, parasympatholytic agents (ipratropium, glycopyrrolate), or xanthine derivatives. If aspiration is suspected, supportive care should be given, and if symptoms or radiographic findings suggest a significant aspiration, reintubation and bronchoscopically directed lavage and removal of particulate material may be indicated. Fortunately, major aspiration events are relatively uncommon in pediatric patients (23).

Pulmonary Edema

Postoperative pulmonary edema of cardiac origin is unusual in otherwise healthy children unless excessive fluids have been administered intraoperatively. Noncardiogenic pulmonary edema may occur, usually in the form of postobstructive pulmonary edema. This may occur after the relief of chronic severe upper airway obstruction or after an episode of postextubation obstruction, as from laryngospasm, with strong inspiratory efforts against a closed glottis (24,25). Noncardiogenic pulmonary edema has also been reported after the bolus administration of naloxone (26). Tachypnea, expiratory grunting, increased oxygen requirements, and rales on auscultation are classic signs of pulmonary edema. A review of the anesthetic record, preoperative history and examination, chest radiograph, and current physical examination will usually point to the cause. If respiratory distress is relatively mild, supportive care and oxygen by face mask may be the only treatment required.

For more severe cases, intubation, pulmonary suctioning, and continuous positive airway pressure with or without additional ventilatory support may be required. Diuretic administration is indicated for treatment of cardiogenic pulmonary edema or if volume overload is suspected. Diuretics are usually unnecessary for treatment of postobstructive or naloxone related-pulmonary edema, although frequently a single dose of furosemide is administered. Postobstructive pulmonary edema usually resolves rapidly, with otherwise healthy patients ready for discharge from the hospital by the the first postoperative day.

Pneumothorax

One final cause of respiratory distress that should always be considered in the postoperative child or in any child who has received positive-pressure ventilation is pneumothorax. Tachypnea, chest pain, asymmetric breath sounds, and hypoxia may be present. Tension pneumothorax may also result in tracheal deviation, jugular venous distention and hypotension, and cardiovascular collapse. A chest radiograph confirms the diagnosis. Immediate decompression and chest tube placement are indicated for the symptomatic patient.

Respiratory Depression

Inhalation agents, narcotic agents, and most other anesthetic agents cause a dose-dependent depression of central respiratory drive. Moderate hypercarbia alone is frequently well tolerated and unless associated with altered CNS status or hypoxemia is not an indication for treatment other than assurance of airway patency and occasional arousal to encourage deep breathing and coughing. Hypoxia secondary to central respiratory depression requires therapy. Arousal, deep breathing, and supplemental oxygen will often suffice. Severe respiratory depression requiring frequent stimulation to prevent apnea needs further therapy. Careful titration of naloxone (1 to 5 μg/kg/dose, IV) will reverse narcotic-induced respiratory depression before reversing analgesia. Flumazenil may be given to reverse the effects of benzodiazepines. Severe and persistent respiratory depression unrelated to narcotics or benzodiazepines may require intubation and mechanical ventilation. This is a particular problem for infants with a history of prematurity **(see Chapter 8)**.

Cardiovascular Instability

Fortunately, dysrhythmias other than extremes of heart rate are uncommon in recovering pediatric patients. Other rhythm disturbance should alert the clinician to the possibility of underlying cardiac pathology, electrolyte imbalance, or autonomic disturbances such as autonomic hyperreflexia. Tachycardia is the most common abnormal rhythm. Tachycardia may be due to many factors including emergence delirium, anxiety, pain, hypovolemia, hypercarbia, parasympatholysis, or hyperthermia. Sinus tachycardia rarely requires specific therapy. Instead, its cause should be determined and appropriate therapy instituted. Tachycardia associated with other indicators of volume depletion such as ongoing blood loss, absent urine output, cool extremities, and hypotension (a late sign in infants) requires immediate volume therapy.

Hypertension

Hypertension may accompany tachycardia when it is due to CNS arousal, pain, or parasympatholysis. Hypertension with a normal or slow heart rate is more common in older children with hypothermia, with α-adrenergic excess, and with increases in intracranial pressure. Hypertension, like tachycardia, frequently does not require specific therapy in pediatric patients. Instead, the cause needs to be determined and appropriate therapy instituted. An exception would be the child at increased risk of hypertensive complications following repair of a coarctation of the aorta or a child in need of afterload reduction to sustain an adequate cardiac output. Hypertension with bradycardia may be the result of an elevation in intracranial pressure, which will require immediate therapy to lower the intracranial pressure, not the systemic blood pressure!

Hypotension

Hypotension is a late sign of volume depletion in infants and is usually preceded by tachycardia. Hypotension may also occur in the PACU after rewarming of a cold, vasoconstricted patient. Hypotension that does not respond to volume administration should raise the possibility of primary cardiac dysfunction or sepsis.

Bradycardia

Bradycardia, especially in an infant, requires immediate attention because it is frequently associated with a profound decrease in cardiac output. Hypoxia-induced bradycardia should be treated by establishing adequate oxygenation first. Bradycardia may also be due to excess parasympathetic tone such as after the administration of acetylcholinesterase inhibitors or after tracheal suctioning, nasogastric tube placement, or ophthalmic pressure. As previously noted, bradycardia may be a sign of intracranial hypertension.

OTHER PACU ISSUES

Nausea and Vomiting

"Nothing you do for children is ever wasted. They seem not to notice us, hovering, averting our eyes, and they seldom offer thanks, but what we do for them is never wasted."
—Garrison Keillor

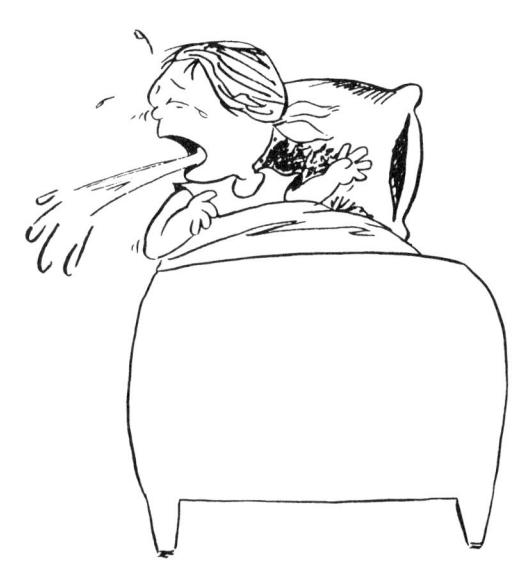

Anything that can be done to minimize nausea and vomiting will win the approval of the patient, the parents, and the nursing staff. The incidence of postoperative nausea and vomiting (PONV) varies from < 10% to >50% depending on the procedure, the anesthetic technique, and the patient population. There are too many studies on the topic to review but some measures can significantly reduce the incidence and severity of PONV including:

- Emptying of gastric contents (especially blood) before emergence
- Propofol (versus inhalation) anesthesia
- Prophylactic administration of antiemetics to patients preceding,[b] during, or

---

[b]Ed Note (JMB): I've always had good luck (i.e., low incidence of vomiting) in strabismus patients by following Jerry Lerman's advice to give the antiemetic before muscle retraction. Jerry now tells us that IV diphenhydramine (Benadryl) works just as well as the more expensive agents.

immediately following high-risk procedures (e.g., strabismus surgery, tonsillectomy). Agents shown to be at least partially effective include the following:

- Droperidol, 10 to 100 µg/kg
- Metoclopramide, 0.15 mg/kg
- Ondansetron, 0.1 mg/kg

Metoclopramide and droperidol may cause extrapyramidal symptoms. Metoclopramide should not be used if gastrointestinal obstruction is suspected. Droperidol may cause excessive sedation. Ondansetron appears to be without significant side effects. As already noted, allowing, *but not requiring*, outpatients to drink clear liquids before discharge will result in less vomiting in the immediate postoperative period. Refractory vomiting is an indication for hospital admission and continued IV hydration.

Pain

Pain management in the PACU is discussed in **Chapter 10.**

Altered CNS Status

"Children seldom have a proper sense of their own tragedy . . . imagining real calamity to be some prestigious drama of their grown up world."

—Shirley Hazzard

Emergence delirium is a term used to describe the patient who, although awake enough to meet extubation criteria, is disoriented and frequently combative in the immediate recovery period. Fortunately, this is usually short-lived. The choice of anesthetic agent, adequacy of analgesia, and the age and disposition of the child all play a role in determining the occurrence of emergence delirium. It is most common in children ages 3 to 9 years (27). In my experience, emergence delirium occurs more frequently after a pure inhalation anesthetic and less frequently if narcotics or propofol have been used. Excessive doses of atropine or scopolamine may cause cholinergic excess and altered CNS status. Ketamine is frequently cited as a cause of emergence delirium, although less frequently in children (28). Any sedative whose effect lasts into the postoperative period (e.g., barbiturates, benzodiazepines) may result in a disoriented, uncooperative child in the PACU.

Emergence delirium needs to be differentiated from more ominous causes of altered CNS status. Hypoxia, severe hypercarbia, hypotension, metabolic disturbances (e.g., hypoglycemia), seizures, and increased intracranial pressure need to be diagnosed and treated. Most frequently, as the child becomes more alert and pain is brought under control, his or her behavior will become more appropriate and docile.

Disorders of Body Temperature Maintenance

Hypothermia

Hypothermia occurs in young pediatric patients if appropriate measures at maintain-

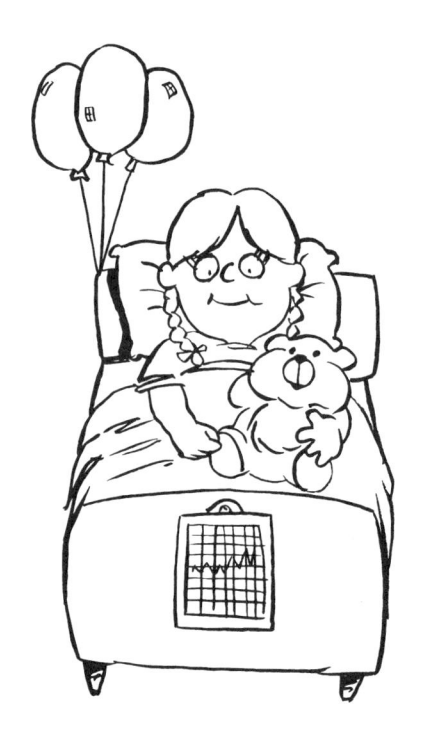

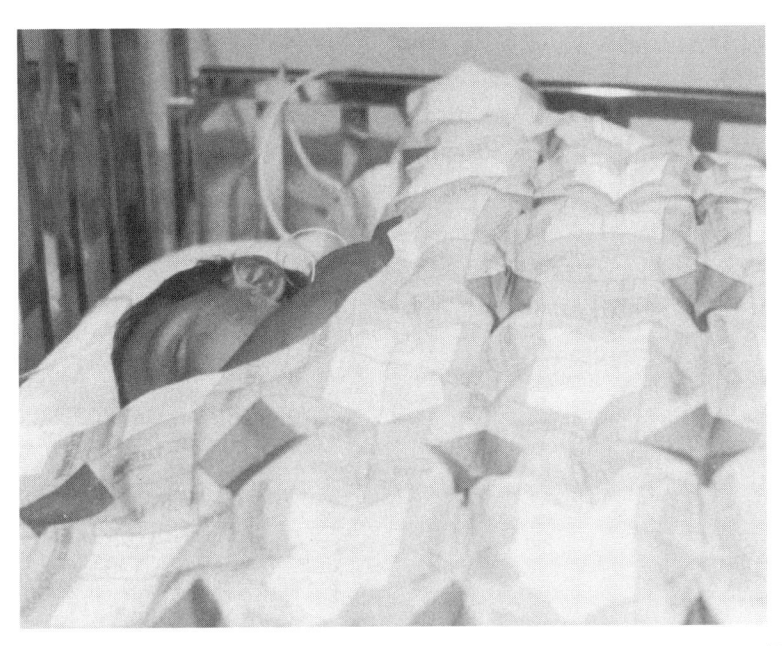

FIG. 3. A sleeping infant in the PACU kept warm with a forced-air warming blanket (Warm-Touch, Mallinckrodt Medical, Inc, St. Louis, MO).

ing normothermia are not carried out in the operating room. Hypothermic infants may become acidotic, bradycardic, hypotensive, or apneic. Hypothermia can potentiate the action of muscle relaxants. Homeostatic efforts on the part of the patient to raise body temperature increase metabolic demands substantially. A profoundly hypothermic child should remain intubated and sedated until the core temperature is at least 35° C. Overhead radiant warmers, heated isolettes, and forced-air warming blankets (Fig. 3) are useful devices to raise or maintain body temperature.

Hyperthermia

Overzealous warming in the operating room is probably the most common cause of hyperthermia in the PACU. This may be exacerbated by the routine administration of atropine to pediatric patients because it interferes with normal heat dissipation (29). This form of iatrogenic hyperthermia requires no therapy other than avoiding overbundling the child in the PACU. A persistently high or rising body temperature requires further investigation **(see Chapter 14)**. Possible causes include intercurrent infection, perioperative sepsis, transfusion reaction, and malignant hyperthermia. If suspected, malignant hyperthermia requires prompt diagnosis and treatment.

SUMMARY

In the PACU, the anesthesiologist is responsible for medically directing patients' return to consciousness and ensuring cardiorespiratory stability and adequacy of pain control (Fig. 4). Proper care and handling of children in the PACU are fundamental components of perioperative medicine and are essential for a rapid and safe recovery.

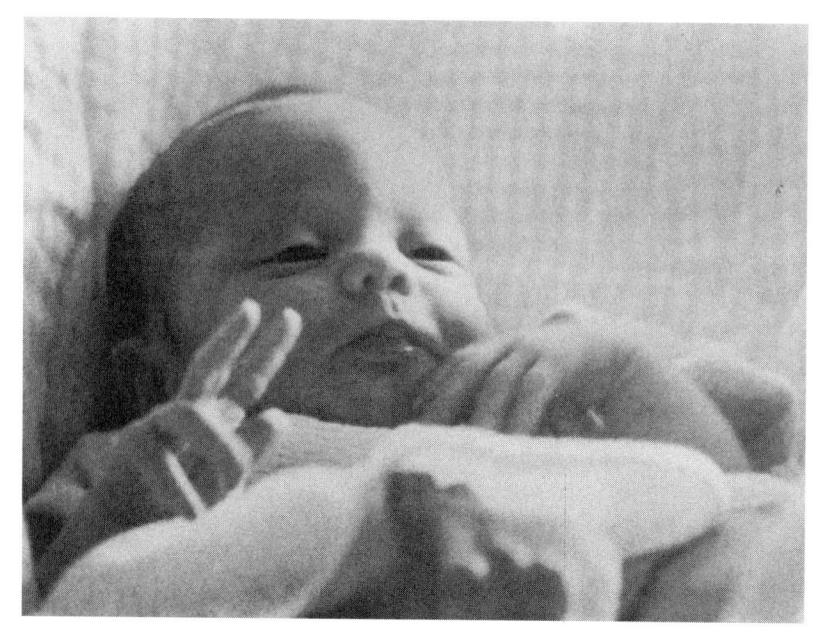

FIG. 4. A happy customer—hernia fixed, pain-free, ready to leave the PACU.

REFERENCES

1. Cohen MM, Cameron CB, Duncan PG: Pediatric anesthesia morbidity and mortality in the perioperative period. *Anesth Analg* 1990;70:160–167.
2. Stoelting RK, Longnecker DE, Eger EI II: Minimum alveolar concentrations in man on awakening from methoxyflurane, halothane, ether, and fluroxene anesthesia MAC awake. *Anesthesiology* 1970;33:5–9.
3. Katoh T, Suguro Y, Ikeda T, et al: Influence of age on awakening concentrations of sevoflurane and isoflurane. *Anesth Analg* 1993;76:348–352.
4. Katoh T, Suguro Y, Kimura T, Ikeda K: Morphine does not affect the awakening concentration of sevoflurane. *Can J Anaesth* 1993;40:9:825–828.
5. Eger EI II, Johnson BH: Rates of awakening from anesthesia with I-653 halothane, isoflurane, and sevoflurane: a test of the effect of anesthetic concentration and duration in rats. *Anesth Analg* 1987;66:977–982.
6. Sjogren D, Sollevi A, Ebberyd A, Lindahl SG: Isoflurane anaesthesia (0.6 MAC) and hypoxic ventilatory responses in humans. *Acta Anaesthesiol Scand* 1995;39: 17–22.
7. Cross KW, Oppe TE: The effect of inhalation of high and low concentrations of oxygen on the respiration of the premature infant. *J Physiol* 1952;117:38–55.
8. Rigatto H, De La Torre Verduzco R, Gates DB: Effects of O_2 on the ventilatory response to CO_2 in preterm infants. *J Appl Physiol* 1975;39:896–899.
9. Rigatto H, Brady JP, Torre Verduzco R: Chemoreceptor reflexes in preterm infants: I. The effect of gestational and postnatal age on the ventilatory response to inhalation of 100% and 15% oxygen. *Pediatrics* 1975;55: 604–613.
10. Rigatto H, Brady JP, De La Torre Verduzco R: Chemoreceptor reflexes in preterm infants: II. The effect of gestational and postnatal age on the ventilatory response to inhaled carbon dioxide. *Pediatrics* 1975;55: 614–620.
11. Soliman IE, Patel RI, Ehrenpreis MB, Hannallah RS: Recovery scores do not correlate with postoperative hypoxemia in children. *Anesth Analg* 1988;67:53–56.
12. Aldrete JA, Kroulik D: A postanesthetic recovery score. *Anesth Analg* 1970;49:924–934.
13. Steward DJ: A simplified scoring system for the post-operative recovery room. *Can Anaesth Soc J* 1975;22: 111–113.
14. Eriksson LI, Lennmarken C, Wyon N, Johnson A: Attenuated ventilatory response to hypoxaemia at vecuronium-induced partial neuromuscular block. *Acta Anaesthesiol Scand* 1992;36:710–715.
15. Eriksson LI, Sato M, Severinghaus JW: Effect of a vecuronium induced partial neuromuscular block on hypoxic ventilatory response. *Anesthesiology* 1993;78: 693–699.
16. Sokoll MD, Gergis SD: Antibiotics and neuromuscular function. *Anesthesiology* 1981;55:148–159.
17. Patel R, Norden J, Hannallah RS: Oxygen administration prevents hypoxemia during post-anesthetic transport in children. *Anesthesiology* 1988;69:616–618.
18. Pullerits J, Burrows FA, Roy WL: Arterial desaturation in healthy children during transfer to the recovery room. *Can J Anaesth* 1987;34:5:470–473.
19. Schreiner MS, Nicolson SC, Martin T, Whitney L: Should children drink before discharge from day surgery? *Anesthesiology* 1992;76:528–533.
20. Koka BV, Jeon IS, Andre JM, et al: Postintubation croup in children. *Anesth Analg* 1977;56:4:501–505.

21. Jordan WS, Graves CL, Elwyn RA: New therapy for postintubation laryngeal edema and tracheitis in children *JAMA* 1970;212:585–588.
22. Goddard JE Jr, Phillips OC, Marcy JH: Betamethasone for prophylaxis of postintubation inflammation: a double-blind study. *Anesth Analg* 1967;46:348–353.
23. Tiret L, Nivoche Y, Hatton F, et al: Complications related to anaesthesia in infants and children. *Br J Anaesth* 1988;61:263–269.
24. Lang SA, Duncan PG, Shephard DA, Ha HC: Pulmonary oedema associated with airway obstruction. *Can J Anaesth* 1990;37:210–218.
25. Mcgowan FX, Kenna MA, Fleming JA, O'Connor T: Adenotonsillectomy for upper airway obstruction carries increased risk in children with a history of prematurity. *Pediatr Pulmonol* 1992;13:222–226.
26. Prough DS, Roy R, Bumgarner J, Shannon G: Acute pulmonary edema in healthy teenagers following conservative doses of intravenous naloxone. *Anesthesiology* 1984;60:485–486.
27. Eckenhoff JE, Kneale DH, Dripps RD: The incidence and etiology of postanesthetic excitement: a clinical survey. *Anesthesiology* 1961;22:667.
28. Sussman DR: A comparative evaluation of ketamine anesthesia in children and adults. *Anesthesiology* 1974;40:459–464.
29. Fraser JG: Iatrogenic benign hyperthermia in children. *Anesthesiology* 1978;48:375.

Clinical Pediatric Anesthesia, edited by J.M. Badgwell. Lippincott–Raven Publishers, Philadelphia © 1997.

PARTING SHOT

J. Michael Badgwell

"I told you butter wouldn't suit the works!" he added, looking angrily at the March Hare. "It was the BEST butter," the March Hare meekly replied.

—Lewis Carroll
Alice in Wonderland

The managment techniques for pediatric cardiac anesthesia described in this book are mostly scientific, yet some remain empiric. Since the majority of methods proposed are drawn from those used by the cited experts, one might assume that these are the methods that will work best every time. Not so. Until you've had the opportunity to compare the "best methods" with each other, along with your own knowledge and experience, you'll continue to be guided by uncertainties. Awareness of this uncertainty makes us better clinicians. We hope this book serves to stimulate you and your colleagues in anesthesia to continue the search for improved care techniques and the "best methods" for your pediatric patients. Please give us a call and let us know what you've come up with. Or, better yet, just give us a call to chew the fat.

"What really knocks me out is a book that, when you're all done reading it, you wish the author that wrote it was a terrific friend of yours and you could call him up on the phone whenever you felt like it. That doesn't happen much, though."

—J.D. Salinger
The Catcher in the Rye

J. Michael Badgwell, M.D.
(702) 671-2262
mikebadg@aol.com

We, like Robert Frost, believe that the key to understanding and enlightenment is through direct communication.

"Something there is that doesn't love a wall, and wants it down"

—Robert Frost

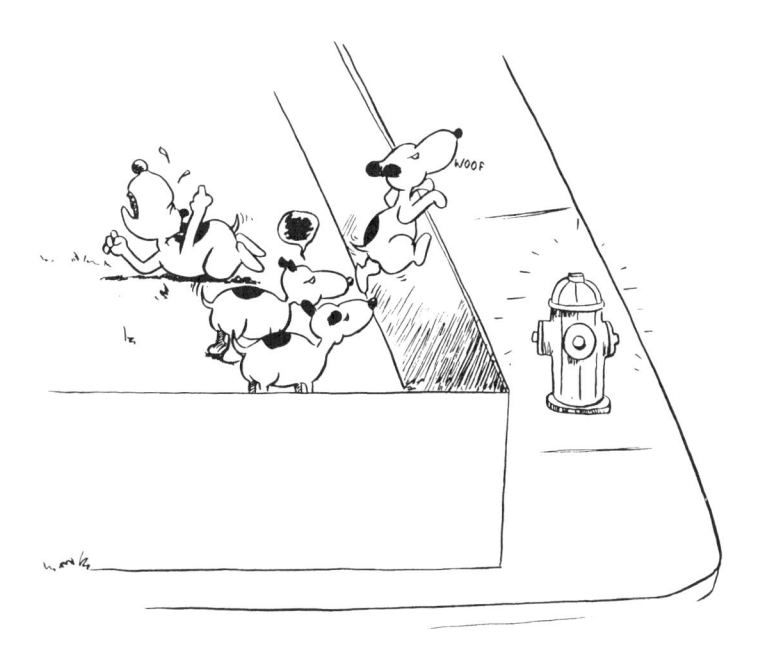

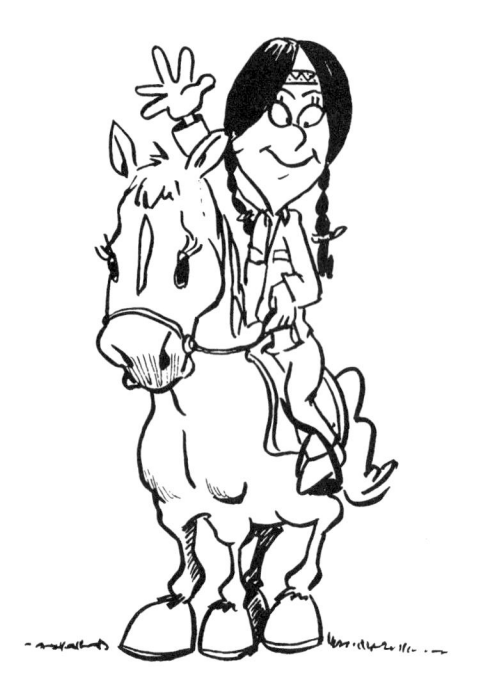

"Come children, let us shut up the box and the puppets, for our play is played out."
– William Makepeace Thackeray

Subject Index

Page numbers followed by *t* and *f* indicate tables and figures, respectively

A

AAP guidelines, 438, 446
Aaron Medical Lighted Intubation Stylet, 100*t*
Abdominal trauma, 426–427
Abscess, peritonsillar, 276
Accurate aspirating capnography, 131–135
Accurate flow-through capnography, 135
Acetaminophen, 235*t*
Acetazolamide, 341
Activated partial thromboplastin time (aPTT), 319
Acute chest syndrome, 397
Acute dilutional hyponatremia, 223–224
Adenoidectomy, 267
    anesthesia for, 270–273
        extubation after, 272–273
        preoperative considerations for, 267–270
    complications of, 273–274
    inpatient guidelines for, 273*t*
Adult ventilator, conversion of, 114
Advanced Cardiac Life Support protocol, 262
Age(s), 262
    cerebral metabolic and blood flow rates by, 339*t*
    induction of anesthesia and, 24
    local anesthetic agent toxicity and, 262
    minimum alveolar concentration versus, 146*t*
    postconceptual, postoperative apnea and, 204*f*
    relationship of: blood pressure to, 19*t*
        heart rate to, 17*t*
    size and type of laryngoscope blades for, 82*t*
Air, intravenous fluid filters and, 49
Air-oxygen mixer, 123*f*
Air-Shields Ventimeter, 138*f*
Airway(s). *See also* Laryngeal mask airway
    anatomic differences of, 82
    difficult, 44
        induction of anesthesia and, 93
        management of, 88, 90
        micrognathia and, 98*f*
        pediatric light wands and, 97–98
        preanesthetic assessment of, 90, 92
        premedication and, 92–93
        Steward's algorithm for, 108–111
        two-person technique and, 93, 96–97
    difficult access for, 6*f*
    emergency with, 282
    emergency surgical, 105–106
        after major trauma, 420, 431–432
    nasopharyngeal, 81*f*
    oral, 79*f*
        appropriate-sized, 80f
    pitfalls of insertion of, 96*f*
    plastic oral, 78*f*, 81*f*
        in position, 80*f*
    preoperative evaluation of, 5–6
    routine, management of: endotracheal tubes and, 79
        laryngoscope blades and, 79
        masks and, 77, 79
        nasal insertion of, 85–86
        oral insertion of, 81–85
        suction apparatus and, 79–80
        tracheal tube placement and, 80
    suspected cervical injury and, 106, 108
Airway CO_2 aspiration sampling device, 134*f*
Airway equipment in trauma room, 418*f*
Airway obstruction
    complete, treatment algorithm for, 40*f*
    incomplete, treatment algorithm for, 41*f*
    upper and lower causes of, 284*f*
Airway patency, 25*f*, 158*f*
    computed tomography and, 80*f*
    difficult, David Steward's algorithm for, 109*f*
    elevation of shoulders and, 454*f*
    improved, 38*f*
    maintenance of, 31*f*
    sniff position pillow and, 454*f*
Albuterol, 384
Aldrete Postanesthesia Recovery Score, 461*t*, 467
Alfentanil, 150–151
    suggested doses for, 151*t*
    target concentrations for, 152*t*
Allen's test, 66*f*
Allergies
    laser, 401–404
    preoperative evaluation and, 3–4
Alveolar gas, 135*f*
Alveolar ventilation. *See also* Specific type of ventilation
    controlled: conclusions about, 126, 128
        effect of fresh gas flow on, 125
    delivery of, 113–114
        anesthesia machine and, 114
        controlled, 114
        volume-controlled, 114–117
    monitoring adequacy of, 113, 128–129
        pediatric capnography and, 131–137, 139–140
        pulse oximetry and, 129–131
        relation of capnography and pulse oximetry and, 140–141
    positive-pressure, through LMA, 125–126
American Academy of Pediatrics (AAP) Committee on Drugs, 436
American Society of Anesthesiologists (ASA) patients
    class I and II, 436, 437
    class III, 437
Aminocaproic acid, 320
Aminophylline, 4*t*, 384*t*
Amoxicillin, 335*t*
    in endocarditis prophylaxis, 8*t*
Ampicillin, 8*t*, 335*t*
Amrinone, 311*t*

SUBJECT INDEX

Analgesia, 232t
  for painful or frightening procedures outside operating room, 435–438
  preemptive, 231
Anatomic airway differences, 82
Anatomic airway obstruction, 37–38
Anemia, 3t
  in neonate, 167
Anesthesia. *See also specific type of anesthesia*
  anatomic airway obstruction during, 37–38
  art of inhalation induction and, 29–30
  asthma and, 382–385
  caudal, 206f
  cerebral palsy and, 386–388
  choice of agents for, 34
  for congenital heart disease. *See under* Congenital heart disease
  congenital hypertrophic pyloric stenosis and, 189–190
  for congenital stridor, 284–285
  cricoid pressure during induction of, 43f
  cystic fibrosis and, 385–386
  deep, 455f
  difficult airway and open-eye, full-stomach considerations and, 44
  emergence from, 152
    blue but well-ventilated child and, 152–153
    sundown sign and, 152
  epidermolysis bullosa nad, 394–396
  for ex-ECMO. *See under* Ex-ECMO patient
  for ex-premature. *See under* Ex-premature
  face mask application and, 30–34
  for foreign body aspiration, 285–287
  full-stomach, no open-eye considerations and, 42
  full-stomach, open-eye considerations and, 42–44
  hemophilia and, 398–399
  increasing inspired concentrations of halothane and sevoflurane and, 34
  induction of, 15
    age and, 24
    atracurium and, 21, 23
    automated blood pressure measurement in neonate and, 19
    blood pressure monitoring and, 17, 19
    child sitting up during, 26f
    difficult airways and, 93
    distraction during, 27f
    drugs and, 21
    electrocardiogram and, 16–17
    by endotracheal intubation, 199
    esophageal stethoscope and, 16
    fasting before, 23
    in frightened infant or child, 28f
    by inhalation in ex-premature, 198–199
    by laryngeal mask airway, 199–200
    midazolam and, 23–24
    monitors applied before, 27f
    muscle relaxants and, 21, 23
    in neonates, 169
    neuromuscular blockade monitoring and, 17
    nondepolarizing muscle relaxants and, 21, 23
    noninvasive monitoring in pediatric patient for, 15–17, 19
    oral transmucosal fentanyl citrate and, 24
    parents in operating room and, 25f
    precordial stethoscope and, 15–16
    premedication before, 23–24
    preparing room for, 15
    rocuronium and, 23
    succinylcholine and, 21
    surrogate mommy figure during, 28f
    temperature monitoring and maintenance during, 19, 21, 23
    vecuronium and, 23
  induction characteristics of halothane versus sevoflurane and, 34–35
  induction procedure for: bringing patient to operating room and, 25–26
    induction room and, 24
    mask application and, 26–29
    operating room and, 24–25
    placing child on surgical bed and, 26
  intravenous induction of, 45
    rapid-sequence, 42–44
    routine for, 41–42
  for juvenile laryngeal papillomatosis, 278–280
  laryngospasm and, 38
    etiology of, 39
    management of, 39–41
    pathophysiology of, 38–39
  latex allergy and, 401–404
  local, maximum recommended dosages of, 241t
  maintenance of: alfentanil and, 150–151
    desflurane and, 147
    fentanyl and, 149–150
    halothane and, 146–147
    with intravenous agents, 145
    isoflurane and, 147
    minimum alveolar concentration and, 145–146
    morphine and, 149
    narcotic-based anesthetics and, 151–152
    in neonate, 169
    opioids and, 148–151
    sevoflurane and, 147–148
    sufentanil and, 151
    with volatile agents, 145–148
  malignant hyperthermia and, 390–393
  Masseter muscle rigidity, 393–394
  medications affecting management of, 4t
  muscular dystrophy and, 388–390
  narcotic-based, 151–152
  neuroblastoma and, 404–405
  for neonate, 163
    cardiovascular system and, 166
    congenital diaphragmatic hernia and, 171–172
    congenital lobar emphysema and, 187–189
    fluid and blood and, 167–168
    monitoring of, 168
    necrotizing enterocolitis and, 185–187
    omphalocele and gastroschisis and, 180–185
    premedication and fasting and, 168–171
    preoperative evaluation and preparation for surgery and, 164–165
    pulmonary system and congenital diaphragmatic hernia, 172–176
    respiratory system and, 165–166
    tracheoesophageal fistula and, 176–180
  for open heart surgery, 312–314
  outside operating room, 449–456
  osteogenesis imperfecta and, 408–412

for painful or frightening procedures outside operating
    room, 435–438
previous experience with, 4–5
Prune-belly syndrome and, 406–408
recovery from, 461–465
regional. *See under* Regional anesthesia
relation of recovery time and solubility of, 463f
risks of, 5
science of inhalation induction of, 34–35
sickle cell anemia and, 396–398
survival position and, 38
for tonsillectomy and adenoidectomy, 267–273
tracheal extubation and, 153–154
    in children who are awake, 158–159
    in deeply anesthetized children, 154–155
    technique for, 155, 157–158
Trisomy 21: Down's syndrome and, 399–401
upper airway obstruction during induction of, 37–41
upper respiratory infection and, 381–382
use of muscle relaxants during inhalation induction of,
    36f
volatile, 262
    avoiding overdose of, 35–37
Wilm's tumor/nephroblastoma and, 405–406
Anesthesia exhalation valve, 120f, 121f
Anesthesia machine, 114, 119f, 202, 449
    vapor-free, 391
900D Anesthesia Machine/Ventilator, 121
Anesthesia ventilator, 118–124
Anesthetic gas, 120f
Anesthetic implications of Down's syndrome, 400t
Anesthetic monologue, 30f
Angiotensin II, 214–215
Ankle, electrode placement for neuromuscular
    stimulation at, 18f
Antecubital fossa, 52–53
Anterior commissure laryngoscope, 104–105
Anterior mediastinal mass, 291–292
Anticholinergic agent, 382
Anticoagulant therapy (ACT), 315
Anticonvulsant, 4t
Antidiuretic hormone, 214, 215
Aortic arch, most common double, 328f
Aortic coarctation, resection of, 326–327
    repair of vascular rings and tracheomalacia and, 327,
    329
Aortic isthmus, 325f
Aortopexy, 329
Apert's syndrome, 7t
Apnea. *See also* Sleep apnea
    of neonate, 165–166
    postoperative: management of, 205
        postconceptual ages and, 204f
        prevention of, 205
Arnold-Chiari malformation
    type I, midsagittal NMR of, 360f
    type II, 368, 369
Arterial catheter, insertion of, 65–67, 69
Arterial hemoglobin oxygen desaturation, 130
Arterial locating technique, 67
Arterial monitoring, 57f
Arytenoid cartilage, 85f
ASA Closed Claims Project, 5
ASA Standards for Basic Anesthetic Monitoring, 5
Aspirating capnography, 131

Aspiration catheter, 134f
Aspirin, 4t
Asthma, 382–385
    drugs in, 384t
Astrocytoma, 359
Atlantoaxial instability, 276–277
Atracurium, 21–23, 425
Atrial septal defect (ASD), 299
Atropine, 40f, 44, 382
    congenital heart defects and, 296
Autoregulation, 288
AVPU, 421
Awake, deep extubation and, 156t
Awake intubation, 199
    endotrachial, 169
Awakening, imminent, sundown sign of, 152
Axial computed tomography (CT)
    of acute epidural hematoma, 372f
    of frontal depressed skull fracture, 370f
    of gross ventriculomegaly and hydrocephalus, 352f
Axillary approach to brachial plexus, 250–252
    continuous brachial plexus nerve block with, 252–253
Axillary artery, 252f
Axillary sheath, 252f
    radiopaque dye injected into, 253f
Ayre's T-piece, Jackson-Rees modification of, 115, 116f

B

Bacterial endocarditis, prevention of, 333, 335t, 336
Bain circuit, 116f, 117f, 119f, 134f
Bain circuit adaptor, 119f
Bain system with Narkomed anesthesia machine, 127f
Balanced salt solution, 217
Barbiturates for neuroanesthesia, 343
Barotrauma, 281f
Baseball grip, 52f
Beaten copper sign, 346
Beckwith-Wiedemann syndrome, 180, 405
Benjamin suspension laryngoscope, 280
Benzodiazepines for neuroanesthesia, 343–344
β_2-agonist, 384, 385
Bier block, 258
Biliary tract, implications of cystic fibrosis on,
    385t
Birth history of neonate, 164
Blade(s)
    for endotracheal intubation, 169
    laryngoscopic, 82
Blalock-Hanlon operation, 329–331
Blalock-Taussig shunt, 299
Bleeding
    excessive treatment of, 319–320
    NSAIDs and, 236
Bleomycin (Blenoxane), 4t20
Blind nasal intubation, 86
Blood
    intravenous fluid filters and, 49
    of neonate, 167
    supplies of, of congenital heart disease, 299
    surgery to decrease pulmonary flow of, 331–332
    surgery to increase pulmonary flow of, 329–330
    treatment for loss of, 220–224
Blood component(s), 183–184
    therapy with, 221, 426
Blood flow rate (CBF) by age, 339t

Blood pressure
  relationship of age to, 19t
  sedation and, 448-449
Blood pressure monitoring, 178
  automated, in neonates, 19
  during induction of anesthesia, 17, 19
  intra-arterial, 69, 75
  necrotizing enterocolitis and, 186
Blue subcutaneous nodule (blueberry muffin), 405
Body temperature, disorders of, in PACU, 472
Body weight, tidal volume delivery and, 115t
Bolus dose, calculation for, 152
Bone marrow needle, 59f
Bowel obstruction, 425
Brachial plexus
  axillary approach to, 250-252
  continuous nerve block of, 252-253
  interscalene block of, 247-249
  parascalene block of, 249-250
  position of child for block of, 250f, 251f
  supraclavicular approach to, 249
Bradycardia
  in PACU, 471
  rapidly developing, 220
  slowly developing, 219
Brain tumor, pediatric, classification of, 355t
Brainstem, radiation of, 451f
Brainstem glioma, 359
Breath rate, 128f
Breathing after major trauma, 420
Breathing circuit, 114, 202
  extra long, for use in MRI, 117f
  Mapleson classification of, 116f
  semiclosed circle, 138f
Breathing circuit volume (V_{bc}), 132
Bronchopulmonary disease in ex-premature and ex-ECMO patients, 196-198
Bronchopulmonary dysplasia (BPD), 141f, 196, 197f
  intraoperative pulmonary care with, 201t
Bronchoscopy, fiberoptic, 102f
Bronchospasm, refractory, 469
Broselow's tape, 413, 418f
Brown fat, 183
Bucking, history of, 469
Bullard (fiberoptic) laryngoscope, 100-104
  insertion of blade of, 103
Bupivacaine, 261f
  with epinephrine, 261f
  maximum recommended dosage of, 241t
Burn from air entry nozzle, 20f
Burn dressing change, deep sedation/anesthesia for, 455-456
Busulfan (Myleran), 4t
Butterfly needle technique, 239

C

Calcium chloride, 311t
Calcium gluconate, 311t
Canadian Standards Association, 443
Cannula material, 69, 75
Cannulation
  central vascular, potential complications of, 63f
  central vein, 58, 61-62
  femoral vein, 54, 58
  internal jugular vein, 60f, 61
  subclavian vein, 61, 62f
Capnograph, human, 158f
Capnographic baseline elevation, 136-137
Capnographic waveform, 136f, 137f, 139f, 141f
  in 6.9-kg, 9-month-old infant, 132f
  measurement of: by flow-through capnography, 140f
    by infrared analysis, 138f
    by mass spectrometry, 138f
Capnography, pediatric, 131, 136, 178
  accurate aspirating, 131
    position of heat and moisture exchanger and, 133
    sample flow rate and, 133-134
    sampling and smoke line and, 132-133
    spontaneously breathing nonintubated patients and, 134-135
  aspirating, 131
  flow-through, 131, 135, 140f
    peritracheal gas leak and, 135
    plateaus and arterial to end-tidal CO_2 differences and, 139-140
    waveform interpretation and, 137, 139
  inaccuracy in, 135f
  at rapid respiratory rates, 136
  relation of pulse oximetry and, 140-141
Capnometry, 131
Carbon dioxide (CO_2)
  effect of, on cerebral blood flow, 341f
  end-tidal, 132f
  plus of, 137f
Cardiac catheterization, 332, 333
Cardiac failure, 366f
Cardiac murmur, innocent versus pathologic, 7t
Cardiac support for congenital diaphragmatic hernia, 173
Cardiopulmonary bypass
  cardiac tamponade and, 320
  coming off, 317-318
  failure to wean from, 318
  management of, 315-319
  restoration of coagulation and, 319
  treatment of excessive bleeding and, 319-320
Cardiopulmonary dysfunction, residual, in ex-ECMO, 209
Cardiotonic drug, doses and effects of, 311t
Cardiovascular symptom from local anesthetic toxicity, 260f
Cardiovascular system
  defects of, in children with Down's syndrome, 400t
  evaluation of, during preoperative evaluation, 7-8t
  of neonate, 166
Cardioversion, 333
Carmustine (BCNU), 4t
Catecholamine, 215, 311t
Catheter(s)
  arterial, insertion of, 65-67, 69
  femoral artery and, 67
  floating of, 56f
  percutaneous placement of, 65-66
  pulmonary arterial flotation, 63, 65
  pulmonary artery data about, 64t
  radial artery and, 66-67
  standard length of, 61t
  surgical cutdown and, 67, 69
Catheter size, pulmonary artery, 65t
Catheterization
  femoral artery, 72f

percutaneous radial artery, 68*f*
radial artery, alternative technique for, 70*f*
Caudal anesthesia, 206*f*
Caudal block, 236, 241*f*
 techniques for, 238–240, 242–243
 anatomic differences between infant and adult and, 237*f*
 during injection of local anesthesia in, 240*f*
 placement of, 237*f*
 proper technique for placement of, 239*f*
Caudal catheter, placement of, for continuous infusion, 242*f*
Caudal epidural blockade, 205
Caudal epidural space, 206*f*
Cellular pump mechanism, failure of, 221*f*
Central core disease, 391
Central nervous system (CNS), 464, 472
Central neuroepithelial tumor, 355*t*
Central shunt, 329
Central vascular cannulation, potential complications of, 63*f*
Central vein cannulation, 58
 complications of, 61–62
 insertion methods for, 58, 61
 internal jugular vein cannulation and, 61
 subclavian vein cannulation and, 61
Central venous pressure (CVP), 340
 monitoring of, 62
Cerebellar astrocytoma, 359
Cerebellar tonsil, 360*f*
Cerebral blood flow (CBF), 340
 effect of CO_2 and O_2 on, 341*f*
 relation between cerebral perfusion pressure and, 340*f*
Cerebral blood flow velocity (CBFV), logarithmic relation between end-tidal CO_2 and, 341*f*
Cerebral blood volume (CBV), 340
Cerebral metabolic rate ($CMRO_2$), 340
 by age, 339*t*
Cerebral palsy, 386–388
Cerebral perfusion pressure (CPP), 340
 barbiturates reduction of, 343
 relation between cerebral blood flow and, 340
Cerebral spinal cord injury, 375–376
Cerebrovascular anomalies, 363–367
Cervical injury, suspected, 108*f*
 airway management in, 106, 108, 428–429, 431
Cervical spine
 high-velocity fracture of, 375*f*
 suspected injury of, 430
Cervicospinal syringomyelia, 360*f*
Chemotherapeutic agent, 4*t*
Chest of neonate, 165
Chest radiography
 inspiratory, 281*f*
 during preoperative evaluation, 11
Child. *See under* Pediatric patient
 concerns of, during preoperative evaluation, 5
 psychological preparation of, during preoperative evaluation, 1–2
 with runny nose, 9–10
Children's Hospital of Eastern Ontario Pain Scale, 230
Children's Memorial Hospital Chicago, 444
Chloral hydrate, 439–440, 443
2-Chloroprocaine, maximum recommended dosage of, 241*t*

Chronic hyponatremia, 224
Chronic lung disease, 141*f*
 infant with, 197*f*
Circle system, 115–117
Circulatory arrest, profound hypothermia with, 321–324
Circumcision, 247
Citrate toxicity, 184
Clindamycin, 8*t*, 335*t*
Clivus, 359*f*
Coagulation screening during radiographic evaluation, 11–12
Coarctation of aorta, 299
Coccyx, 238*f*
Codeine, 232*t*
Cold, preoperative evaluation and, 9-10
Colonoscopy, HSC anesthetic technique for, 452
Compensatory mechanisms for fluid loss, 214–215
Compensatory polycythemia, 295
Computed tomography (CT)
 airway patency maintained by, 80*f*
 axial: of acute epidural hematoma, 372*f*
  of frontal depressed skull fracture, 370*f*
 congenital stridor and, 284
 midsagittal, of lumbosacral spine, 367*f*
Congenital anomalies, association of
 with CDH, 172–173
 with tracheoesophageal fistula, 176
Congenital aqueductal obstruction, 359*f*
Congenital arteriovenous connection, 366*f*
Congenital diaphragmatic hernia (CDH)
 anesthetic management of, 173–174
 clinical presentation of, 172–173
 control of F_IO_2 and, 175
 endotracheal intubation and, 174
 extracorporeal membrane oxygenation and nitrous oxide and, 175
 hyperventilation and, 175
 incidence and etiology of, 171–172
 postoperative management of, 174–176
 prognosis for, 176
 pulmonary system and, 172
 supplemental oxygen and, 174
 treatment of pulmonary hypertension and, 174–175
Congenital heart disease(s) (CHD), 295–301
 abbreviations in, 297*t*
 anesthesia for, 302, 312–314
 anesthesia for noncardiac surgery in child with, 333
 bacterial endocarditis prophylaxis and, 333, 336
 cardiac catheterization and, 332–333
 management of cardiopulmonary bypass and, 315–321
 types of, 296*t*
Congenital hypertrophic pyloric stenosis, 189
 anesthetic management of, 189–190
 special anesthetic problems with, 189
Congenital left ventricular outflow obstruction, considerations for, 310*t*
Congenital lobar emphysema (CLE), 187–188
 anesthetic management of, 188–189
 1-month-old infant with, 188*f*
Congenital pulmonary hypoplasia, 407
Congenital stridor, 284, 285
Conscious sedation
 controversies about, 435–436
 drug dosages for, 443–444
Contact dermatitis, 402

Continuous positive airway pressure (CPAP), 123f, 317
Controlled ventilation, 114, 179, 290
    conclusions about, 126, 128
    effect of fresh gas flow on, 125
    history of, 186
    for open heart surgery, 312
Cook intraosseous infusion needle, 59f
Cooperative Study of Sickle Cell Disease Group, 10
Cor pulmonale, 269–270
Cornua, 238f
Coronal plane, 241f
CPRAM technique, 136f
Craniofacial deformity, 7t
Craniopharyngioma, 358f
Crawford needle, 253f
Creatine phosphokinase (CPK), 391
Creighton (two-person) technique, 110
    expanded version of, 81
Cricoid cartilage, 85f
Cricoid pressure, 108f, 431f
    application of, 43f
Cricothyroid membrane, identification of, 106f
Cricothyrotomy, 105–107f
Crossover from controlled to spontaneous ventilation, 154f
Crouzon's disease, 7t
Cryotherapy, surgery for, of retinopathy of prematurity, 202
Crystalloid, 220–221
Cuff maximum inflation, testing and deflation of, 94f
Curare cleft, 141f
Cushing triad, 372, 374
Cyanotic patient, 299
Cyclophosphamide (Cytoxan), 4t
Cystic fibrosis, 385–386
    implications of, 385t

D

Dantrolene, 392
Daunorubicin (Daunomycin), 4t
Dead space of head mask, 33f
Deep extubation, awake versus, 156t
Dental procedure, 335t
Dermatitis, contact, 402
Desflurane, 146t, 147, 392
    for neuroanesthesia, 343
    solubility of, 463f
Desmopressin acetate (DDAVP), 275, 359
Diabetes insipidus, 358
Diagnostic imaging
    deep sedation/anesthesia and, 453–454
    sedation for, 445–447
Diagnostic Imaging Sedation Committee, 446
Diaphragmatic hernia, 3t
Diazemule, 443
Diazepam, 443
Digitalis, 296
Digoxin, 311t
Disability after major trauma, 421
Diuretics for reduction of intracranial pressure, 349–350
Dobutamine, 311t
Dopamine, 311t
Doppler imaging, transtracheal, 301
Dorsal penile nerve block, 247, 248f
Dorsal spinous precesses, 107f

Dosage considerations in ex-premature, 200
Down's syndrome, 399–401
    anesthetic implications of, 400t
    cardiovascular defects in children with, 400t
Doxorubicin (Adriamycin), 4t
    for Wilms' tumor, 406
DPT/CM3, 440
Droperidol for neuroanesthesia, 343
Drug(s)
    in asthma, 384t
    dosages of, for conscious sedation, 443–444
    emergency, 301t
    monitoring and maintenance of temperature and, 21
    prepartion of, for CHD, 301–302
    titration of, 170
Drug history, congenital heart disease and, 298
Duchenne's muscular dystrophy (DMD), 388
Duodenal atresia, 400
Dural sac, 241f

E

Ear surgery, 277–278
Elbow adaptor, 134f
Elective surgery
    determining whether to proceed with, 383t
    oral intake of fluids before, 215
Electrocardiogram (ECG)
    during combined light general anesthesia and regional analgesics, 261f
    during induction of anesthesia, 16–17
    of piglets receiving drugs, 261f
    sedation and, 448
Electrode placement for neuromuscular stimulation at wrist, 18f
Electrolyte(s)
    basic requirements of, in infants and children, 213–214
    in bypass patients, 323
Embolism, venous air, 350–351
Emergence from anesthesia, 152
    blue but well-ventilated child and, 152–153
    of neonate, 171
    sundown sign and, 152
Emergence delirium, 472
Emergency drug(s), 301t
Emergency room
    preparation of, 413–414
    sedation in, 444–445
Emergency surgical airway, 105–106
Encephalocele, occipital, 368f
Endocardial cushion effect, considerations for, 304t
Endotracheal extubation in ex-premature, 202–203
Endotracheal intubation, 169, 416f
    blades and tubes for, 169
    for congenital diaphragmatic hernia, 174
    in ex-premature, 199
    juvenile laryngeal papillomatosis and, 279–280
    after major trauma, 442–425
    of newborn with TEF, 178–179
    for open heart surgery, 302
    position of head during, 86f
    with suspected cervical injury, 108f
    useful technique for, 102f
Endotracheal tube, 79, 89f
    adult-sized, 103f

gas leak around, 135f
Endotracheal tube adaptor, 134f
End-tidal CO_2, 132f
   cerebral blood flow velocity and, 341f
   detector for, 414, 419f
Endocarditis prophylaxis, 8t
   indications for, 334t
Endogenous vasopressor, 214
Enflurane, 392
Ependymoma, 359
Epidermolysis bullosa, 394–396
Epidural anesthesia, complications of, 259–264
Epidural hematoma, 371–372
   acute, 372f
Epiglottis, 85f
   pushing down of, into glottic opening, 79f
Epiglottitis, 282–283
Epinephrine, 261f, 311t
   bupivacaine with, 261f
   lidocaine with, 261f
   in local anesthetic, 207
Equipment
   for major trauma, 413
   preparation of, for congenital heart disease, 299–301
   for tracheal tube placement, 82
Erythromycin, 335t
Esophageal atresia, 3t
Esophageal stethoscope, 16
Esophagus, 85f
Ethmoid sinus, 85f
Etomidate for neuroanesthesia, 343
Ex-ECMO (extracorporeal membrane oxygenation) patient, 166, 175, 177, 195, 207
   anesthetic considerations for, 207–210
      difficult venous access and, 210
      fluids and, 210
      hematologic concerns for, 209–210
      narcotic dependency and, 210
      neurologic concerns for, 209
      renal concerns for, 209–210
      residual cardiopulmonary dysfunction and, 209
Expiratory jet ventilation, 281f
Exposure after major trauma, 422
Ex-premature patient, 195. See also Prematurity
   bronchopulmonary disease and, 196–198
   caudal anesthesia in, 206f
   dosage considerations for, 200
   endotracheal extubation and, 202–203
   fentanyl and, 200
   induction of general anesthesia in: by endotracheal intubation, 199
      by inhalation, 198–199
      by laryngeal mask airway, 199–200
   intraoperative pulmonary care and, 201
   patent ductus arteriosus and, 324
   postanesthetic respiratory complications of, 203–205
   preoperative assessment of, 196–198
   regional anesthesia and, 205–207
   retinopathy of prematurity and, 201–202
   tracheal intubation in, 199t
   typical, 195–196
External nares, 81f
Extracorporeal membrane oxygenation (ECMO), 166, 177, 207. See also Ex-ECMO patient

Extremely low birth weight, definition of, 195
Extubation. See also Tracheal extubation
   in children who are awake, 158–159
   deep technique of, 155, 157–158
   in deeply anesthetized children, 154–155
   omphalocele and gastroschisis and, 184
   recovery of patient and, 465
   TEF and, 179
   after tonsillectomy, 272–273

F

Face mask
   acceptance of, 30f
   application of, 31, 32, 34
   appropriate application of, 32f
   belly full of gas after routine induction by, 33f
   Patil-Syracuse, 101f
   pillow, 33f
   proper application of, for maintenance airway patency, 31f
   Rendell-Baker-Soucek, 33f
   size of, 92t
Faces Pain Rating Scale, 230
Factor replacement requirement, 399t
Family, psychological preparation of, during preoperative evaluation, 1–2
Family history, 5
Fascia iliaca compartment block, 256–257
Fasting
   controversies about, 437–438
   guidelines for, 215
   before induction of anesthesia, 23
   neonate and, 168–171
Femoral area, anatomic relations of, 255f
Femoral artery, 67
   catheterization of, 72f
   pulsation of, 256f
Femoral nerve block, 255, 256
   femoral artery pulsation and, 256f
Femoral vein, 57f
   cannulation of, 54, 58
Fentanyl, 149–150, 232t, 357
   cardiovascular stability and respiratory depression and, 150
   chest wall rigidity and, 150
   in ex-premature, 200
   oral transmucosal, 456
   suggested doses for, 151t
   target concentrations for, 152t
Fetal circulation, transition from, 181
Fiberoptic bronchoscopy, 102f
Fiberoptic Intubation Stilette AMS, 100t
Fiberoptic laryngoscope, 100
   Bullard, 102f, 103f
Fiberoptic Medical Products, 100t
FiO_2, 123f
   control of, 175
Fixation, 67
   of peripheral IVs, 54
Flagg blade, 82f
   C-shaped flange of, 83f
Flexible fiberoptic laryngoscope, 101f
Floating-the-catheter, 56f
Flow-through capnography, 131, 140f
Flow-volume loop, 284

Fluid(s)
    basic requirements for, in infants and children, 213–214
    in bypass pat;ients, 323
    compensatory mechanisms for loss of, 214
    in ex-ECMO, 210
    guidelines for administration of, 217t
    management of, in head-injured patients, 431
    intracranial pressure control and, 348–349
    intraoperative, choice and quantitiy of, 216–217
    intraoperative replacement of, 215–217
        omphalocele and gastroschisis and, 183–184
    maintenance of balance of, 314–315
    of neonate, 167–168
    perioperative management of, 213, 215–217, 224–225
        changes related to volume status and, 219–220
        glucose and, 217–219
        treatment of hypovolemia and blood loss and, 220–224
    postoperative problems with, 223–224
    rapidly occurring loss of, 219
    slowly developing loss of, 219
Flumazenil, 442, 443
Foramen magnum, 360f
Forced-air warming blanket, 20f, 473f
Foreign body aspiration, 285
    anesthetic management of, 286–287
    induction techniques for, 287
    maintenance of, 287–291
    preoperative evaluation of, 285–286
Fourth lumbar vertebra, 254f
Fracture. *See also specific type of fracture*
Fresh frozen plasma (FFP), 223
Fresh gas flow (FGF), 136f
Fritz Berry (top-gun) grip, 45f
Frontoparietal burr hole, 353f
Full-stomach, no open-eye considerations about intravenous induction, 42
Full-stomach, open-eye considerations about intravenous induction, 42–44

G

Gas
    fresh flow of, controlled ventilation and, 125
    leak of: around endotracheal tube, 135f
        peritracheal, 135
Gastric distention, 33f
Gastroenterology patients, deep sedation/anesthesia for, 452–453
Gastrointestinal procedure, 335t
Gastrointestinal side effects of NSAIDs, 236
Gastroschisis, 3t, 180–181
    anesthetic management of, 183–185
    hypotension and, 181–183
    preoperative evaluation of, 181
    prognosis for, 184–185
General anesthesia, light, 261f
Genitourinary procedure, 335t
Gentamicin, 335t
Germ cell tumor, 355
Gestational age, 164–165
Glasgow Coma Scale, 373, 413, 421
    accurate estimate of ICP by, 428
    for infants and children, 422t
Glenn procedure, 329

Glossoptosis, 284f
Glottic opening, 31f, 89f, 91f
    LMA and, 95f
    push epiglottis down into, 79f
    visualization of, 104f
Glucose
    in fluids, 217–219
    harm of, in IV solutions, 218–219
Glycopyrrolate, 382, 469
Goldenhar's syndrome, 7t, 90
Great vein of Galen, 363
Great vessels, considerations for transposition of, 306t
Gross ventriculomegaly, 352f
Guidelines, 436
Guidewire, 71f, 72f
    in endotracheal intubation, 102f
Gunshot wound victim, 422

H

Haemophilus influenzae type B, 282
Halothane, 146–147, 392
    increasing inspired concentrations of, 34
    induction characteristics of sevoflurane versus, 34–35
    for neuroanesthesia, 342
    solubility of, 463f
Hand
    position of, for Bullard laryngoscope, 103f
Head
    of infant cadaver, 85f
    neutral position of, 86f, 88f, 91f
Head injury, 371, 428–431
    epidural hematoma and, 371–372
    fluid management in patients with, 431
    intracerebral hematoma and, 372–374
    subdural hematoma and, 372
Heart
    abbreviations for congenital disease of, 297t
    sympathetic innervation of, 181–182
    types of congenital defects of, 296t
    volar aspect of, 52
Heart rate, relationship of age to, 17t
Heart surgery, 301t
    open, 313f
Heat and moisture exchanger (HME), 415
    position of, 133
Helmet head deformity, 409
Hematocrit, acceptable, 223t
    guidelines for, 222–223
Hematologic concerns in ex-ECMO, 209–210
Hematology patient, deep sedation/anesthesia for, 450–452
Hematology procedures, sedation for, 447
Hematoma
    epidural, 371–372
    intracerebral, 372–374
    subdural, 372
Hemifacial microsomia, 7t
Hemoglobin concentration during preoperative evaluation, 10–11
Hemoglobinopathy
    Down's syndrome and, 399–401
    hemophilia and, 398–399
    sickle cell anemia and, 396–398
Hemophilia, 398–399
Hemorrhagic shock, 221f

SUBJECT INDEX

interstitial fluid translocation and, 222f
Hemothorax, 427
Heparinization, 315
Hernia, diaphragmatic, 3t
Herniorraphy, 208f
High-velocity cervical spine fracture, 375f
Hirschsprung's disease, 400
History of patient
    elective surgery and, 383t
    neuroanesthesia and, 345–346
Hopkins rod lens telescope, 105
Hospital for Sick Children (HSC), 447
    Department of Anesthesia guidelines from, 436
    Sedation Protocol 1995 from, 443–444
Human immunodeficiency virus (HIV), hemophilia and, 399
Hydrocortisone, 384t
Hydrocephalus, 352f–353, 359f
    induction and intubation for, 353
    maintenance of, 353–354
    postoperative management of, 354
Hypercarbia, 262
Hypertension in PACU, 471
Hyperthermia, 473
Hyperventilation, congenital diaphragmatic hernia and, 175
Hypopituitarism, 358
Hypotic agent, 463
Hypotension in PACU, 471
Hyponatremia
    acute dilutional, 223–224
    chronic, 224
Hypoplastic left heart syndrome, considerations for, 308t
Hypotension
    neonate and, 170
    in newborn with omphalocele or gastroschisis, 181–183
    rapidly developing, 220
    slowly developing, 219
    systemic, 139f
Hypothermia, 472–473
    hypotension and, 182–183
    major trauma and, 415
    prevention of, 415
    profound, with circulatory arrest, 321–324
Hypotonic replacement fluid, 216
Hypovolemia, treatment of, 220–224
Hypoxia, 262
Hysteresis of cerebral vasculature, 342

I

Ibuprofen, 231, 235t
Induction of anesthesia. *See under* Anesthesia, induction of
Induction room, 24
Iliohypogastric nerve block, 245
Ilioinguinal nerve block, 245, 246f
Imaging evaluation of congenital diaphragmatic hernia, 172
Improved vision (IV) MacIntosh blade, 84f
Infant. *See also* Ex-premature patient
    basic fluid and electrolyte requirements in, 213–214
    causes of upper and lower airway obstruction in, 284f
    with chronic lung disease, 197f
    fully awake, 203t
    with lumbosacral myelomeningocele, 364f
    with no chin, 98f
    well-secured saphenous vein IV in, 57f
Infant cadaver, sagittal section of head and neck in, 85f
Infant respiratory distress syndrome (IRDS), 167
Infrared analysis, capnographic waveform measured by, 138f
Infratentorial compartment pressure, 359f
Inguinal herniorrhaphy, 205
Inguinal ligament, 72f, 256f
Inguinal paravascular nerve block, 255f
Inhalation anesthesia
    neuroanesthesia and, 342–344
    recovery from, 462–463
Inhalation induction, 151t
    art of, 29–30
    choice of agents for, 34
    in ex-premature, 198–199
    increasing inspired concentrations of, 34
    science of, 34–35
    use of muscle relaxants during, 36f
Initial assessment after major trauma, 420–422
In-line stabilization, 108f, 430f, 431f
Insertion (methods)
    of arterial catheters, 65–67, 69
    for central vein cannulation, 58, 61–62
    intraosseous, 58
    laryngeal mask airway and, 86–88
    nasal, of tracheal tube, 85–86
    oral, of tracheal tube, 81–85
    for pulmonary arterial flotation catheters, 65
Inspiratory chest radiograph, 281f
Inspiratory cycle, inflation hold and, 128f
Intensive care unit
    cardiopulmonary bypass and, 321
    initial management of post-bypass patients in, 322
Internal carotid artery, lateal view of injection of, 366f
Internal jugular vein, 60f
    cannulation of, 61
Interscalene block of brachial plexus, 247–249
Interstitial fluid, translocation of, 222f
Intestinal tract, implications of cystic fibrosis on, 385t
Intra-arterial blood pressure monitoring, 69
    cannula materials and, 69, 75
    contraindications against, 69
    indications for, 69
Intra-arterial mixing, surgery for, 331
Intracardiac shunting, 297
    control of, 314–315
Intracellular water excess, 221f
Intracerebral edema, 372f
Intracerebral hematoma, 372–374
Intracerebral pressure, 345
Intracranial cortical cerebrovascular malformation, 363f
Intracranial pressure (ICP), 340
    control of, 348–349
    diuretics for reduction of, 349–350
    high, 352f
    pathophysiology of, 344–345
    relation between volume and, 345f
Intracranial tumor, 354–355
Intramuscular induction of anesthesia, 45
Intramuscular (IM) injection, 227
Intraoperative considerations for TEF, 179
Intraoperative pain, management of, 227, 229

Intraoperative pulmonary care, 201
　with bronchopulmonary dysplasia, 201t
Intraosseous needle, 59f
　insertion of, 58
Intravenous analgesics
　continuous infusion of, 232–233
　intermittent injections of, 231–232
　patient-controlled analgesia and, 233–234
Intravenous (IV) cannulation, 145
　baseball grip for, 52f
　for major trauma, 424
　neuroanesthesia and, 343–344
　recovery from, 463–464
　successful, more helpful hints for, 51–52
　two-person technique of, 54f
Intravenous equipment kidney basin, 50
Intravenous induction, 41–42, 151t
　rapid-sequence, 42–44
Intravenous infusion pump, 49–50
Intravenous regional block, 258–259
Intravenous solution flush, 44
Intubation. *See also* Endotracheal intubation;
　　Nasopharyngeal intubation
　awake, 199
　difficult, two-handed laryngoscopy in, 99f
　endotracheal, 416f
　　for CDH, 174
　　of newborn with TEF, 178–179
　lighted stylet, 99t, 100t
　rigid bronchoscopic, with Hopkins rod lens telescope, 105
Ipratropium, 469
Isocapnic ventilation, 136f
Isoflurane, 146t, 147, 392
　neuroanesthesia and, 342–343
　solubility of, 463f
Isoproterenol, 311t
Isotonic replacement fluid, 215–216

J

Jackson-Rees modification of Ayre's T-piece, 115, 116f
Jackson-Rees circuit, 117f, 157f
Jaw thrust, 32f, 37f
Jet ventilation, 281f
Juvenile laryngeal papillomatosis
　airway emergence and, 282
　airway management for, 279–280
　anesthetic maintenance for, 280
　epiglottitis and, 282
　industrial anesthesia for, 278–279
　laryngotracheobronchitis and, 283–284
　laser considerations for, 280, 282
　preoperative considerations for, 278
　ventilation techniques for, 279–280

K

Keep vein open (KVO) rate, 316
Ketamine, 45f, 227, 384, 440–441
　for neuroanesthesia, 344
Ketorolac, 231, 235t
Kidney, transition and maturation of, 213
Kidney basin, IV equipment, 50
King-Denborough syndrome, 391
Kuhlenkampf method, 249

L

Laboratory evaluation
　of neonate cardiovascular system, 166
　neuroanesthesia and, 346
　during preoperative evaluation, 10–12
Laryngeal mask airway (LMA), 93f, 94f
　in ex-premature, 199–200
　fiberoptic laryngoscopy through, 100
　insertion of, 86–88, 102f
　pitfalls of insertion of, 96f
　positive-pressure ventilation through, 125–126
Laryngeal web, 284f
Laryngomalacia, 284f
Laryngoscope
　anterior commissure, 104–105
　Bullard, 101–104
　　blade of, 104f
　　hand position for, 103f
　flexible fiberoptic, 101f
Laryngoscope blade(s), 79, 82, 104f
　after placement of, 88f
　before placement of, 87f
　insertion of, 89f
　size and type of, for age, 82t
Laryngoscopy
　direct oral, 108f
　fiberoptic, 100–101, 103–104
　oral, 91f
　two-handed, algorithm for proper use of, 99f
Laryngospasm, 38, 157, 469
　etiology of, 39
　in infant, 38, 57f
　management of, 39–41
　pathophysioilogy of, 38–39
　prevention of, 159f
Laryngotracheobronchitis (LTB), 283–284
Larynx, 31f, 89f
Laser, juvenile laryngeal papillomatosis and, 280–281
LAST (latex allergosorbent test), 403
Lateral femoral cutaneous nerve block, 255–256
Lateral position, 157f, 237f
Lateral ventricle, 353f
Latex allergy, 401–402
　anesthetic management of, 402–403
　anesthetic technique and, 403–404
Latex precaution, 403
Left thoracotomy, 325f
Lidocaine, 41f, 44, 261f
　with epinephrine, 261f
　maximum recommended dosage of, 241t
　topical, 247
Ligamentum arteriosum, 328f
Light wand, pediatric, 97–98
Lighted stylet(s)
　features, advantages, and disadvantages of, 100t
　indications and advantages of intubations with, 99t
Lindholn laryngoscope, 280
Line placement for open heart surgery, 312
Local anesthetic
　plasma concentration of, progression of symptomatology and, 260f
　postcircumcision pain relief with, 247
　toxicity of, 260–262
　　treatment of, 262–263
Loop diuretics, 350

Lower extremity block, 254–258
Lower respiratory problems in PACU, 469–470
Lumbosacral myelomeningocele, 364f
Lumbosacral spine, midsagittal CT scan of, 367f
Lung(s)
    chronic disease of, 197
    implications of cystic fibrosis on, 385t
    of neonate, 165

M
MAC-awake of inhalation agent, 462
    levels of, 464
MacIntosh blade, 84f
Magill's forceps, 91f
Magnetic resonance imaging (MRI)
    adaptation of Mapleson D for use in, 117
    congenital stridor and, 284
    extra long breathing circuit in, 117f
    sedation during, 448
Maintenance infusion rate (MIR), calculation for, 152
Maldevelopmental tumor, 355t
Malignant hyperthermia (MH), 389–393, 409
    treatment of, 392t
Malignant hyperthermia Association of United States (MHAUS), 392
Mandible, 38f, 85f
    ascending ramus of, 85f
Mandibular hypoplasia, 6f
Mannitol for reduction of intracranial pressure, 349–350
Manual-controlled ventilation, 117f
Manual ventilation, 202
Mapleson classification of breathing systems, 116f
Mapleson D circuit, 116f, 132f, 202
    adaptation of, for use in MRI, 117
    ventilation controlled through, 136f
Mapleson E system, 116f
Mapleson F system, 116f
Mask, 77, 79
    application of, 26–29
Mass spectrometry, capnographic waveform measured by, 138f
Masseter spasm, 36f
Masseter muscle rigidity, 393–394
Mastoid surgery, 277–278
Maternal history, 164
Mean arterial pressure (MAP), 340
Measured end-tidal CO_2 ($P_{ET}CO_2$), 131
Mechanical-controlled ventilation, 117f
Medial malleolus, 56f
Median nerve, 252f
Medical history, 2–5
Medical problems in neonatal intensive care unit, 3t
Medication(s)
    administration of, 416f, 417f
    preoperative evaluation and, 3–4
Medulloblastoma, 359
Memorial Sloan-Kettering Cancer Center in New York, diagnostic procedures of, 450
Meningeal tumor, 355t
Meperidine, 232t
Mepivacaine, maximum recommended dosage of, 241t
6-Mercaptopurine (6-MP), 4t
Metaproterenol, 384t
Methylprednisolone, 384t
Micrognathia, 98f, 284f

Midazolam, 23–24, 441–443
Middle cerebral artery, 341f
Middle ear surgery, 277–278
Miller blade, 82f
Minimum alveolar concentration (MAC), 145–146, 195
    age versus, 146t
    desflurane and, 147
    halothane and, 146–147
    isoflurane and, 147
    in neonate, 169
    relation of surgical events with, 154f
    sevoflurane and, 147–148
Minute ventilation (V_e), 136f
Minute volume, expired, 128f
Mivacurium, 22t, 280, 425
Moebius sequence, 7t
Monitor(s), application of, before induction of anesthesia, 27f
Morphine, 149, 232t, 443
Motor evoked potential, 374
Moyamoya disease, 364
Murphy eye, 103f
Muscle relaxant(s), 290
    atracurium and, 21, 23
    during inhalation induction of anesthesia, 36f
    intracardiac shunting and, 314
    for major trauma, 424–425
    monitoring and maintenance of temperature and, 21, 23
    nondepolarizing, 21–23
    for neuroanesthesia, 344
    rocuronium and, 23
    succinylcholine and, 21
    vecuronium and, 23
    wearing off of, 141f
Muscular dystrophy, 388t
Musculocutaneous nerve, 252f
Musculoskeletal system
    cerebral palsy and, 386–388
    epidermolysis bullosa and, 394–396
    malignant hyperthermia and, 390
    Masseter muscle rigidity and, 393–394
    muscular dystrophy and, 388–390
Myelodysplasia, 3t, 367–369
    emergence and, 371
    maintenance of anesthesia for, 369–371
    postoperative management of, 371
Myelomeningocele, 367f, 368f
Myocardium of neonate, 166, 181
Myringotomy, 277

N
Naloxone, 443
Narcotic-based anesthetic, 151–152
Narcotic dependency in ex-ECMO, 210
Nares, 91f
Narkomed anesthesia machine, Bain system with, 127f
Nasal insertion of tracheal tube, 85–86
Nasopharyngeal airway, 77, 81f
Nasotracheal intubation, 91f, 92f
Nausea in PACU, 471–472
Neck
    of infant cadaver, 85f
    neutral position of, 88f, 91f
Neck extension, 87f, 88f

Neck injury, 430f
Necrotizing entercolitis (NEC), 3t, 185–186
    anesthetic management of, 186–187
Neonatal intensive care unit
    potential medical problems associated with admission to, 3t
Neonate
    anemia of, 167
    anesthesia for, 163
    apneic spells of, 165–166
    automated blood pressure measurement in, 19
    birth history of, 164
    cardiovascular system of, 166
    congenital diaphragmatic hernia and, 171–172
    congenital hypertrophic pyloric stenosis and, 189–190
    congenital lobar emphysema and, 187–189
    emergence and postoperative care for, 171
    endotracheal intubation and, 169
    gestational age of, 164–165
    hypotension and, 170
    induction of anesthesia and, 169
    laboratory tests on, 166
    lungs and chest of, 165
    maintenance of: anesthesia and, 169–171
        normothermia for, 167–168
    maternal history of, 164
    minimum alveolar concentration and, 169
    myocardium of, 181
    necrotizing enterocolitis and, 185–187
    omphalocele and gastroschisis and, 180–185
    opioids and, 169–170
    pain management and, 170
    patent ductus arteriosus and, 324
    precordial stethoscope and, 168
    premedication and fasting in, 168–171
    pulmonary system and congenital diaphragmatic hernia and, 172–176
    renal metabolism of, 167
    retinopathy of prematurity and, 170–171
    standard monitors and, 168
    total body water of, 167
    tracheoesophageal fistula and, 176–180
    transfusion therapy and, 171
    upper airway of, 165
Nephroblastoma, 405–406
Nerve block. *See also specific type of nerve block*
    dorsal penile, 248f
    ilioinguinal iliohypogastric, 246f
Neuraxial opioid, complications related to, 263
Neuroanesthesia, 339
    cerebrovascular anomalies and, 363–367
    cervical spinal cord injury and, 375–376
    craniopharyngioma and, 358–359
    craniosynostosis and, 351–352
    diuretics for reducing intracranial pressure and, 349–350
    fluid management and, 348–349
    head injury and, 371–374
    history and physical exam and, 345–346
    hydrocephalus and, 352–354
    induction of, 347–348
    intracranial pressure control and, 348–349
    intracranial tumors and, 354–355
    laboratory tests and, 346
    maintenance of, 348
    monitoring of, 347
    myelodysplasia and, 367–371
    pathophysiology of intracranial pressure and, 344–345
    patient positioning and, 346–347
    pharmacology of, 342–344
    posterior fossa surgery and, 359–362
    premedication and, 346
    spinal cord surgery and, 374–375
    supratentorial craniotomy and, 355–358
    temperature homeostasis and, 350
    venous air embolism and, 350–351
Neuroblastoma, 404–405
Neurocognitive defects in OSA, 270
Neurologic concerns in ex-ECMO, 209
Neurologic disease, 437
Neuromuscular blockade monitoring, 17
Neuromuscular function, recovery of, 464–465
Neuromuscular stimulation at wrist or ankle, 18f
Neurophysiology, 339–342
Neuroplaque, 368f
Neutral position, 86f, 88f, 91f
Newborn
    myocardium of, 166
    pulmonary vasculature of, 166
Nitroprusside, 311t
Nitrous oxide, 175, 442–443
    for neuroanesthesia, 342
Nitrous oxide/oxygen, 444
Noncatecholamine, 311t
Nondepolarizing muscle relaxant, 21–23
Noninvasive monitoring in pediatric patient
    blood pressure monitoring and, 17, 19
    electrocardiogram and, 16–17
    esophageal stethoscope and ,16
    neuromuscular blockade monitoring and, 17
    precordial stethoscope and, 15–16
Nonopioid analgesics, 235t
Nonpump case, 299
Nonsteroidal anti-inflammatory drug (NSAIDs), 4t, 227, 231, 235–236
    bleeding and NSAIDs and, 236
    gastrointestinal side effects of, 236
    renal side effects of, 236
Norepinephrine, 311t
Normothermia, maintenance of, 167–168
North American Drager Narkomed, 121–123
    2B anesthesia machine of, 126f
    2C, control panel and bellows of, 124f
Nose
    implications of cystic fibrosis on, 385t
    surgery on, 277–278
Nuclear magnetic resonance (NMR), midsagittal
    of Arnold-Chiari type I malformation, 360f
    of high-signal mass lesion, 358f
Nursing care in PACU, 467

O

Objective pain-discomfort scale, 244t
Obstruction, upper airway physiology of, 269
Obstructive sleep apnea, 268–269
    management of, 270f
Occipital encephalocele, 368f
Odontoid process, subluxation of, 375f
Ohmeda anesthesia ventilator, 123–124
    model 7800, 128f

model 7810, 138f
model 7900, 129f
Oligohydramnios, 407
Omphalocele, 3t, 180–181
   anesthetic management of, 183–185
   hypotension and, 181—183
   preoperative evaluation of, 181
   prognosis for, 184–185
Oncology patient
   deep sedation/anesthesia for, 450–452
   sedation for, 447–448
Open heart surgery, 301t
   anesthesia for, 302, 312–314
   line placement sites and vascular equipment for, 313t
Operating room
   anesthesia outside, 449–456
   bringing patient to, 25–26
   induction of anesthesia and, 24–25
   parents in, 25f
Opioid(s), 148–149, 232t
   alfentanil and, 150–151
   choice of, for intravenous infusion, 233
   fentanyl and, 149–150
   morphine and, 149
   for neonate, 169–170
   neuraxial, complications and, 263
   for neuroanesthesia, 344
   sufentanil and, 151
   suggested doses for, 151t
   target concentrations for, 152t
Oral airway, 77, 79f
   appropriate-sized, 80f
Oral insertion of tracheal tube, 81–82
   anatomic airway differences and, 82
   equipment for, 82
   technique for, 83–85
Oral laryngoscopy, 91f
   direct, 108f
Oral transmucosal fentanyl citrate (OTFC), 24, 456
Organ systems, preoperative evaluation and, 2–5
Orophangeal axis, 86f, 87f
Oropharynx, 93f
Osmotic demyelination syndrome, 224
Osteogenesis imperfecta, 408–409
   anesthetic management of, 410
   anesthetic technique for, 410, 412
   clinical manifestations of, 409–410
Otoplasty, 6f
Outflow obstructive lesion, 297–298
Oximetry, sedation and, 449
Oxycodone, 232t
Oxygen (O_2)
   cerebral blood flow and, 341f
   inspired concentration of, 128f
   supplemental, for CDH, 174
Oxyscope, 169

P

Packed red blood (PRBC) cell, 299
Pain
   Faces Pain Rating Scale and, 230f
   mechanism of, 231
   objective pain-discomfort scale and, 244t
   ten-point objective pain-discomfort scale and, 231t
Pain management
   in bypass patients, 323–324
   in children vs. adults, 229–231
   complications of epidural and spinal anesthesia and, 259–264
   intraoperative, 227, 229
   in neonate, 170
   perioperative, 227, 228f
      caudal block and, 236, 238–240, 242–243
      continuous postoperative caudal analgesia and, 243–245
      ilioinguinal and iliohypogastric nerve block and, 245
      intravenous regional blocks and, 258–259
      lower extremity blocks and, 254–258
      splash block and, 245, 247
      upper extremity blocks and, 247–253
   postcircumcision with local anesthetics, 247
   postoperative, 229
      pharmacologically, 231–236
Pancreas, implications of cystic fibrosis on, 385t
Pancuronium, 22t, 44, 296
   hypertension and, 314
Panting respiratory pattern, 347
PAR score, 461
Paradoxical respiration, 468
Parascalene block of brachial plexus, 249–250
Parasympatholytic agent, 469
Parent(s)
   concerned, during preoperative evaluation, 5
   in operating room, 25f
   presence of, in induction room, 24
Partial thromboplastin time (PTT), 399
Patent ductus arteriosus (PDA), 166, 295, 298
   ligation of, 324
   neonatal, surgeon's perspective of, 325f
Patient-controlled analgesia (PCA), 233–234
Patil-Syracuse mask, 100, 101f
   fiberoptic laryngoscopy through, 100
PDA ligation, 299
Peak inspiratory pressure (PIP), 114
Pediatric bellows, 127f
Pediatric Advanced Life Support (PALS), 421
Pediatric difficult airway, David Steward's algorithm for, 109f
Pediatric light wand, 97–98
Pediatric patient(s)
   application of mask on, 26–30, 32, 34
   awake: extubation in, 158–159
      progression of symptomatology and, 260f
   basic fluid and electrolyte requirements in, 213–214
   blue but well-ventilated, during emergence, 152–153
   bringing of, into operating room, 25–26
   classification of skull fractures in, 371t
   deeply anesthetized, extubation in, 154–155
   differential diagnosis of wheezing in, 383t
   guidelines for fluid administration in, 217t
   noninvasive monitoring in: blood pressure monitoring and, 17, 19
      electrocardiogram and, 16–17
      esophageal stethoscope and, 16
      neuromuscular blockade monitoring and, 17
      precordial stethoscope and, 15–16
   pain of, 230–231
      versus adult pain, 229–230
   placing of, on surgical bed, 26

Pediatric patient(s) *(contd.)*
  size of, mask size and, 92*t*
  spontaneously breathing nonintubated, 134–135
  traumatized, airway management in, 106, 108
  weight, medication dosage, and equipment for, 418*f*
Pediatric trauma room, 416*f*
Pentobarbital, 441, 443
Percutaneous placement of arterial catheter, 65–67, 69
Percutaneous radial artery catheterization, 68*f*
Perioperative considerations about congenital hypertrophic pyloric stenosis, 189–190
Perioperative pain management. *See under* Pain management, perioperative
Peripheral intravenous access, 49
  antecubital fossa and, 52–53
  femoral vein cannulation and, 54, 58
  fixation of, 54
  intraosseous needle insertion and, 58
  IV equipment kidney basin and, 50
  IV fluid filters and, 49
  IV infusion pumps and rate controllers and, 49–50
  saphenous veins and, 53–54
  techniques for, 50–54
  two-person dorsal hand technique for, 52
  volar aspect of hand for, 52
Peritonsillar abscess, 276
Peritracheal gas leak, 135
Perivascular approach, 251*f*
Periventricular edema, 352*f*
Pfeiffer's syndrome, 7*t*
Phenylephrine, 311*t*
Physical examination
  of cardiovascular system of neonate, 166
  elective surgery and, 383*t*
Physical signs of congenital diaphragmatic hernia, 172
Pierre Robin anomaly, 7*t*, 81, 90
Piglet, ECG of, after drugs, 261*f*
Pillow face mask, 33*f*
Plasma, fresh frozen (FFP), 223
Plastic oral airway, 78*f*
  in position, 80*f*
  tongue depressor and, 81*f*
Plateau on capnographic waveform, 139–140
Platelet, 223
Pneumomediastinum, 281*f*
Pneumothorax, 425, 427
Polycythemia, compensatory, 295
Positive end-expiratory pressure (PEEP), 123*f*, 201, 288, 351
  high levels of, 175
Positive-pressure ventilation (PPV), 32
  avoidance of, 33*f*
  through laryngeal mask airway, 125–126
Postanesthetic respiratory complications in ex-premature, 203–205
Postanesthesia care unit (PACU), 147, 156*t*, 157*f*, 461–465
  analgesics in, 229
  cardiovascular instability and, 470–471
  child before transporting to, 466*f*
  discharge criteria for, 462*t*, 467–468
  pain while in, 472
  pediatric discharge criteria for, 462*t*
  routine care in, 465–468
  sleeping infant in, 473*f*

Posterior fossa surgery, 359–360, 362*f*
  maintenance of anesthesia and, 361–362
Posterior iliac crest, 238*f*
Posterior superior iliac spine (PSIS), 254*f*
Posterior vertebral body, 107*f*
Postoperative apnea, 203–205
  incidence of, postconceptual ages and, 204*f*
  management of, 205
  prevention of, 205
Postoperative care
  congenital diaphragmatic hernia, 174–176
  congenital hypertrophic pyloric stenosis, 190
  necrotizing enterocolitis and, 187
  of neonate, 171
  TEF and, 180
Postoperative nausea and vomiting (PONV), 471
Postoperative pain, management of, 229
  intravenous analgesics and, 231–234
  nonsteroidal anti-inflammatory drugs and, 235–236
Potter facies, 407
Potts operation, 329
Practice of Anesthesia guidelines, 443
Preanesthetic assessment of difficult airway, 90, 92
Precordial stethoscope, 15–16, 168
Prednisolone, 384*t*
Prednisone, 384*t*
Preemptive analgesics, 231
Pregnancy testing, 11
Premature ventricular contraction, 288
Prematurity, 3*t*. *See also* Ex-premature patient
  problems associated with NEC and, 185–186
Premedication
  algorithm for use of, 456*f*
  difficult airways and, 92–93
  before induction of anesthesia, 23–24
  of neonate, 168–171
Preoperative evaluation, 1
  airway evaluation and, 5–6
  cardiovascular evaluation and, 7–8*t*
  chest radiographic exam and, 11
  child and parental concerns and, 5
  coagulation screening and, 11–12
  colds and, 9–10
  about congenital hypertrophic pyloric stenosis, 189
  family history and, 5
  hemoglobin concentration and, 10–11
  medical history and, 2–5
  medications and allergies and, 3–4
  of neonate, 164–165
  pertinent laboratory evaluation during, 10–12
  pregnancy testing and, 11
  previous experience with anesthesia and, 4–5
  psychological preparation of child and family and, 1–2
  review of organ systems and, 2–5
  risks of anesthesia and, 5
  serum electrolytes and, 11
  urinalysis and, 11
Preoperative pain management, 227
Preoperative Transfusion in Sickle Cell Disease Study Group, 10
Preset tidal volume (V$_{t\,set}$), 115
Probe patent foramen ovale (PPFO), 152, 153
Procaine, maximum recommended dosage of, 241*t*
Prone position, 451*f*
  for posterior fossa surgery, 362*f*

SUBJECT INDEX

Prophylaxis, endocarditis, 333, 336
    indications for, 334t
Propofol, 384, 463
    intravenous, 451f
    neuroanesthesia and, 343
    outside ooperating room, 449–450
Prostaglandin E_1 (PGE_1), 298
Protamine, 319
Prothrombin time (PT), 319
Prune-belly syndrome, 406–408
Pseudosubluxation of C2–C3, 107f
Pseudotachycardia, 389
Psoas compartment block, 254f–255
Psychological preparation of child and family, 1–2
Pulmonary arterial flotation catheter(s), 63
    complications of, 65
    contraindications against, 63, 65
    indications for, 63
    insertion methods for, 65
    sites of insertion of, 65
Pulmonary artery catheter
    data from, 64t
    size of, 65t
Pulmonary blood flow, 329–332
Pulmonary care, intraoperative, 201
    with bronchopulmonary dysplasia, 201t
Pulmonary disease, 437
Pulmonary function testing, 284
Pulmonary hypertension, treatment of, 174–175
Pulmonary system, 381–386
    congenital diaphragmatic hernia and, 172
Pulmonary vasculature of newborn, 166
Pulmonary vascular resistance (PVR), 182
    sudden increases in, 166
Pulmonary ventilation, preoperative facilitation of, 362f
Pulmonic stenosis/atresia, 309t
Pulse oximetry, 129
    accuracy of, 130
    accuracy during arterial hemoglobin oxygen
        desaturation and, 130
    clinical uses of, 130–131
    complications of, 131
    effect of physiologic factors on, 129–130
    relation of capnography and, 140–141
    tracheoesophageal fistula and, 177–178
Pump case, 299

Q
Quinsy tonsil, 276

R
Radial artery
    alternative technique for catheterization of, 70f
    occlusion of, 66f
    percutaneous catheterization of, 66–68f
    surgical cutdown of, 73f, 74f
Radial nerve, 252f
Radiation of brainstem, 451f
Radiographic imaging
    neuroanesthesia and, 346
    sedation during, 448
Radiopaque dye, 253f
RAE tube, 134f
RAST (radioallergosorbent test), 403
Rate controller, 49–50

Recovery
    from anesthesia and surgery, 461–465
    cardiovascular, 464
    central nervous system, 464
    extubation and, 465
    from inhalation anesthesia, 462–463
    from intravenous agents, 463–464
    of neuromuscular function, 464–465
    rate of, 462
Red blood cell, 221–222
Refractory bronchospasm, 469
Regional analgesia, 205–207, 261f
Regional anesthesia
    caudal block and, 236, 238–240, 242–243
    continuous postopeative caudal analgesia and,
        243–245
    iliohypogastric nerve block and, 245
    ilioinguinal block and, 245
    intravenous, 258–259
    lower extremity blocks and, 254–258
    splash block and, 245, 247
    upper extremity block and, 247–253
Remote sedation location, 444–447
    monitoring children in, 448–449
Renal concerns in ex-ECMO, 209–210
Renal metabolism of neonate, 167
Renal side effects of NSAIDs, 236
Rendell-Baker-Soucek mask, 33f
Repair pump case, 299
Reperfusion, 67f
Residual pulmonary involvement, abnormal pulmonary
        findings with, 198t
Respiratory distress syndrome (RDS), 195, 324, 326
Respiratory problem in PACU, 468
Respiratory rate, rapid, capnography at, 136
Respiratory system of neonate, 165–166
Resuscitation, initial, for major trauma, 415
Retinopathy of prematurity (ROP), 170–171, 201–202
Retropharyngeal abscess, 276
Rigid bronchoscopic intubation with Hopkins rod lens
        telescope, 105
Rigid collar, 430f
Rocuronium, 22t, 23, 44, 424
Runny nose
    differential diagnosis of, 382t
    preoperative evaluation and, 9–10

S
Sacral hiatus, 238f
    palpation of, 242f
Sacrococcygeal ligament, 206f
Sample flow rate, 133–134
Sampling catheter, 137f
Sang multi-institutional survey, 263
Saphenous vein, 53–54, 56f
    cutdown of, 54
    proper positioning for cannulation of, 56f
    well-secured IV of, 57f
Sciatic nerve block, 257–258
Sechrist Infant Ventilator, 118–120, 140f
Sechrist IV-100B ventilator, 118f–120
Sechrist IV-200, 120, 121f
    control panel of, 122f–123f
Secondary brain insult, 349
Secondary survey after major trauma, 422

Sedation
   assessment before, 436–438
   chloral hydrate and, 439–440
   conscious, 435–436
      during dosages for, 443–444
   deep, 438, 455f
   DPT/CM3 and, 440
   drug dosages for, of children according to weight, 447t
   fasting controversies and, 437–438
   flumazenil and, 442
   ketamine and, 440–441
   midazolam and, 441–442
   nitrous oxide and, 442–443
   for painful or frightening procedures outside operating room, 435–438
   pentobarbital and, 441
   remote location for, 444–447
      monitoring of children in, 448–449
Sedation/anesthesia vehicle, transportable, 450f
Sedatives, current dosages of, 446t
Seimens-Elema 900C Serva Ventilator, 121
Seldinger technique, 57f
Sellick maneuver (cricoid pressure), 373
Sepsis, 298
   hypotension and, 183
Serum electrolytes during radiographic evaluation, 11
Sevoflurane, 146t-148, 392
   increasing inspired concentrations of, 34
   induction characteristics of halothane vs., 34–35
   for neuroanesthesia, 343
   solubility of, 463f
Short-bevel needle, 239f
Short gut syndrome, 3t
Shoulders, elevation of, 454f
Sickle- -thalassemia, 396
Sickle C disease, 396
Sickle cell anemia, 396–398
Sickle cell disease (SCD), 10
Sickle trait, 396
Silastic catheter, 353f
Skin, 386
Skin prick test, 402
Skull fracture(s)
   classification of, in children, 371t
   frontal depressed, 370f
Slack brain, 361
Sleep apnea, obstructive, 268–269. See also Apnea
   management of, 270f
Small-channel aspiration catheter, 134f
Small for gestational age, definition of, 195
Smoke line, 132–133
Sniff position pillow, 453, 454f
Soft palate, 85f
Solubility of anesthetic agent, 463f
Somatosensory evoked potential, 374
Spasm, Masseter, 36f
Spinal anesthesia, complications of, 259–264
Spinal cord, blood flow of, 341–342
Spinal cord surgery, 374–375
   cervical, 375–376
Spinal subarachnoid anesthesia, 264
Splash block, 245, 247
Spontaneous respiratory activity, 141f
Spontaneous ventilation, 117f, 179, 287–290

Spontaneously breathing nonintubated patient, 134–135
Spring guidewire, 71f
Stage 1 and 2 recovery, 466–467
Status post lower abdominal incision, 233f
Steeple sign, 283
Sternocleidomastoid muscle, 60f
Sternum, 85f
Steroid, 384t
Stethoscope
   esophageal, 16
   precordial, 15–16
Steward's algorithm for pediatric difficult airway, 108–111
Steward's postanesthesia scoring system, 462t, 467
Stress
   hypotension and, 182
   psychological, 298
Strip craniectomy, 351
Subclavian vein cannulation, 61, 62f
Subcutaneous ring block, 247
Subdural hematoma, 372
Subglottic stenosis, 284f
Subluxation, 107f
   of odontoid process, 375f
Succinylcholine, 387, 392
   child with major trauma and, 424
   inhalation induction of anesthesia and, 36f
   intravenous, 40f, 57f
   monitoring and maintenance of temperature and, 21
Suction (apparatus), 79–80, 416f, 417f
Sufentanil, 151
   suggested doses for, 151t
   target concentrations for, 152t
Sugar water nipple, 208f
Sundown sign of imminent awakening, 152
Sunset sign, 345
Superimposed pneumonia, 197f
Superior vena cava (SVC) pressure, 317
Supraclavicular approach to brachial plexus, 249
Supratentorial craniotomy, 355
   emergence and, 357
   induction and intubation and, 356
   maintenance and, 356–357
   postoperative management of, 357–358
   preinduction and, 356
Surgery
   for cryotherapy of retinopathy of prematurity, 202
   elective, determining whether to proceed with, 383t
   recovery from, 461–465
   relation of minimum alveolar concentration with, 154f
   omphalocele and gastroschisis and, 184
   of tracheoesophageal fistula, 177
Surgical cutdown of radial artery, 67, 69, 73f, 74f
Survival position, 37f, 38f, 40f
   modification of, 157f
Sympathetic innervation of heart, 181–182
Syndrome of inappropriate antidiuretic hormone (SIADH), 346, 355
Systemic vascular resistance, 182

T

Tampon, soft, 90f
Technical factor, complications related to, 263–264
Temperature
   drugs and, 21

SUBJECT INDEX

homeostasis of, 350
monitoring and maintenance of, 19
muscle relaxants and, 21, 23
sedation and, 449
Temporamandibular joint, 38*f*
Ten-point objective pain-discomfort scale, 231*t*
Tetracaine, maximum recommended dosage of, 241*t*
Tetralogy of Fallot, considerations for, 307*t*
Thiopental, 44, 384
    intravenous, 40*f*
Thiopentothal, 463
Thoracic trauma, 427–428
Throat surgery. *See under* Adenoidectomy; Tonsillectomy
Thromboelastography, 319
Thymus gland, 85*f*
Tibial plateau, 59*f*
Tidal volume (V$_t$), 124*f*, 132
    adjustment of, 126*f*, 127*f*
    delivery of, body weight and, 115*t*
    expired, 128*f*
    preset, 114–115
Tight brain, 342
Titration of drugs, 170
Tongue, 85*f*
    Flagg blade and, 83*f*
    insertion of laryngoscope blade and, 89*f*
Tongue depressor, plastic oral airway and, 81*f*
Tonsil
    bleeding, 274–275
    Quinsy, 276
Tonsillectomy, 267
    anesthesia for, 270–273
        extubaiton after, 272–273
        preoperative consideration for, 267–270
    complications of, 273–274
    inpatient guidelines for, 273*t*
Total body water, 167
Total intravenous anesthesia (TIVA), 154*f*
Toxicity, local anesthetic
    signs and symptoms of, 260–262
    treatment of, 262–263
Trachea, 85*f*
Tracheal axis, 86*f*, 87*f*
Tracheal dilator, 107*f*
Tracheal extubation, 153–154
    in children who are awake, 158–159
    in deeply anesthetized children, 154–155, 157*f*
    fully awake infant and, 203*t*
    technique of, 155, 157–158
Tracheal intubation, 80, 431*f*
    in ex-premies, 199*t*
    inhalation induction of anesthesia and, 36*f*
    nasal insertion of, 85–86
    oral insertion of, 81–82
        anatomic airway differences and, 82
        equipment for, 82
        technique for, 83–85
Tracheal reintubation, 430*f*
Tracheal stenosis, 284*f*
Tracheal tube, 102*f*
    in bypass patients, 323
    complications in children with, 262
Tracheoesophageal compression, 328*f*
Tracheoesophageal fistula (TEF), 3*t*, 176
    anesthetic management of, 177–179

blood pressure monitoring and, 178
capnography and, 178
clinical presentation of, 176
congenital anomalies associated with, 176
endotracheal intubation and, 178–179
extubation and, 179–180
maintenance of anesthesia for, 179–180
preoperative evaluation of, 176–177
prognosis for, 180
pulse oximetry and, 177–178
surgical repair of, 177
Tracheomalacia, 284*f*, 327
Trachlight Laerdal, 100*t*
Transarterial approach, 250
Transcapillary refill, 215
Transesophageal echocardiography (TEE), 300–301
Transfusion therapy in neonate, 171
Transportable sedation/anesthesia vehicle, 450*f*
Transposition of great vessels, consideration for, 306*t*
Transtracheal Doppler imaging, 301
Transtracheal jet ventilation, 281*f*
Trauma, major, 413–415
    airway trauma and, 431–432
    blood component therapy and, 426
    crystalloid and, 425
    endotracheal intubation and, 422–425
    head injury and, 428–429, 431
    initial assessment and treatment of, 420–422
    initial resuscitation and care of, 415
    intravenous agents and, 424
    maintenance of anesthesia and, 425
    muscle relaxants and, 424–425
    secondary survey and, 422
    suspected cervical injury and, 428–429
    thoracoabdominal trauma and, 426–428
    volume replacement and, 425–426
Trauma room, 414*f*
    airway equipment for any emergency in, 418*f*
    pediatric, 416*f*
Traumatized child, airway management in, 106, 108
Treacher Collins syndrome, 7*t*, 90
Tripod effect, 52*f*
Trisomy 21, 399–401
Truncus arteriosus, considerations for, 305*t*
Tube for endotracheal intubation, 169
Tube-Stat Xomed, 100*t*
T-wave
    change in, 261*f*
    elevation of, 207*f*
Two-handed laryngoscopy, algorithm for proper use of, 99*f*
Two-person technique for IV insertion, 52, 54*f*, 85, 96
    Creighton's, 110
    for difficult airways, 93, 96–97

U

U-bolster, 362*f*
Ulnar artery
    occlusion of, 66*f*
    release of pressure of, 67*f*
Ulnar nerve, 252*f*
Upper airway of neonate, 165
Upper airway obstruction
    during induction, 37–38
    in PACU, 468–469
    physiology of, 269

Upper extremity block, 247–253
Upper respiratory infection (URI), 381–382
   pathophysiologic effects of, 382t
Upper respiratory procedure, 335t
Urinalysis during preoperative evaluation, 11
Urologic precedure, 233f

V

Vancomycin, 8t, 335t
Vaponephrine, 290
Vapor-free anesthetic machine, 391
Vascular ring, 284f
   repair of, 327
Vasopressor, endogenous, 214
Vasospasm, 367
VATER, 176
Vecuronium, 22t, 23, 424
Vein of Galen varix, 366f
Veins, best, in small infants, 55f
Venous access, difficult, in ex-ECMO, 210
Venous air embolism, 350–351
Ventilation, 114. *See also specific type of ventilation*
   congenital diaphragmatic hernia and, 173
   controlled, 290
      in bypass patients, 322–323
      open heart surgery and, 312
   manual, 202
   spontaneous, 287–290
Ventilation tubes, placement of, 277
Ventilator(s)
   anesthesia, 118–124
   North American Drager Narkomed, 121–123
   Ohmeda Anesthesia, 123–124
   pediatric conversion of adult to, 114
   Sechrist-Infant, 118–120
   Seimens-Elema, 121
Ventricular catheter, 353f
Ventricular septal defect (VSD), 295
   considerations for surgery for, 303t
Vincristine (Oncovin), 4t
Visual Analogue Scale, 234
Vocal cord(s), 89f
   paralysis of, 284f
Volar aspect of hand, 52
Volatile anesthetic agent(s), 262
   avoiding overdose of, 35–37
   desflurane and, 147
   for ex-premature, 200
   halothane and, 146–147
   isoflurane and, 147
   maintenance of anesthesia with, 145–148
   minimum alveolar concentration and, 145–148
   sevoflurane and, 147–148
Volume, relation between intracranial pressure and, 345f
Volume-controlled ventilation, 114–115
Volume replacement, 425–426
Vomiting in PACU, 471–472
von Willebrand's disease, 275

W

Wake-up test, 374
Warming blanket, forced-air, 20f, 473f
Water, intracellular excess of, 221f
Waterston procedure, 329
Waveform interpretation, capnography and, 137, 139
Wheezing, differential diagnosis of, 383t
Wilms' tumor, 405–406
Wound debridement, 455
Wrist
   neuromuscular stimulation at, 18f
   volar aspect of, 55f

X

Xanthine, 384, 469
X-linked recessive trait, hemophilia and, 398